Practical Implant Dentistry

# Practical Implant Dentistry
## The Science and Art

### Second edition

By
**Ashok Sethi**
BDS, DGDP (UK), MGDSRCS (Eng), DUI (Lille), FFGDP (UK)
**Thomas Kaus**
Dr Med Dent (FRG), Dip Impl Dent (RCS Eng)

Forewords by Prof Dr H Weber and Raj K Raja Rayan OBE

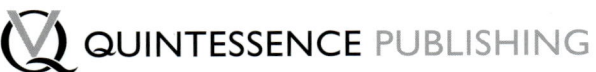

London, Berlin, Chicago, Tokyo, Barcelona, Beijing, Istanbul, Milan, Moscow, New Delhi, Paris, Prague, São Paulo, Seoul, Singapore and Warsaw

*This book is dedicated to friends and family –
past, present and future.
In appreciation of those who made us who we are.
In gratitude to those whose support we have now.
In anticipation of those whose paths we may touch.*

**British Library Cataloguing in Publication Data**
Sethi, Ashok.
 Practical implant dentistry. -- 2nd ed.
 1. Dental implants.
 I. Title II. Kaus, Thomas.

 617.6'93-dc23
 ISBN: 978-1-85097-223-5

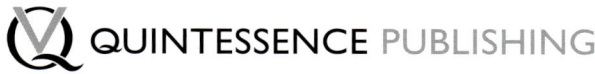

Quintessence Publishing Co. Ltd,
Grafton Road, New Malden, Surrey KT3 3AB,
United Kingdom
www.quintpub.co.uk
Copyright © 2012 Quintessence Publishing Co Ltd

All rights reserved. This book or any part thereof may not be reproduced, stored in a retrieval system, or transmitted in any form or by any means, electronic, mechanical, photocopying, or otherwise, without prior written permission of the publisher.
Editing: Quintessence Publishing Co. Ltd, London, UK
Layout and Production: Quintessenz Verlags-GmbH, Berlin, Germany
Printed and bound in Germany

# Forewords

### Prof Dr H Weber Chairman and Medical Director, Clinic for Dental, Oral and Maxillary Medicine, Tübingen, Germany

It was a desirable expectation that this comprehensive, outstanding book on 'Practical Implant Dentistry – The Science and Art' would be published in a second edition, for several reasons:
- The sold-out first edition, written by practitioners for practitioners, represents a rare combination of practical guidelines for encompassing clinical implant dentistry. Founded on a sound and solid personal clinical experience of the authors on one side, the scientific basis is also provided with an analysis of the relevant literature on the other side. Such a well accepted book must have another edition.
- Implant dentistry has dramatically evolved in past years due to digitalisation in both fields i.e., computer based diagnostics and therapy and restorative laboratory procedures – a state-of-the-art book must include all of this.
- Another edition would enable the authors to utilise the unique chance of presenting follow-ups of patients shown in the first edition, and by doing so shall reflect the value and the reliability of treatment concepts.

The second edition meets all of these three reasons/expectations in an unsurpassed way by reflecting marvellously the developments in our clinical understanding and technology:
- Clinically, we all – by gaining experience – are moving our indications for certain treatments to other levels of complexity and difficulty. In implant dentistry, bone grafts have become more frequent and important because of our personal demands as well as our patients' with regard to what can be, or rather must be achieved aesthetically and functionally by such a treatment.
- Technically, digitalisation has a tremendous impact in both fields – clinically and in the dental laboratory:
  - In diagnostics/therapy, advanced CBT/CT-scans with improved software enhanced our understanding of the individually appropriate treatment, on our surgical possibilities in terms of computer guided surgery, and, last, but not least, by all of this on the safety of our patients.
  - In the dental lab, sophisticated CAD/CAM-technology is steadily widening/enlarging our possibilities with regard to materials, design, and precision. This book introduces these new technologies.

Furthermore, the new edition does not only cover the modern topics mentioned above in a state-of-the-art manner, but by presenting follow-ups of some of the cases shown in the first edition, it confirms the efficacy of the treatment principles described.

In the field of implant dentistry, this book is again a must for beginners as well as for advanced colleagues. Having been involved in surgical as well as restorative implant dentistry clinically and scientifically myself for more than three decades, I do appreciate the enormous input of the authors in this field resulting in an equivalent impact of their book on our profession. I would like to thank the authors for the very successful efforts they invested into this book. Together with my appreciation, congratulations, and my thanks, I would like to state that this book will be another milestone in our University Medical Library.

# Forewords

## Raj K Raja Rayan OBE MSc FFGDP FDS MGDS MRD DRD MA(Clin Ed)
## Past Dean, Faculty of General Dental Practice, Royal College of Surgeons of England

Holland[1] suggested that healthcare career preferences could be mapped in six broad types (RIASEC model) for vocational career choices. They were surgery (realistic), hospital medicine (investigative), psychiatry (artistic), public health (social), administrative medicine (enterprising) and laboratory medicine (conventional).

The greatest innovation in dental treatment and the biggest growth area in dentistry at the beginning of this millennium is the field of implantology. A clinician who embarks upon it will need to embrace all six disciplines of healthcare choices. A clinician who practises implantology is the complete practitioner. The concept of the scientist practitioner (investigative) is now at the core of all dental treatment planning. Evidence-based healthcare, where evidence is based on audit and clinical governance interacting with clinical pathways, makes the professional accountable to the public. Quality assurance is then used to ensure that untoward outcomes are kept to a minimum. Therefore, public health dentistry (social) and practice management (enterprising) have evolved prominently. Those who embark upon dental implantology are engineers of medicine, solving problems at high levels of mechanical and technical excellence, emphasising practical skills and craftsmanship, with immediate and effective results (realistic). Implantology spans almost all aspects of clinical dentistry to include complex surgery and advanced prosthodontics. These practitioners need to have an artistic approach to the subject, seeing, interpreting and responding imaginatively to a range of dental, medical, social, ethical and other problems, including responding to ideas expressed by patients. Evidence-based medicine, where it exists, must be balanced with treatment specific to that unique individual (artistic). Precision technology and attention to detail at the micrometre level in the laboratory will crown the eventual result (conventional).

The authors have mapped this publication to encompass all disciplines required for advancing the complete implant practitioner. Their in-depth understanding of general dental practice and their wide experience in teaching have lent themselves well to their well-rehearsed and structured methodology. This book is a practical and sensible approach to excellence in implantology. It is written in an easy style and is full of beautiful illustrations to help guide the practitioner of implantology through the myriad of choices. I have learnt much from it. This publication is a benchmark in our modern approach to implant dentistry.

1   Holland JL. Making vocational choices: a theory of careers. New York: Prentice Hall, 1973.

# Preface

## Preface to the First Edition

Conceptually the replacement of a missing tooth by means of an implant is attractive for several reasons:
- it is functionally and aesthetically superior to any other form of restoration
- it replaces the tooth in a manner that closely resembles its missing natural predecessor
- the implant-supported restoration can be independent of the adjacent teeth
- it is therapeutically attractive because it will stimulate the bone and induce an increase in density in response to functional load.

This book offers a practical and pragmatic approach to implant dentistry, outlining predictable protocols for each stage. Our aim is to present guidelines to assist the clinician during decision making. The illustrations are designed to facilitate the comprehension of the clinical procedures. The flowcharts are designed to provide an understanding of the procedures and the various available pathways. We hope that the flowcharts will make clear the treatment options available and help in visualising each stage within the overall treatment plan. There are checklists for certain stages to ensure that the relevant points have been adequately addressed before embarking on the next stage.

Coalescing the art and science of implant dentistry, this book aims to eliminate compromise in a rational and methodical manner. It aims to make implant dentistry a predictable field that can be brought within the reach of the clinician. The protocols outlined are based on clinical experience in a practice wholly dedicated to the surgical and restorative aspects of implant dentistry. It is not intended to cover every technique available to the clinician in this field, but rather to present a limited number of options, which are evidence based, efficient in terms of time and predictable in terms of outcome. These protocols, with high success rates and excellent aesthetic and functional outcome, are presented in a manner that simplifies the decision-making process. We are confident that the clinician who follows the protocols outlined here and who has a thorough understanding of their principles will be able to carry out treatment to the benefit of the patient.

For the patient, restoring a gap with an implanted tooth that is aesthetically and functionally close to what nature had intended, has far-reaching benefits. It restores health and function, thus preventing the harm that results from the loss of function. Furthermore, it must not be overlooked that the aesthetics are also restored. The mouth, after all, is the organ that is the centre of communication and, therefore, critical to how we present ourselves to our fellow human beings.

This book hopes to encompass the many disciplines that contribute to implant dentistry. It is not the purpose of this book to teach basic sciences, such as physiology, anatomy or pharmacology. We have assumed that clinicians entering this field will be familiar with both the surgical and restorative aspects of dentistry as well as the basic sciences. Clinicians who hope to practise implant dentistry must not only be familiar with the restorative and surgical aspect of treatment but must also understand the manage-

# Preface

ment of patients. Understanding the needs and expectations of patients within the framework of their general health and well-being is fundamental to the successful outcome of treatment. The general dental practitioner, adequately trained, is well suited for providing patients with implant treatment.

'Medical education is not completed at the medical school: it is only begun' (William H Welch, MD, 1850–1934).

Ashok Sethi
Thomas Kaus
London and Tübingen

## Preface to the Second Edition

Translation of our first edition into 10 languages served as inspiration for us to update. There is merit in what is 'old': established treatment protocols that have stood the test of time and acquitted themselves as valid procedures. Science, however, has at its very core the ongoing mechanism of critical examination and validation of new and existing evidence to accumulate new knowledge and thus elevates our level of understanding. This is change and must be embraced, for that is life itself.

With this in mind, we have introduced treatment protocols that have benefited from advances in technology and our better understanding of biological principles. There are new paradigms that emerge out of these advances and we hope to have embraced them.

Therefore, in updating this book, we have also presented follow-ups of some of the cases to validate treatment protocols described in the first edition. Additional cases using new and described above protocols have also been presented, reflecting our ongoing practice.

'Science has built-in, error-correcting machinery at its very heart.'
'When we are self-indulgent and uncritical, when we confuse hopes and facts, we slide into pseudoscience and superstition' (Carl Sagan, scientist, 1934–1996).

Ashok Sethi
Thomas Kaus
London and Kitchener-Waterloo

# Acknowledgements

A book such as this owes its existence to all those who have laid the foundations for the many facets of this very interesting field, and the work of the following contributors to this field is acknowledged:

Per Ingvar Brånemark, who has brought methodology to this field and whose protocols, which may have been seen as dogma, have enabled the profession to predict the outcome of treatment for their patients.

Willi Schulte, who pioneered the concept of immediate replacement of a failing tooth, introducing the concept of functionally sustaining form. His innovation has led to the recent and rapid development of immediate implants.

Philippe Daniel Ledermann, who recognised the possibility of immediately loading an implant by ensuring stability with the aid of splinting. His innovation has led to the introduction of single-staged implant treatment.

Hilt Tatum Jr, who has contributed greatly to the art of implant dentistry by devising innovative surgical techniques that have made the treatment of so many patients possible and who has given freely and generously of his time and experience.

We are grateful for the contributions made by Peter Sochor, master technician. All the technical work shown in this book (unless otherwise indicated) has been carried out by Peter. He has been responsible for devising many techniques and protocols that have contributed to the art and science of implant dentistry. His innovative mind, his persistence at solving problems and his broad knowledge of the range of techniques available in dental technology has enabled us to provide our patients with the treatment to improve the quality of their lives.

John Cawood has contributed greatly to the treatment of many patients in addition to those described in this book. We are grateful to him for the considerable support he has offered and for the rationale he has brought to the treatment of our patients. His skills as a surgeon are second to none and are enhanced by his understanding of prosthodontics, the facial form and the needs and expectations of the patients.

We are also grateful to Michael Boscoe, consultant anaesthetist, for the support he has provided in evaluating patients who have required anaesthesia or assessment prior to treatment.

We thank Harbhajan Plaha, consultant orthopaedic surgeon, who has generously given of his time to enable us to carry out treatment that has required bone from extraoral sources with the greatest skill and expertise.

All clinical work depends on the support of a highly qualified team. We would like to acknowledge the support of those who made the treatment of the patients possible. The administrative, preoperative and postoperative care and management of the patient was provided by Subir Banerji, Christine Sethi, Siby Boyd, Sarah Jelly, Juliet Teale, Kirstie Swift, Karen O'Shaughnessy, Jo Taylor, Kiersten Piercy and Gill Carlaw, all of whom are based in London, and by Gabi Aßmuß, Jochen Diehl, Jürgen Braunwarth and Eberhard Kober, who are based in Germany, as well as Leslie Waddell, Sue Sims, Terry Steffler, Barbara Bast, Claire Mc Kinley, Julie Kesselring, Jane Ritz and Andrea Stokes who are based in Kitchener-Waterloo.

# Contents

**Section I Introduction and Assessment** ............................................................. 1
Chapter 1 Introduction ........................................................................................ 5
Chapter 2 Patient Selection and Treatment Philosophy .............................. 7
Chapter 3 Patient Assessment............................................................................ 9
Chapter 4 Medical Evaluation and Patient Management........................... 15
Chapter 5 Additional Diagnostic Procedures ............................................... 19
Chapter 6 Anatomical Variations..................................................................... 31

**Section II Implant Placement: Surgery and Prosthodontics**....................... 43
Chapter 7 Immediate Placement and Computer-guided Surgery............. 49
Chapter 8 Delayed Placement in Adequate Bone with Mature Ridge........ 103
Chapter 9 Delayed Loading: Implant Exposure .......................................... 153
Chapter 10 Restorative Phase: Prosthetic Protocols................................... 167

**Section III Augmentation**................................................................................ 201
Chapter 11 Overview......................................................................................... 205
Chapter 12 Bone Expansion............................................................................ 219
Chapter 13 Localised Onlay Bone Grafts ..................................................... 239
Chapter 14 Extensive Bone Grafts ................................................................. 261
Chapter 15 Posterior Maxilla.......................................................................... 301
Chapter 16 Posterior Mandible...................................................................... 333
Chapter 17 Corrective Soft Tissue Surgery .................................................. 353

References........................................................................................................... 381
Glossary of Terms.............................................................................................. 391
Index..................................................................................................................... 393

# SECTION I

# Introduction and Assessment

*'Health is a state of complete physical, mental and social well-being and not merely the absence of disease or infirmity'*

(Preamble to the Constitution
of the World Health Organization, 1948)


*'I will follow that system of regimen which, according to my ability and judgement, I consider for the benefit of my patients, and abstain from whatever is deleterious and mischievous… While I continue to keep this oath unviolated, may it be granted to me to enjoy life and the practice of the art, respected by all men, in all times'*

(Extract from the Hippocratic Oath,
Hippocrates, 460–377 BC)


*'To acquire knowledge, one must study; but to acquire wisdom, one must observe'*

(Marilyn vos Savant)

# Chapter 1

# Introduction

The primary focus of attention in implant dentistry has shifted from the achievement of osseointegration, since this can be achieved so predictably,[1–11] and has now become centred on the creation of aesthetic implant-supported restorations that mimic the tooth being replaced. A host of supplementary treatment options has been devised in an aim to achieve this goal. Many of these techniques are supported by research that documents a high degree of predictability. Others, however, are mainly based on case studies without any long-term clinical follow-up.

Clinicians, therefore, need to be able to discriminate between those techniques that will be of benefit to patients with a minimal risk of failure. Furthermore, the clinician needs to function within a framework that offers him or her clear-cut options which can be followed when presented with a problem that needs to be solved. The assessment of the patient is, therefore, critical and should accurately define the problem, which will, in turn, make the ideal treatment self-evident.

The ultimate goal of the treatment is to produce teeth that are aesthetically and functionally acceptable. It is, therefore, appropriate to start any treatment planning by first determining the desired tooth position. This must logically be followed by the assessment of the hard and soft tissues that are present to support the implant-borne restoration. Finally, the predetermined tooth position must be related to the supporting tissues to assess whether any augmentation or manipulation of those tissues is necessary. The treatment format that has been developed has well-defined stages, which enable information to be transferred from one stage to the next.

- Tooth size, form and position can be decided upon by means of a diagnostic preview, which may be functionally assessed by the patient by construction of a provisional restoration.
- The hard and soft tissues can be assessed in terms of both quantity and quality by using the appropriate range of diagnostic imaging techniques available and establishing whether there is a need to augment or manipulate the supporting tissues. The tooth position, as determined by the diagnostic preview, will play an important part in deciding whether augmentation is necessary.
- The implant must be placed in the correct anatomical position within the available bone without violating surgical or biological principles. The position of the implant and the abutment should be determined with the aid of a template based on the diagnostic preview.

# Introduction and Assessment

- The next stage is to decide whether loading should be immediate or delayed.
- Completion of the restorative phase is achieved by reproducing the tooth size, form and position that was determined at the beginning of the treatment and which had subsequently been confirmed and approved.

Understanding and working within these principles will establish a framework within which treatment can be completed predictably with a successful outcome.

In light of the developing digital computer-aided design and computer-aided manufacturing (CAD/CAM) technologies, the goal will evolve towards constructing the definitive prosthesis prior to surgery. This will require the use of increasingly accurate diagnostic imaging for interactive planning. The execution of the treatment using digitally generated surgical guides for osteotomy preparation and implant seating will, therefore, require accurate cross referencing between clinical imaging and laboratory phases. The taking of impressions to generate casts will in time be replaced by digital scanning and computer-generated models.

The principles outlined above will form the basis of this natural evolution for the benefit of the patient.

# Chapter 2

# Patient Selection and Treatment Philosophy

The range of treatment that is available in the field of implant dentistry is vast, varying from the simple immediate replacement of a tooth carried out over a short span of time to extensive hard and soft tissue reconstruction coupled with fixed implant-supported restorations. The selection of patients must, therefore, take into account several factors when assessing the benefit that the patient will derive from the treatment against the extent and invasiveness of the treatment proposed for that patient.

The factors that need to be taken into consideration are numerous, and none should be overlooked when deciding on the course of action. Clearly, any treatment that is carried out should not compromise the medical condition of the patient. The age of the patient is relevant because the healing process takes longer with advancing biological age. Chronological age must, therefore, be considered in light of the patient's physical and mental well-being.

Benefit in terms of lifespan is a difficult judgement to make, as the improvement in the quality of life has to be evaluated in view of the discomfort and indignity that a patient may suffer if deprived of treatment. This is particularly true for patients who have undergone ablative surgery for the treatment of neoplasms.[12–16]

## Financial Considerations

Funding of the treatment must also be taken into account. Direct funding by the patient makes the assessment of benefit versus cost easier for the clinician as the patient is involved directly in the decision-making process. Third party funding, either by the state or by insurance companies, brings additional factors into this equation, particularly when considering the long-term outcome. These may not necessarily be in the best interests of the patient. The clinician must, therefore, understand the benefits of implant therapy with respect to future investments that would otherwise have to be made for alternative reparative or prosthetic treatment.

## Patient Expectations

Patient expectations must be very clearly defined early on during the selection and assessment process. It is well known that the loss of a tooth has a psychological effect on the patient.[17–19] However, this must not be mistaken for a patient holding tooth loss responsible for any unrelated psychological problems. Patient expectations with respect to aesthetic outcome must be addressed early during the treatment through the use of

## Introduction and Assessment

diagnostic previews or provisional restorations to define in practical terms what can be achieved.

## Record Keeping

Detailed records of all clinical procedures form a part of good clinical practice. This should include description of the procedure carried out, which is enhanced by the use of digital imaging and photography. Detailed records of all biomaterials should be kept in the patient's notes and in a central database to facilitate retrieval.

Established protocols should be followed in recording manufacturers, batch numbers and so on. In particular, the dimensions of the component parts must be recorded to facilitate management of any future maintenance.

Accurate and detailed record keeping becomes even more important in this field, where the need for sharing information is increasing. The longevity of the treatment and the demographic changes that naturally take place require the information to be shared with other clinicians for ongoing management and maintenance.

Records of any discussions that have taken place form the basis of the ongoing decision-making and consent process.

## Tele-medicine

The extensive use of digital records and the availability of a global computer network with high bandwidth enables clinical data to be shared and greatly facilitates additional opinions as well as a multidisciplinary approach. Remote consultation, therefore, is an integral part of the practice of medicine today and in the future.

## Informed Consent

The patient must be given a realistic account of what the treatment involves in terms of success rate, complications, specific risks, costs and commitment to maintenance, as well as the alternatives and the consequences of not undergoing treatment. It is essential that the patient understands the proposal for treatment and formally consents to it.

## Benefit Assessment

The benefit to the patient must be measured not only in terms of the improved ability to masticate, with its attendant benefits of adequate nutrition, but also in terms of the improvement to his or her quality of life.[20-24] The ability of a patient to communicate adequately, with stable, aesthetically acceptable dentition, is of immeasurable benefit, as it impacts on personal relationships as well as on his or her performance at work. The benefits to society from the contribution of such individuals, who are not simply free from disease but are in a state of well-being, must not be overlooked.

# Chapter 3

# Patient Assessment

Patients undergoing implant dentistry should be sufficiently healthy to be able to withstand oral surgical procedures. The healing potential of patients should be such that adequate soft and hard tissue healing may progress to enable osseointegration to take place. Furthermore, systemic factors should allow the continuing health of the implant. Bone metabolism should be such that a positive response to functional loading takes place by an increase in bone density around the implant. The soft tissue response should be judged to be such that adequate permucosal health can be maintained. Adequate preoperative assessment must be carried out for all patients. The outcome of such an examination should give the clinician an indication of the possible clinical response to the treatments available. The assessment of biotypes in conjunction with all the above factors will also be an indicator to the outcome. The following requirements should be considered before prescribing implants.

## General Health

Dental implant therapy constitutes elective treatment, and consequently the patient must not be put at risk. Assessment of general health must be carried out carefully.[25–27] A detailed medical history questionnaire should be filled out by patients, followed by verbal personal verification.

The American Society of Anaesthesiologists (ASA) classifies patients in terms of the risk imposed by their medical condition (Table 3-1). It may be interpreted as follows, and these guidelines are recommended:

- ASA 1: no systemic disease – patients may be treated taking appropriate care that is consistent with the surgical procedure
- ASA 2: mild systemic disease – patients may be treated in consultation with the patient's general or specialist medical practitioner
- ASA 3–4: Moderate or severe systemic disease – elective treatment is generally not recommended for patients assessed as posing a moderate or severe anaesthetic risk.

**Table 3-1** American Society of Anaesthesiologists: classification

| ASA 1 | Healthy with no systemic disease |
|---|---|
| ASA 2 | Mild systemic disease responding to treatment |
| ASA 3 | Moderate systemic disease partially corrected by treatment |
| ASA 4 | Severe systemic disorder threatening the survival of the patient |
| ASA 5 | Moribund |

# Introduction and Assessment

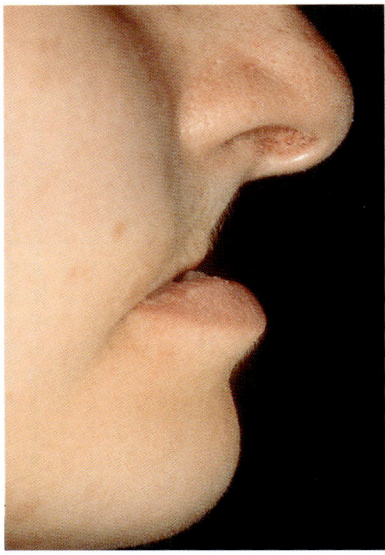

**Fig 3-1** Lateral view of a patient who has undergone severe maxillary atrophy following tooth loss with total loss of support for the upper lip.

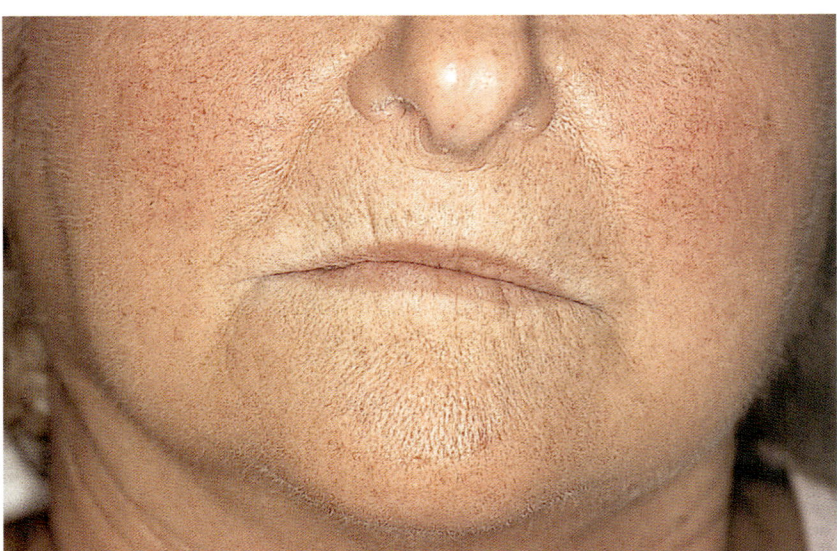

**Fig 3-2** Frontal view of the lower part of the face showing an asymmetry of the lips and the mandible. The angle of the mandible can be seen to have an asymmetry, with the right angle being more prominent and more superiorly placed.

Where appropriate, further medical examinations should be carried out. These may be undertaken either by the dental surgeon or by through referral to a physician.

## Intraoral/Extraoral Examination

A standard format should be followed during the clinical examination of patients to ensure that no aspect is overlooked.

### Skeletal Pattern

The skeletal pattern should be observed and recorded according to Angle's classification. A normal intermaxillary relationship is categorised as Class I, a prominent maxilla as Class II and a prominent mandible as Class III.

### Facial Profile

For edentulous patients and those who have multiple missing teeth the facial profile should be observed with and without the prostheses in place. This provides an indication of the amount of atrophy that has taken place. The naso-labial angle, the fullness of the lips and the prominence of the mandible are indications of the loss of support for the circumoral musculocutaneous and mucosal tissues (Fig 3-1).[28] Facial symmetries and proportions must also be observed, using specific landmarks (e.g. the pupils) as reference points (Fig 3-2). Where appropriate, this can be recorded graphically on the consultation form (Fig 3-3).

### The Masticatory Muscles

Palpation to evaluate the size and activity of the masticatory muscles (masseter, lateral and medial pterygoids and temporalis) is carried out to provide an indication of the forces of mastication as well as the presence of parafunctional activity, such as clenching, grinding and posturing.[29,30] The masseter and the temporalis muscles are observed visually and palpated for size and activity. The lateral and medial

**Table 3-2** Muscle tenderness

| Right | Muscle | Left |
|---|---|---|
|  | Medial pterygoid |  |
|  | Lateral pterygoid |  |
|  | Temporalis |  |
|  | Sternomastoid |  |

# 3 Patient Assessment

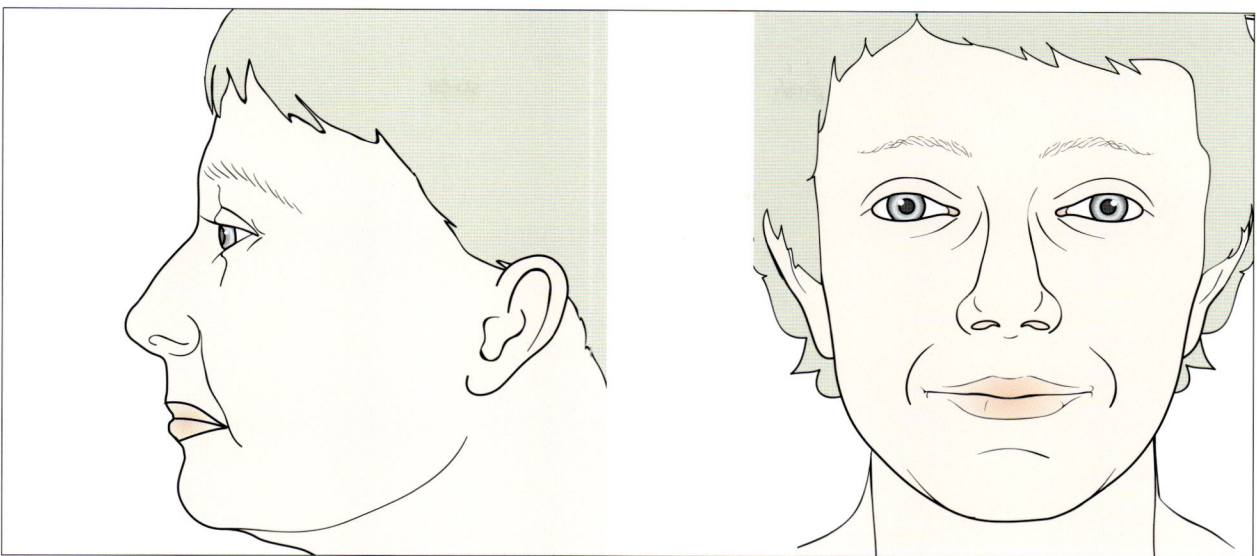

**Fig 3-3** The lateral facial profile may be used to sketch indicators of atrophy, such as an increased naso-labial angle, indicating a loss of maxillary ridge, or the protrusion of the chin, indicating a loss of vertical dimension. It may also be used to record disproportions of the face. The anterior view may be used to record facial asymmetries or discrepancies in the proportions of the midface.

pterygoid muscles and other muscles are palpated for tenderness to observe the presence of parafunctional activity (Table 3-2).

## Temporomandibular Joints and Occlusion

The temporomandibular joints are examined externally by palpation for pain, clicks or crepitus during opening and closing movements. Palpation is completed by placing the index fingers into the external auditory canal to evaluate the movement of the condyle in the glenoid fossa during opening and closing of the jaws (Table 3-3).
Deviations of the mandible in the sagittal plane should be noted. Premature contacts during closure should also be noted (Table 3-4).

The area of maximum opening between the incisors is recorded to give an indication of the amount of access for surgery. The occlusal scheme should be recorded whenever possible according to the following categories:
- canine/anterior guidance
- group function
- anterior open bite/posterior guidance
- non-working side contacts and interferences.

## Teeth

A complete chart of the teeth should be drawn up and should include:
- missing teeth
- incidence of caries

Table 3-3  Temporomandibular joint: symptom

| Right | Symptom | Left |
|---|---|---|
|  | Pain |  |
|  | Clicking (opening/closing) |  |
|  | Crepitus (opening/closing) |  |

Table 3-4  Mandibular deviation

| Right | Left |
|---|---|
|  |  |

# I Introduction and Assessment

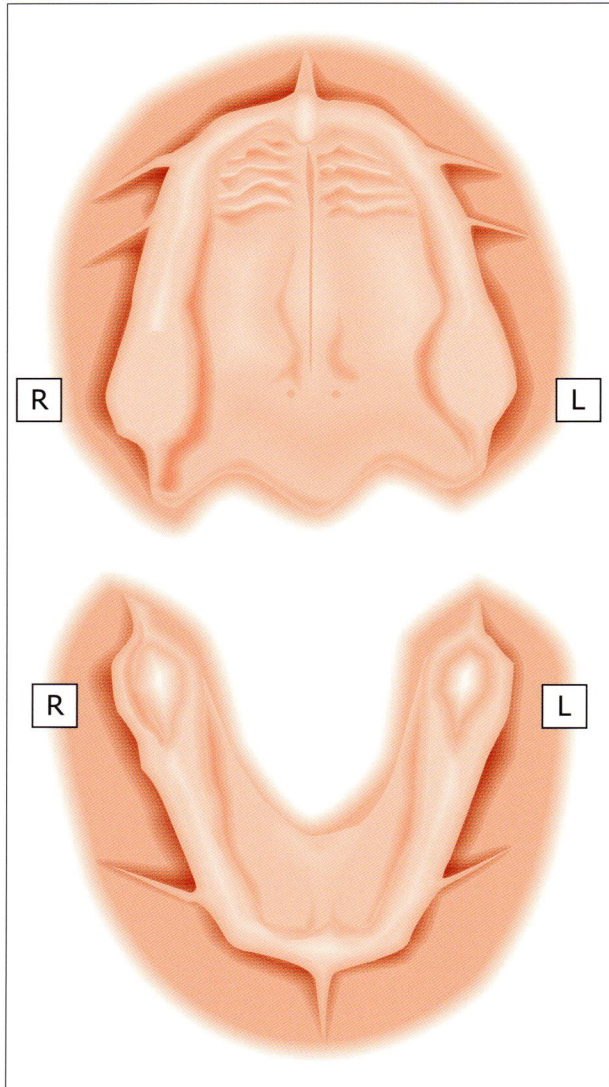

**Fig 3-4** The amount of attached keratinised tissue may be measured and recorded in millimetres in the region of concern. The presence and position of frenae may also be recorded.

- the structural status of the teeth, including the endodontic status, the presence and size of restorations and the presence of posts.

These assessments can be corroborated by information from radiographs taken during the primary clinical examination appointment and should be updated during the treatment period.

## Tooth Wear

The four components of tooth wear (attrition, abrasion, abfraction and erosion) are used to provide an indication of the degree of parafunction as well as the typical occlusal loads that the patient would have exerted.[31–33]

## Periodontal Tissues

Probing depths should be recorded in all cases. Two-point charting (mesial and distal) of all the teeth should be carried out. For patients who show evidence of periodontal disease (probing depths greater than 6 mm with bleeding) the use of six-point charting is recommended. Points at which bleeding occurs should be recorded as possible indicators of active periodontal disease.

All patients who are compromised periodontally should be assessed and should receive periodontal therapy before implant treatment is started. They should be reassessed throughout the course of the treatment and post-operatively.

## Soft Tissues

The presence of attached keratinised gingival tissue should be noted, particularly in areas of muscle attachments. Frenum attachments are of concern, as are mobile non-attached mucosa (Fig 3-4). Examination of the soft tissues for any pathological lesions should always be carried out. Lymph nodes should also be examined by palpation.

## Residual Ridges

The residual ridges are examined for height and width, and a preliminary impression is gained of their position relative to the planned prosthetic tooth. Observations of the current prostheses, adjacent teeth and measurements of the interarch distance are valuable in determining this.

Assessing the teeth for prediction of resorption may be carried out by observing the thickness and contour of the alveolar bone around the roots of the teeth. Greater resorption of the labial plate has been observed in patients where the vestibular contours of the roots are palpable due to the very thin alveolar bone around the labial aspects of these roots and deep depressions between roots. Furthermore, whenever more than one or multiple adjacent teeth are removed, greater loss of

Table 3-5 Assessment of hard and soft tissue biotype
(a) Soft tissue biotype

| Thickness | Thin | Medium | Thick |
|---|---|---|---|
| Form | Scalloped | Normal | Flat |

(b) Bone biotype

| Clinical assessment | Prominent roots | Thick ridge, non-palpable roots |
|---|---|---|
| 3D imaging | Thin labial bone, interdental depression | Thick flat labial bone |
| Likely treatment outcome | Recession | Stability |

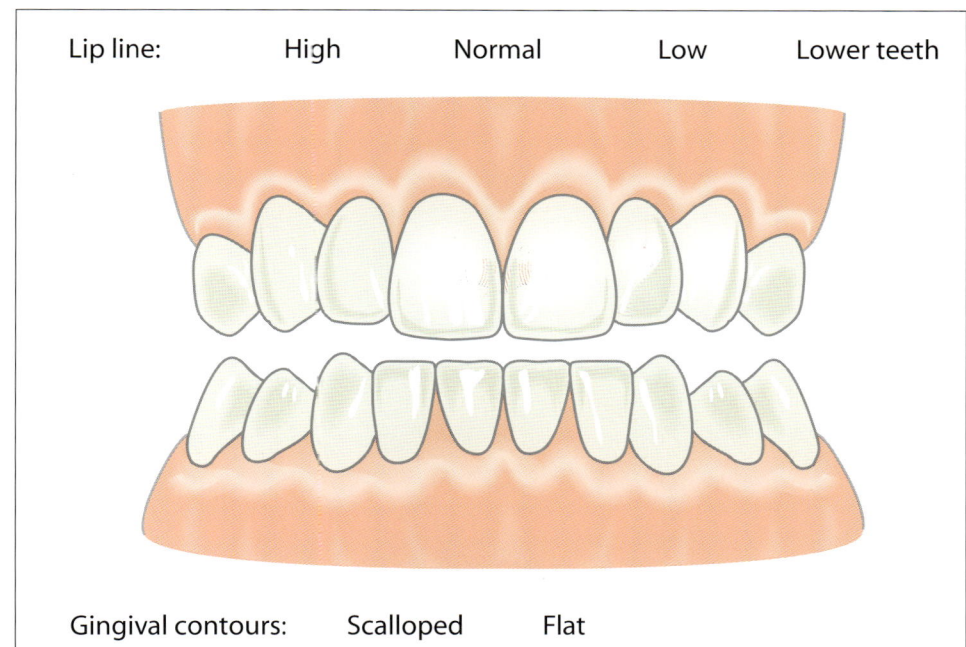

Fig 3-5 A sketch depicting the lip line and other relevant details, such as the length and width of teeth, diastemas, gingival form, etc., provides good visual summary and record of observations.

height and width of bone takes place, and there is also a loss of attached keratinised tissue.

## Assessing Hard and Soft Tissue Biotype

Clinical assessment of the hard and soft tissue biotype is carried out during the consultation and further supplemented at a later stage should three-dimensional (3D) imaging be available. Assessment is carried out visually and by palpation of the labial aspect of the alveolar ridge. The data are recorded in the table as well as photographically. Table 3-5 helps to evaluate the treatment outcome based on hard and soft tissue biotype.

## Lip Line

The lip line, which is examined with the patient smiling naturally and during speech, is recorded graphically. The length and width of the teeth should be measured, and the presence of diastemas should be recorded along with the width of space available for any tooth that needs to be replaced. The type of gingival contour should be assessed as being either flat or scalloped because of the difficulty in reproducibility of contours of fine scalloped tissues. Exposure of the gingival tissues during smiling is, therefore, considered of importance, as the gingival contours have to be harmonious (Fig 3-5).

# Chapter 4

# Medical Evaluation and Patient Management

## Introduction

It is not the remit of this book to cover the vast field of medical assessment but merely to provide a philosophy for the safe management of patients before, during and after treatment. The clinician should be sufficiently trained in the assessment of patients and must refer to texts and training programmes designed to impart such information. There is a paucity of established data on the impact of medical condition on the well-being of implants. Clinical judgement and experience are valuable, and consultation with specialist physicians and surgeons is strongly advised during the assessment. There are numerous publications that arbitrarily list absolute and relative contraindications. These must be viewed in light of risks and benefits as well as the facilities that are available to safely manage the patient.

The life expectancy of patients has greatly increased and many patients attending treatment have disorders that are being medically treated. The disorder being treated might well have comorbidities, and the drugs that are used to contain the disorder will invariably have an impact on the patient's physiology. Consequently, a thorough working knowledge of medical conditions and currently used drugs is necessary. Numerous conditions require surgical intervention, which may require precautions and are indicative of an underlying susceptibility.

## Medical Evaluation

Implant dentistry is an elective procedure that is carried out to enhance the patient's well-being. It is not a life-saving procedure, and the patient should, therefore, not be put at unnecessary risk. A medical history form should be completed by the patient and discussed in detail with the clinician to ensure that all aspects of the patient's health have been covered. This provides an opportunity to address conditions not covered directly within the medical history form. The format of the medical history form should be such that it is easy for the patient to complete and for the clinician to assess. A broad range of medical history forms is available. The main topics that should be addressed are:
- medical care, present or past (including current medication)
- current or past illnesses (e.g. cardiovascular, respiratory, neurological, gastrointestinal, endocrine, renal, hepatic or haematopoietic problems)
- psychological profile
- infectious diseases

# Introduction and Assessment

- allergies
- social profile (for example, smoking, drinking).

## Aim

Assessment of the medical condition of the patient should consider the factors affecting the short-, medium- and long-term well-being of the patient. The treatment process and outcome should be considered along these timescales, which are arbitrary and overlapping. A process of risk assessment and risk containment should be taken with the seriousness it deserves.

## Short-term Issues

This period refers to the perioperative time and the key concern is that the patient should first survive and, second, not suffer any complications that require emergency resuscitation or remedial action.

A number of conditions that are potentially harmful need to be identified. Typically these would affect those systems fundamental to life support. Therefore, assessment of medical conditions that would typically result in life-threatening incidents should be considered, for example:

- cardiovascular system – acute myocardial infarction or a stroke
- respiratory system – respiratory distress as may be caused by asthma, emphysema, or obstruction
- endocrine system – diabetic crisis (normally caused by hypoglycaemia)
- haematopoietic system – bleeding disorders (factor VIII, haemophilia)
- nervous system – epilepsy.

## Medium-term Issues

The medium term refers to the immediate post-operative period including the primary healing phase and leading up to the period when the implants are brought into function. Obvious overlaps with short-term issues exist with respect to bleeding disorders, which may be drug induced. Other examples of potential problems in this period are:

- post-operative haemorrhage
- ischaemia of the healing tissues, which may be iatrogenic or patient induced (e.g. smoking or excessive alcohol intake)
- infection due to susceptibility initiated by any number of factors that result in a deficiency of the immune system, such as immunosuppressant drugs or Acquired Immune Deficiency Syndrome (AIDS) caused by HIV infection
- unstable diabetes, resulting in infection or flap breakdown
- health consequences of treatment such as infection of valvular prosthesis leading to long-term compromise of the patient's health.

## Long-term Issues

Long term arbitrarily covers the period following the completion of initial healing and the maintenance phase. Recognition of diseases that leave the patient compromised with respect to disease susceptibility or metabolic imbalances requires judgement in the absence of established clinical data, for example:

- smoking
- osteonecrosis – induced by drugs (e.g. bisphosphonates) or radiation therapy
- neurological, social or psychiatric disorders that compromise patient compliance
- endocrine metabolic disorders such as unstable diabetes or thyroid disorders.

## Further Investigations

In cases where more complicated procedures are necessary, particularly those requiring a general anaesthetic or if the patient is uncertain about any aspects of his or her general health, additional investigations may be carried out. These should include blood tests to provide information about the blood cells and the biochemical components. Any irregularity that warrants further investigation should be followed up by a specialist physician.

## Specialist Referral

Referral to a specialist physician should be considered for all patients whose mental or physical well-being is in question. This would include those

- who are already under the care of a health professional
- who have irregularities in their medical history

- who show abnormal results in medical investigations.

Letters to the specialist should describe the procedure that is to be carried out. Details should be given of the length of the planned procedure, the drugs that need to be used and the type of anaesthetic (local, general or sedation) required. The physician should also be informed of any post-operative medication that is likely to be prescribed so that the specialist is able to advise on the suitability of the procedure and whether any variation in the drug regimen is advised.

## Patient Management

In modern surgery, the conditions under which any procedure is carried out must be without pain and anxiety and with the reduction of risks to a minimum. Typically treatment may be carried out under
- local anaesthesia
- sedation and local anaesthesia
- general anaesthesia.

### Local Anaesthesia

Local anaesthesia is suitable for minor procedures of short duration. However, with good patient management, longer procedures can be carried out with local anaesthesia without adjunctive management of anxiety. Longer procedures require larger amounts of local anaesthetic agent and the patient's ability to metabolise the anaesthetic agent must be assessed to prevent systemic compromise.

### Conscious Sedation and Local Anaesthesia

Inhalation sedation or oral sedation may be used employing established protocols and guidelines.

Intravenous sedation offers distinct advantages. When used responsibly as an incremental drug it offers control over the level of sedation. The use of an indwelling canula is, therefore, necessary. Current guidelines require blood pressure, pulse and oxygen saturation to be monitored. All vital signs need to be recorded along with the dosages, timing and batch numbers of all drugs used. A nasal oxygen canula is also recommended.

Where there is a single operator/sedationist, a single sedative drug is recommended. The most commonly used single drug is midazolam.

There are other distinct advantages of having an intravenous line. Additional drugs may be administered, including:
- antibiotics – administration of an antibiotic 30 min prior to surgery ensures the drug will reach soft and hard tissues
- steroids – for reduction of post-operative discomfort and oedema[34,35]
- non-steroidal anti-inflammatory drugs or analgesics
- atropin – reduction in salivary flow and secretions
- anti-fibrinolytic agents such as tranexamic acid
- sedative antagonist such as flumazenil
- antiemetics such as metoclopramide or ondansetron.

Intravenous access is also useful for any other remedial or emergency drug that may need to be administered.

Most patients have a higher level of anxiety prior to surgery, often resulting in an increased blood pressure ('white-coat effect'). The use of a sedative agent reduces blood pressure and associated bleeding. Additional benefits are a reduced likelihood of any hypertension-related incidents. Most importantly the amnesia caused by the sedative drug results in a less unpleasant experience.

Longer procedures can, therefore, be carried out always bearing in mind that the threshold of the local anaesthetic required is not exceeded.

Adequate training of the operator as well as the assistant is essential. The procedure must be supported by adequate monitoring of the patient, with appropriate emergency drugs and equipment available, as well as recovery facilities. A non-anxious healthy patient (ASA 1 or 2) may well be managed by a trained operator–sedationist.

Anxious and phobic patients are more safely treated by a dedicated sedationist, who is able to use supplementary drugs to provide deeper conscious sedation. The sedationist is also able to monitor the level of consciousness of the patient more closely. A number of short-acting drugs may be used. The most common is propofol, a strong hypnotic drug that does not have analgesic effects and, therefore, is often used with fentanyl, an opioid and a very powerful analgesic.

Patients who have medical problems that are controlled but who need more close systemic monitoring should also be treated by a dedicated sedationist.

## General Anaesthesia

General anaesthesia is indicated in a variety of circumstances, which may relate to the management of the patient, the length and invasiveness of the procedure or the medical condition.

Patients who require extensive surgery such as iliac crest grafts, inferior alveolar nerve repositioning or even simultaneous treatment of both jaws are most comfortably treated under general anaesthesia. Anxious and phobic patients can be treated without any concerns regarding cooperation.

Current practice requires intubation to protect the airway. The hospital environment with extensive recovery, resuscitation and intensive care facilities is often chosen for the management of patients with more extensive systemic disease (ASA 3).

The anaesthetist must assess the patient preoperatively, prescribing any special investigations that may be necessary. Communication with specialist physicians and surgeons may be used to influence the management of the patient. General anaesthesia is a well-established and safe method of treatment.

# Chapter 5

# Additional Diagnostic Procedures

## Diagnostic Imaging

Radiographic examination appropriate to the proposed treatment should be carried out in order to establish the presence or absence of pathology, the assessment of the hard tissues and as an aid to planning treatment.[36,37]

Implant dentistry requires specific information from diagnostic imaging additional to that required for other branches of dentistry involving advanced restorative treatment. These are listed below.

- **Bone volume**.
  - **Bone height**. This is usually measured from the crest of a ridge to the opposing border of the jaw or relevant anatomical structure. It includes alveolar and basal bone. Selection of the implant length is based on this.
  - **Bone width**. This refers to the bucco-lingual width. Selection of the diameter of implant is based on this.
  - **Length of the edentulous ridge**. This refers to the distance between two adjacent teeth and of their roots in a bound gap or the length along the crest of an edentulous ridge. This determines the number of implants and the distance between the implants and adjacent teeth.
- **Bone quality**. This refers to the density and thickness of the cortical portion as well as the trabecular density in the cancellous portion. This will influence the success of treatment or the method by which osteotomy preparation may be carried out. It may be used for the assessment of bone for immediate loading.
- **Ridge orientation**. This is the inclination of the edentulous ridge to the adjacent teeth and the proposed restoration. It will influence the angulation at which the implant is placed.
- **Spatial relationship of bone to the proposed restoration**. This provides information relating tooth position to the bony ridge in horizontal (bucco-lingual and mesiodistal) and vertical (corono-apical) dimensions. It, therefore, relates the proposed tooth position to the proposed implant position.
- **Relationship to anatomical structures**. Implant dentistry requires the precise identification and location of anatomical structures in order to prevent damage during hard and soft tissue surgery.

The diagnostic imaging techniques currently available are outlined with some of the benefits specific to implant dentistry.

# I Introduction and Assessment

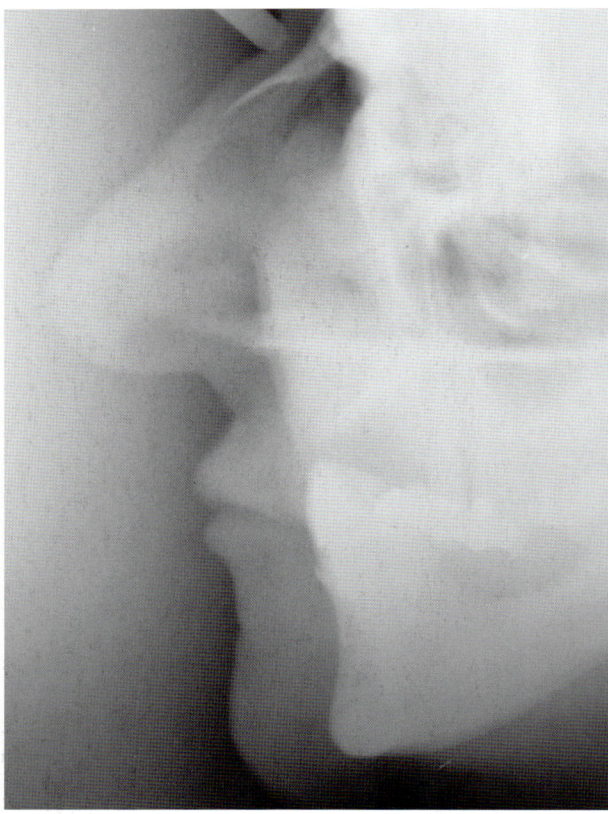

**Fig 5-1** Lateral cephalograph using soft tissue filter prior to treatment. The soft tissue contours can be seen with the patient's mandible in an overclosed position due to an absence of the maxillary denture.

## Dental Panoramic Tomography (Orthopantomography)

A good diagnostic dental panoramic tomograph (DPT), otherwise known as orthopantomograph, provides the clinician with a good overview of the mouth.

The presence of teeth, any pathology and related anatomical structures, as well as bone heights, all on one image makes it an invaluable treatment planning aid. Judicious measurement of the magnification of each section will provide the clinician with a reasonably accurate assessment of bone height available for implant placement. It is indicated for patients requiring implant treatment as a screening and planning aid.

## Periapical Radiography

Periapical radiographs provide details of the region being investigated. The structure, periodontal and endodontic status of the teeth can be established. The level of bone in the edentulous ridge and its level of attachment to the adjacent teeth can be measured accurately, and residual roots and pathology within the ridge can be seen in detail.

## Lateral Cephalography

Lateral cephalography provides excellent information regarding the facial profile (using soft tissue filters; Figs 5-1 and 5-2), the relation of the jaws and some indication about the width of bone in the midline (Fig 5-3).

## Conventional Tomography

Conventional tomography provide cross-sectional information about the area being investigated. However, it should be used with caution, as the magnification and mesiodistal positioning may lack accuracy,[38] and multiple exposures increase the radiation dose significantly. They do not have a place anymore in imaging in implant dentistry.

## Computed Tomography

Computed tomography (CT) scans provides the implant clinician with a substantial amount of valuable information (Figs 5-4–5-8). The CT scan (and cone beam CT) is the only investigation that ideally provides the information that the implant surgeon requires for the planning of treatment. This includes bone volume and density, ridge orientation and spatial relationship to the proposed prosthesis, opposing jaw and anatomical structures. It is, therefore, the ideal investigation from the point of view of data provision. Accurate measurements can be made, which is particularly important when working within the posterior mandible.

Considerable advances have taken place in the development of scanners as well as software. Multi-slice and spiral CT scanners and their advancement in

## 5  Additional Diagnostic Procedures

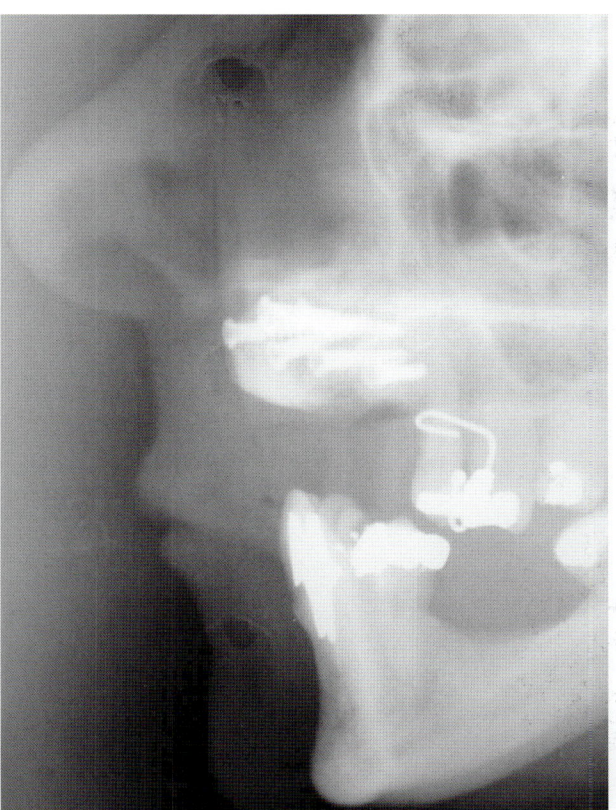

**Fig 5-2** Lateral cephalograph after augmentation. Same patient as Fig 5-1. The onlay graft can be seen with its effect on lip support.

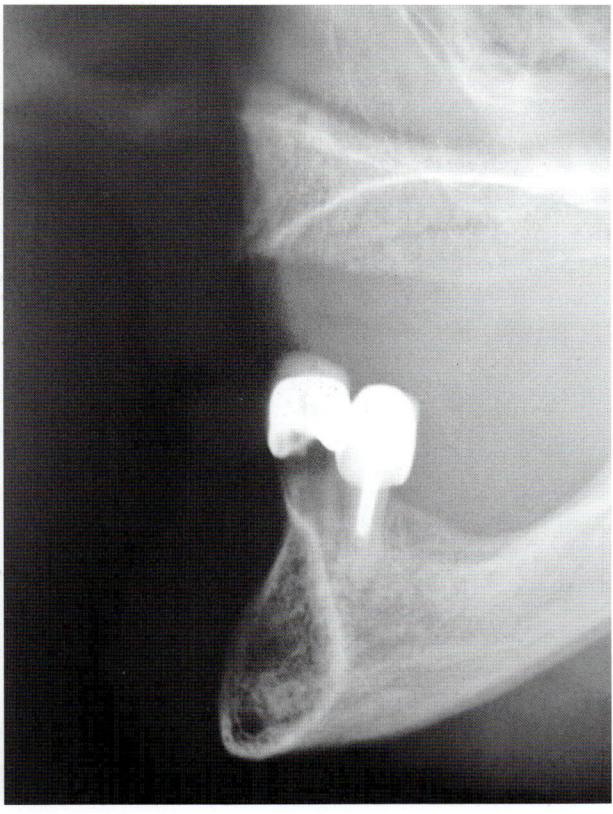

**Fig 5-3** The lateral cephalograph may be used to provide an indication of bone availability in the midline, both in the maxilla and the mandible. It will also provide information about the intermaxillary relationship.

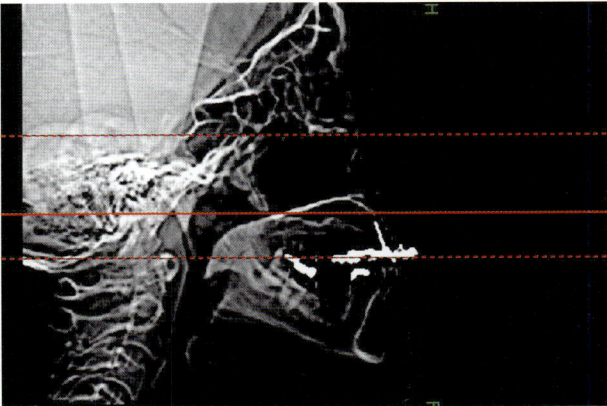

**Fig 5-4** CT Scan in scout view (lateral view of the skull). This is used to determine the area to be scanned (between red lines).

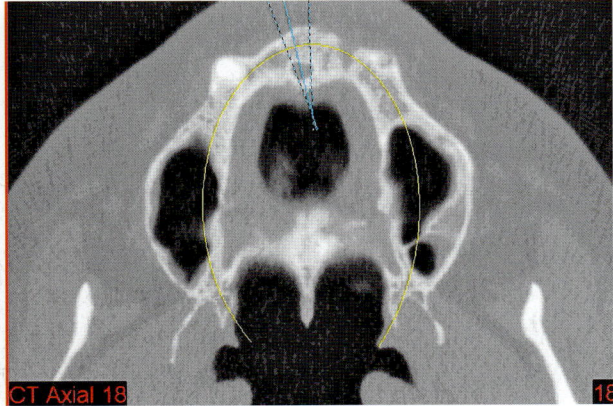

**Fig 5-5** CT scan in axial section through the maxilla passing through the canine teeth and depicting the maxillary sinuses. The mandibular rami and the pterygoid plates as well as the surrounding soft tissues are visible. The greater density of the muscles is discernible. The yellow line indicates the position of the panoramic section (Fig 5-7) and the blue lines the position of the cross-sectional reformations of the alveolar ridge (Fig 5-6).

21

I | Introduction and Assessment

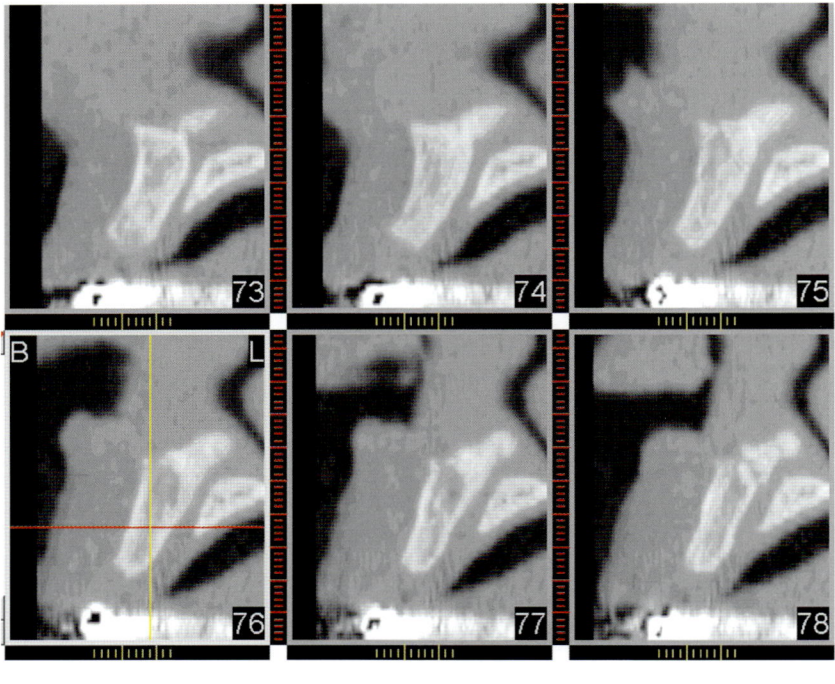

**Fig 5-6** Cross-section of the maxilla in the midline showing the ridge width, density and inclination. The naso-palatine foramen and canal can be seen. The buccal aspect is on the left of each section and the palatal on the right. The radiopacity at the bottom of each image is due to the metal framework of the provisional fixed partial denture.

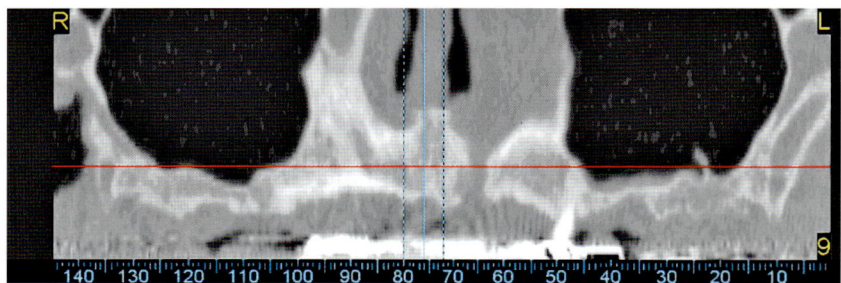

**Fig 5-7** A panoramic section through the maxilla depicting the structures within that section: one root can be seen, on the left-hand side, the nasal cavities, and both maxillary sinuses with a small septum in the left sinus. A bony deficiency in the region of the left lateral incisor can also be noted.

detector and data acquisition technology have greatly improved accuracy and reduced radiation dosage as well as scanning time.

CT scans can provide information regarding the density of the cortical and cancellous components of the ridge (Fig 5-9). The bone density is measured using the Hounsfield unit (HU), which is an X-ray attenuation (density) measurement used to describe voxel (volume element in a 3D image) values in CT scanning.

Voxels are normally represented as 12-bit binary numbers and, therefore, have 4096 possible values. These values are arranged on a scale from minus (-) 1.024 HU to plus (+) 3.071 HU and calibrated so that -1.024 HU is the attenuation produced by air and 0 HU is the attenuation produced by water.

Cancellous bone is normally between 200 and 700 HU, depending on the trabecular density, but can be lower depending on the quality of the bone and the quantity of fat.[39] Fatty soft tissues range from approximately -100 to -20 HU, and water-based soft tissue, such as muscle, ranges from +20 to +80 HU. Cortical bone has a range in the region of 1000 HU, but metals used in the construction of dental prostheses will have a greater density, usually of more than 2000 HU, which may lead to artefacts that make it difficult to interpret the image.

## Cone Beam Computed Tomography

Cone beam CT differs from conventional CT in the manner in which data is acquired. Instead of multiple slices, the source of radiation is a tube generating a

## 5  Additional Diagnostic Procedures

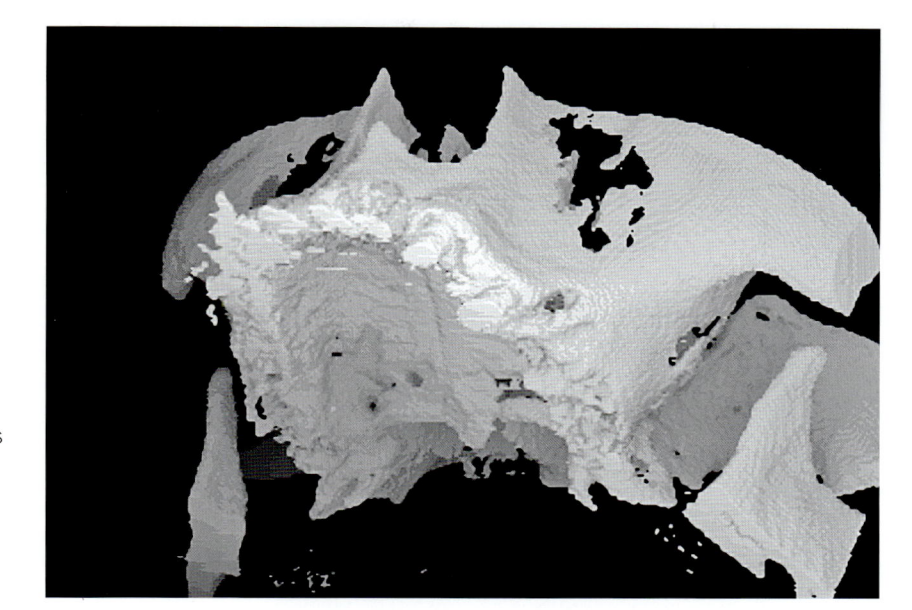

**Fig 5-8**  A 3D view of the bony structures of the maxilla observed obliquely from the left inferior aspect. The zygomatic process, anterior nasal spine, the roots on the left-hand side as well as the deficiency in the left lateral incisor region are all visible. The thin wall of the maxillary sinus appears to be incomplete and the algorithm used for the 3D reconstruction causes this phenomenon.

**Fig 5-9**  Cross-sectional image of maxillary ridge with implant placed between the cortical plates (red). The abutment has been attached and is angled to connect the implant to the projected tooth position as depicted by the provisional restoration. The overall density of the bone surrounding the implant is on the right-hand side outlined by the bar chart showing the variation of density in Hounsfield units along the implant length. The mean bone density can be seen to be 457 HU. (Simplant, Materialise, Leuven, Belgium.)

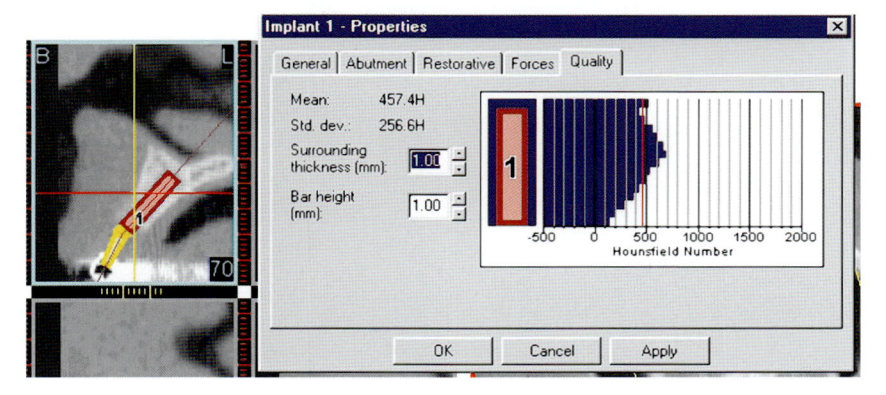

cone beam and the detection is carried out by means of a flat panel detector (FPD) or a charge-coupled device (CCD) performing one part or complete rotation. The net result of this is a lower radiation dose, with resultant reduced artefacts from heavy metal objects. The data can be acquired using a smaller field of view, thus leading to a further reduction in radiation dosage. However, reducing radiation dose affects the quality of the image.[40]

Cone beam CT scanners are smaller and less expensive than conventional medical CT scanners and can, therefore, be installed within a dental practice.

Technology in this field is developing fast; however, presently data about bone density cannot be accurately extracted.[41]

### Three-dimensional Interactive Software and Rapid Prototyping

Data from both conventional multislice and cone beam CT scanners is stored by using digital imaging and communications in medicine (DICOM) as file format and can, therefore, be converted to be used with commercially interactive planning software programs for implant dentistry.

The ability to interactively plan treatment by means of a computerised graphic simulation facilitates surgical procedures (Fig 5-9). Simulating treatment on the computer can now be transferred into the surgical field by using templates fabricated from these data (Figs 5-10 and 5-11).[42,43] Implants can then be accurately positioned using these templates (Figs 5-12 and 5-13).

I | Introduction and Assessment

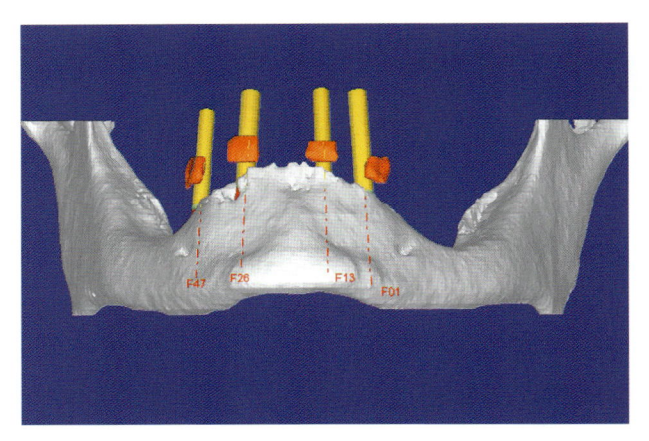

**Fig 5-10** Three-dimensional view of the mandible from the anterior aspect with four implants placed interactively in the interforaminal region (yellow bars). The red markers represent radiopaque markers placed within the patient's denture in the region of the lateral incisors and first premolars. This information will be transferred to a surgical guide (Simplant).

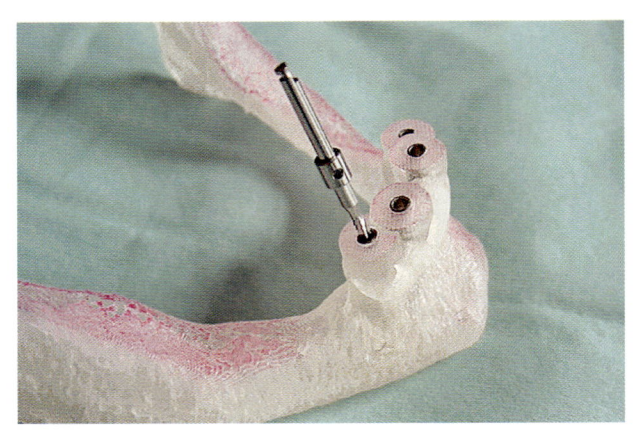

**Fig 5-11** Three-dimensional model of jaw and CT data-based surgical template fabricated by means of stereolithography. The pilot bur is directed by the titanium tubes positioned from the treatment planned on the computer, positioning the implants precisely in the ideal position. (Same patient as in Fig 5-10.)

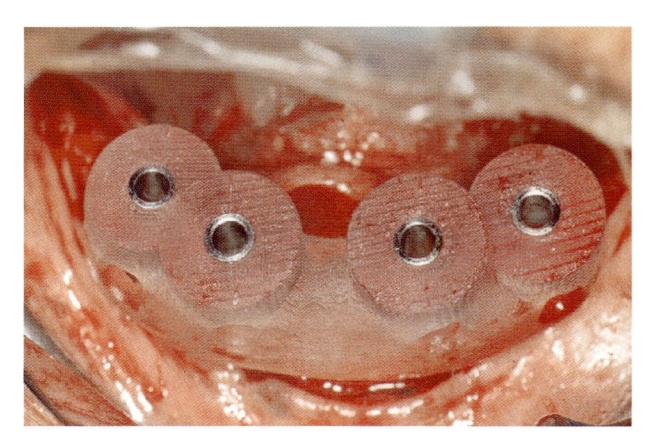

**Fig 5-12** Surgical template constructed from the treatment planning data fits precisely onto the bony ridge to enable implants to be placed accurately as planned. (Same patient as in Fig 5-10.)

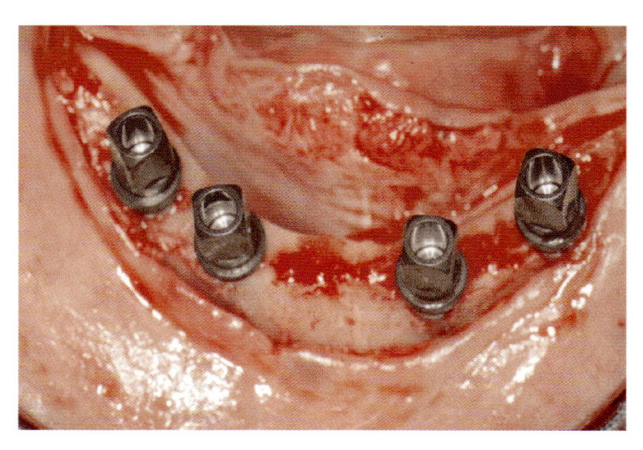

**Fig 5-13** Implants after placement, using CT data-based surgical template. (Same patient as in Fig 5-10.)

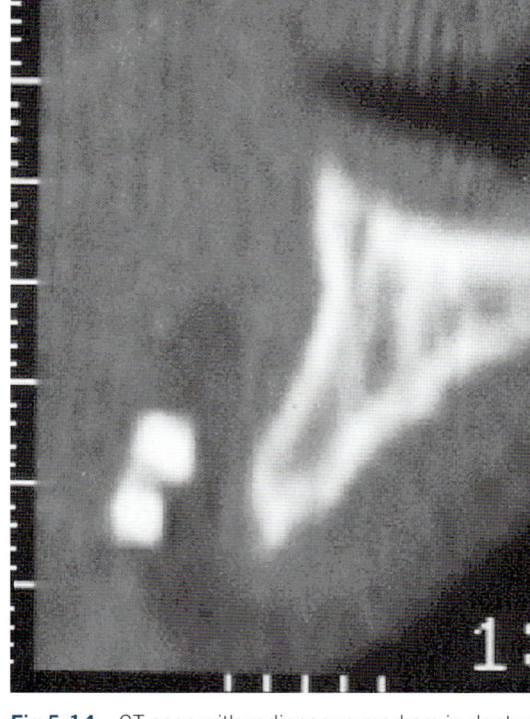

**Fig 5-14** CT scan with radiopaque markers in denture flange indicating tooth position. The two markers denote the lateral incisor position adjacent to a narrow ridge.

5   Additional Diagnostic Procedures

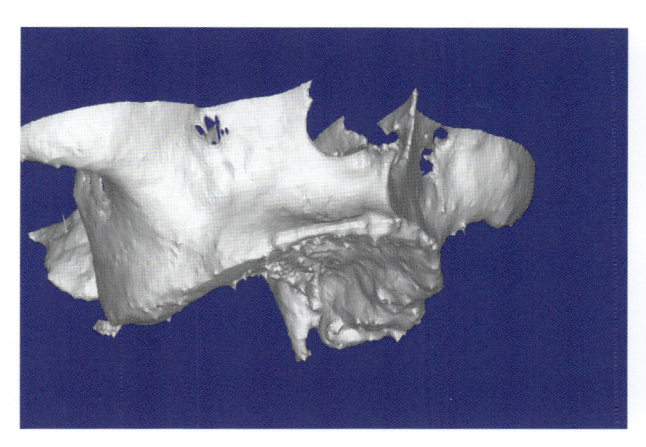

**Fig 5-15** Preoperative 3D reconstruction of maxilla. The severe resorption of the anterior maxilla is evident.

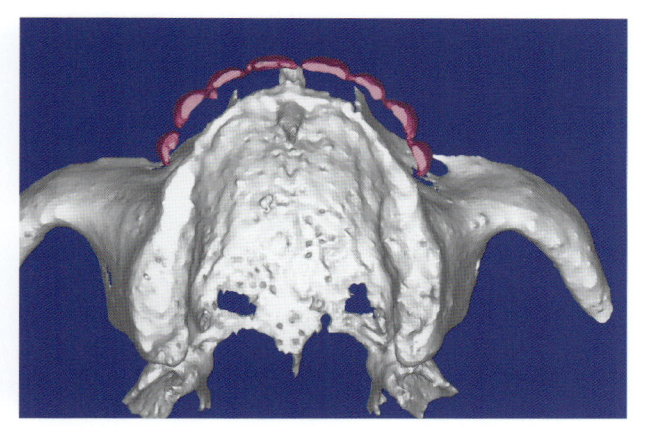

**Fig 5-16** Occlusal view of the 3D reconstruction in Fig 5-15 with the radiopaque markers defining the labial surfaces of the planned teeth. The bucco-lingual discrepancy is evident, clearly demonstrating the labial resorption.

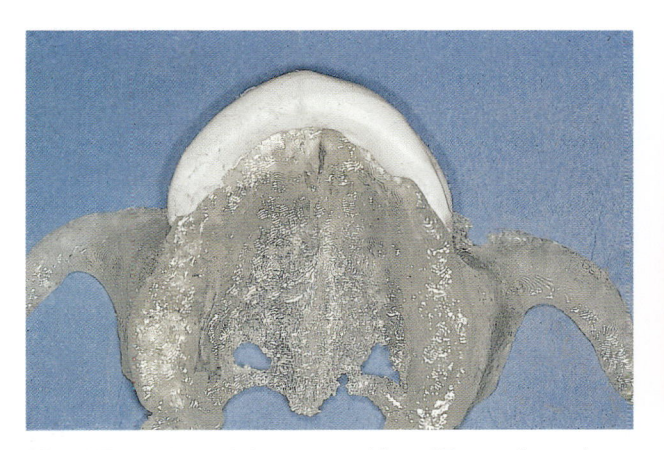

**Fig 5-17** Resin model constructed from CT scan data using stereolithography, with a silicone template fabricated to provide the information about the size and shape of the bone graft required for reconstruction to enable implants to be inserted according to the planned tooth position.

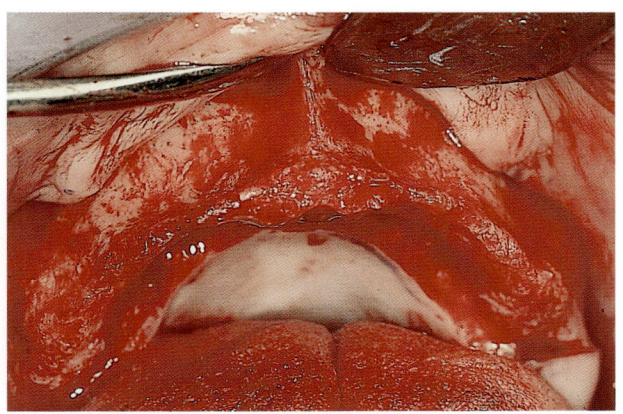

**Fig 5-18** Clinical view of the exposed ridge at augmentation surgery which can be related to the preoperative 3D reconstruction (see Fig 5-15).

The use of radiopaque markers enables the clinician to relate the diagnostic tooth position to the available bone (Fig 5-14).[44]

The advent of interactive planning in conjunction with 3D visualisation further refines treatment planning, particularly in being able to relate tooth position to the implant–abutment complex, as well as the available bone, which may need to be augmented. The software is sophisticated enough to be able to distinguish between the bone graft and the original bone as well as any markers of distinct radiopacity (Figs 5-15–5-25).

Software to assess the consequences of treatment and proposed treatment on the soft tissue contours of the face is available and being refined further.

The evolving process of prefabricating prostheses to be fitted onto implants planned interactively will be addressed in greater detail in the appropriate section (Chapter 7).

**I** Introduction and Assessment

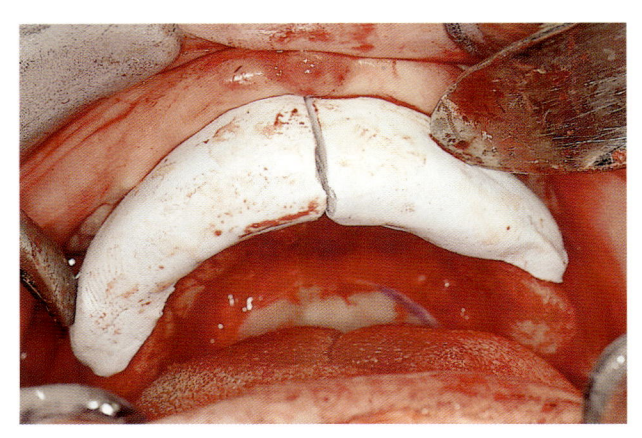

**Fig 5-19** Clinical view of silicone template being tried in to plan soft tissue closure.

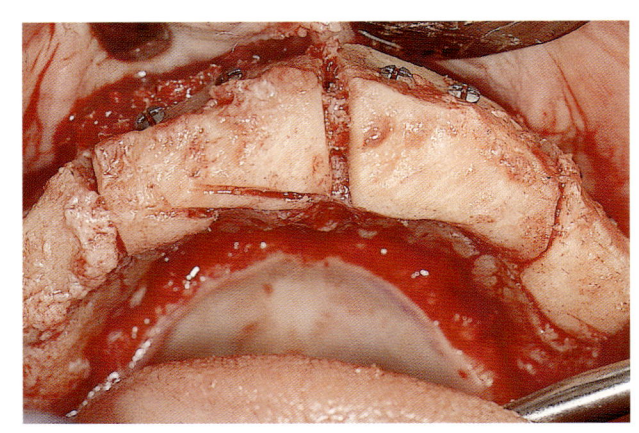

**Fig 5-20** Cortico-cancellous block bone graft obtained from the iliac crest fixed with screws reconstructing the ridge in width and height to the prescribed dimensions.

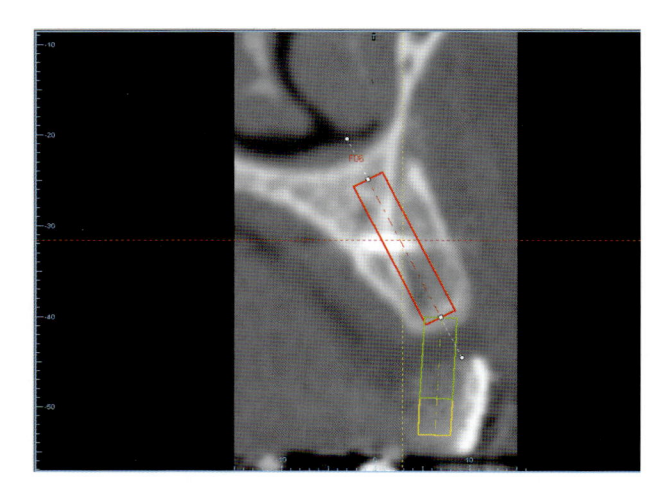

**Fig 5-21** Interactive planning on the cross-sectional view of the augmented ridge based on a CT scan taken prior to implant placement. The grafted bone is visible and can be differentiated from the original ridge. The fixation screw is partly visible, as is the labial outline of the prosthetic envelope depicted by the radiopaque marker on the template, which was worn by the patient during the scan. The future implant position is planned and selected to engage the grafted bone and maxillary ridge. Its dimension is outlined in red; the angled abutment (37.5 degrees) is selected at the same time to fit within the prosthetic envelope and can be seen in green with the prosthetic space visible in yellow.

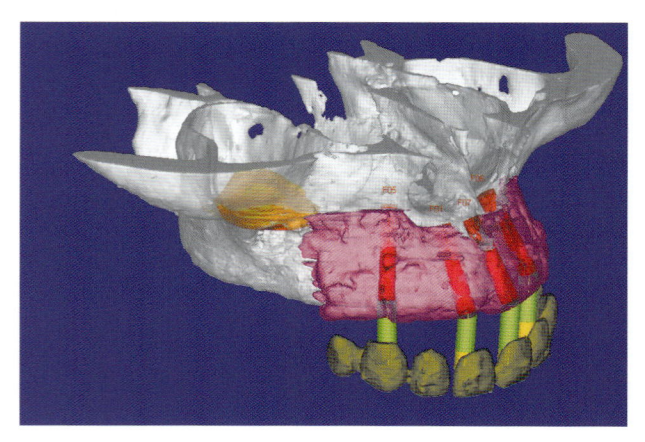

**Fig 5-22** The implants planned in central incisor and canine position are visible in the oblique 3D reconstruction. The alignment of the abutments (green) within the prosthetic envelope (brown) is visible. The augmented bone (purple) has been rendered translucent to enable the future implant position and orientation to be seen in 3D (red).

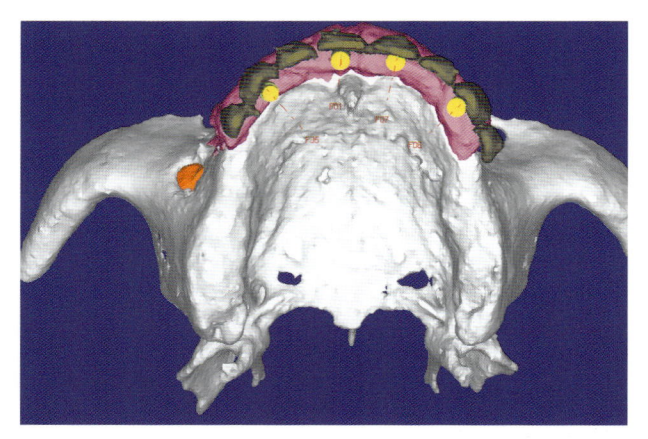

**Fig 5-23** Occlusal view of the 3D planning image indicating the parallel abutments (yellow) within the buccal aspect of the prosthetic envelope (brown).

**5** Additional Diagnostic Procedures

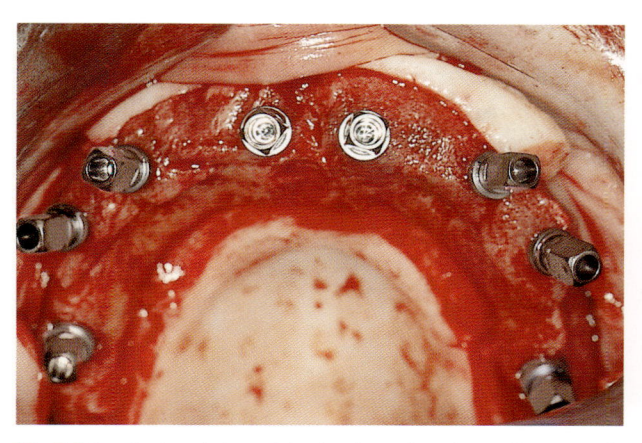

**Fig 5-24** Occlusal view of the implants (carriers still attached) inserted into positions determined by the template. The alignment of the implants according to the planned positions can be seen.

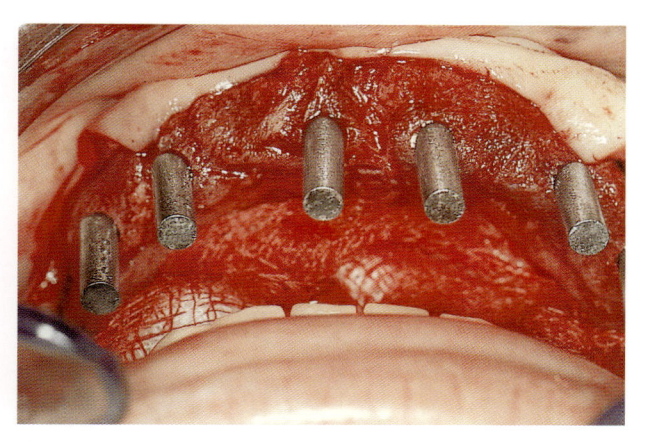

**Fig 5-25** Direction indicators used to confirm the abutment angle that has been selected interactively. Additional implants not shown on the above images for the sake of image clarity were also planned and can be seen with their abutments aligned.

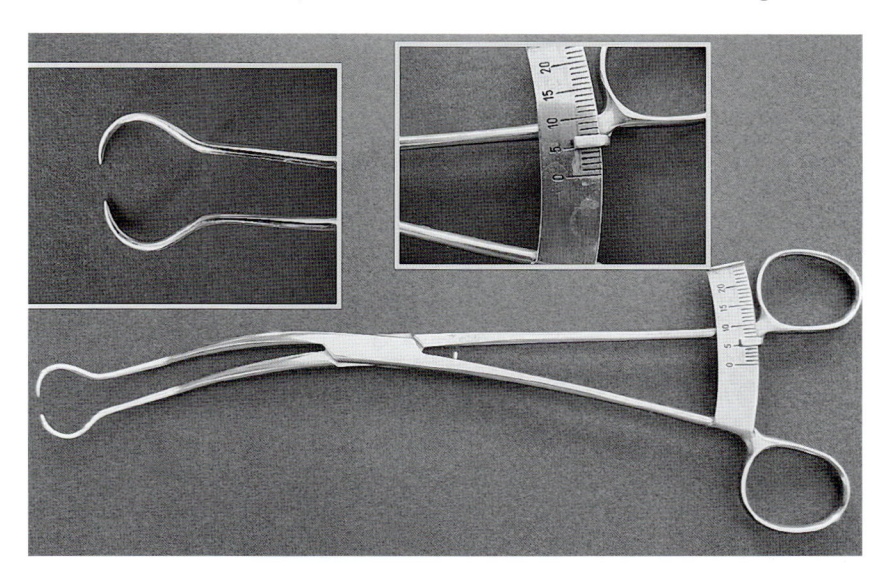

**Fig 5-26** Original ridge-mapping calipers designed by Wilson.

## Magnetic Resonance Imaging

Magnetic resonance imaging (MRI) is useful for depicting the soft tissues but is not commonly used during the planning of implant treatment, because hard tissues are difficult to assess with this technique.[45,46] Future refinements and development of software holds promise for this technique.

## Ridge Mapping

Ridge mapping is a means of direct measurement of the ridge width through the soft tissues.[47] The procedure is carried out under local anaesthetic using a pair of sharp calibrated calipers (Fig 5-26). Measurements are carried out at several points along the ridge at each proposed implant site. The first measurement is taken approximately 3 mm from the soft tissue crest, which is often at the edge of the bony crest. Several other measurements taken at approximately 3 mm intervals

27

**I** Introduction and Assessment

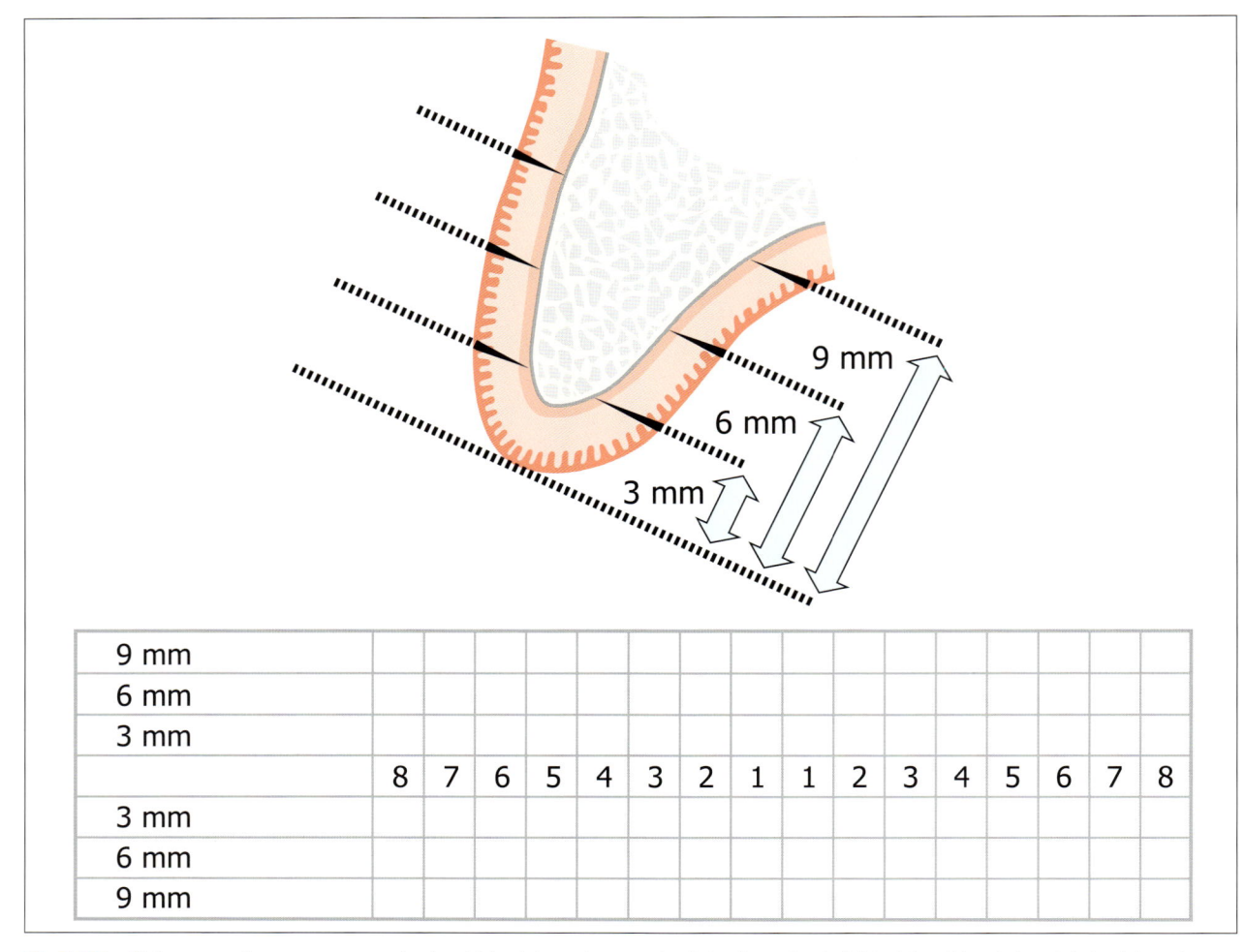

|   |   |   |   |   |   |   |   |   |   |   |   |   |   |   |   |   |
|---|---|---|---|---|---|---|---|---|---|---|---|---|---|---|---|---|
| 9 mm |   |   |   |   |   |   |   |   |   |   |   |   |   |   |   |   |
| 6 mm |   |   |   |   |   |   |   |   |   |   |   |   |   |   |   |   |
| 3 mm |   |   |   |   |   |   |   |   |   |   |   |   |   |   |   |   |
|   |   | 8 | 7 | 6 | 5 | 4 | 3 | 2 | 1 | 1 | 2 | 3 | 4 | 5 | 6 | 7 | 8 |
| 3 mm |   |   |   |   |   |   |   |   |   |   |   |   |   |   |   |   |
| 6 mm |   |   |   |   |   |   |   |   |   |   |   |   |   |   |   |   |
| 9 mm |   |   |   |   |   |   |   |   |   |   |   |   |   |   |   |   |

**Fig 5-27** Ridge-mapping measurements should be taken at several points along the height of the ridge to be able to determine the outline of the bony ridge. This should be recorded for each site that has been selected for implant placement. A typical chart for such records can be seen. Additional measurements at 12 or 15 mm from the ridge crest may sometimes need to be made.

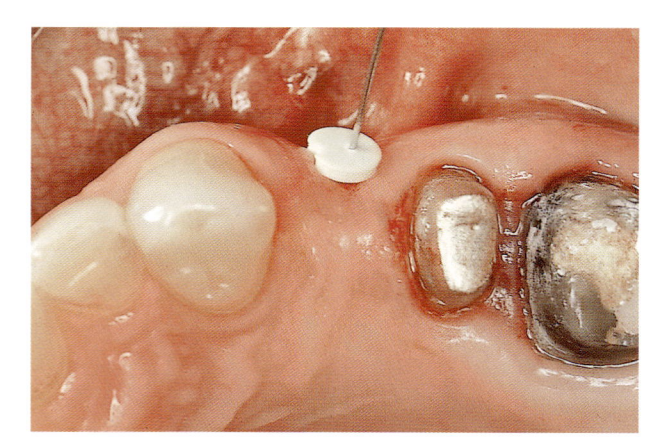

**Fig 5-28** Ridge mapping with a sharp probe and a rubber stop. The probe is inserted until it contacts bone and the measurement of tissue depth is transferred to the cast.

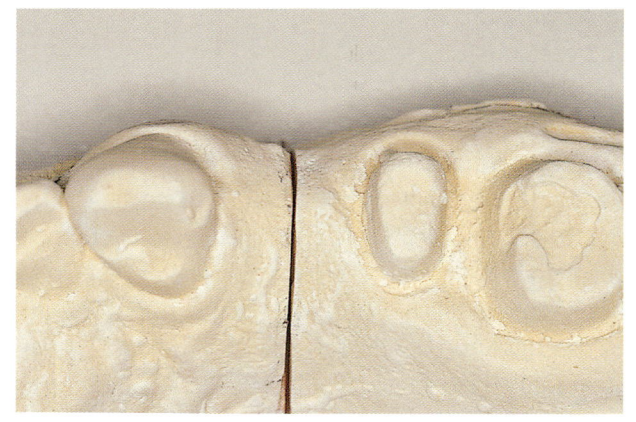

**Fig 5-29** A plaster cast is sectioned in the region of interest, where the measurements have been made.

**5** Additional Diagnostic Procedures

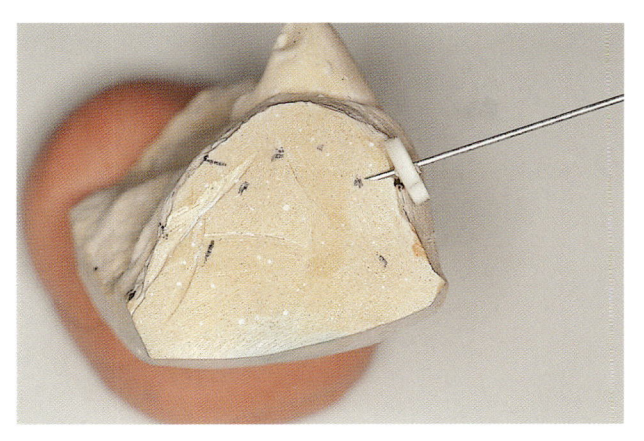

**Fig 5-30** Transfer of measurement to the cast made at the same distance from the ridge crest.

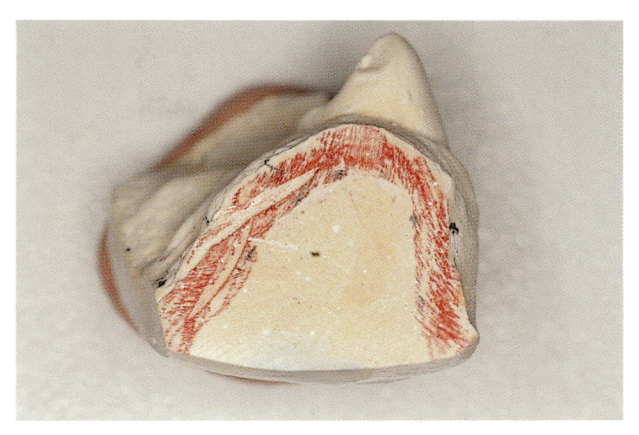

**Fig 5-31** Sectioned cast showing bony ridge as identified by ridge mapping. The soft tissues are shaded in red.

are used to provide cross-sectional information about the ridge at that particular point (Fig 5-27). The technique using calipers merely provides the width of the ridge, and clinical judgement has to be used about its relationship to the tooth position. Alternatively, a sharp probe with a rubber stop can be used for ridge mapping. Measurements are then transferred to a sectioned cast of the ridge, and the bony profile can be outlined indicating its position within the ridge (Figs 5-28–5-32). However, the advent of 3D low-radiation and low-cost imaging techniques, which offer much greater information, has made ridge mapping a less common technique.

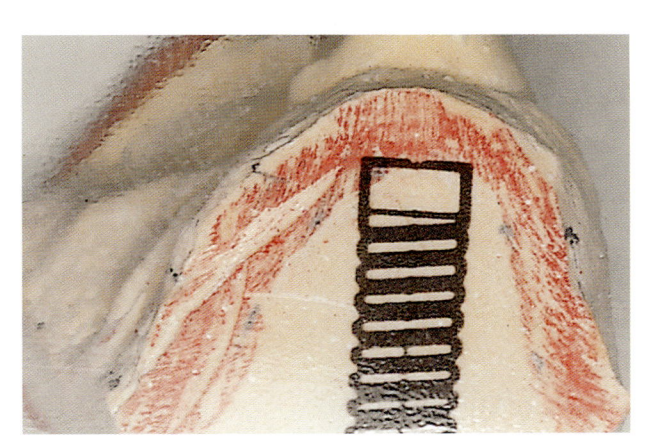

**Fig 5-32** The prepared cast can be used to select the implant of the correct width. Angulation of the implant can also be estimated.

## Study Casts and Diagnostic Preview

Impressions of the jaws using irreversible hydrocolloids and cast in plaster should be articulated using a semi-adjustable articulator in the intercuspal position. Facebow records may be used to transfer the relationship between the maxilla and the temporomandibular joints. Recording the relationship of the jaws to one another may be achieved by using occlusal registration pastes or wax for patients in stable occlusions. Wax registration blocks constructed on acrylic resin baseplates should be used for edentulous patients or for those who require changes in the occlusal vertical dimension.

These articulated study casts provide information about both the static and the dynamic positions of the jaw. This enables a diagnostic preview to be carried out by arranging acrylic resin teeth in wax in the ideal tooth position. Functional viability may be established and aesthetic acceptance of the arrangement confirmed by transferring the preview to the mouth for patient approval. Further confirmation can be achieved by the use of a provisional restoration that transfers the diagnostic preview data into the patient's mouth.

# Chapter 6

# Anatomical Variations

Surgical procedures designed to alter the form of the jaws or their function require the existing structures to be quantified in light of aesthetic and functional needs. Sufficient quantity of bone of adequate quality is required to provide appropriate support to withstand functional and parafunctional loads. Additionally, the position of the bone should be such that it allows implants to be placed in positions permitting normal function with the opposing jaw.

This should enable the prosthesis to be constructed in a manner that ensures that the aesthetic needs are met both in terms of the facial form and the emergence profile; this, in turn, will enhance the ability of the patient to carry out good oral hygiene.

## Atrophy

Pathology, dysfunction or disuse atrophy may result in deficient ridges. These have been classified by numerous authors based on observation and quantification or treatment possibilities.[48–52] The aim of this section is not to elaborate on these but to focus on variations resulting from the different locations within the mouth.

## Bone Quality

Bone quality has been described by a number of authors. Lekholm et al.[51] divided bone density into four classes based on the proportions of cortical and cancellous bone. Misch described the four qualities of bone according to their resistance to drilling.[53,54]

The clinical distinction between the two middle grades of bone in both these systems is often difficult to make and is of doubtful significance in clinical practice. A number of authors have addressed this issue and based their conclusions both on clinical and radiological observations.

Clinical perception of bone density is considered to be most accurately made using hand instruments.[55] Clinical classification of the bone density was compared with histomorphometric analysis, and no significant differences could be found between the two middle classifications in the above systems.[55] Analysis of bone density using modern imaging techniques (interactive CT) also showed the two middle grades to be difficult to differentiate.[39]

Other clinicians have adjusted their clinical approach based on the quality of bone. Nentwig has a specific protocol that relates to the surgical and prosthodontic management of three different bone quali-

# I  Introduction and Assessment

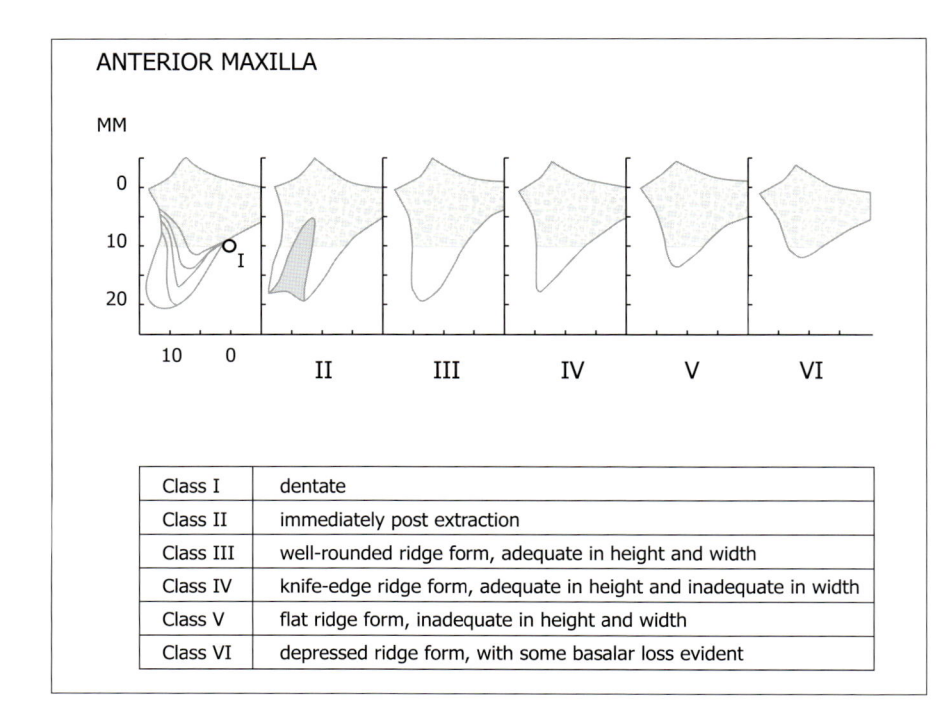

|  | |
|---|---|
| Class I | dentate |
| Class II | immediately post extraction |
| Class III | well-rounded ridge form, adequate in height and width |
| Class IV | knife-edge ridge form, adequate in height and inadequate in width |
| Class V | flat ridge form, inadequate in height and width |
| Class VI | depressed ridge form, with some basalar loss evident |

**Fig 6-1** Cawood and Howell classification for the anterior maxilla.[50] Class IV is the form of ridge that is most commonly found. It often has separate cortical plates with intervening cancellous bone (IVa), but on occasion the two cortical plates may be fused (IVb).

ties: hard, medium and soft. His assessment of bone quality is made clinically and ultimately by the type of hand instrument required to complete the osteotomy and bone tapping.[9]

The density of bone encountered is used to moderate the manner in which the implants are brought into function, based on the concept of progressive loading as introduced by Misch.[53,54]

## Anterior Maxilla

The factors significant to the anterior maxilla are outlined below.

### Bone Quantity

Following tooth loss, a reduction in ridge width takes place, which will vary from person to person, depending on numerous factors. Typically, the reduction takes place at the expense of the labial bone. A reduction in height is also observed. Within the first year of tooth loss, approximately 3 to 4 mm of height is lost where adjacent teeth are not present to sustain bone height.[56] This, of course, has a significant effect on the aesthetic outcome in patients who have a high smile-line. The resorption pattern of the anterior maxilla is depicted in Fig 6-1.

### Bone Quality

The alveolar ridge in the anterior maxilla most commonly consists of a thin and malleable cortical plate on the labial aspect and a dense and thicker cortical plate on the palatal aspect. There is often intervening cancellous bone of varying density (Cawood and Howell classification IVa). The quality of bone most prevalent in the anterior maxilla is of medium density, lying between the dense cortical bone of the anterior mandible and the sparsely trabeculated cancellous bone of the posterior maxilla.

### Ridge Orientation

The maxillary ridge typically flares labially, with its crest describing a larger circumference than its base (Fig 6-2). This is of significance in the placement of implants, which must be positioned at an angle to the longitudinal axis of the proposed restoration in keeping with the sound surgical principles of positioning the implants between the cortical plates. As a result, the coronal portion becomes labially inclined and frequently requires angular correction, with the abutment lingually inclined in relation to the implant (Figs 6-3–6-5).

# 6 Anatomical Variations

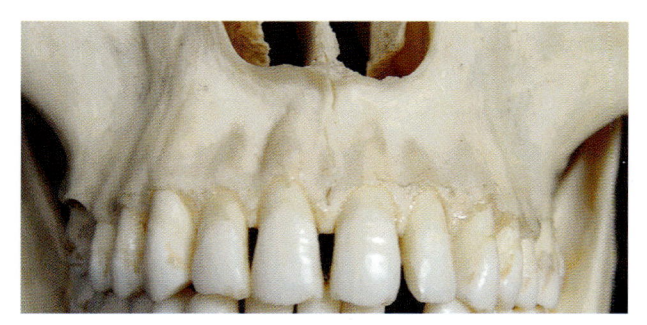

**Fig 6-2** Labial view of a dentate skull showing proclination of teeth and flare of maxilla. Note the thin cortical bone overlying the roots of the teeth, which is likely to resorb following tooth loss.

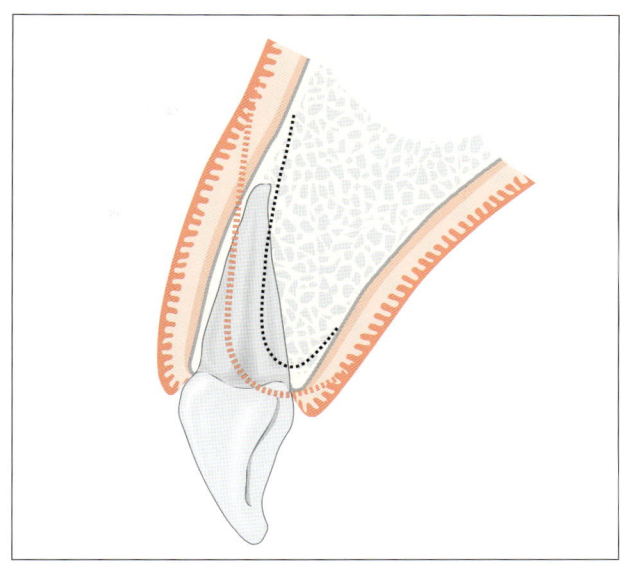

**Fig 6-3** Cross-sectional diagram of maxillary incisor showing thin cortical labial socket, with the possible resorption pattern outlined.

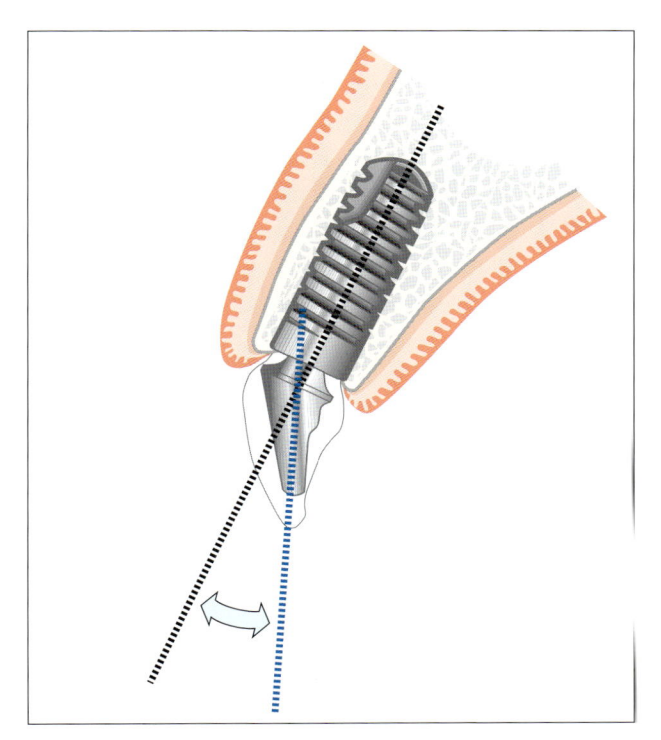

**Fig 6-4** Implant placed between cortical plates following ridge remodelling, depicting a difference in the angles between the implant and the long axis of crown.

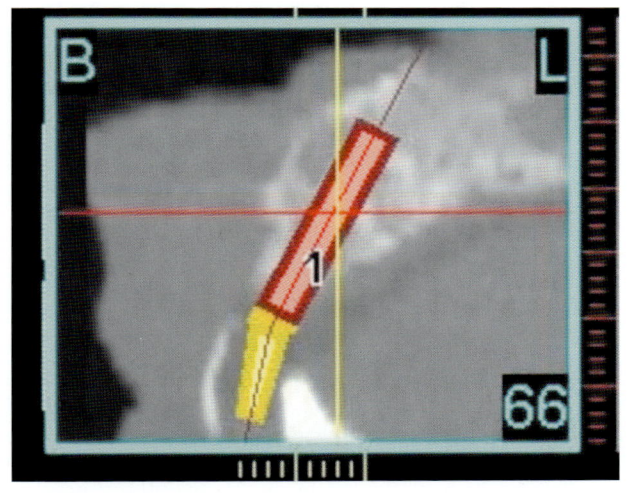

**Fig 6-5** CT scan showing angulation between the abutment determined by the future tooth position and the planned implant positioned ideally within the available bone. The labial aspect of the proposed restoration is identified by the radiopaque marker. The palatal aspect of the prosthetic envelope is identified by the position of the mandibular incisor.

## Special Clinical Considerations

Aesthetics are of utmost importance, particularly in patients with high smile-lines. The emergence profile, gingival margin and interdental papilla become disproportionately important.

Adequate assessment of the type of gingival–alveolar complex becomes quite important. Patients with thick alveolar ridges, where the roots are not palpable and not prominent, are less difficult to treat. This is because the collapse of the labial plate is less likely following tooth loss. It is often associated with flat, thick gingival margins (Fig 6-6).

This is in contrast with those patients who have prominent roots that are palpable and protrude from interdental depressions. The cortical plate surround-

33

**I** Introduction and Assessment

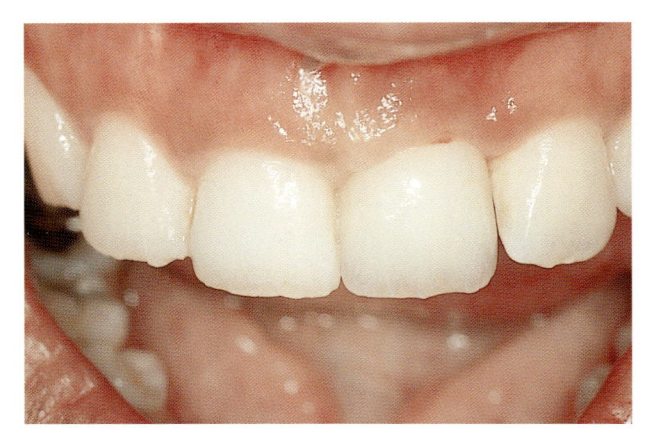

**Fig 6-6** Patient with flat gingival margins and low papillary height.

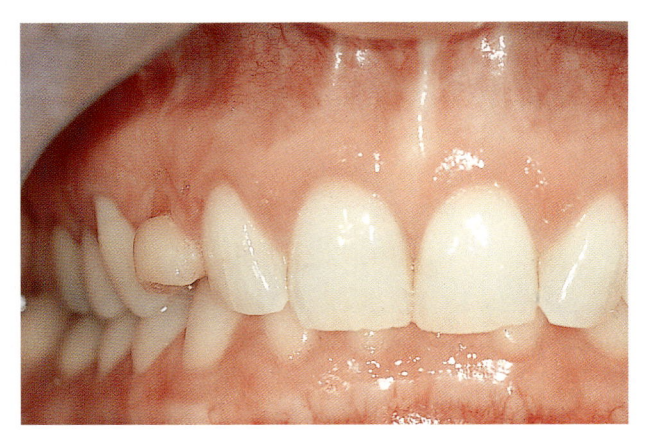

**Fig 6-7** Patient with scalloped gingival margins and significant papillary height.

ing the vestibular aspect of the roots is thin or non-existent and resorbs rapidly to the level of the interdental bone once the supporting tooth is lost. These patients are more difficult to treat because some form of re-contouring is often required. Caution should also be exercised if immediate implants are being considered because of the risk of resorption. Scalloping of the gingival margin is associated with this type of patient with prominent roots and is indicative of high interdental levels of bone and recession of the vestibular bone (Fig 6-7; see also Fig 6-2).

Support of the upper lip is also a consideration where multiple tooth replacement is necessary. The position of the naso-palatine canal becomes significant when replacing central incisors. It is in this area that bone expansion is most commonly carried out, to enable implants to be placed in the narrow ridges resulting from labial bone loss and to re-contour the labial plate to re-establish an aesthetic ridge form for the emergence profile. Autogenous onlay bone grafts are commonly used, with aesthetics being the primary indication even in situations where adequate bone is present for functional support. CT scans provide an opportunity to examine the underlying morphology and assist in making clinical decisions regarding possible future remodelling of bone (Figs 6-8–6-13).

## Posterior Maxilla

The factors significant to the posterior maxilla (defined as extending distally from the canines) are outlined below.

### Bone Quantity

Bone loss takes place at the expense of the labial plate and ridge height. However, this is not always significant because aesthetics are not usually critical in this region. The resorption pattern of the posterior maxilla is depicted in Fig 6-14. It is rarely the loss of alveolar bone that causes limitation in the height of the available bone, except in cases where extensive periodontal destruction has taken place. It is the enlargement of the maxillary sinus that is most commonly responsible for inadequate bone being present. The pneumatisation of the sinus varies and most commonly restricts the height in the area of the first molar but can extend from the pterygoid plate in a mesial direction as far as the central incisor, with the floor and lateral wall being reduced to a thin cortical shell.

### Bone Quality

Very thin cortical bone and very sparsely trabeculated cancellous bone are the hallmarks of the posterior maxilla, with bone quality deteriorating towards the distal area from medium density bone in the premolar region (Fig 6-15).

### Special Clinical Considerations

Implants are invariably positioned towards the palatal aspect as a result of the centripetal resorption resulting from labial bone loss. This may influence the intermaxillary relationship and speech. Access to the posterior maxilla is easily gained from the bucco-mesial aspect. An implant may need to be positioned at an angle in

6  Anatomical Variations

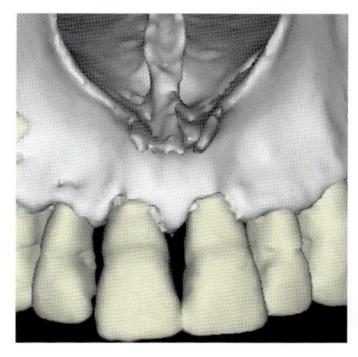

**Fig 6-8** Three-dimensional reconstruction of a CT scan showing minimal scalloping of labial bone. It is possible that less remodelling will be noted in this case.

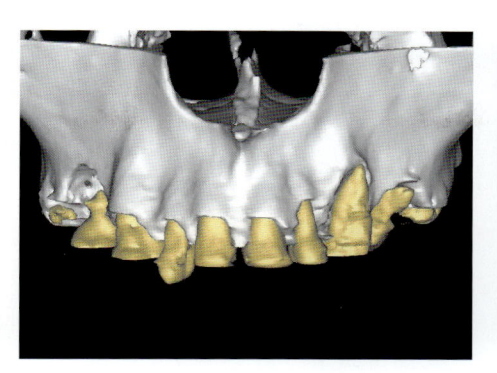

**Fig 6-9** Three-dimensional reconstruction of a maxilla showing severe interdental depressions indicating likelihood of possible extensive remodelling.

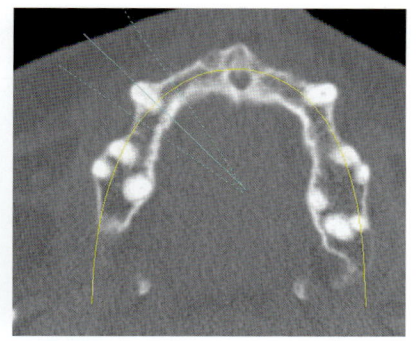

**Fig 6-10** Axial view of CT scan depicting very prominent roots in the maxillary canine region (Fig 6-11), healing socket in the right central incisor region (Fig 6-12) and healed sites in the lateral incisor regions (Fig 6-13). The loss of width can be predicted.

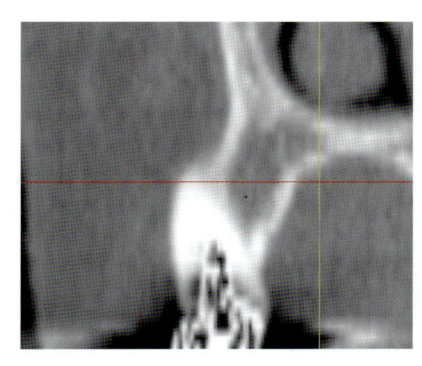

**Fig 6-11** Cross-sectional image through the canine region showing very thin labial bone overlying the prominent root.

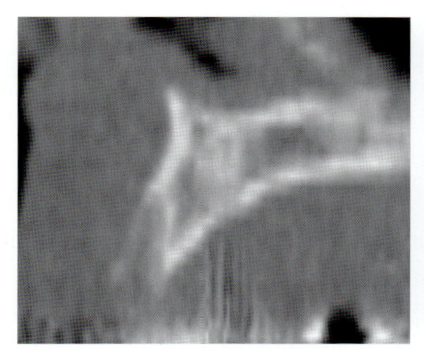

**Fig 6-12** Cross-section through the right central extract on site, which demonstrates the process of resorption taking place with the loss of the labial plate.

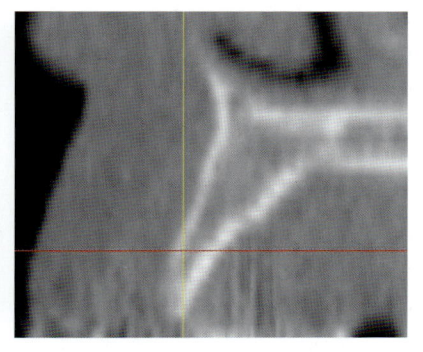

**Fig 6-13** Cross-section through the lateral incisor region depicting extremely narrow residual ridge following resorption after extraction.

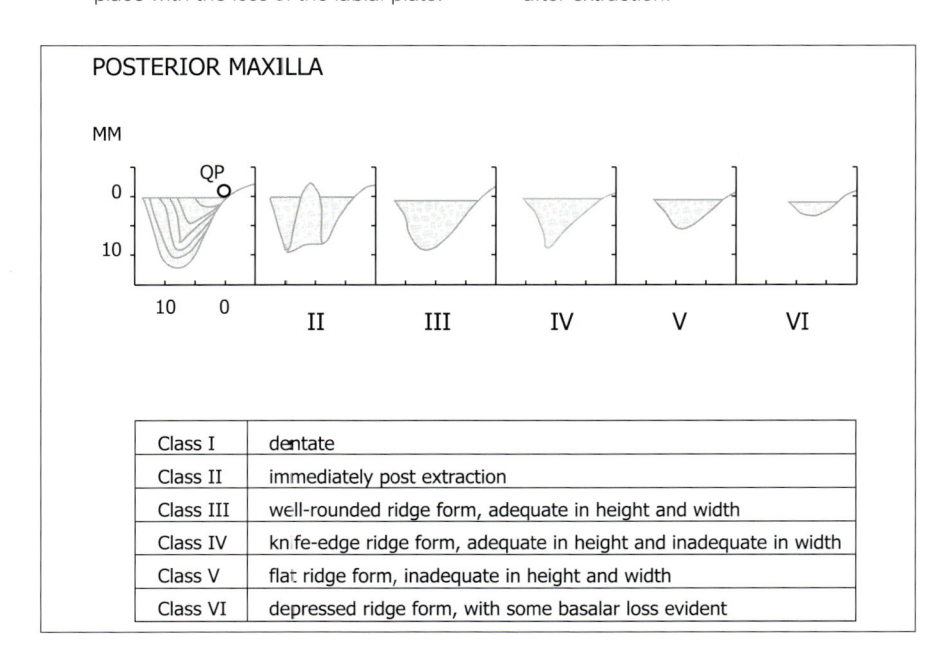

**Fig 6-14** Cawood and Howell classification for the posterior maxilla.[50] The most significant factor affecting bone availability is the enlargement of the sinus.

| Class I | dentate |
|---|---|
| Class II | immediately post extraction |
| Class III | well-rounded ridge form, adequate in height and width |
| Class IV | knife-edge ridge form, adequate in height and inadequate in width |
| Class V | flat ridge form, inadequate in height and width |
| Class VI | depressed ridge form, with some basalar loss evident |

**I** Introduction and Assessment

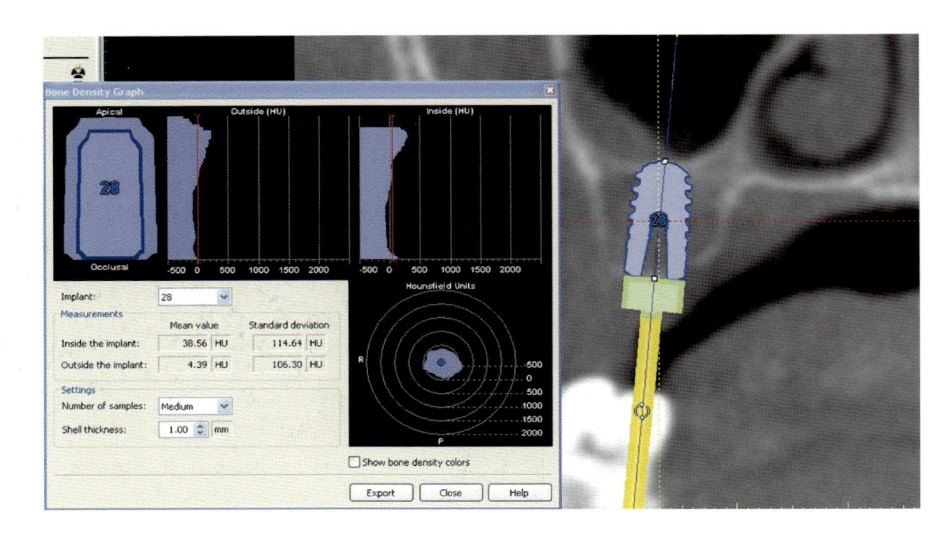

**Fig 6-15** Bone density in the posterior maxilla can be seen to be very low and just above that of water, which is 0 HU.

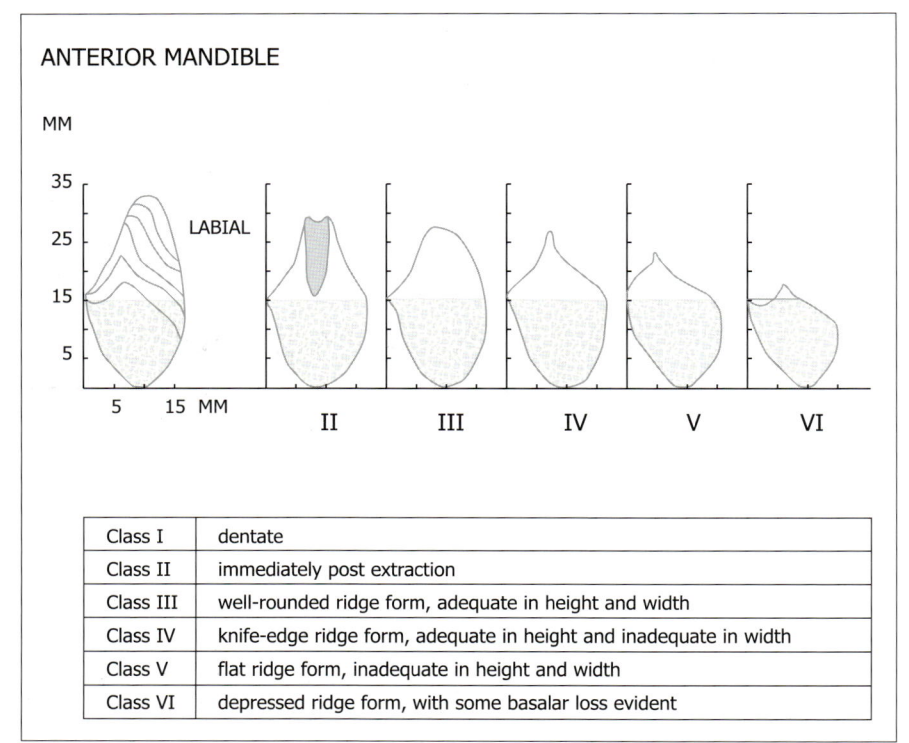

| Class I | dentate |
| Class II | immediately post extraction |
| Class III | well-rounded ridge form, adequate in height and width |
| Class IV | knife-edge ridge form, adequate in height and inadequate in width |
| Class V | flat ridge form, inadequate in height and width |
| Class VI | depressed ridge form, with some basalar loss evident |

**Fig 6-16** Cawood and Howell classification for the anterior mandible.[50]

order to avoid the maxillary sinus. Pterygoid and zygomatic implants have been developed to cope with the presence of the maxillary sinus.

Increasing the height of the available bone becomes critical in the positioning of implants. Manipulating the floor of the sinus at the time of implant placement enables larger implants to be used, as long as sufficient bone is present for primary stability (more than 7 mm). When there is a reduced amount of bone present, the sinus lift procedure carried out as a one- or two-stage approach has made the treatment of the posterior maxilla feasible, enabling large implants to be placed in a region where bone quality is normally poor and the occlusal loads are high. Severe alveolar destruction is occasionally the indication for an onlay bone graft, but the intermaxillary distance limits the bone height that can be gained by onlay grafts. Furthermore, the use of onlay bone grafts is rare because aesthetics are not

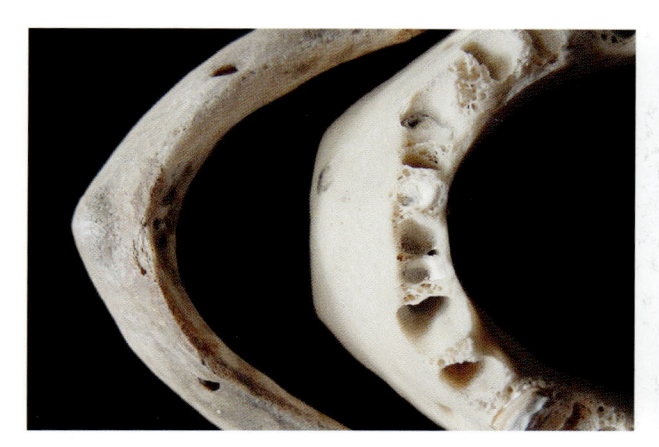

**Fig 6-17** Mandible immediately after extraction (right) and after atrophy has taken place (left). The loss of height results in the greater apparent circumference of the mandible caused by the centrifugal movement of the ridge crest.

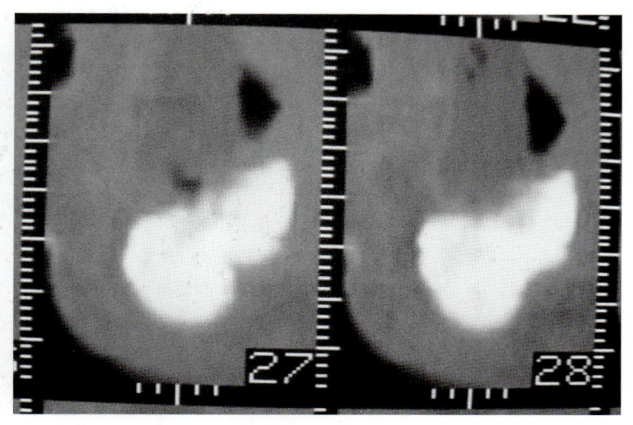

**Fig 6-18** CT scan of anterior mandible showing severe atrophy. The high density of the bone is evident. The labial aspect is on the left of the image and the peak seen on the top right-hand side is the genial tubercle, which is now positioned superiorly to the ridge crest.

critical in this region, and biomechanical criteria can be met by creating bone using the sinus lift procedure, which is very predictable in gaining a substantial volume of bone.

## Anterior Mandible

The anterior mandible may be defined as the area anterior to the mental foramina. The factors significant to this region are described in the following sections.

### Bone Quantity

The amount of bone available in the anterior mandible is almost invariably sufficient for implant placement. It should be borne in mind, however, that the pattern of resorption can often lead to the need to reduce the height of alveolar bone in order to utilise the remainder of the basal bone. Following the loss of the teeth, resorption typically takes place at the expense of the labial plate, which is thinner than the lingual plate. This is followed by a progressive loss of height. A typical resorption pattern can be seen in Fig 6-16. As height is lost the mandible increases in diameter (Fig 6-17).

### Bone Quality

The anterior mandible consists of two distinct portions, the alveolar ridge and the basal bone. There is intervening cancellous bone of varying density. The labial cortical plate is thinner than the lingual cortical plate and is not generally malleable, thus making it difficult to manipulate. The density and width of the cortical plates varies considerably. On occasion, the cortical bone can thicken to the point where little trabecular bone remains (Fig 6-18).

### Inclination of the Alveolar and Basal Bone

The alveolar process is commonly inclined labially, with the circumference of the crest wider than the base. The basal bone is also inclined labially, with the circumference of the mandible along the lower border generally being broader than the junction of basal and alveolar bones (Fig 6-19). Considerable care needs to be taken while preparing the osteotomy within the alveolar bone because of its inclination. Complete resorption of the alveolar ridge often leaves sufficient width and height of bone to allow for the placement of the implants. The osteotomy preparation in the basal bone requires the burs to be inclined, with the apical portion directed labially towards the tip of the chin.

### Special Clinical Considerations

The placement of implants within the basal bone is often at an angle, with the implant apex pointing in the labial direction. The implant is often at an angle to the longitudinal axes of the proposed restoration; the abutment therefore needs to be inclined labially (Fig 6-20). Whenever an implant is placed in the alveolar process,

# Introduction and Assessment

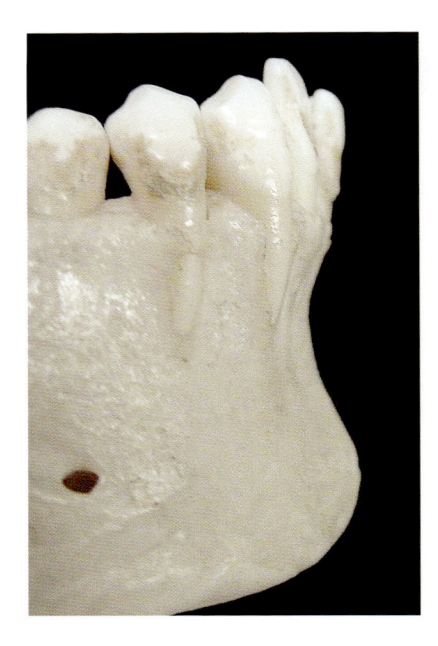

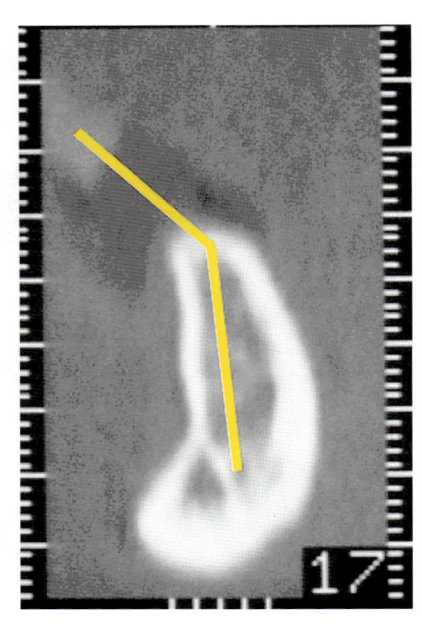

**Fig 6-19** (left) Lateral view of mandible showing inclination of alveolar and basal bone and, therefore, the position and inclination of the teeth.

**Fig 6-20** (right) CT scan showing optimum implant and abutment angulation. The tooth visible as a radiopaque marker on the left-hand side of the image is positioned for ideal lip support.

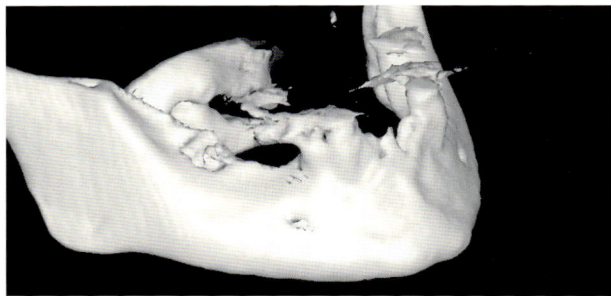

**Fig 6-21** Three-dimensional reconstruction of the mandible showing bone loss in the anterior region, leading to a narrow ridge. The inclination of the symphysis in relation to that of the tooth is also evident.

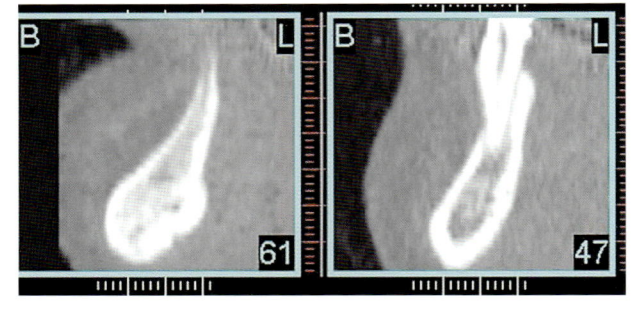

**Fig 6-22** Oblique section of anterior region. Ridge reduction would result in substantial loss of height. Augmentation on the labial aspect of the lost bone would provide the ideal ridge for implant placement. The image on the right shows a section through an adjacent site with a tooth in position. (Same patient as in Fig 6-21.)

care needs to be taken in order to ensure that the lingual plate is not perforated.

In edentulous patients it is possible to reduce the height of a narrow alveolar ridge. However, in patients where some of the teeth are present in the anterior region, it may be more suitable to use augmentation procedures to build up the bone in order to ensure that the emergence profile of the implant-borne crown is at the same level as the adjacent teeth (Figs 6-21 and 6-22).

Incisor teeth are narrow and, therefore, care needs to be taken to ensure that the adjacent teeth are not damaged and that the implant is in the tooth position when required (Fig 6-23). However, the focus is normally to place as many implants as possible in this interforaminal region without damaging the mental nerve.

The dense nature of bone in this region requires the osteotomy to be prepared with great care, using internal irrigation to prevent overheating (Fig 6-24). Osteotomy site preparation almost invariably should be completed with the threads being tapped into the site, which will prevent the use of excessive force when seating the implant.

## Posterior Mandible

The posterior mandible is located distal to the mental foramina.

**6  Anatomical Variations**

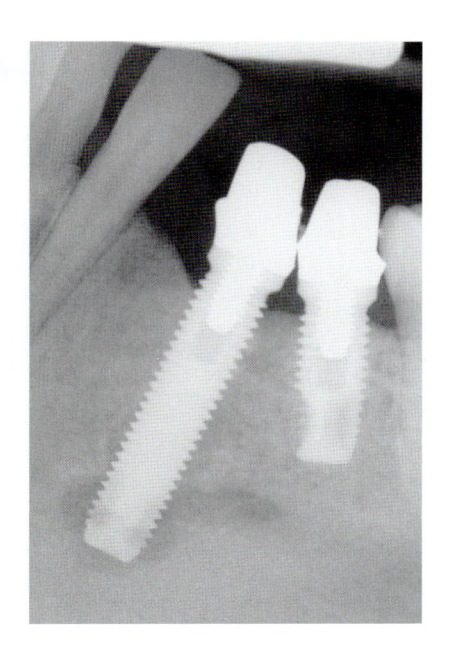

**Fig 6-23** (left) Periapical radiograph of anterior area with narrow teeth. Placement of an implant is restricted by the availability of space between the roots.

**Fig 6-24** (right) Radiograph of implant showing apical radiolucency resulting from overheating of bone. The osteotomy burs of this system are externally cooled, thus increasing the risk of overheating.

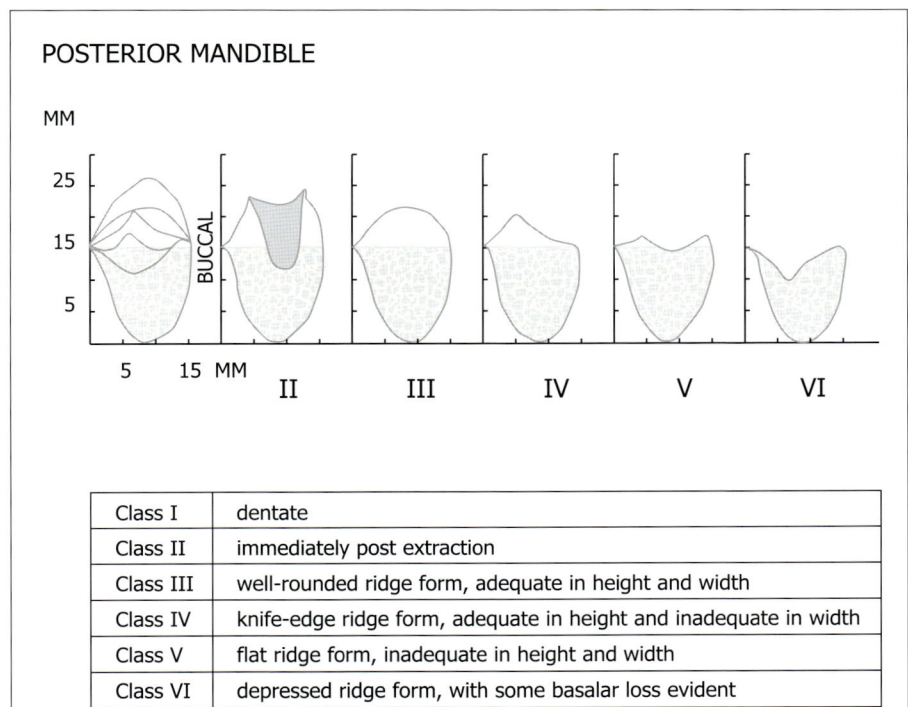

**Fig 6-25** Cawood and Howell classification for the posterior mandible.[50] The inferior alveolar nerve is the primary restriction to the placement of implants in this region.

| Class I | dentate |
|---|---|
| Class II | immediately post extraction |
| Class III | well-rounded ridge form, adequate in height and width |
| Class IV | knife-edge ridge form, adequate in height and inadequate in width |
| Class V | flat ridge form, inadequate in height and width |
| Class VI | depressed ridge form, with some basalar loss evident |

## Bone Quantity

The height of bone available for implants is limited by the position of the inferior alveolar neurovascular bundle. Tooth loss results in loss of height. The pattern of resorption is initially the loss of the labial alveolar plate, resulting in a narrow ridge, followed by reduction in height (Fig 6-25). This loss of height results in the widening of the arch measured along the middle of the alveolar crest, reflecting a centrifugal resorption pattern. The junction between the alveolar and basal bone may be arbitrarily defined as

I Introduction and Assessment

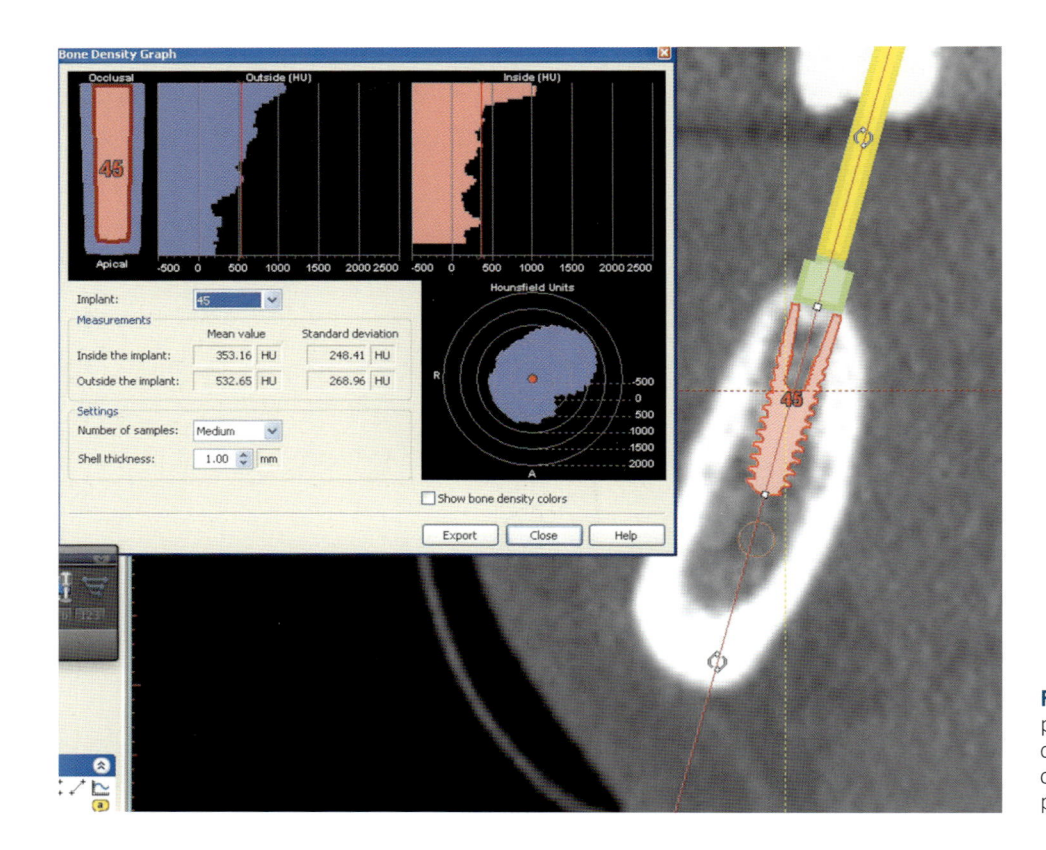

**Fig 6-26** CT section with proposed narrow implant, depicting trabecular bone density (Hounsfield units) in posterior mandible.

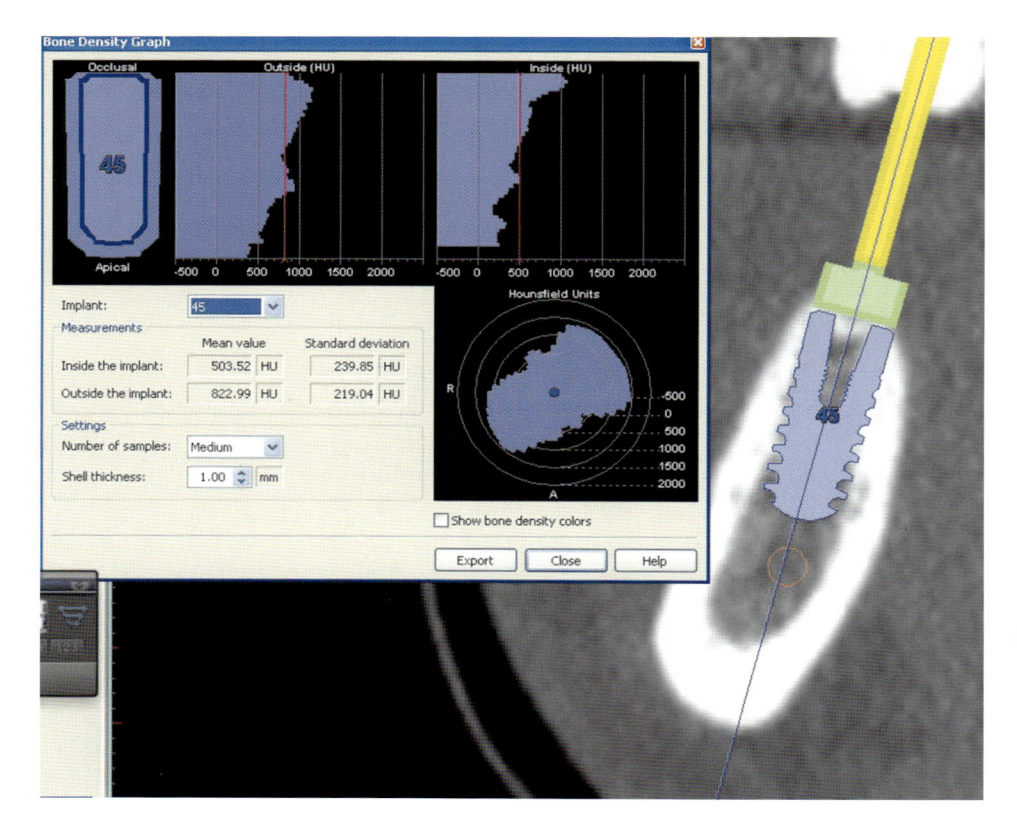

**Fig 6-27** CT section with proposed wide implant (same section as Fig 6-26). Note the higher density resulting from the engagement of the buccal and lingual cortical plates.

the point of insertion of the buccinator muscle, which may coincide with the location of the inferior alveolar canal.[50,57] There is considerable individual variation with respect to the local anatomy. The consequence of damage to anatomical structures in this region is such that the location of all anatomical structures particular to the patient in this region is even more critical than in other regions.

## Bone Quality

The posterior mandible is characterised by dense cortical bone of varying thickness surrounding cancellous bone whose trabecular density may also vary considerably (Figs 6-26 and 6-27).

## Inclination of Residual Ridge

The alveolar ridge is inclined in the lingual direction, reflecting the support of the molars in articulation with the maxillary teeth along the curves of Spee and Wilson. The inclination of the ridge is generally less steep in the premolar region than in the second molar region, where the effective inclination is greater, as influenced by the submandibular fossa below the mylohyoid ridge (Fig 6-28).

Interactive 3D treatment planning permits the placement of an implant within the alveolar ridge as well the selection of an abutment in the cross-sectional view (Fig 6-29) and permits its confirmation in the 3D view (Fig 6-30).

## Special Clinical Considerations

Accurate location of the inferior mandibular nerve is mandatory for the safe practice of implant dentistry in this region. The height of the canal below the ridge as well as the bucco-lingual position of the neurovascular bundle should be located accurately. The magnification of the imaging technique must be taken into consideration. The mesiodistal position of the implant site must be selected accurately, since the location of the neurovascular bundle varies in height mesiodistally. A clearance of 2 mm must be allowed above the canal to minimise the risk of damage to the nerve. Bypassing the inferior alveolar nerve should not be considered because of the inherent risk of paraesthesia.[58]

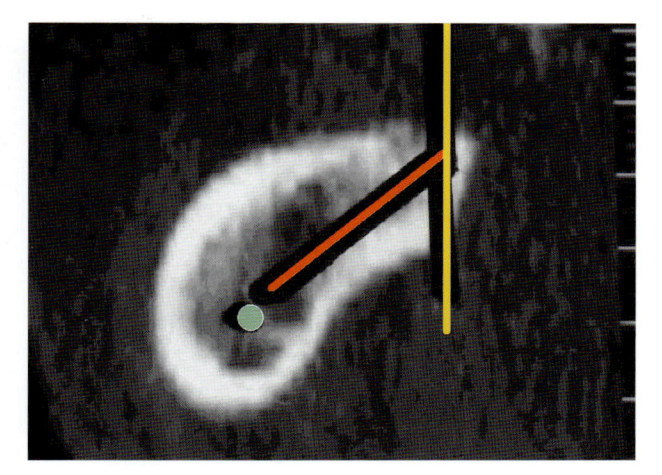

**Fig 6-28** CT cross-section of the posterior mandible indicating the angulation between the longitudinal axis of the abutment and the implant. The submandibular fossa below the mylohyoid ridge results in accentuating the inclination of the posterior mandible.

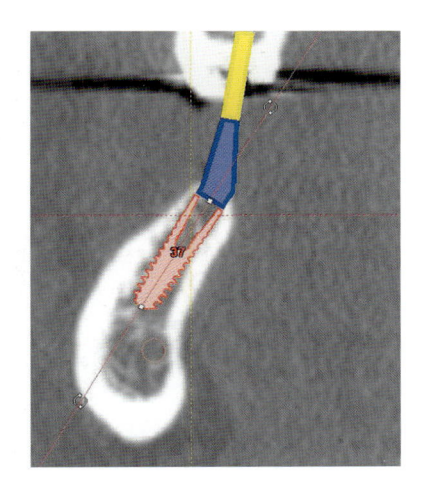

**Fig 6-29** Cross-sectional view of alveolar ridge of CT scan showing interactive selection of implant and corresponding 22.5-degree angled abutment.

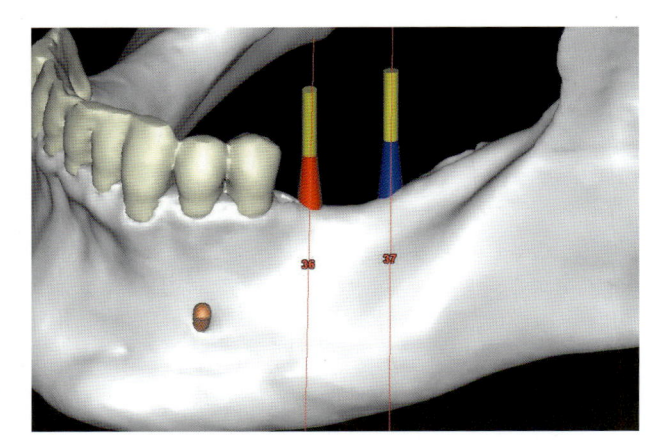

**Fig 6-30** Verification of abutment selection in the 3D view.

**I** Introduction and Assessment

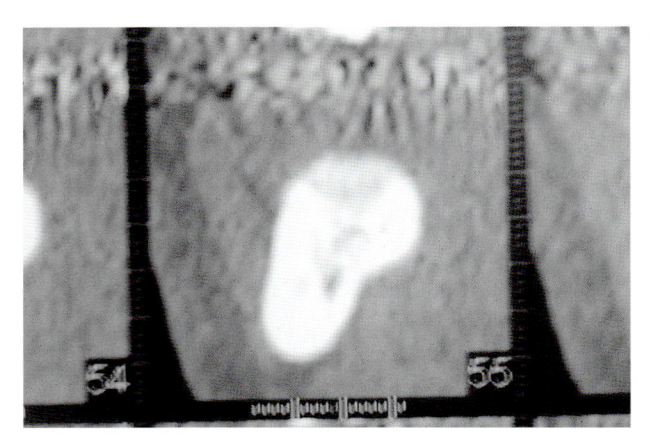

**Fig 6-31** CT cross-section of the posterior mandible showing good bone density and adequate width, even though the bone height above the canal is limited. Note the outline of the submandibular fossa.

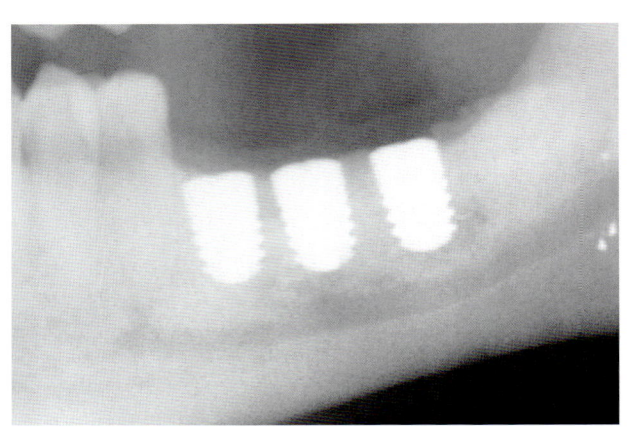

**Fig 6-32** Post-operative panoramic tomograph (same patient as in Fig 6-31) with three short (9.5 mm), wide-bodied (5.5 mm) Ankylos implants (Dentsply Friadent, Mannheim, Germany) in situ with adequate clearance above the inferior dental nerve.

Implants often have to be positioned at an angle, with the drill inclined from the palatal aspect of the maxillary teeth to compensate for the very poor access in this region.

The loss of ridge width results in insufficient bone, which can be augmented using autogenous onlay block bone grafts. A reduction in height is more difficult to correct in this manner because of the limited intermaxillary distance available for the restoration. Consideration should, therefore, be given to repositioning the inferior alveolar nerve, taking the benefits and risks into account.

The occlusal loads are greater in this area than in the anterior region, and yet the amount of available bone is often limited. Shorter multiple implants with larger diameters may often improve the biomechanics (Figs 6-31 and 6-32).

# SECTION II

# Implant Placement: Surgery and Prosthodontics

*'To overturn orthodoxy is no easier in science than in philosophy, religion, economics, or any of the other disciplines through which we try to comprehend the world and the society in which we live.'*

(American biologist Ruth Hubbard)


*'Science is based on experiment, on a willingness to challenge old dogma, on an openness to see the universe as it really is. Accordingly, science sometimes requires courage – at the very least the courage to question the conventional wisdom.'*

(American scientist Carl Sagan)


Planning for implant placement will depend on whether a tooth is present or missing. Different sets of criteria are required for the assessment and planning of treatment, depending on the condition the patient presents with. Flowcharts provide an ideal way to visualise the sequence of diagnostic and treatment steps that may be required. A general overview is provided by the master flowchart (Flowchart II-1), which addresses the pathways that may be taken for the treatment of either a missing tooth with a healed residual ridge or a tooth that is failing. This flowchart addresses all the options, from the diagnostic stages to the restorative phase. More detailed flowcharts will supplement each treatment modality and may be referred to in the appropriate section.

This section covers the decision-making processes and clinical treatment sequences for those cases where no augmentation is required. It addresses the diagnostic, surgical and restorative aspects.

II   Implant Placement: Surgery and Prosthodontics

**Missing tooth** → Residual ridge → Diagnostic imaging / Diagnostic preview / Ridge mapping → Provisional restoration / Diagnostic template → Adequate hard & soft tissues

Inadequate hard tissues– Augmentation / morphological manipulation

- bone expansion
- bone grafts
- sinus lift
- GTR
- Ti mesh
- distraction osteogenesis

Delayed placement

Immediate loading

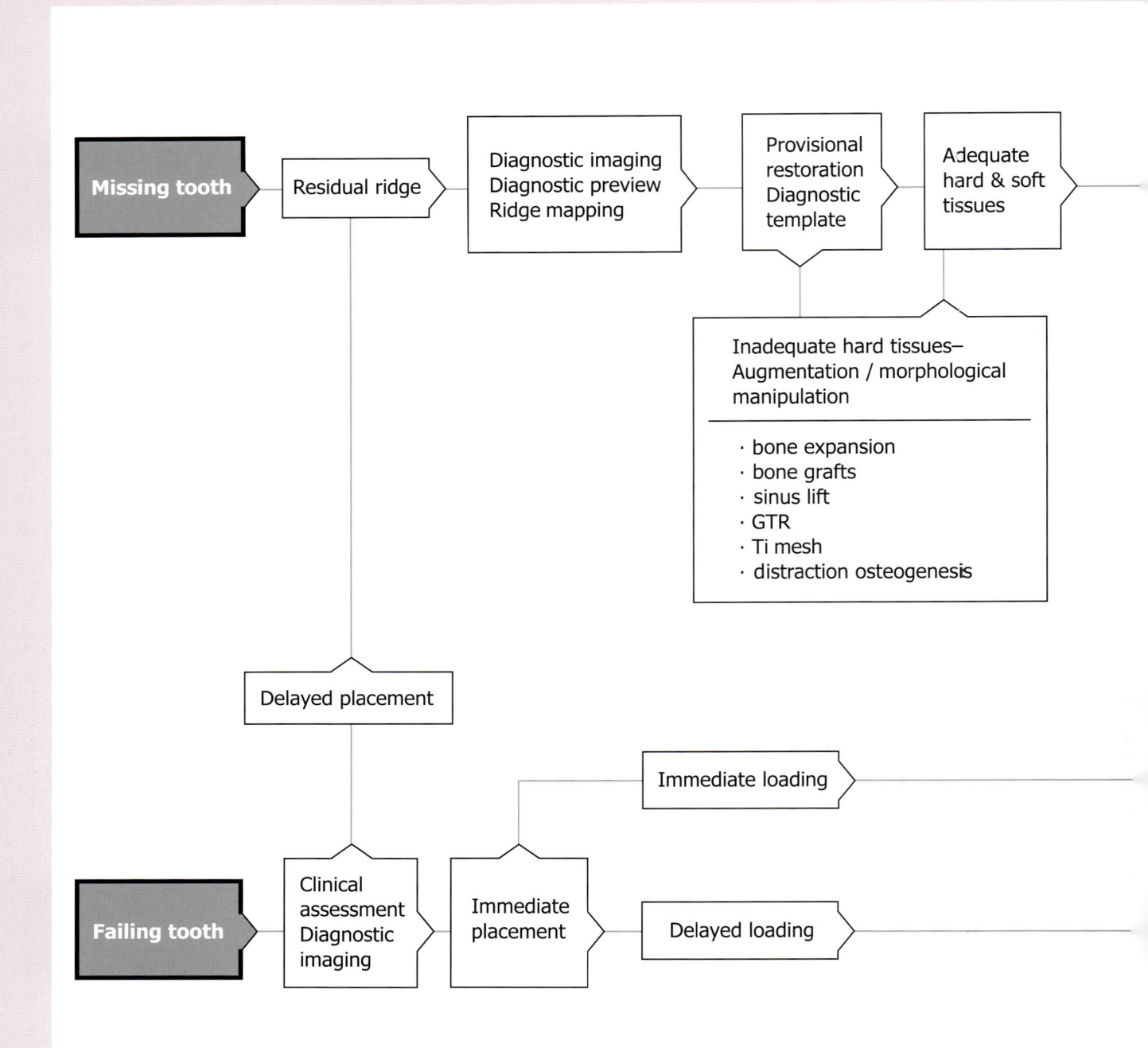

**Failing tooth** → Clinical assessment / Diagnostic imaging → Immediate placement → Delayed loading

**Flowchart** II-1   Assessment for immediate or delayed placement.

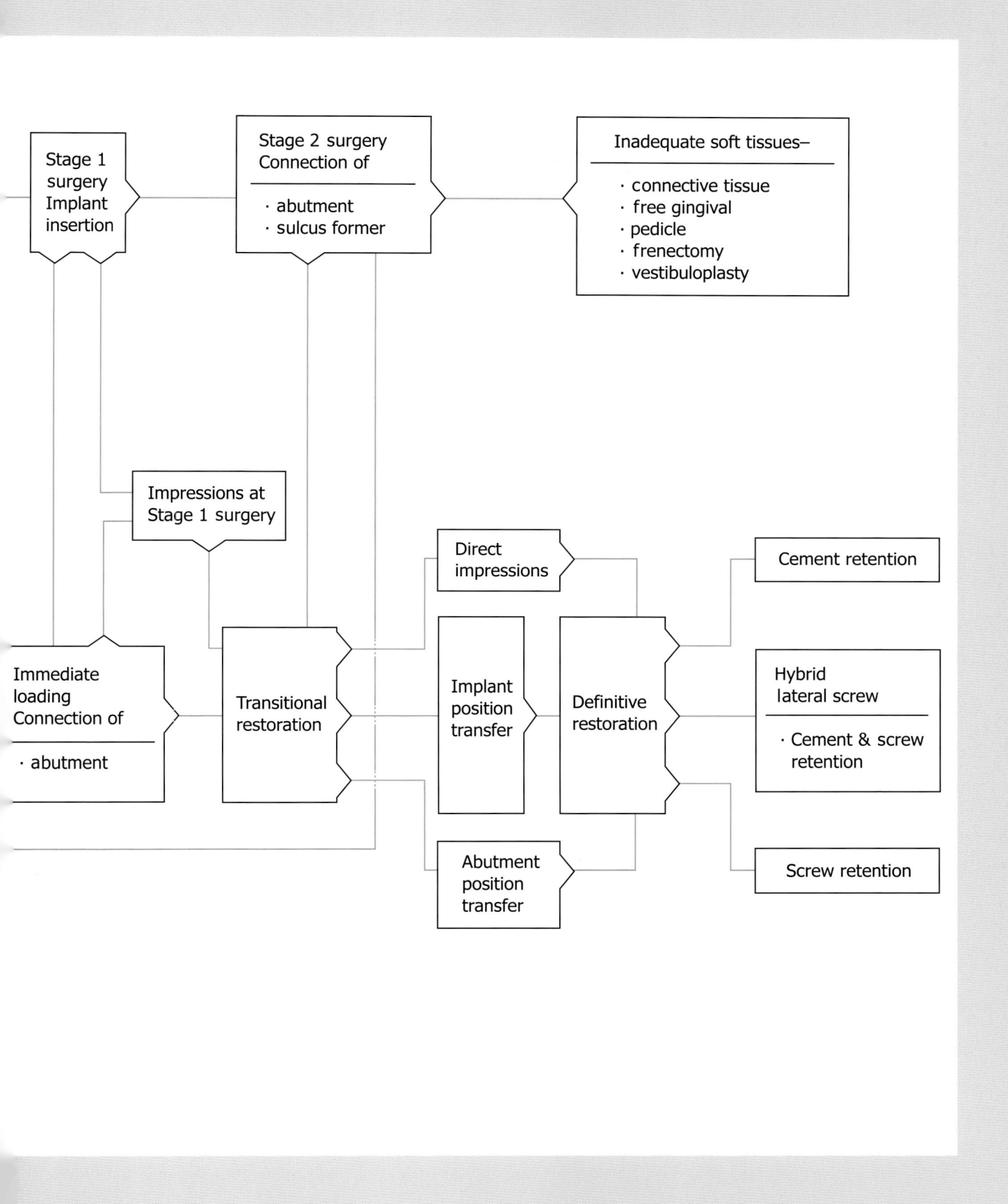

```
┌─────────────┐   ┌─────────────────┐        ┌──────────────────────┐
│ Stage 1     │   │ Stage 2 surgery │        │ Inadequate soft tissues– │
│ surgery     │──▶│ Connection of   │───────▶│ ──────────────────── │
│ Implant     │   │ · abutment      │        │ · connective tissue  │
│ insertion   │   │ · sulcus former │        │ · free gingival      │
└─────────────┘   └─────────────────┘        │ · pedicle            │
                                             │ · frenectomy         │
                                             │ · vestibuloplasty    │
                                             └──────────────────────┘

              ┌──────────────────┐
              │ Impressions at   │
              │ Stage 1 surgery  │
              └──────────────────┘
                                      ┌──────────────┐
                                      │ Direct       │──┐   ┌──────────────────┐
                                      │ impressions  │  │   │ Cement retention │
                                      └──────────────┘  │   └──────────────────┘
┌─────────────┐   ┌──────────────┐                      │
│ Immediate   │   │              │    ┌──────────────┐  │   ┌──────────────────┐
│ loading     │   │ Transitional │    │ Implant      │  │   │ Hybrid           │
│ Connection of│─▶│ restoration  │───▶│ position     │─▶│──▶│ lateral screw    │
│ ─────────── │   │              │    │ transfer     │  │   │ ──────────────── │
│ · abutment  │   └──────────────┘    └──────────────┘  │   │ · Cement & screw │
└─────────────┘                                         │   │   retention      │
                                      ┌──────────────┐  │   └──────────────────┘
                                      │ Abutment     │  │
                                      │ position     │──┘   ┌──────────────────┐
                                      │ transfer     │      │ Screw retention  │
                                      └──────────────┘      └──────────────────┘
                                                    │ Definitive  │
                                                    │ restoration │
```

## Chapter 7

# Immediate Placement and Computer-guided Surgery

## Introduction

The concept of removing a tooth that is failing and replacing it with an implant that is brought into function immediately has tremendous attraction. Delayed loading of immediately placed implants is a very well-established technique that has a high success rate.[4,5,59–61] The most obvious benefits of this technique to the patient are the reduction in treatment time and considerable convenience in comparison with conventional implant treatment. Another reported benefit of immediate placement is the preservation of bone.[62]

Immediate loading of implants placed in healed sites is also well established and depends on absence of micro-movement (primary stability) during the healing phase.[63–65] It has recently been shown that bone healing around immediately loaded implants results in greater bone density and more mature bone.[66–70] The procedure is minimally invasive, allowing the tooth socket to be used for the implant. It is a predictable technique as long as the assessment is carried out accurately. In assessing the benefits and risks of such a procedure, the clinician should bear in mind the remedial steps that would be required to rectify the situation in the event of any complications. Flowchart 7-1 describes the factors that need to be considered in assessing a failing tooth. This will enable the clinician to make a decision and provide a rationale for planning treatment.

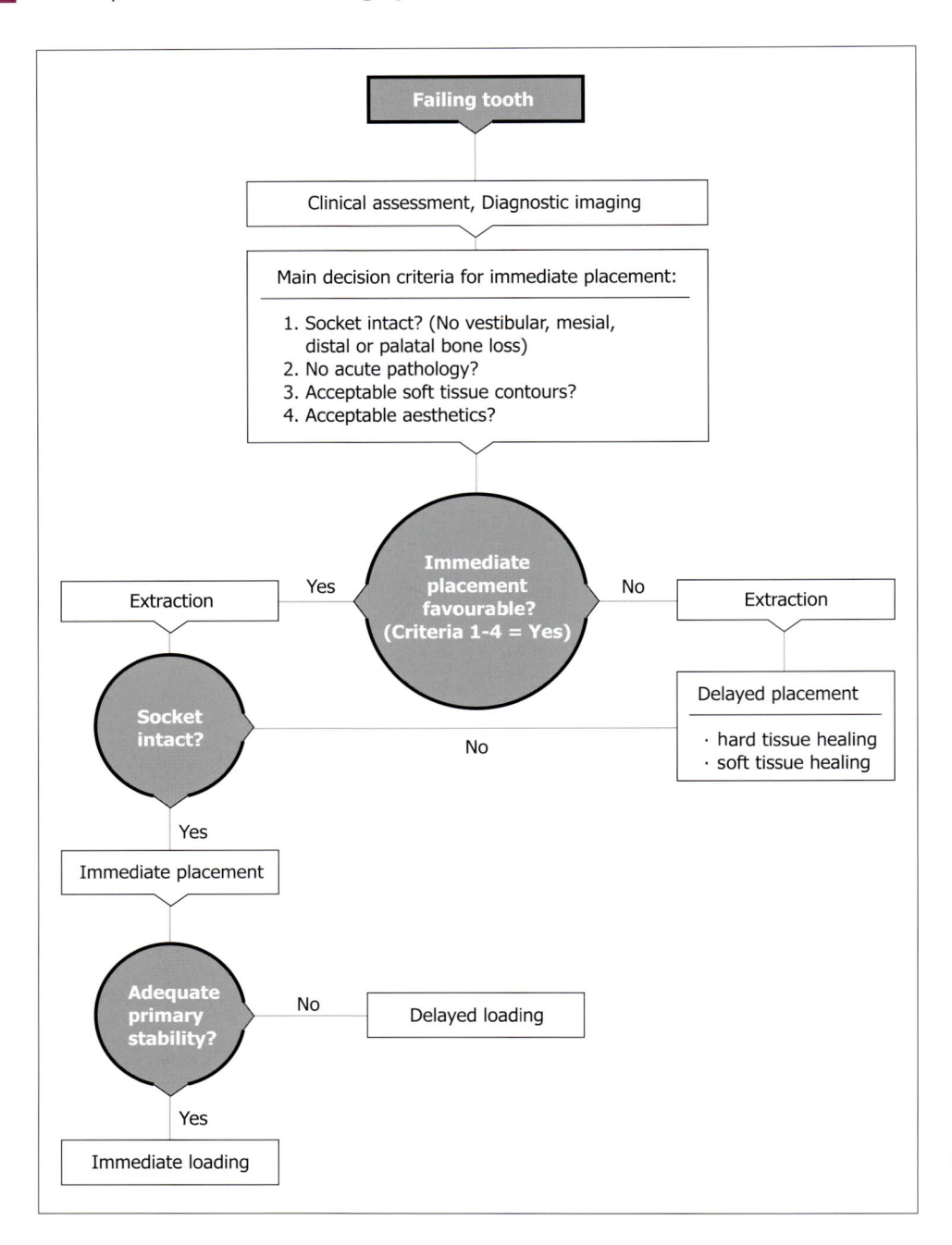

II  Implant Placement: Surgery and Prosthodontics

```
                    Failing tooth
                         │
         Clinical assessment, Diagnostic imaging
                         │
      Main decision criteria for immediate placement:
      1. Socket intact? (No vestibular, mesial,
         distal or palatal bone loss)
      2. No acute pathology?
      3. Acceptable soft tissue contours?
      4. Acceptable aesthetics?
                         │
                    Immediate
      Yes ←── placement favourable? ──→ No
               (Criteria 1-4 = Yes)
       │                                  │
   Extraction                         Extraction
       │                                  │
   Socket                            Delayed placement
   intact? ─── No ────────────────→  · hard tissue healing
       │                              · soft tissue healing
      Yes
       │
   Immediate placement
       │
   Adequate
   primary  ── No ──→ Delayed loading
   stability?
       │
      Yes
       │
   Immediate loading
```

**Flowchart 7-1** Assessment for immediate or delayed placement.

## Assessment

### Clinical Assessment

#### Absence of Pathology

There should be no acute pathology present in either the periodontal tissues or in the periapical region (Figs 7-1 and 7-2). There should be no sign of symptoms, although it may be acceptable to proceed prudently where chronic well-contained lesions are present.[71–76] Vertical root fractures of teeth that have been restored by means of post-crowns should be assessed carefully to ensure that the labial plate of bone has not been compromised (Figs 7-3–7-6).

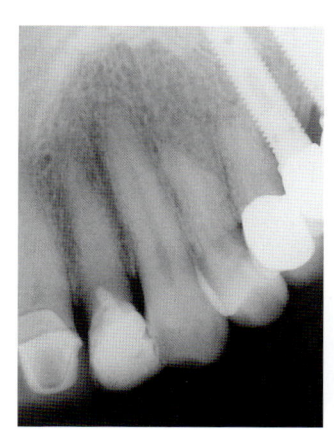

# 7  Immediate Placement and Computer-guided Surgery

**Fig 7-1** Periapical radiograph of lateral incisor with obliterated root canal and almost complete destruction of the coronal portion. No pathology is evident and tooth replacement is for restorative reasons.

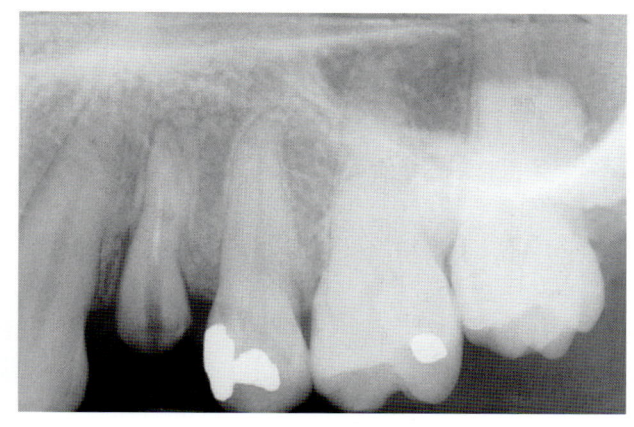

**Fig 7-2** Radiograph of first premolar with dislodged post-crown and clinical signs of a fine vertical fracture with no signs of acute pathology. An ideal candidate for immediate replacement with an implant.

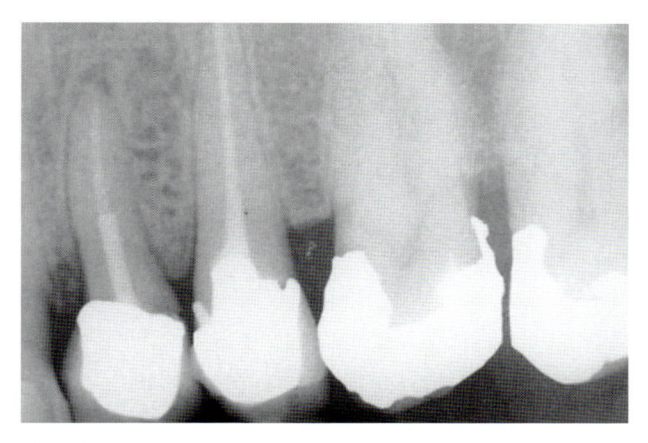

**Fig 7-3** Radiograph of first premolar restored with a post-retained crown and a vertical root fracture with a well-contained periapical lesion, ideal for immediate replacement with an implant.

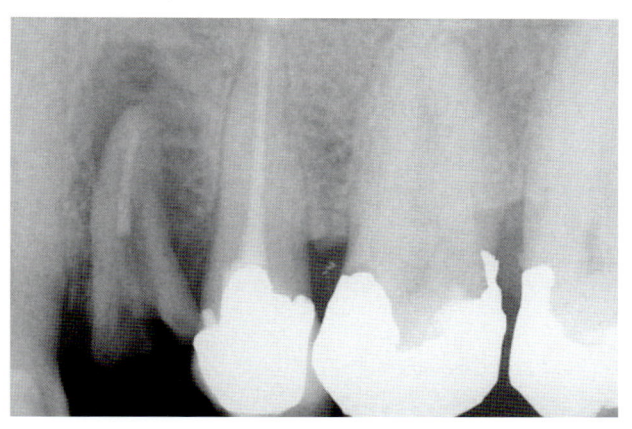

**Fig 7-4** Periapical radiograph of the tooth shown in Fig 7-3 3 months later. A delay in treatment has led to the propagation of the fractured root and extensive bone loss resulting from the inflammatory process. Active lesions such as these are not predictable to treat with immediate implants.

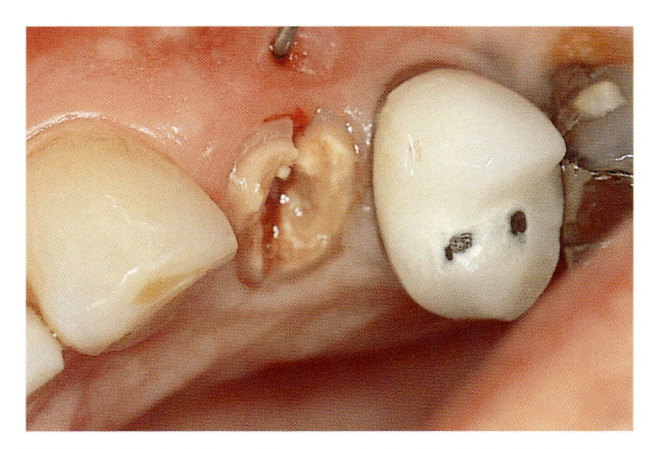

**Fig 7-5** Clinical view of the same tooth (Fig 7-4) with labial fistula indicating labial bone loss.

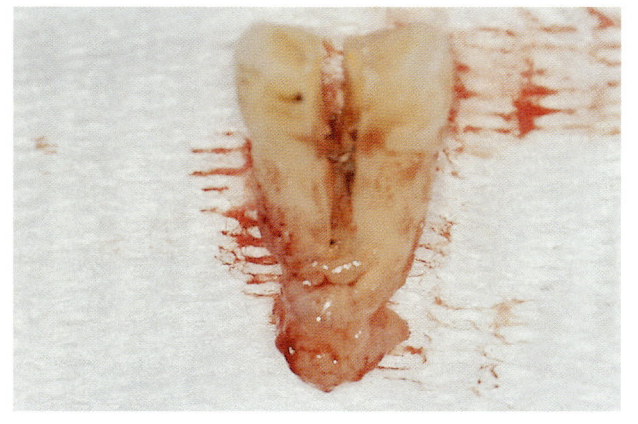

**Fig 7-6** The extracted fractured root of the premolar (as shown in Fig 7-5) with associated periapical lesion. This has resulted in the destruction of the entire labial plate as well as considerable periapical bone loss.

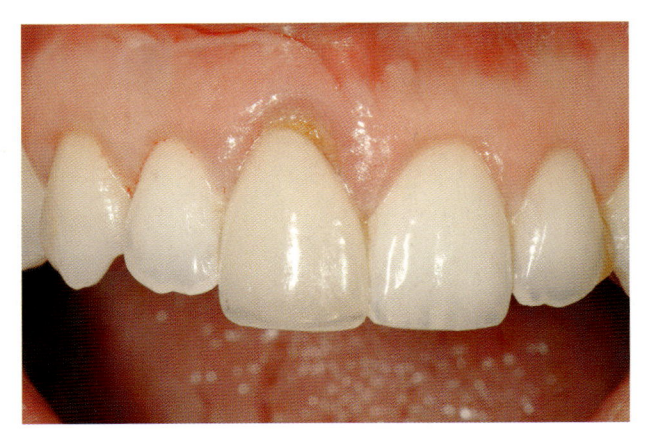

**II** Implant Placement: Surgery and Prosthodontics

**Fig 7-7** Tooth with labial gingival recession in a patient with a high lip line. Satisfactory aesthetics can not be easily achieved without supplementary augmentation procedures.

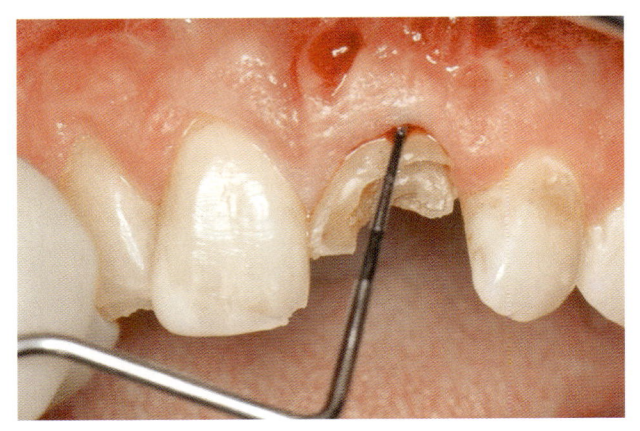

**Fig 7-8** Fractured central incisor being assessed for immediate placement with a periodontal probe to assess the likely level of the labial aspect of the bony socket.

### Soft-Tissue Health and Aesthetic Contours

The contours of the soft tissues around the tooth to be extracted should be such that they will appear acceptable around the intended restoration. It should be borne in mind that augmentation of the hard and soft tissues in such situations is complex, reducing the predictability and defeating the purpose of a procedure designed to simplify treatment (Fig 7-7). It should also be borne in mind that the soft tissues will remain stable as long as the hard tissues are present to support them.

### Socket Integrity

It is of benefit to have a socket that is intact.[59] Preoperatively this can be checked by means of periodontal probing (Fig 7-8). Loss of bone around the tooth to be replaced may result in the bone healing to a level that is not predictable. The level of bone that exists in contact with the adjacent teeth is critical because it will be responsible for the maintenance of the papillary height (Figs 7-1–7-3).

Anatomical variations of the teeth make some teeth better candidates for immediate implant placement. Typically the central incisors and canines are more likely to have dehiscent roots (Fig 7-9), whereas the lateral incisors are positioned in a more palatal direction (Fig 7-10).

## Radiographic Assessment
### Periapical Radiograph

Periapical radiographs are valuable for disclosing any periapical pathology and establishing interdental bone levels. They may also provide an idea of the available bone height beyond the apex, the mesiodistal dimensions of the roots and the space available between the adjacent roots. They also indicate the mesiodistal orientation of the roots (see Chapter 8 and Figs 7-1–7-3).

### Orthopantomograph (OPG)/ Dental Panoramic Tomograph (DPT)

DPT provides an excellent overview of the jaws, confirming the information obtained from the periapical radiographs, in particular the availability of bone beyond the apex.

### Computed Tomography

CT provides very useful 3D information regarding the spatial position of the root in relation to the ridge. The orientation of the root in the bucco-lingual plane enables the direction of the projected osteotomy to be determined accurately. The cross-sections provide valuable information regarding the integrity of the lingual and labial plates of bone (Figs 7-9 and 7-10). The unique contribution of the CT scan is to provide a method for measuring bone density (in Hounsfield units). However, care needs to be taken to exclude

# 7  Immediate Placement and Computer-guided Surgery

**Fig 7-9** (left) Cross-sectional CT image of central incisor showing the inclination of the root, the thin labial cortical plate and the ample bone available on the palatal aspect of the root to achieve primary stability for an implant of adequate dimensions. Implant placement in the direction of the root would clearly lead to a labial fenestration, independent of the shape of the implant used.

**Fig 7-10** (right) Cross-sectional CT image of lateral incisor showing the inclination of the root, which is more favourable for implant placement with a reduced risk of fenestration of the labial plate. Selection of the implant site will need to be on the palatal aspect of the socket apex depending upon the diameter of the implant, which may be selected using an interactive treatment planning program.

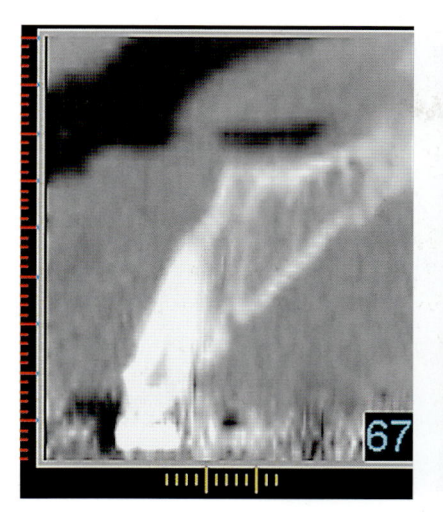

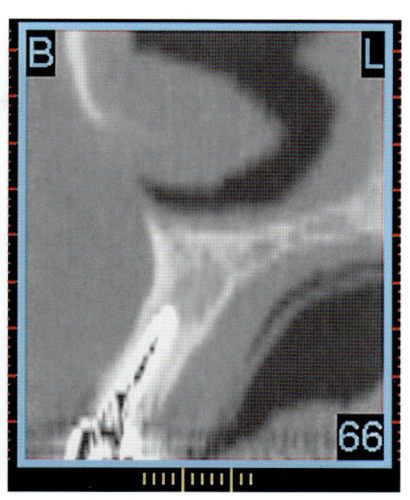

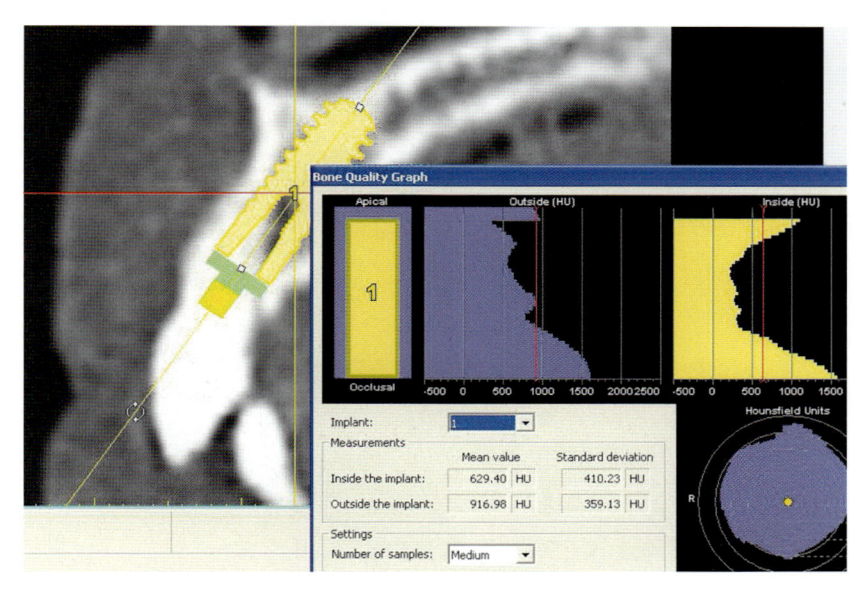

**Fig 7-11** Interactive treatment planning showing the bone density in Hounsfield units in the region of the implant site. The high density resulting from the tooth root should be ignored. The density around the apical portion of the implant (<500 HU) indicates that bone condensers may well be needed in order to achieve the primary stability required for immediate loading.

the high density of the roots. This, therefore, allows the decision regarding immediate loading to be made preoperatively. It also specifies the likelihood of using the series of instruments available for ensuring the primary stability of the implant by altering bone density (Fig 7-11).

## Treatment Sequence

The assessment made prior to the immediate replacement of a tooth (Figs 7-12–7-14) with an implant can be carried out with the assistance of the checklist outlined in Table 7-1. Once the decision has been made to place

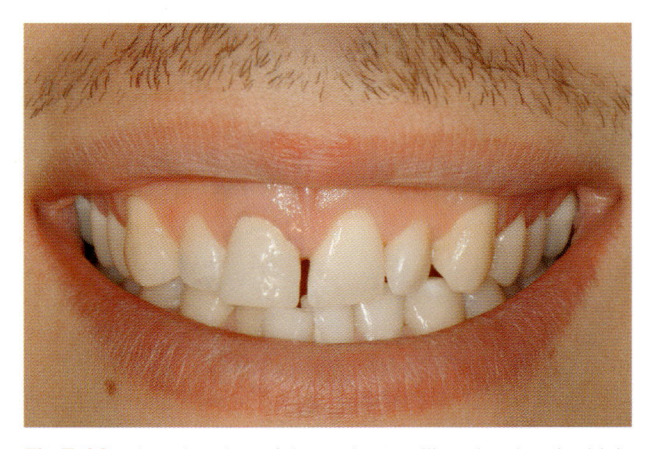

**Fig 7-12** Anterior view of the patient smiling showing the high lip line and failing central incisor (No. 11).

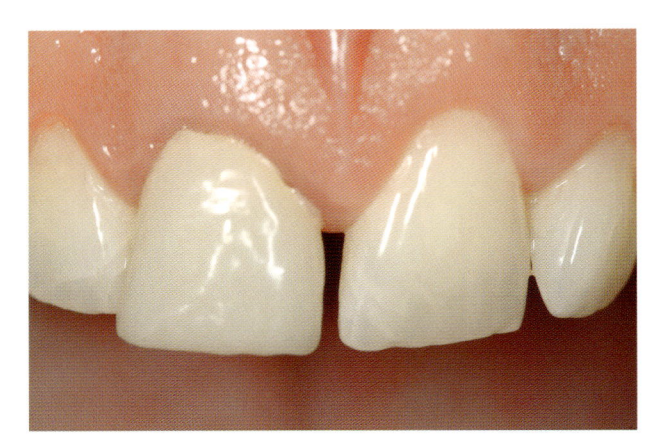

## II  Implant Placement: Surgery and Prosthodontics

**Fig 7-13**  Labial view of the maxillary right central incisor area showing an acceptable level of soft tissue.

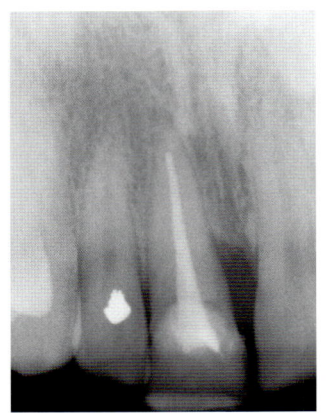

**Fig 7-14**  Periapical radiograph showing the previously root canal-treated failing central incisor, with a mesial bony defect visible. Abundant bone beyond the apex is visible and is sparsely trabeculated. Labial probing depths indicated an intact socket with a deeper pocket on the mesial aspect. The bone level adjacent to the left central incisor is adequate.

**Table 7-1**  Checklist for assessing a failing tooth prior to implant placement and loading

| For immediate placement | |
|---|---|
| Symptoms | |
| Pathology | |
| Aesthetics | |
| **Socket integrity:** | |
| Probing | |
| Fistulae | |
| Dehiscences | |
| **Bone level**<br>• mesial<br>• distal<br>• buccal<br>• palatal<br>• bone beyond apex | |
| Density | |
| Root anatomy | |
| Root inclination | |
| Interdental space | |
| Root width | |

an implant immediately at the time of extraction and bring it into function a sequence of clinical and laboratory stages needs to be planned. These are outlined in Flowchart 7-2 (see page 56–57).

### Preoperative Stage

Preoperative impressions are taken for the construction of a provisional restoration (Figs 7-15–7-17). Upper and lower alginate impressions are taken in addition to the registration of the relationship of the jaws in maximum intercuspation. Facebow recordings are recommended, where appropriate, to transfer information relating to the position of the condyles, as well as condylar and tooth guidance.

### Extraction

During extraction of a tooth, the integrity of the socket must be maintained. Extraction forceps with fine beaks may be used in addition to root elevators. However, these are often used in conjunction with a periotome, whose fine blade enables the tooth to be separated from the socket by severing the periodontal ligament.[61,77] Access for the periotome to the mesial and distal part of the root is facilitated by removing the interdental contact point (Fig 7-18). Care must always be taken to avoid damaging the labial plate, which is often most fragile in the anterior region (Fig 7-19). Access for the application of extraction forceps can be facilitated by removing excessive contours of the clinical crown. This prevents damage to the soft tissues caused by the deflection of the forceps

**7** Immediate Placement and Computer-guided Surgery

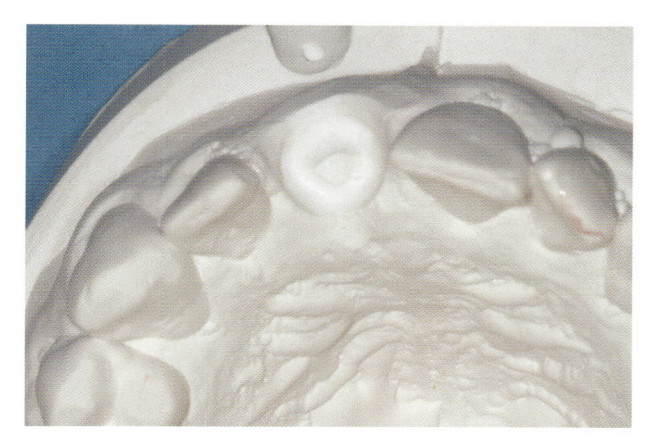

**Fig 7-15** Model with the right central incisor removed and socketed to a depth of 2 mm for the fabrication of the transitional restoration, which will fit within the socket of the extracted tooth.

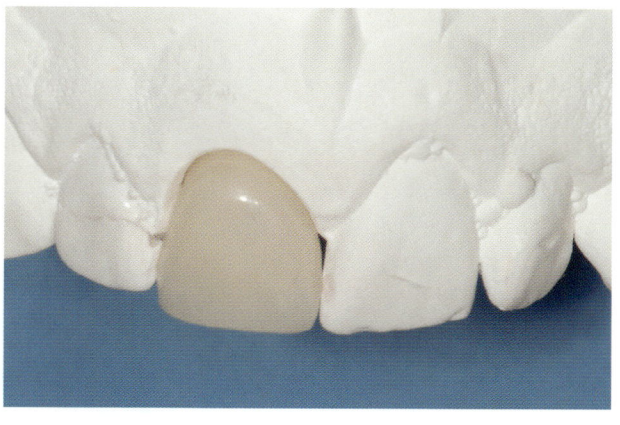

**Fig 7-16** Hollow transitional restoration made out of acrylic resin, which will also be used to define the prosthetic envelope to select the abutment during implant placement.

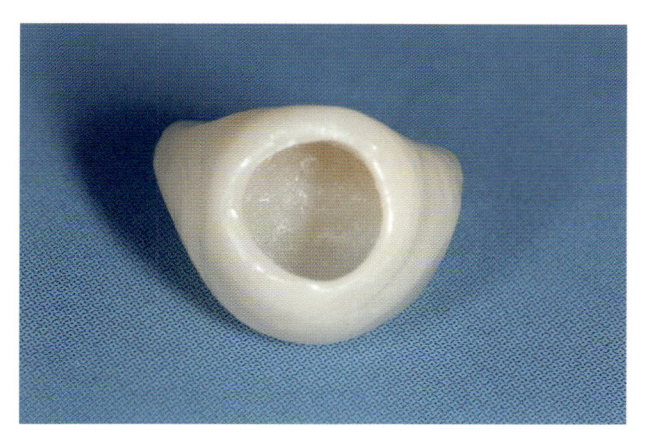

**Fig 7-17** View of fit surface of the hollow transitional restoration, which will seal the extraction socket after adaptation to the abutment.

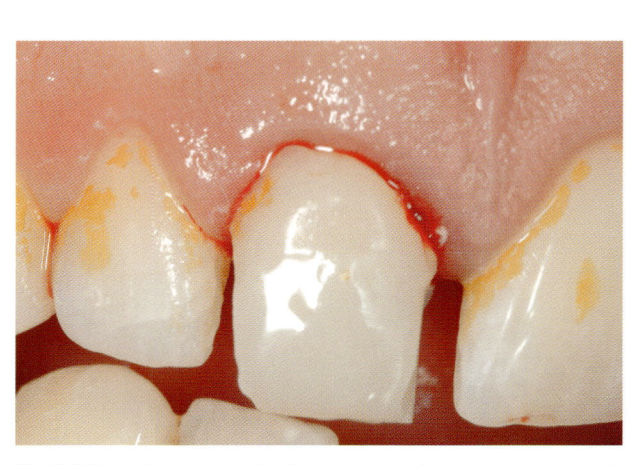

**Fig 7-18** Labial view of tooth to be extracted showing removal of contact points for easy access of periotome.

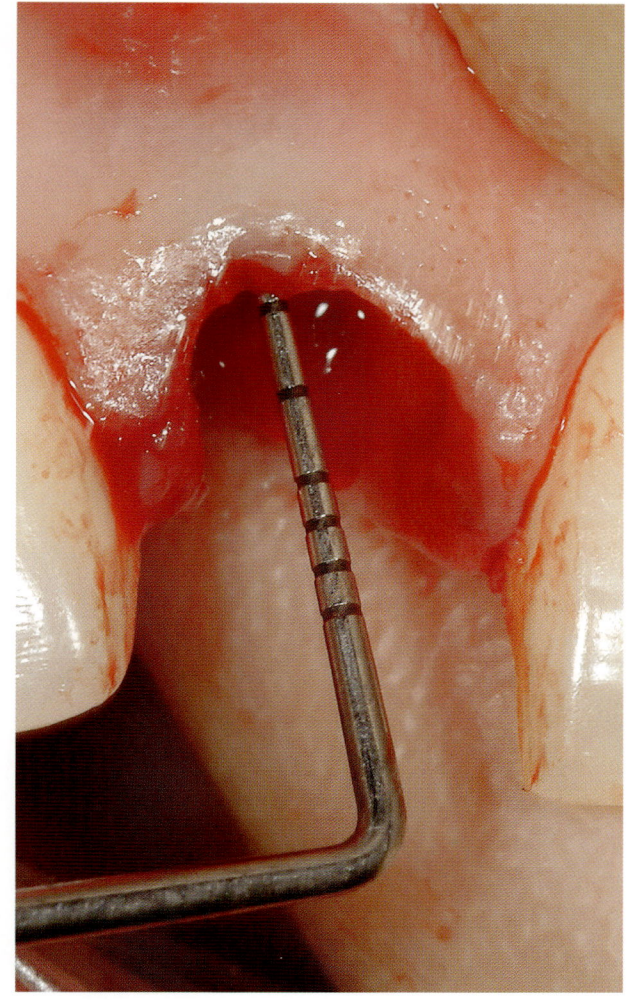

**Fig 7-19** Periodontal probe being used to check the integrity of the socket. The bony socket margin is positioned less than 3 mm away from the gingival margin.

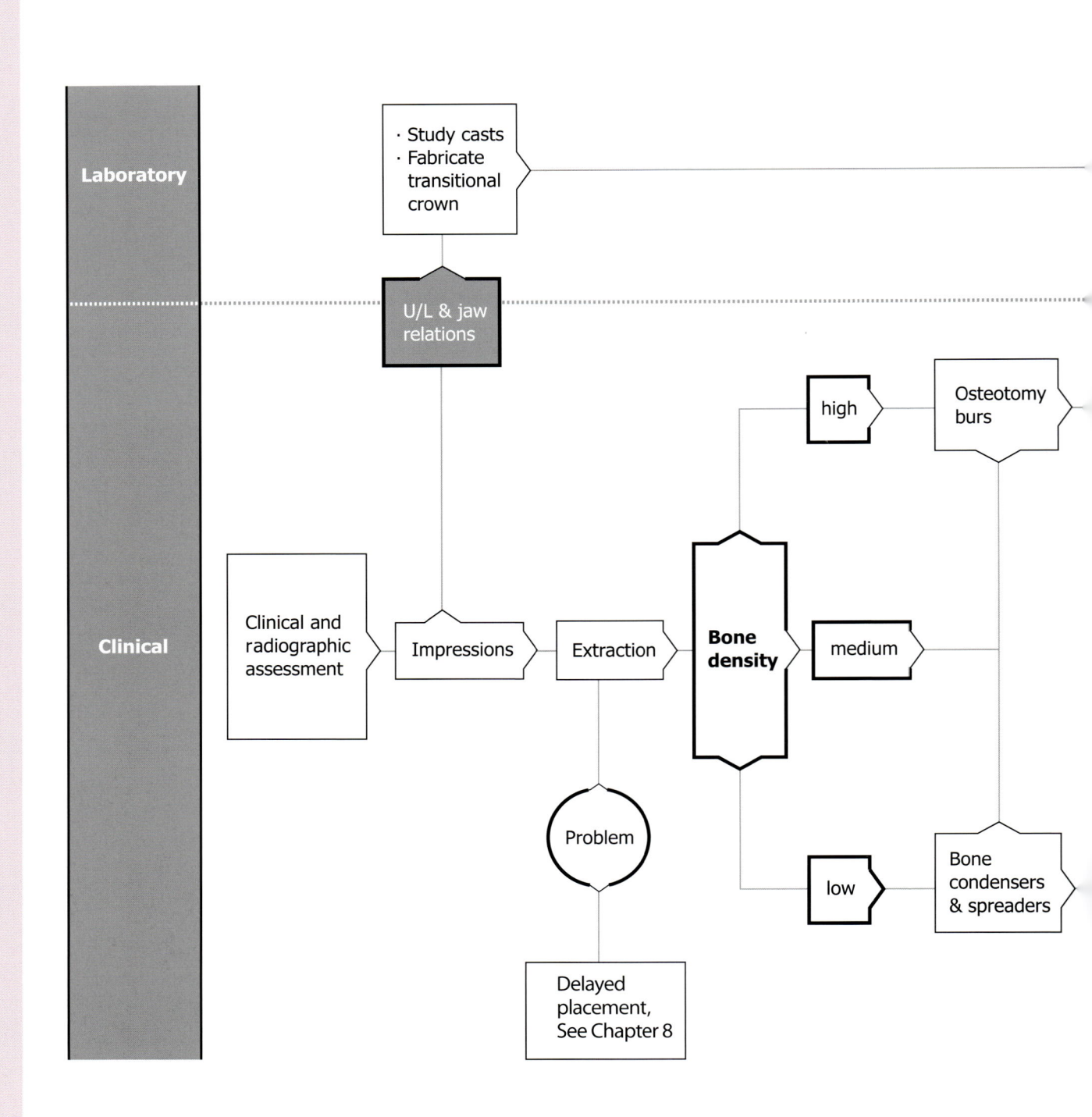

## II  Implant Placement: Surgery and Prosthodontics

**Laboratory**
- Study casts
- Fabricate transitional crown

**Clinical**
- Clinical and radiographic assessment → Impressions → Extraction → **Bone density**
- U/L & jaw relations
- Bone density: high → Osteotomy burs; medium → Osteotomy burs / Bone condensers & spreaders; low → Bone condensers & spreaders
- Problem → Delayed placement, See Chapter 8

**Flowchart 7-2**  Immediate placement and loading: Clinical stages

**7** Immediate Placement and Computer-guided Surgery

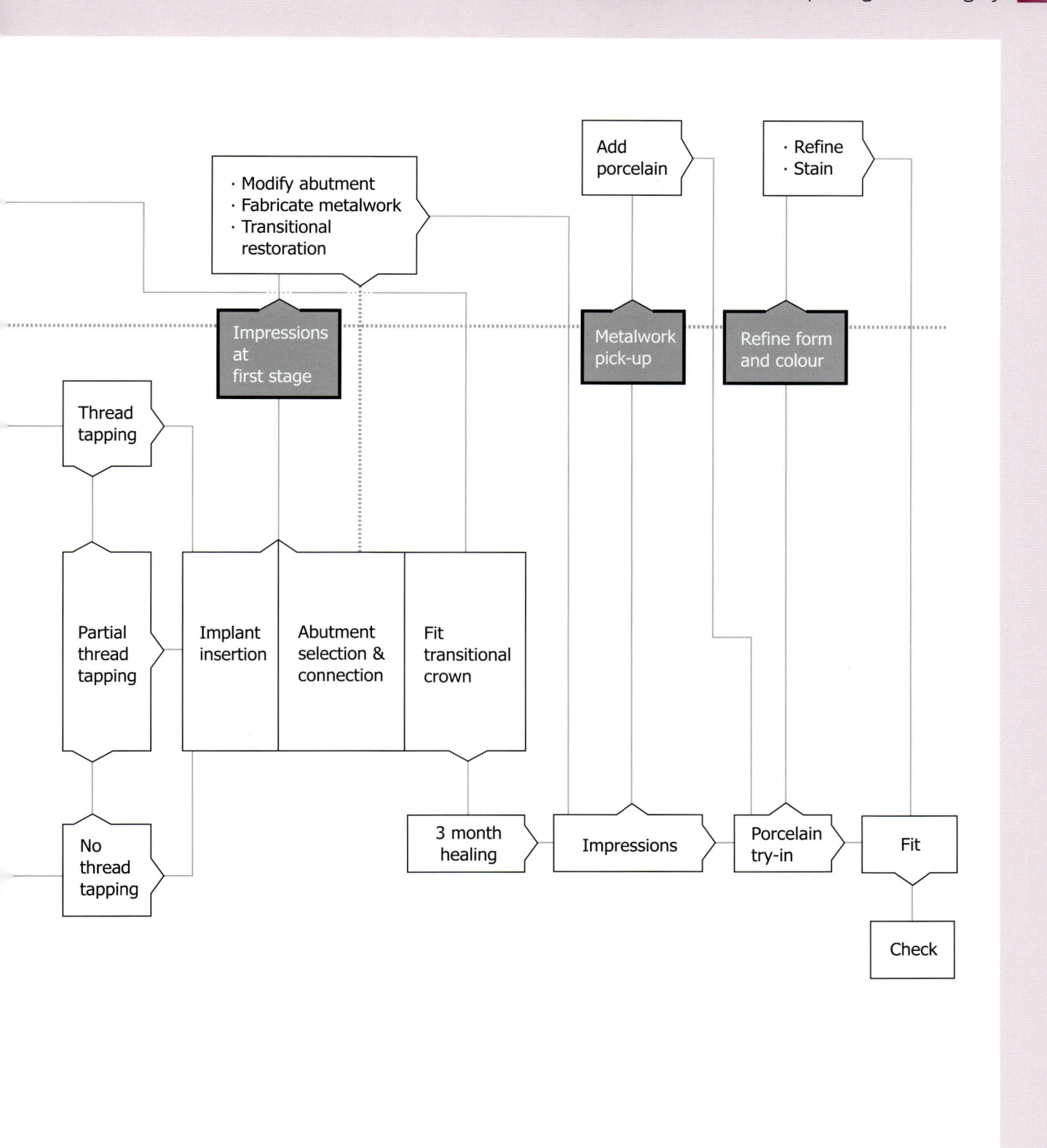

- Modify abutment
- Fabricate metalwork
- Transitional restoration

Add porcelain

- Refine
- Stain

Impressions at first stage

Metalwork pick-up

Refine form and colour

Thread tapping

Partial thread tapping

No thread tapping

Implant insertion

Abutment selection & connection

Fit transitional crown

3 month healing

Impressions

Porcelain try-in

Fit

Check

57

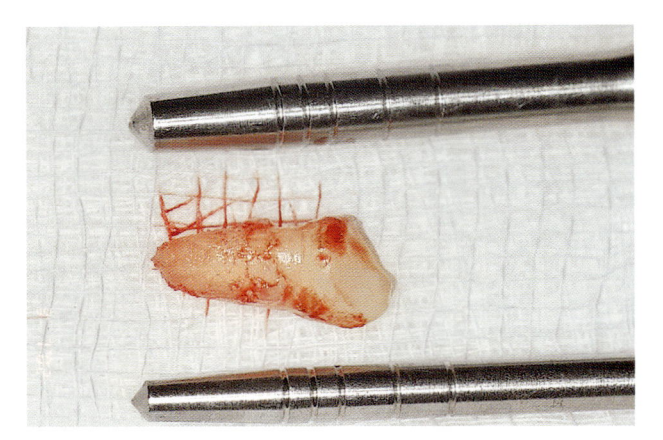

# II  Implant Placement: Surgery and Prosthodontics

**Fig 7-20**  The extracted tooth alongside the bone condensers to determine the diameter of implant that will be required. The implant diameter should be wide enough to maximise the space available within the socket to gain primary stability, be one millimetre away from the labial aspect of the socket and yet avoid perforation of the cortical plates.

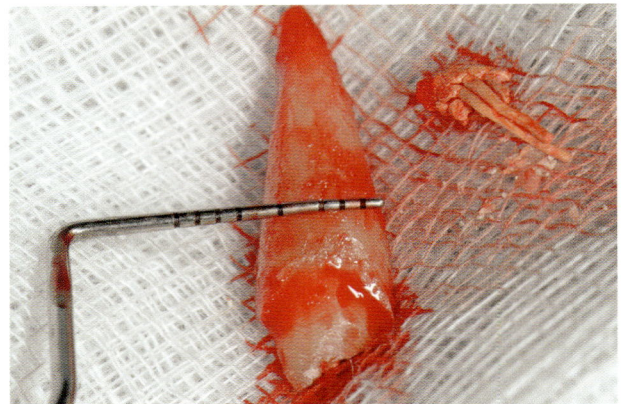

**Fig 7-21**  Periodontal probe measuring the root width along the height of the bony crest of the socket to estimate the implant diameter and residual space.

by excessive coronal contours. Single teeth with a root form resistant to removal, such as a bulbous tip or a curve, may have to be removed by sectioning the root mesiodistally in the longitudinal plane or bucco-lingually if damage to the labial plate can be prevented. In elevating the sectioned root, care must be taken not to damage the socket or interstitial bone. Teeth with multiple roots should be divided and each of the roots removed separately, using the techniques outlined above.

## Implant Placement
### Site Selection

The implant site must be selected by projecting the point where the final position of the implant is required. The aim is to obliterate as much of the socket as possible with the implant without perforating the labial or the lingual plate and without damaging any of the adjacent teeth (Figs 7-20–7-22). Typically, in the anterior maxilla, the implant site may be positioned approximately one-third of the way along the palatal wall of the socket from the apex (Fig 7-23). This will enable the osteotomy to be prepared without any dehiscence. The direction of the osteotomy should be determined using the adjacent teeth and the alveolar cortical plates as direction guides. Use of 3D imaging is particularly helpful in identifying the available bone and its relationship to the socket for accurate implant placement.

### Osteotomy Preparation

A small round bur or a position marker is used at the beginning of the procedure to determine the centre of the osteotomy (Fig 7-24). The position marker may now be used to extend the osteotomy to the predetermined depth based on radiographic measurements. Alternatively, a pilot bur (Lindemann bur) may be used. This will provide an indication of the density of the bone or may confirm the results of a previous CT scan. The diameter of the osteotomy is then enlarged until it matches the core diameter of the implant (Figs 7-25 and 7-26). In bone of low density in the maxilla it is preferable to use bone condensers to ensure that the osteotomy is carried out with a minimal risk of perforation of the labial or lingual plates. Furthermore, the use of bone condensers increases bone density and the bone-to-implant contact during the early phase of healing, at which stage stability and the prevention of excessive micro-movement is critical.[78,79] The use of bone condensers is not recommended in the mandible. However, bone spreaders may be used for the same purpose. If resistance is met during the initial stages of osteotomy preparation, it is preferable to use osteotomy burs. Palpation of the buccal and palatal tissues gives an early indication of any inadvertent perforation by a misdirected osteotomy bur. The osteotomy is prepared to a depth that allows the selected implant to be placed

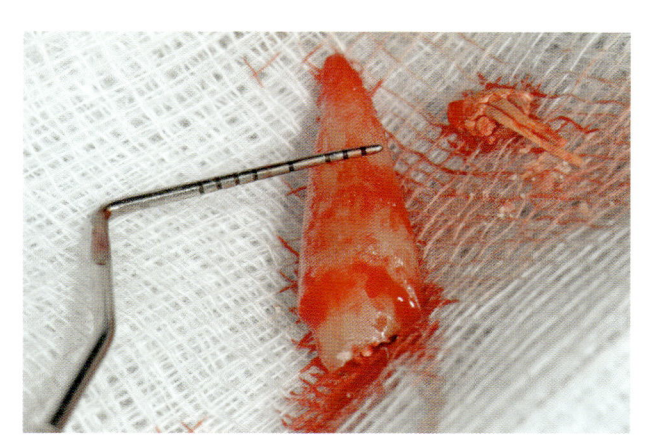

## 7   Immediate Placement and Computer-guided Surgery

**Fig 7-22**  Measurement of the root diameter midway along its length establishing implant diameter to be 4.5 mm for adequate primary stability and sufficient space to prevent damage to the labial plate at the crest.

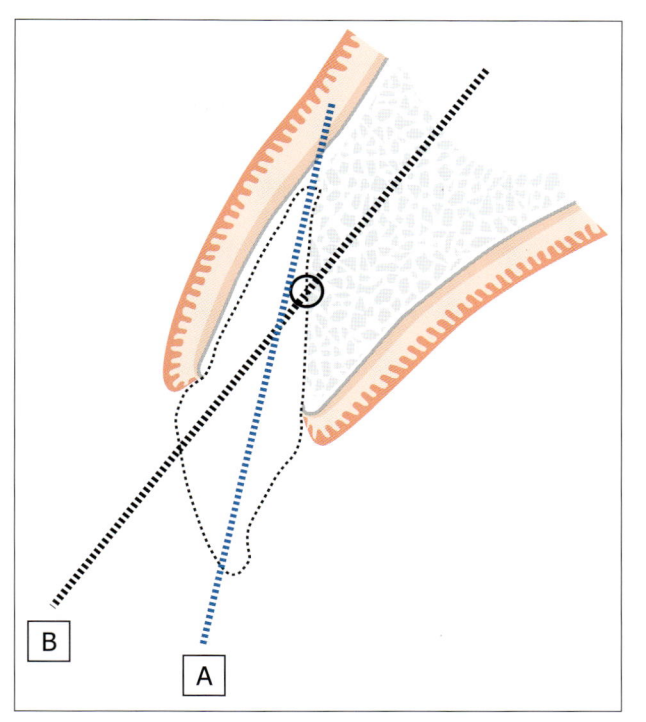

**Fig 7-23**  Immediate implant placement following the extraction of central incisor. Diagram depicts the ideal point of entry into the extraction socket at a point one-third to one-half from the apex. The direction of line B depicts the direction of osteotomy. Line A demonstrates the inevitable perforation through the labial plate if the osteotomy is directed through the apex.

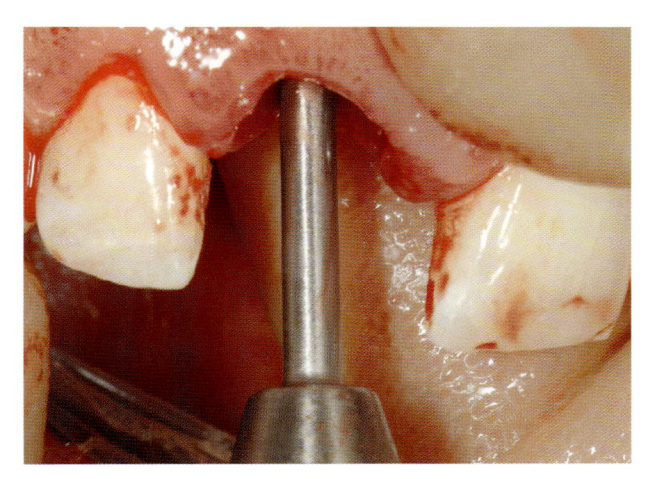

**Fig 7-24**  Position marker being used to select site and direction of the future implant.

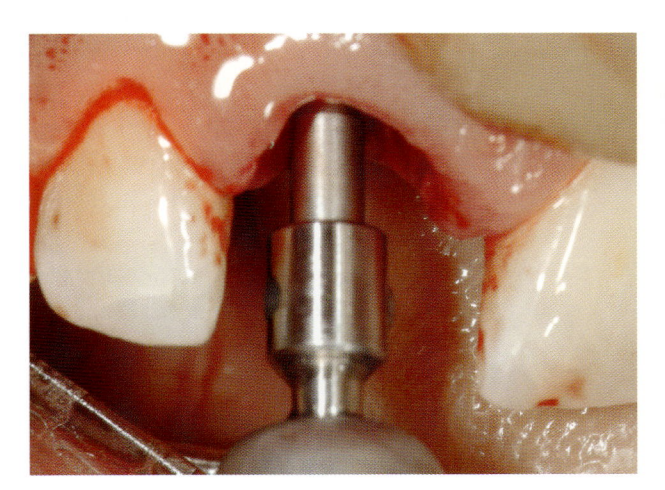

**Fig 7-25**  Lindemann bur used to establish direction and confirm density of residual bone beyond the socket.

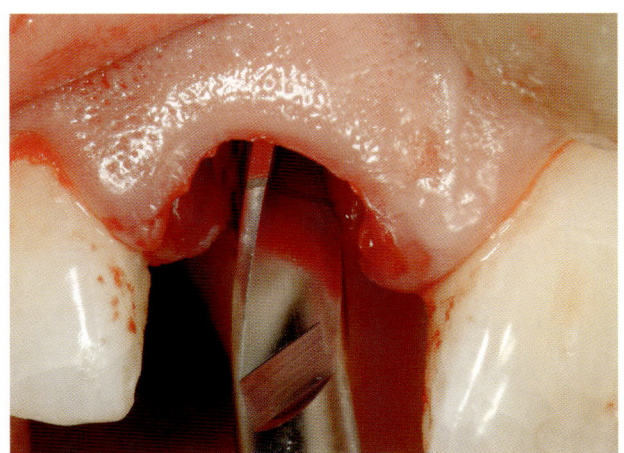

**Fig 7-26**  Final osteotomy bur (4 mm diameter for 4.5-mm implant) following the sequential enlargement of the osteotomy.

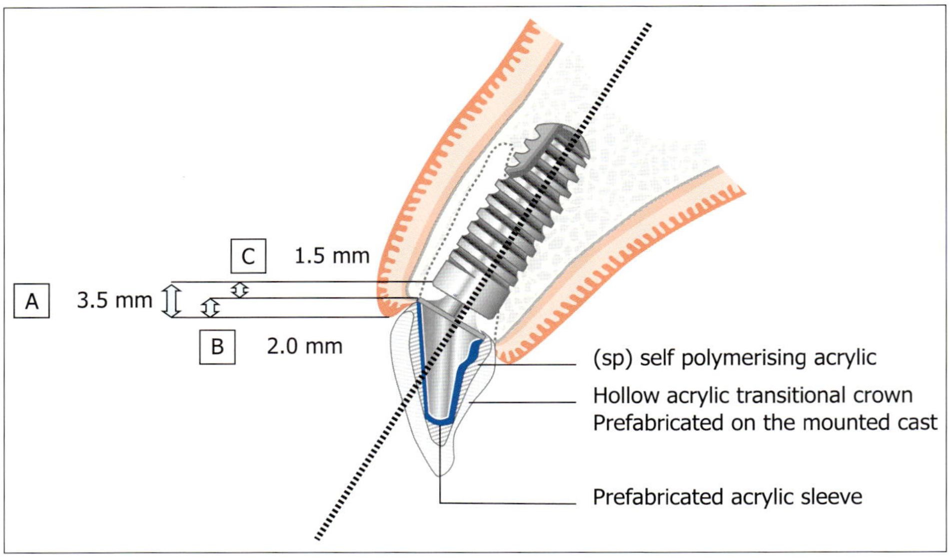

II  Implant Placement: Surgery and Prosthodontics

**Fig 7-27** Example of positioning of implant. Depth of implant placement (A = 3.5 mm) below the labial gingival margin is given by B (gingival thickness determined by probing depth) plus C (depth of implant placement below the labial bony socket crest).

approximately 1.5 mm below the level of the labial wall of the socket (Fig 7-27). Variations in preparation will occur depending on the bone density.

- **Low-density bone.** The implant may be inserted without any further development of the osteotomy. If excessive resistance is met during the insertion of the implant, the implant should be unscrewed and inserted after partial tapping of the threads.
- **High-density bone.** The bed for the implant must be formed completely. This may involve the use of any hand reamers and bone taps required by the implant system that is being used.
- **Moderate-density bone.** A hand reamer may be used and the osteotomy partly threaded with a bone tap before insertion of the implant.

This variation in osteotomy preparation will ensure that adequate primary stability for the implant can be achieved for immediate loading.

## Implant Insertion

The implant is inserted using the clinical experience and judgement of the operator to ensure that there is no damage to the implant, bone or insertion device from using excessive force, and yet the implant is secure enough to be able to withstand immediate loading (Fig 7-28). This will vary from system to system. The depth to which the implant is inserted should be sufficient to allow the creation of an emergence profile that is aesthetically acceptable (Fig 7-29). The required depth can be estimated by measuring the thickness of the labial gingiva from the margin to the level of the bone and adding it to the depth to which the implant should be inserted below the bony crest (1.5 mm). With the Ankylos implant system (Dentsply Friadent, Mannheim, Germany) the implant carrier with its circumferential ring and other features can be used as a gauge to estimate the depth of the implant insertion.

It is well known that bacteria can induce inflammatory bone loss depending on local and systemic factors.[80–85] We believe that if the implant is to be placed below the level of the bone the connection between the implant and abutment should be sufficiently tight to prevent leakage of microbial endotoxins and other virulent factors. Most of the known interfaces between implant and abutment carry the risk of microbial leakage, which may be a contributory factor to inflammatory bone loss.[86–89]

Leakage can be prevented or minimised by the use of silicone sealants or cements. However, they may deteriorate or dissolve.[90,91] Alternatively, a high-precision conical connection (Fig 7-30) can provide a tight seal, which may prevent micro-leakage, as demonstrated by vacuum tests of preassembled components.[92] This should be maintainable under functional load to prevent the loss of bone in an area that is critical for

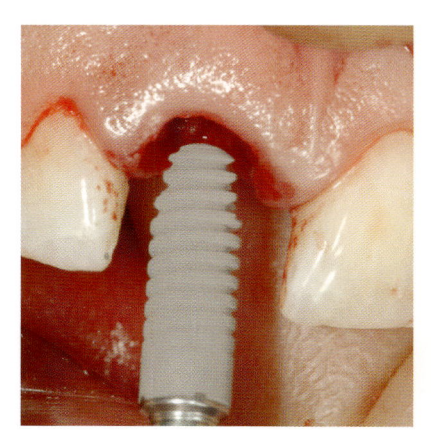

# 7 Immediate Placement and Computer-guided Surgery

**Fig 7-28** A 14-mm implant being inserted after the use of the final osteotomy bur. A precisely fitting self-tapping implant will provide high primary stability for immediate loading.

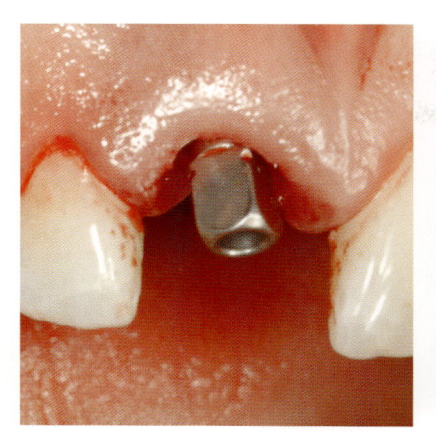

**Fig 7-29** The implant is seated. The depth and angulation to which it has been placed can be seen from the structure and orientation of the implant carrier.

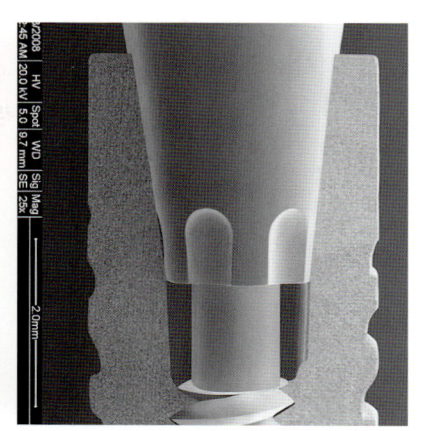

**Fig 7-30** Scanning electron microscope shows the seal between abutment and implant provided by the high accuracy of the component parts. This seal prevents microbial leakage, which is significant because of the positioning of the junction below the level of the bone. Please note the presence of an index on the abutment, which may or may not be used as an index, can limit the number of positions of engagement. However, the tight conical connection still is functional for anti-rotation as well as acting as an antibacterial seal.

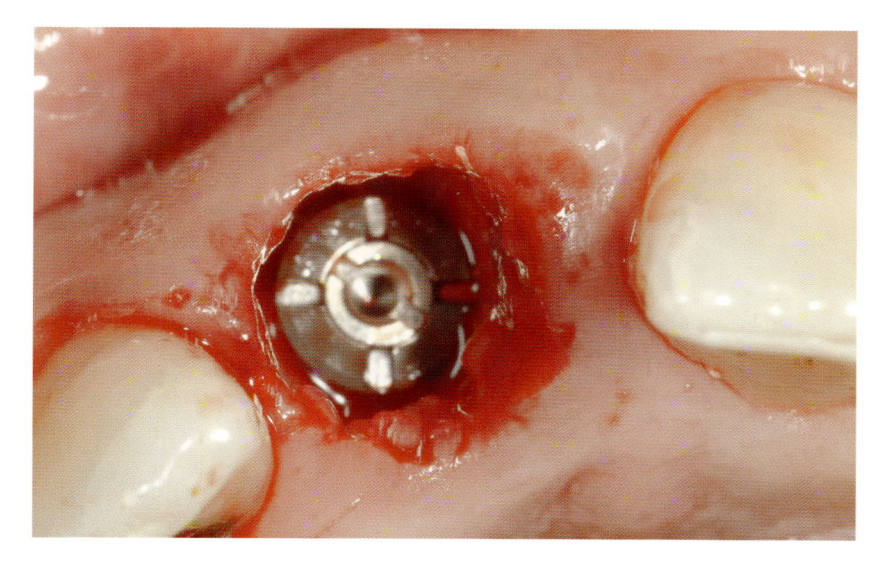

**Fig 7-31** Occlusal view of the implant in situ, showing its position in relation to the socket walls, particularly to the labial plate. The formation of a blood clot is the first stage in bone regeneration and will need to be retained by the transitional restoration.

aesthetics.[93] Mechanical load testing demonstrates a significant superiority of a conical connection, which acts by preventing gap formation caused by movement between implant and abutment.[94] Tests to demonstrate leakage must be properly conceived. Inoculation or penetration tests are only valid if a preassembled abutment–implant complex is tested.[87] Inoculation and subsequent assembly of the implant–abutment complex has the obvious drawback of overspill during assembly or contamination of internal or external surfaces of the connection. This may lead to fallacious conclusions with regard to penetration tightness.[95,96]

The implant should ideally be positioned to maximise on a good aesthetic outcome. A space of approximately 1 mm from the labial surface is desirable (Fig 7-31). This will compensate for any remodelling that may take place. The use of a micro-structured implant surface enables contact osteogenesis and improves bone-to-implant contact in comparison with machined surfaces.[97–99]

Figures 7-31 to 7-45 demonstrate the clinical management of an implant placed subcrestally and restored using a tight conical connection with a zirconium oxide abutment.

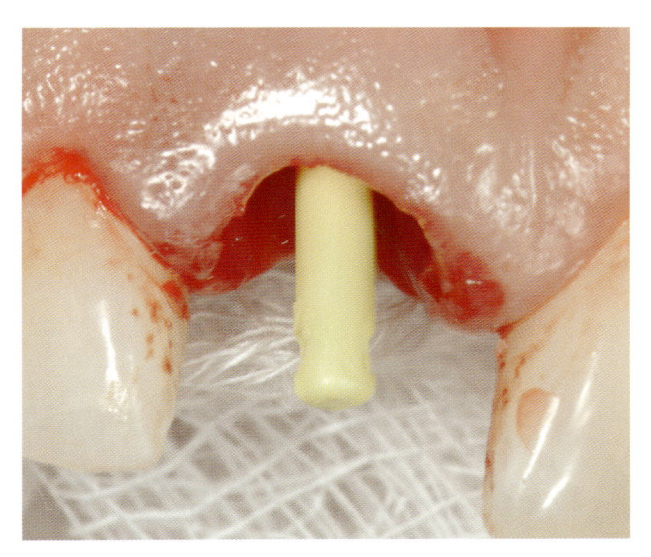

## II  Implant Placement: Surgery and Prosthodontics

**Fig 7-32**  Direction indicator being used to select the abutment. Alternatively a trial abutment can be used to estimate the angle (e.g. Ankylos CX implant).

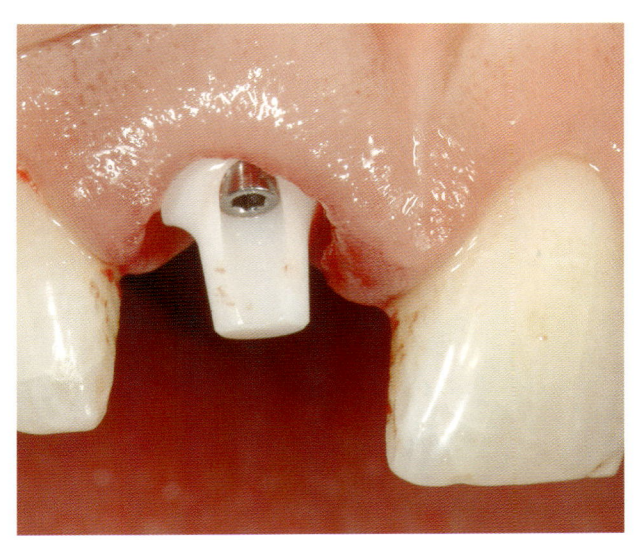

**Fig 7-33**  A 15-degree zirconium oxide abutment is selected and tried in. It is tightened with light finger pressure and disengaged to assess any interference with the alveolar socket. Rapid engagement on tightening combined with sudden disengagement following loosening of the screw is indicative of an absence of interference with the socket.

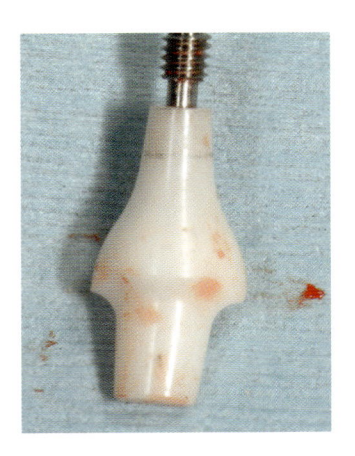

**Fig 7-34**  Following disengagement of the ceramic abutment, it is removed from the mouth and examined for a continuous grey line around the margin, which will signify that it was indeed properly seated without any deflection caused by the tooth socket. If the grey line is incomplete, seating of the abutment was prevented by interference adjacent to the region where the grey line is missing, and this will require modification of the abutment until the ring is complete.

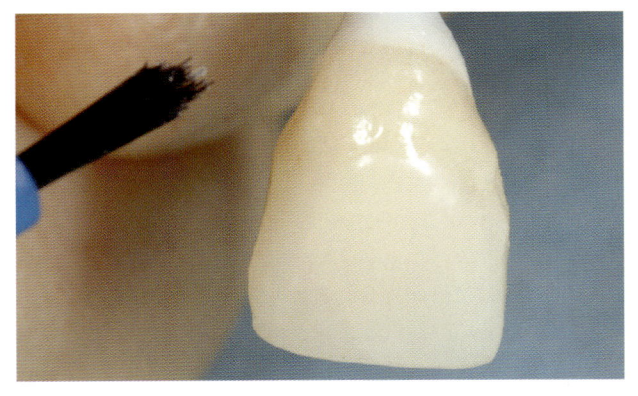

**Fig 7-35**  The transitional restoration is adapted using autopolymerising acrylic resin with the abutment in situ. The abutment is removed and any minor discrepancies can be corrected extraorally.

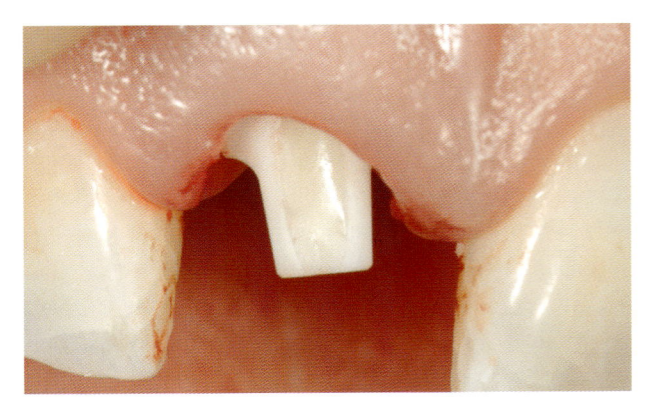

**Fig 7-36**  The abutment is then seated and its orientation confirmed using the transitional restoration. Wax is used to seal the hex of the screw followed by a glass-ionomer cement to occlude the screw access hole. This allows a predictable amount of cement to be used to avoid excess.

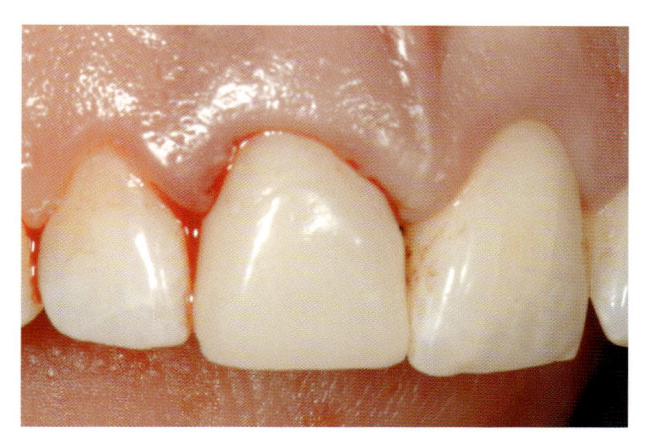

# 7  Immediate Placement and Computer-guided Surgery

**Fig 7-37** The transitional restoration cemented with a soft cement (Temp Bond; Kerr, West Collins, CA, USA). The transitional restoration has been constructed on a study cast to fit to 1 mm below the gingival margin and in contact with the soft tissues. This provides support and prevents the soft tissues from collapsing.

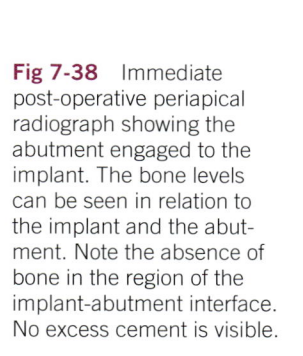

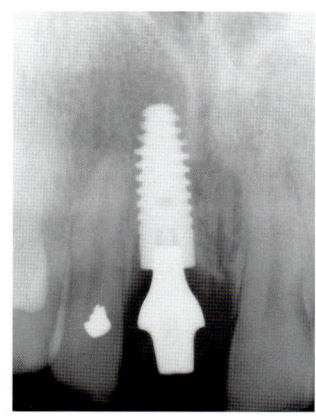

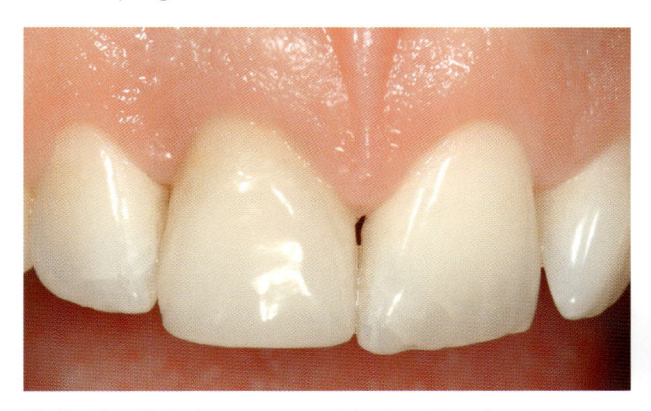

**Fig 7-38** Immediate post-operative periapical radiograph showing the abutment engaged to the implant. The bone levels can be seen in relation to the implant and the abutment. Note the absence of bone in the region of the implant-abutment interface. No excess cement is visible.

**Fig 7-39** Clinical appearance of the transitional restoration at three months after insertion showing stable healed and healthy soft tissues. Note the transitional restoration has been constructed shorter to avoid contact in protrusive excursions.

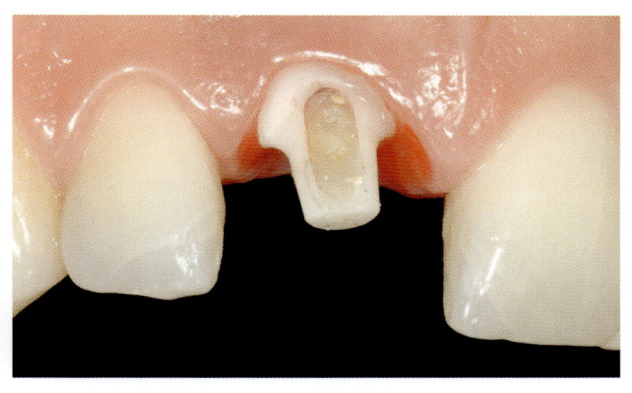

**Fig 7-40** Labial view of the abutment after removal of the transitional restoration prior to conventional impression taking using fine retraction cord and addition cured impression material. Note the proximity of the margin to the soft tissues resulting from the use of a larger and scalloped ceramic abutment.

**Fig 7-41** Periapical radiograph taken three months following implant insertion showing clearly the development of bone above the implant and approximating the abutment. This is indicative of a tight implant-abutment connection and the absence of micro-leakage.

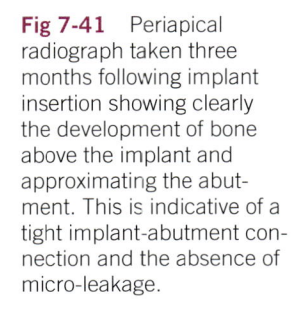

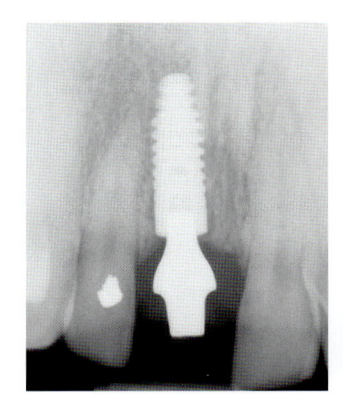

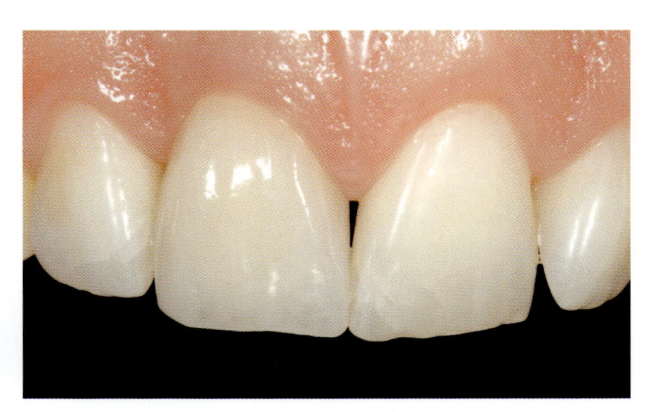

**Fig 7-42** Definitive restoration in situ 6 months following implant insertion showing harmonious soft tissue contours and excellent reproduction of tooth form and colour using a zirconium oxide coping veneered with porcelain.

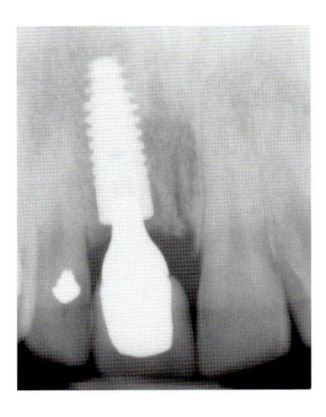

II  Implant Placement: Surgery and Prosthodontics

**Fig 7-43** Periapical radiograph taken six months after insertion showing further development of bone above the implant and in apparent contact with the abutment. Note the maturation of bone around the adjacent central incisor.

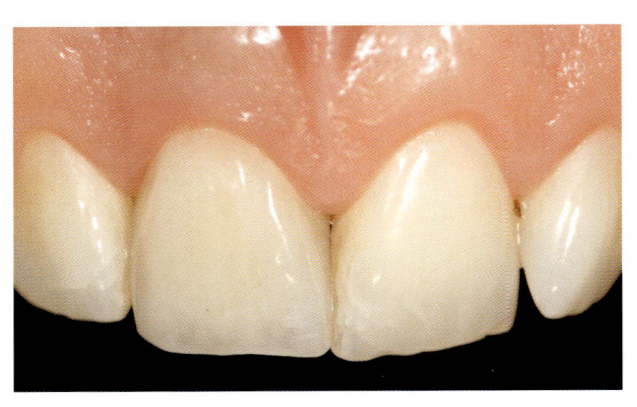

**Fig 7-44** Clinical appearance two years after the procedure showing stable soft tissue contours. In addition the development of the interdental papilla can be seen.

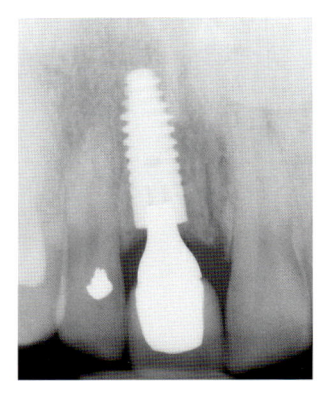

**Fig 7-45** Periapical radiograph taken two years after the procedure. Note the increase in bone overlying the implant and in contact with the abutment. Further development of bone adjacent to the left central incisor can be seen and could be assumed to have provided support for the generation of the papilla. Stable bone levels are fundamental to stable soft tissue contours and may be contributed to a micro-textured implant surface in combination with a tight conical connection between implant and abutment.

Where there is a thin bone biotype, the addition of a biomaterial may be considered. The choice of a non-resorbable or slowly resorbing material is likely to provide stability and support for the soft tissues.[100]

### Impressions at First Stage

Impressions at first-stage surgery can be taken to transfer the implant position to the laboratory for the restorative phase (Figs 7-46–7-50). The clinical and laboratory details of this technique will be addressed in the appropriate section. This impression can also be used for the fabrication of the transitional restoration in the surgery to be fitted at the same visit. Impressions at first-stage surgery are particularly indicated in cases of delayed loading. It enables the clinician to prepare for second-stage surgery.

## Delayed Loading: Clinical Management

If primary stability is not considered sufficient to load the implant immediately, some measures must be taken to minimise the risk of failure or complications.

### Preserving Soft Tissue Architecture

The use of a pontic to maintain and support the soft tissue contours is the primary method of choice. This requires an accurately fitting pontic, which will obliterate the margin of the socket, providing a seal for the protection of the blood clot. Ideally a fixed restoration such as a metal-acrylic resin Rochette bridge may be used. Attachment of a sulcus former or healing abutment will facilitate location of the implant at the time of loading. Alternatively, in a non-aesthetic region, the clinician may choose to use a sulcus former that has been modified to contain the blood clot.

### Wound Closure

Several methods to close the wound over immediately placed implants are available. These are described below.

### Vascularised Pedicled Flaps

Because vascularised pedicled flaps have a blood supply they have a relatively low chance of breakdown.

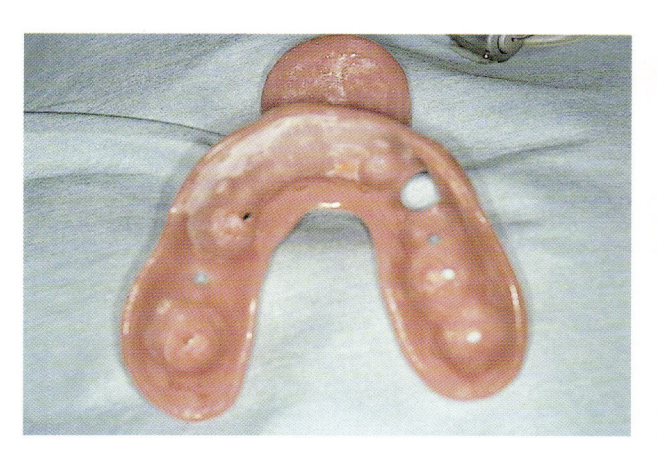

**7   Immediate Placement and Computer-guided Surgery**

**Fig 7-46**   A customised impression tray for an open-tray technique.

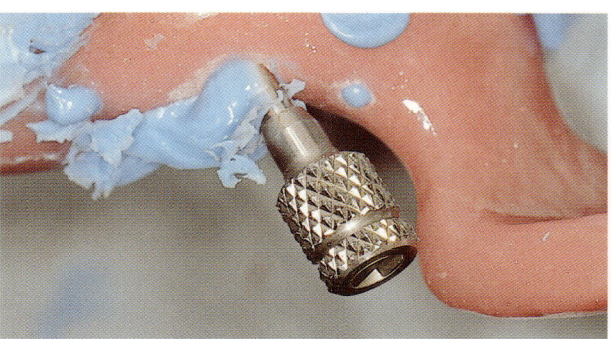

**Fig 7-48**   The impression tray in situ with the handle attached to the hex driver prior to disengagement of the implant carrier.

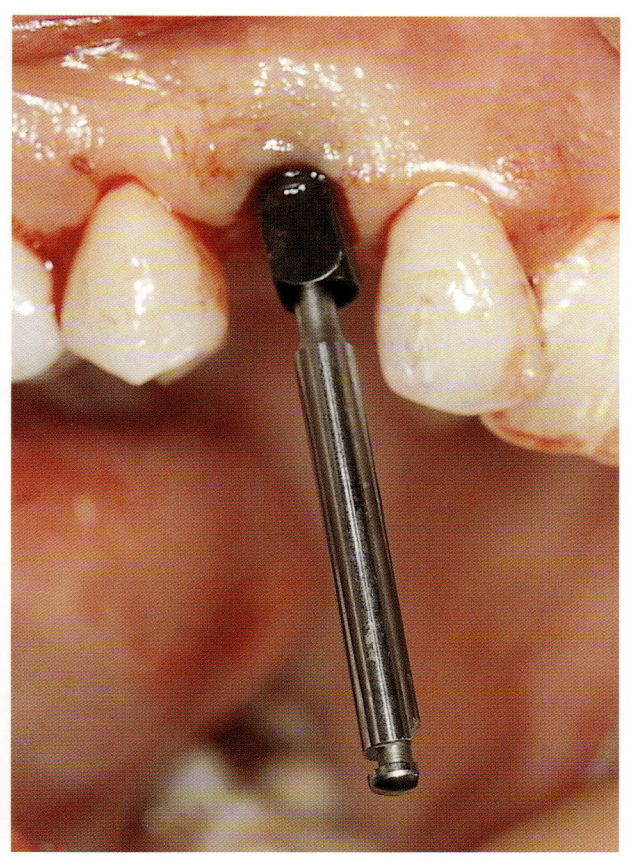

**Fig 7-47**   A hex driver inserted into the implant carrier prior to seating of the impression. The design of the carrier is suitable for transferring the implant position using an open-tray impression technique.

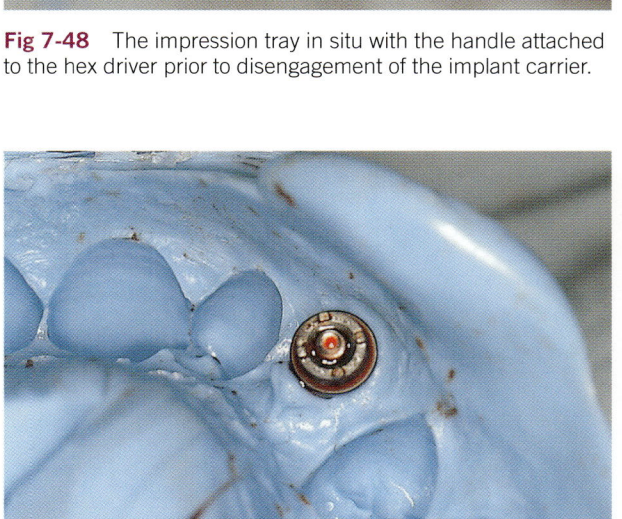

**Fig 7-49**   Impression tray after removal from the mouth. The implant carrier is visible secure within the impression, avoiding the need for reinsertion inaccuracies.

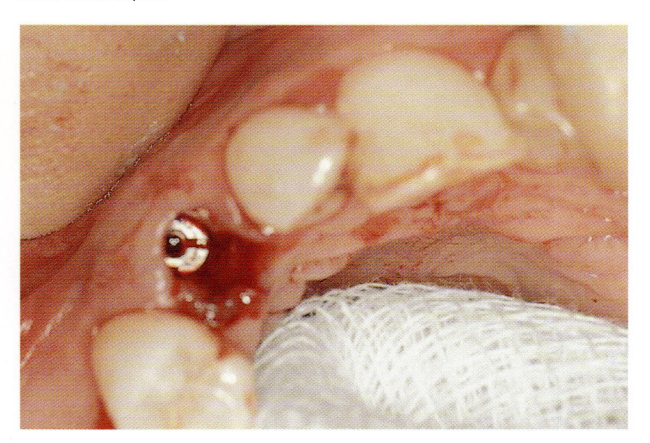

**Fig 7-50**   The implant is visible within the socket following the removal of the implant carrier. The decision as to how to proceed can be implemented. Immediate loading using a provisional abutment can be carried out. Alternatively soft tissue closure can be performed. A further option is to seal the blood clot in the socket and support the soft tissues using a provisional restoration such as a Rochette bridge. A modified sulcus former may be used to provide ease of access at the time of bringing the implant into function.

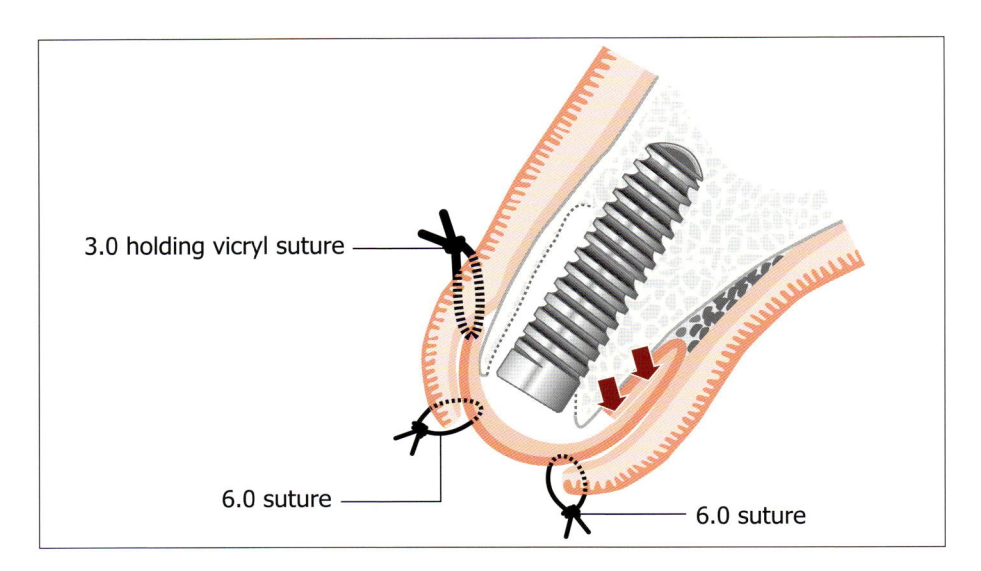

**Fig 7-51** Pedicled flap from the palate may be used to close over the socket (see section on soft tissue surgery).

- **The palatal pedicled flap.** This is the flap of choice for closure of an immediate implant site in the anterior maxilla. Its vascularised nature makes it very predictable. Furthermore, it may be used to increase the amount of soft tissue bulk in this region without compromising the amount, texture or colour of the attached keratinised gingiva (Fig 7-51).
- **The labial coronally advanced flap.** This has the disadvantage of advancing the buccal attached gingiva to close the wound, resulting in a reduction of the attached keratinised gingiva around the implant.

### Free Non-vascularised Grafts

Grafts that are non-vascularised are less predictable and more prone to breakdown.

- **Composite grafts.** These include gingival and connective tissue and may be used as a plug to cover the implant. They are designed to fit exactly into the socket and derive their blood supply from the socket margins. They retain the colour and texture of the epithelial tissue of origin (Fig 7-52).
- **Connective tissue grafts.** These do not have the epithelial component and are generally placed underneath the partially mobilised margins of the surrounding soft tissue, which provides the blood supply for the graft (Fig 7-53).

### Occluding Membranes

Occluding membranes are non-permeable and are placed over the socket and tucked under the socket margins. They permit connective tissue to form underneath the membrane; they are removed after approximately four weeks, enabling epithelialisation of the underlying connective tissue to proceed. Resorbable membranes (collagen based) may be used in a similar manner and permit epithelialisation onto the membrane.

## Immediate Loading: Clinical Management

It is not intended to provide a specific prescription for the assessment of primary stability. The decision to carry out immediate loading will depend upon the clinical judgement, understanding and experience of the clinician. Factors to be considered will be discussed later within this chapter under 'Immediate Loading: Primary Stability'.

### Abutment Selection and Attachment

After removal of the implant carrier, the appropriate abutment can be selected. Some implant systems offer direction indicators or trial abutments to facilitate this. The hollow transitional restoration can be used to confirm the angulation and sulcus depth of the required abutment based on the depth of the implant (Fig 7-54, see also 7-32). The definitive abutment is selected,

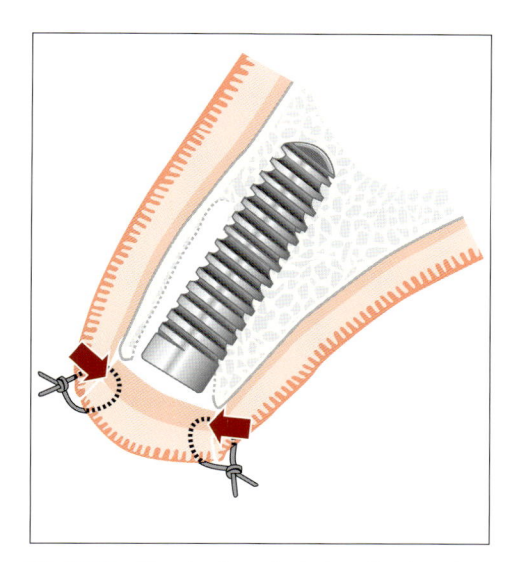

# 7 Immediate Placement and Computer-guided Surgery

**Fig 7-52** Circular free gingival graft sutured to socket soft tissue margins. The source of reestablishment of blood supply is indicated by the arrows.

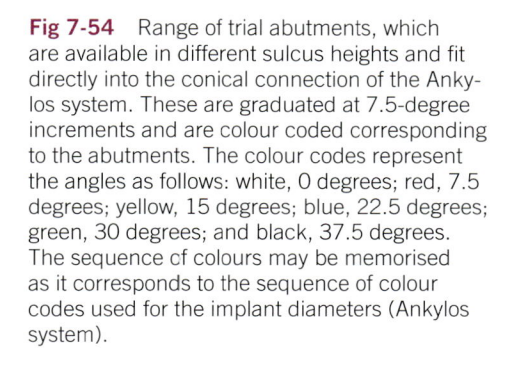

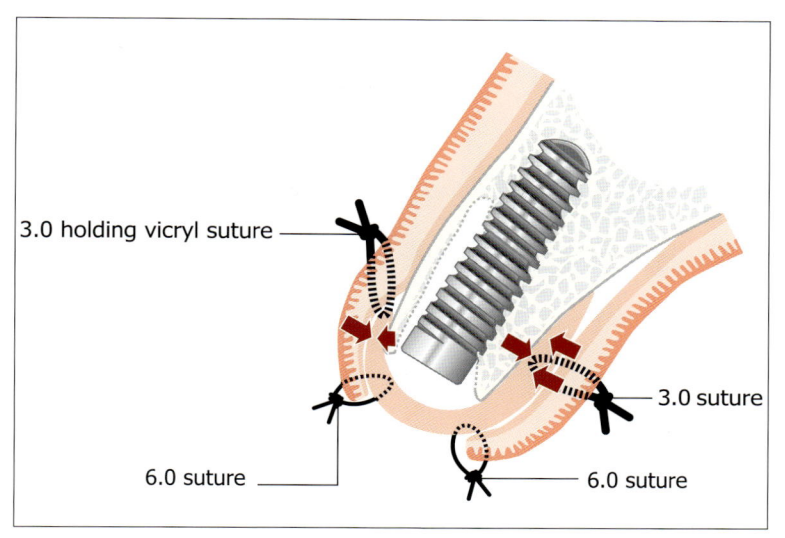

**Fig 7-53** Subepithelial connective tissue graft may be used as described in the section on soft tissue surgery. Re-establishment of the blood supply will depend on the contact area indicated by arrows. Occlusive membranes (for instance, TefGen, Lifecore Biomedical, Chaska, MN, USA) may also be used in a similar way.

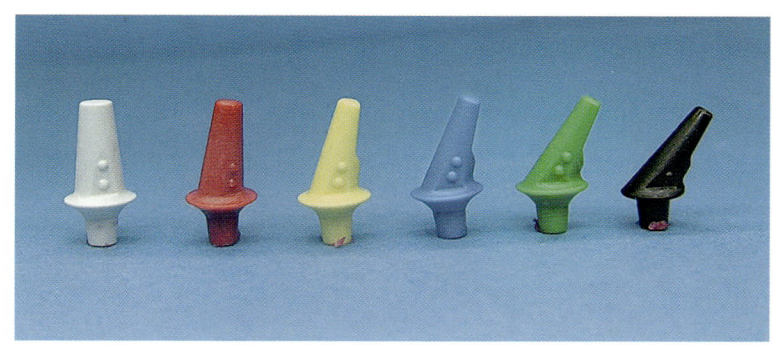

**Fig 7-54** Range of trial abutments, which are available in different sulcus heights and fit directly into the conical connection of the Ankylos system. These are graduated at 7.5-degree increments and are colour coded corresponding to the abutments. The colour codes represent the angles as follows: white, 0 degrees; red, 7.5 degrees; yellow, 15 degrees; blue, 22.5 degrees; green, 30 degrees; and black, 37.5 degrees. The sequence of colours may be memorised as it corresponds to the sequence of colour codes used for the implant diameters (Ankylos system).

modified if necessary and then attached to the implant using the recommended torque.

## Prefabricated Angled Titanium Abutments

The availability of a range of prefabricated angled titanium abutments is particularly well suited to the selection of the correct abutment and its attachment to the implant without substantial modifications. The availability of six angles and four sulcus depths enables most clinical needs to be met. The considerable advantage of a narrow abutment is the ease with which it can be attached to the implant without interfering with the socket. At the same time, it will readily fit within the prosthetic envelope.

This concept requires the discrepancy between the abutment and the transitional restoration to be filled directly at the time of surgery with autopolymerising acrylic resin. This offers tremendous flexibility and ease of operation and is most significant when multiple implants are placed, which require the abutments to be positioned within the prosthetic envelopes and at the same time aligned to each other.

The disadvantage of this approach is the dependence upon acrylic resin for the guidance of the soft tissue contour development and the resultant deeply placed margin of the restoration.

Figures 7-55 to 7-81 illustrate the use of a prefabricated angled titanium abutment in the aesthetic zone in conjunction with a biomaterial at the time of implant placement and loading immediately following extraction of a failing tooth.

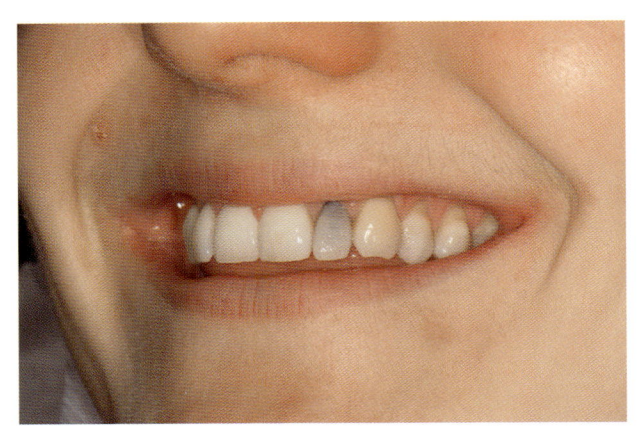

II    Implant Placement: Surgery and Prosthodontics

**Fig 7-55**  Preoperative view of a patient with a failing discoloured lateral incisor.

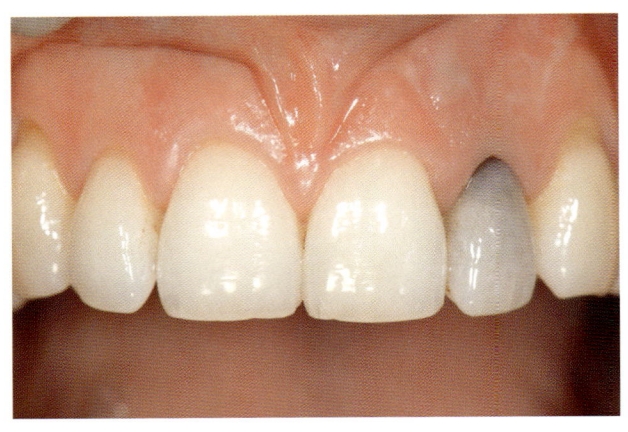

**Fig 7-56**  Intraoral view of anterior maxilla recording the soft tissue contours. Gingival margins, papillary height as well as the thickness of the overlying tissues should be noted (namely soft tissue biotype relating to contours and thickness).

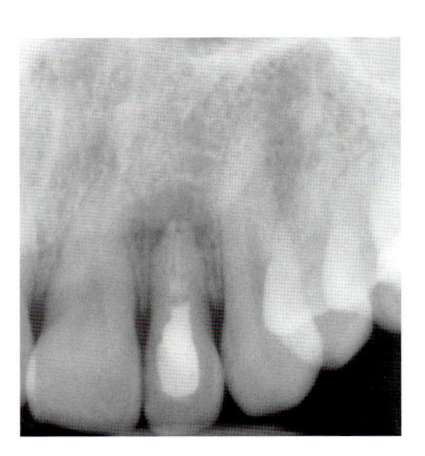

**Fig 7-57**  Preoperative periapical radiograph of inadequately restored failing lateral incisor demonstrating bone loss and root resorption.

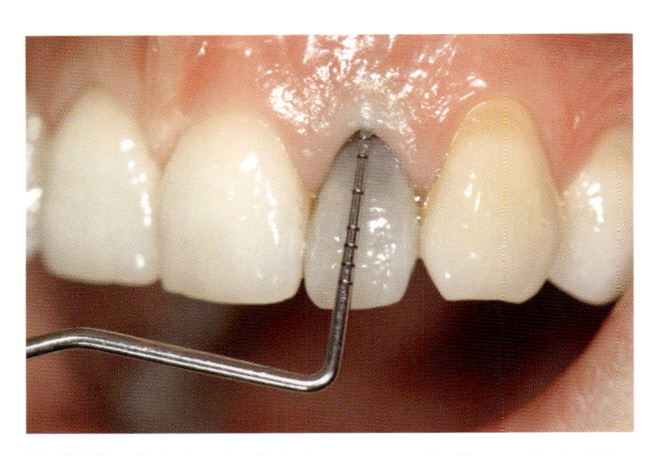

**Fig 7-58**  Sulcular depth being measured with a periodontal probe to assess the possible level of bony socket. The 2 mm reading is indicative of 3 mm distance to the bony socket.

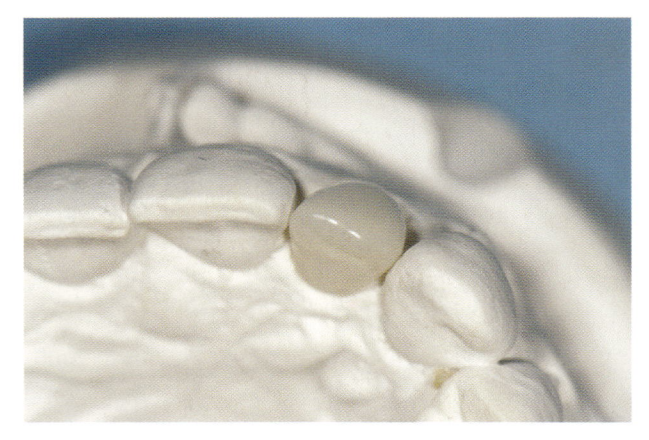

**Fig 7-59**  Occlusal view of hollow acrylic resin transitional restoration designed to provide support to the soft tissues following extraction and immediate implant placement and loading.

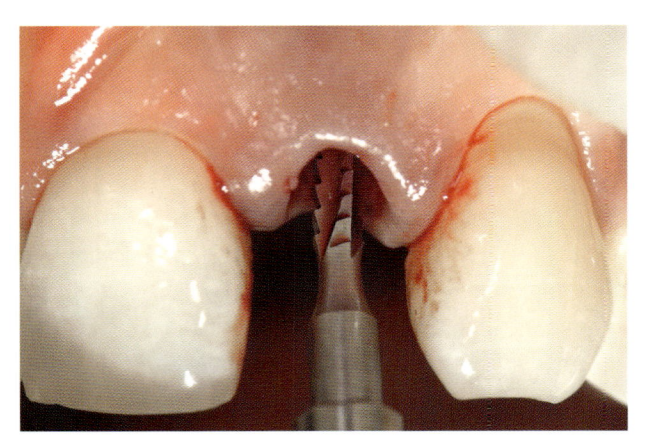

**Fig 7-60**  Pilot osteotomy bur (Lindemann bur) being used to commence an osteotomy on the palatal aspect of the socket apex.

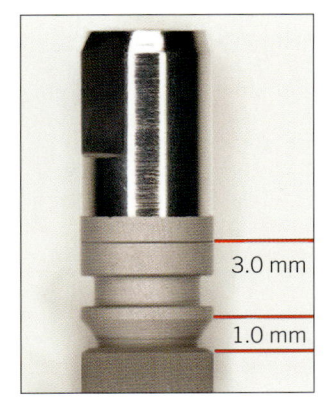

# 7  Immediate Placement and Computer-guided Surgery

**Fig 7-61** Intraoperative radiograph using a radiopaque indicator to confirm direction of the pilot osteotomy. This ensures avoiding damage to the adjacent teeth.

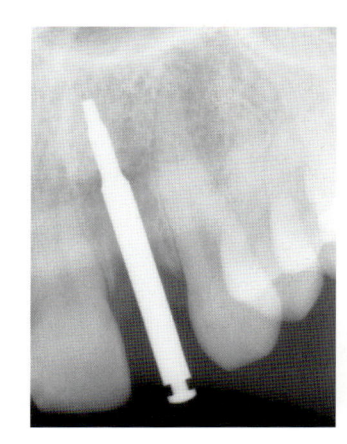

**Fig 7-62** Internally irrigated osteotomy drill being used to enlarge the osteotomy to receive a 3.5-mm diameter implant.

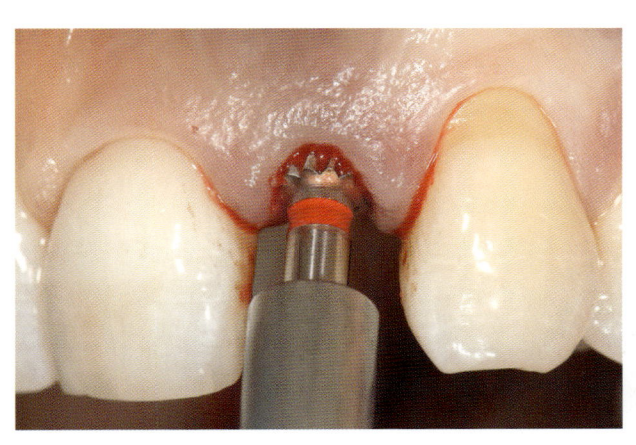

**Fig 7-63** Tapered reamer being used to confirm implant diameter and osteotomy depth as well as to establish the bed for the tapered body of the implant.

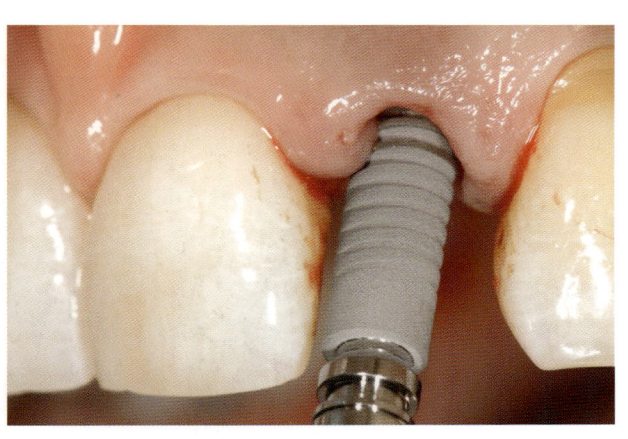

**Fig 7-64** The insertion of a titanium implant as a self-tapping device to maximise primary stability in medium-density bone.

**Fig 7-65** Implant carrier with calibrations to facilitate correct depth of placement of implant from gingival margin.

**Fig 7-66** Implant being inserted to the estimated depth of 1.5 mm below the crest of the alveolar socket. The implant is, therefore, inserted to 4.5 mm below the labial gingival margin. The dots on the insertion instrument are oriented towards the buccal to permit the use of an indexed abutment should that be the clinicians choice. The final position of the index would have to be confirmed using an abutment of the correct angulation and sulcus depth to confirm the correct rotational alignment of the implant.

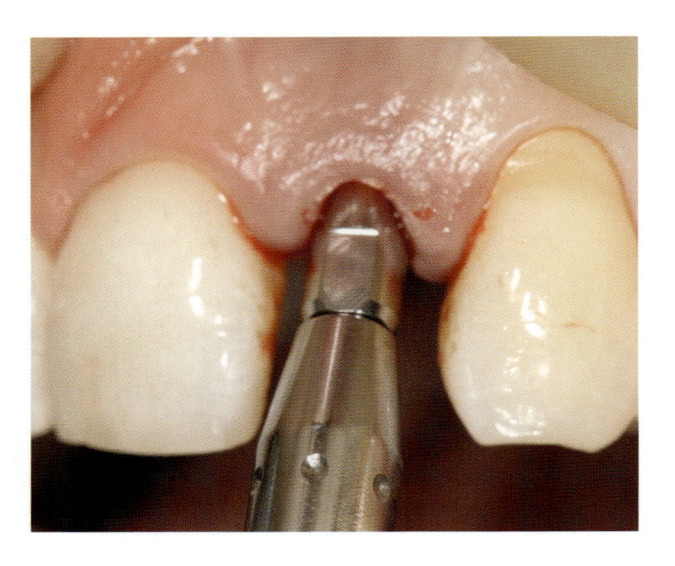

69

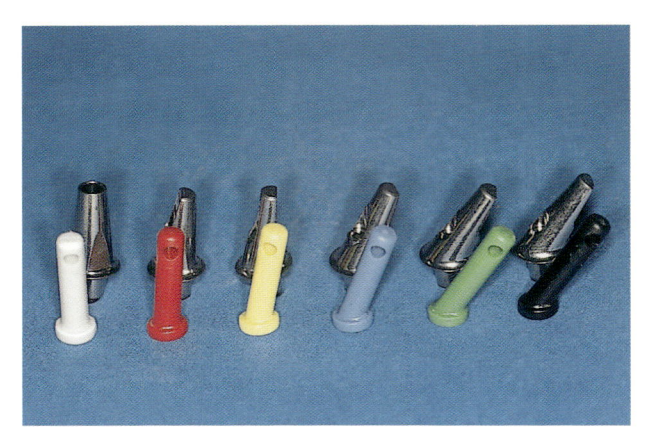

## II  Implant Placement: Surgery and Prosthodontics

**Fig 7-67**  Range of direction indicators with matching abutments. These are graduated at 7.5-degree increments and are colour coded corresponding to the abutments. The colour codes represent the angles as follows: white, 0 degrees; red, 7.5 degrees; yellow, 15 degrees; blue, 22.5 degrees; green, 30 degrees; and black, 37.5 degrees.

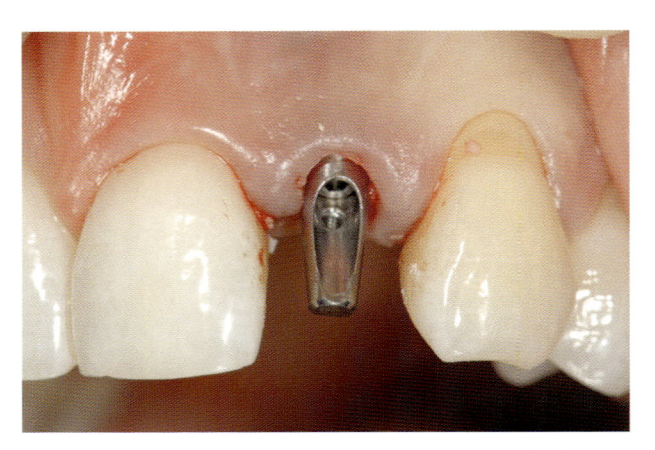

**Fig 7-68**  The definitive titanium abutment in situ following selection using direction indicators, which require the cover screw to be inserted after removal of the implant carrier. Any biomaterial, if indicated, must be inserted with the cover screw in situ to prevent ingress into the internal connection of the implant.

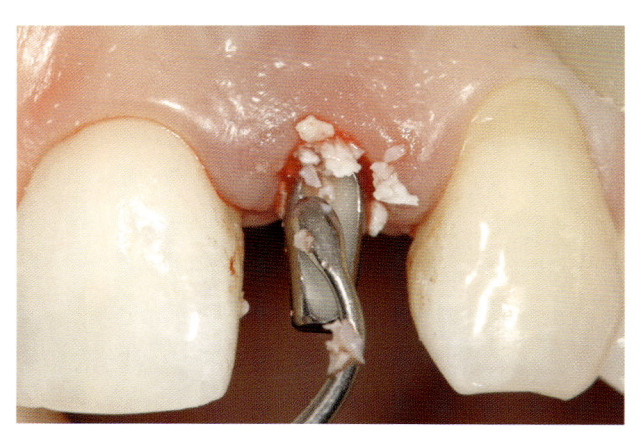

**Fig 7-69**  Any further biomaterial that may be required for tissue support should be inserted prior to cementation of the transitional restoration. Note that the screw access hole has been sealed with wax and glass-ionomer cement as previously described allowing control of the cement quantity to prevent excess.

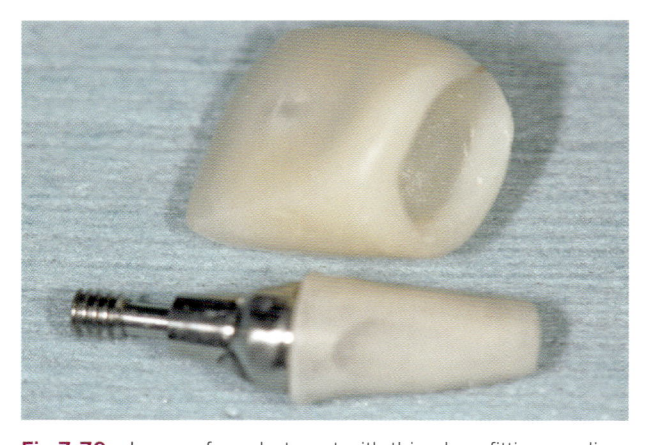

**Fig 7-70**  Image of an abutment with thin close-fitting acrylic resin sleeve and a hollow transitional crown. Note that the abutment has been modified by the removal of the shoulder to prevent interference with the socket. The tight-fitting sleeve requires the very minimum amount of cement during cementation. The hollow acrylic resin crown is attached to the sleeve using cold-curing acrylic resin and, therefore, prevents excess resin from extruding below the abutment margin. This technique greatly facilitates the management of patients with excellent predictability.

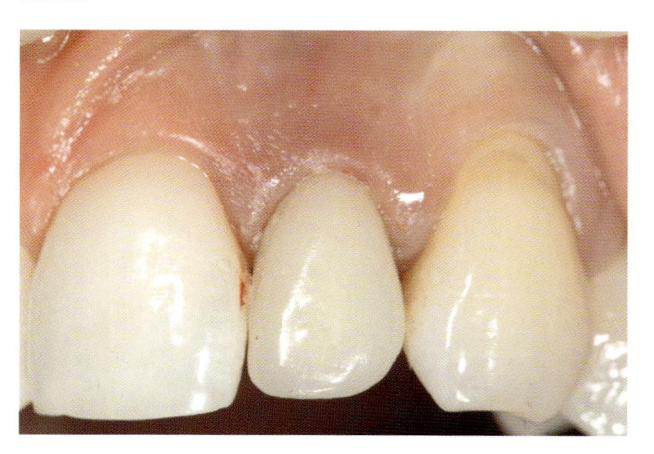

**Fig 7-71**  Transitional restoration cemented in place. Minimum cement is essential. The outside of the transitional restoration is coated with an antibiotic paste (auramycin or dentamycin) to facilitate the removal of any excess cement, should there be any. It further may serve to reduce the risk of a possible infection of the biomaterial.

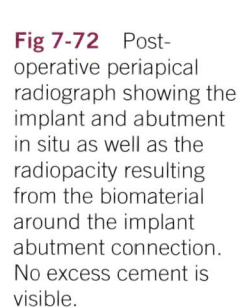

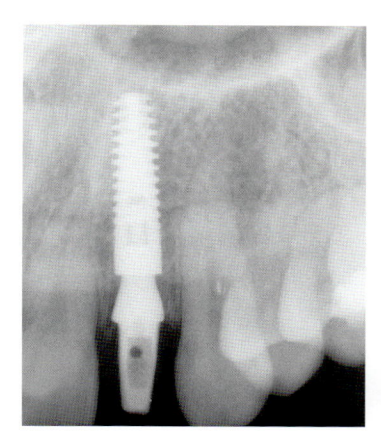

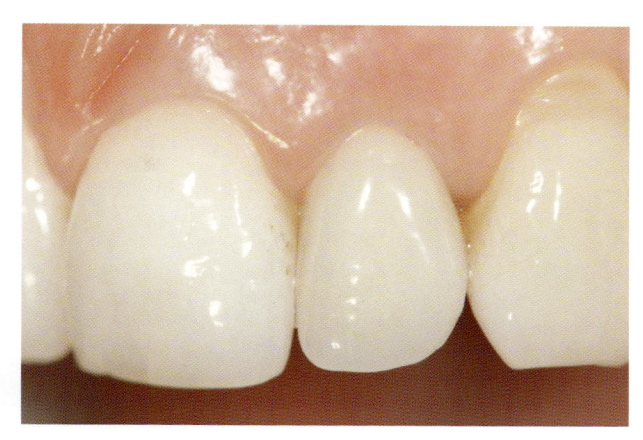

## 7  Immediate Placement and Computer-guided Surgery

**Fig 7-72** Postoperative periapical radiograph showing the implant and abutment in situ as well as the radiopacity resulting from the biomaterial around the implant abutment connection. No excess cement is visible.

**Fig 7-73** Labial view of transitional restoration three months after surgery showing healthy well-contoured soft tissues.

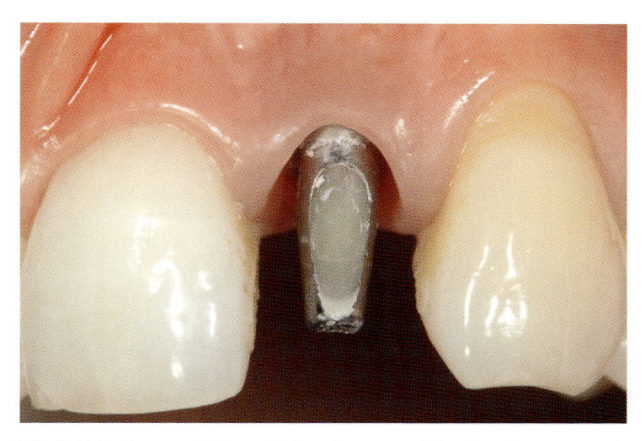

**Fig 7-74** Intraoral view of the abutment following the removal of the transitional restoration prior to impression taking at three months after insertion.

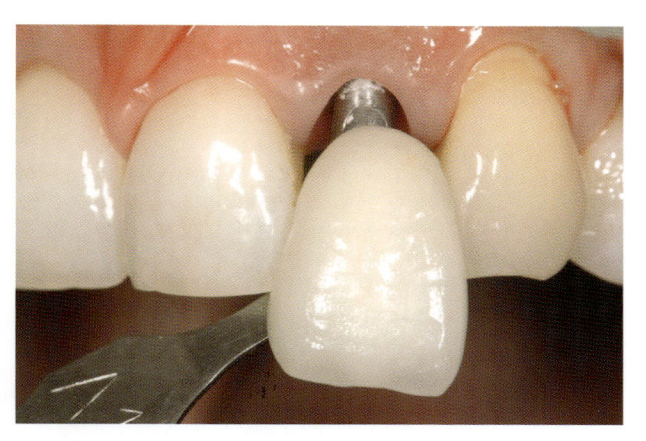

**Fig 7-75** Shade taking using a custom-made shade guide with porcelain fused to bonding alloy of choice. Communication of the shade with the dental technician, via a photograph as well as a drawing of specific stains and translucencies, facilitates the construction of an aesthetically acceptable restoration. Alternatively the technician can take the shade directly.

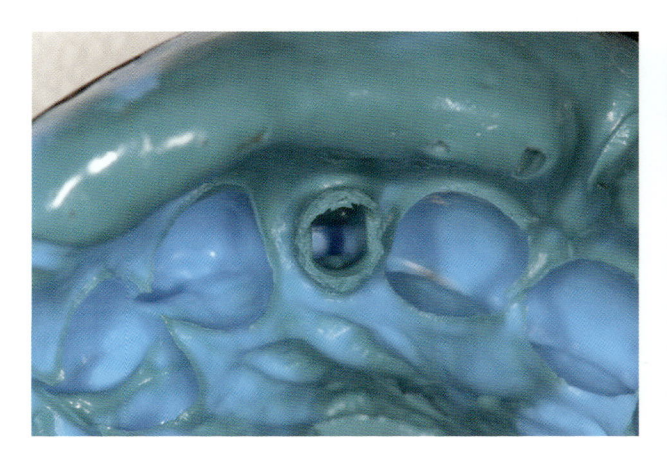

**Fig 7-76** Conventional impression of abutment taken using retraction cord to capture the abutment margin as well as the soft tissue contours.

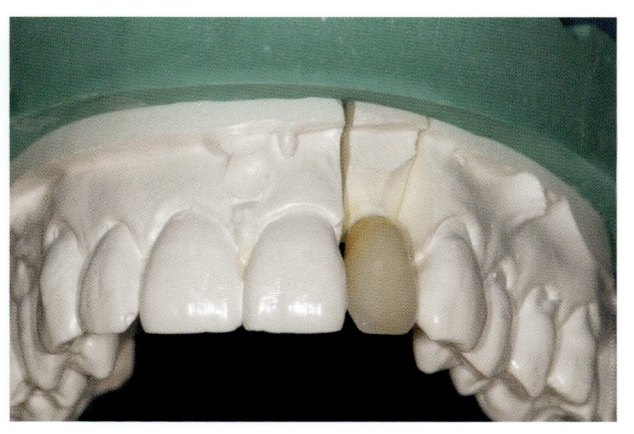

**Fig 7-77** Finished crown on cast fabricated from an epoxy resin. The porcelain is built up on an untrimmed cast, which depicts the soft tissue contours.

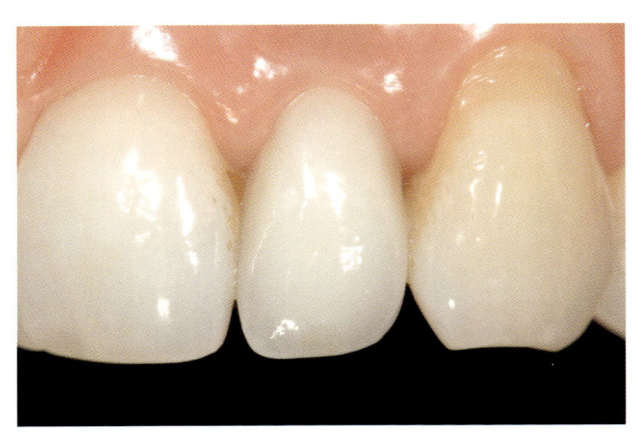

II  Implant Placement: Surgery and Prosthodontics

**Fig 7-78** Definitive restoration emerging from naturally contoured tissues mimicking the adjacent teeth.

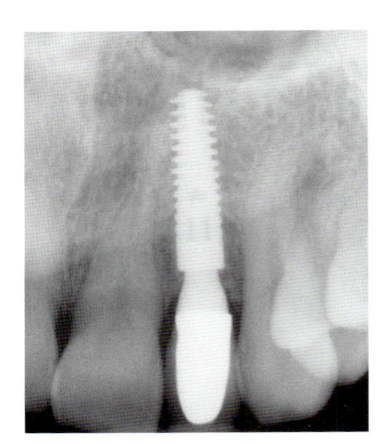

**Fig 7-79** Periapical radiograph showing bone levels and confirming no presence of excess cement following cementation. The use of Vaseline (petroleum jelly) on the outer surface of the crown prior to cementation and dental floss in conjunction with air–water spray ensures that any excess is predictably removed.

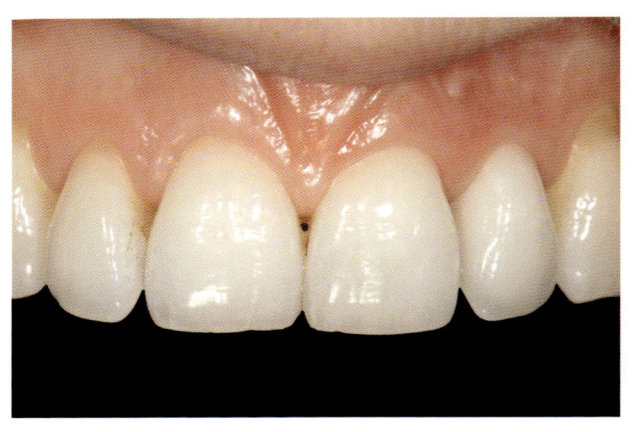

**Fig 7-80** Labial view showing the maintenance of gingival contours and harmony.

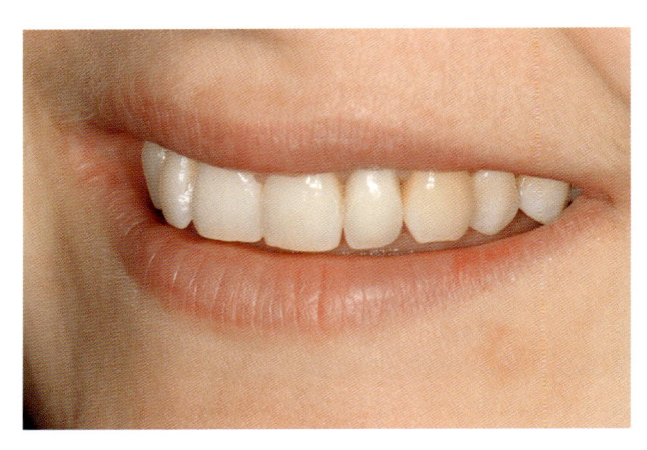

**Fig 7-81** Post-treatment view of patient smiling.

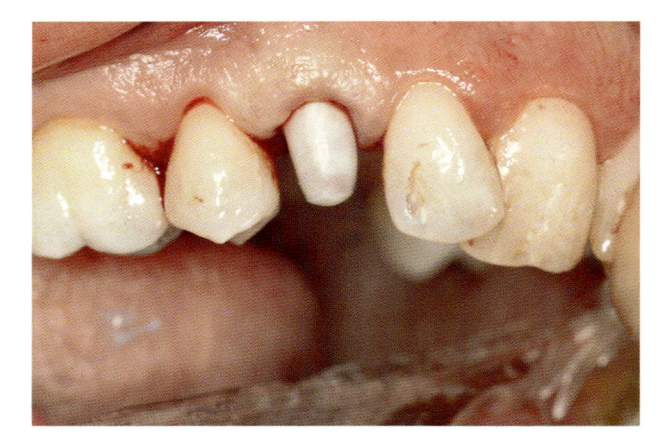

**Fig 7-82** The accurately fitting acrylic resin sleeve in situ prior to connection to the transitional restoration. The sleeve prevents the extrusion of the auto-polymerising resin into the socket.

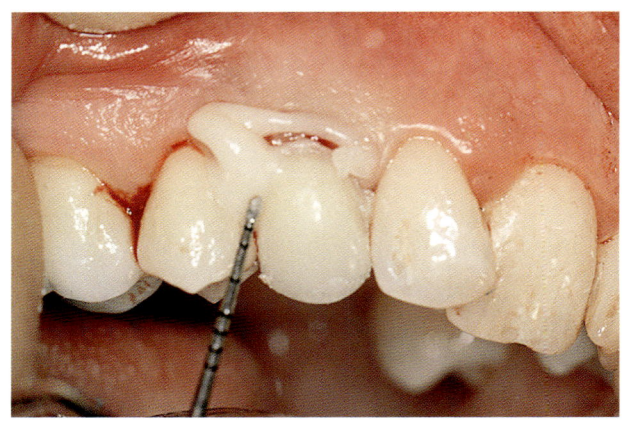

**Fig 7-83** The transitional restoration can be seen seated, and superfluous resin is removed prior to the removal of the transitional crown for trimming and polishing.

# 7  Immediate Placement and Computer-guided Surgery

## Prefabricated Angled Ceramic Abutments

Prefabricated angled ceramic abutments are generally much bulkier and are presently available in a limited number of sizes and angles.

Their relatively large size may not fit within the alveolar socket as well as the prosthetic envelope. The use of these abutments, therefore, requires modification of the abutment to ensure that the socket does not prevent the abutment from seating properly and engaging the implant to establish connection and a seal.

Similarly the limited range of angles available requires modifications to fit within the transitional crown. The biocompatibility of the zirconium oxide offers better soft tissue adaptation and acceptance. Furthermore, once it has been appropriately modified, the cement margin is usually closer to the gingival margin, thus facilitating cement removal.

Most importantly its white or dentine colour avoids the potential greying that may arise should thin soft tissues overlay a titanium abutment.

Figures 7-31 to 7-45 describe the use of a prefabricated angled ceramic abutment in conjunction with an immediate implant.

## Transitional Restoration: Clinical Adaptation

The prefabricated acrylic resin sleeve is fitted onto the abutment and the transitional hollow restoration is tried in and checked functionally and aesthetically (Fig 7-82). The transitional restoration should be seated until it is in contact with the soft tissues around the socket margin, avoiding excess pressure. The hollow transitional restoration is then attached to the acrylic resin sleeve using auto-polymerising resin (Fig 7-83). A single strip of gauze may be used as a spacer, with the patient in the intercuspal position to provide sufficient clearance.

Care must be taken to use the correct consistency of resin to ensure that no material extends beyond the abutment. The transitional restoration is removed, allowed to polymerise until hard and trimmed following the correction of any deficiencies. The restoration is then polished and cemented with a minimal amount of temporary cement (Fig 7-84). The occlusal clearance is checked and the restoration adjusted to ensure that there are no contacts during excursions.

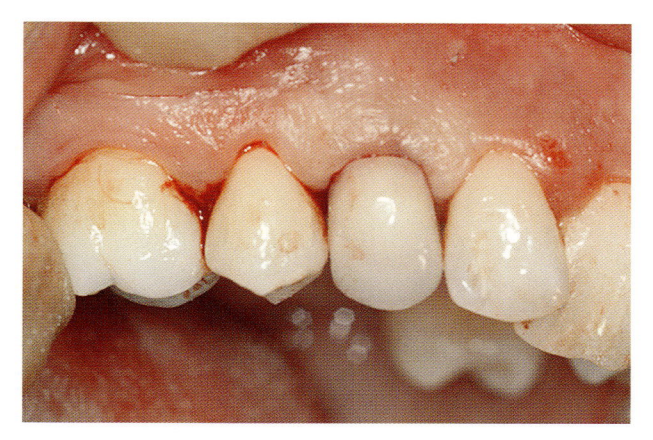

**Fig 7-84** Finished transitional restoration in situ, cemented with a minute amount of temporary cement to avoid extrusion of any cement.

A post-operative radiograph is taken to ensure that there is no excess cement and to provide a baseline record of the level of bone in relation to the implant (Figs 7-38 and 7-72).

## Restorative Phase

After a healing period of approximately three months, the restorative phase is started on the basis that soft tissue levels will have stabilised (see Figs 7-39, 7-40, 7-73 and 7-74). This is confirmed by observing the gingival margin and papillary levels using the transitional restoration as a reference. Continuing changes within the soft tissue indicate that the restorative phase should be delayed.

Any of the techniques described for taking impressions may be used to transfer information to the laboratory for the fabrication of the definitive restoration:
- pick-up impressions after first-stage impression (Figs 7-85–7-90)
- conventional impressions (Figs 7-74–7-78)
- implant transfer (open tray or closed tray)
- abutment transfer (Figs 7-91 and 7-92).

A more detailed description of different techniques will be covered in Chapter 10.

## II  Implant Placement: Surgery and Prosthodontics

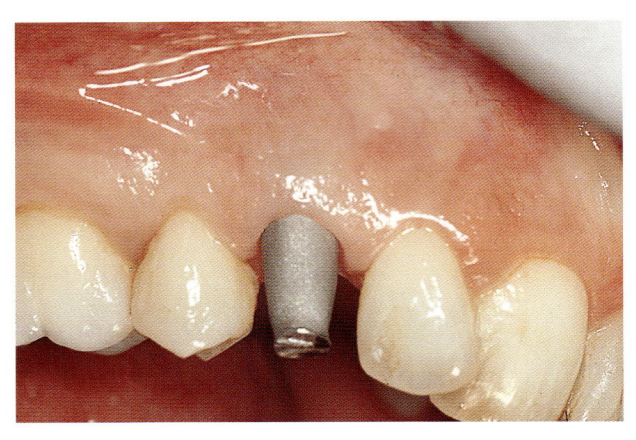

**Fig 7-85**  Metalwork can be seen in situ prior to pick-up impression. This will transfer the soft tissue contours to the laboratory for the addition of porcelain.

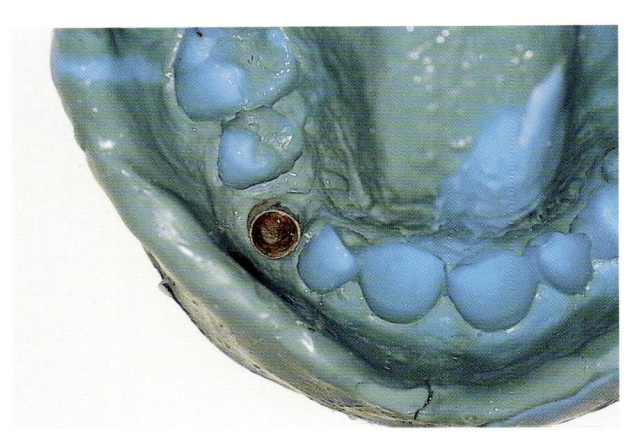

**Fig 7-86**  The metalwork picked up using an addition cured heavy and light-bodied impression material.

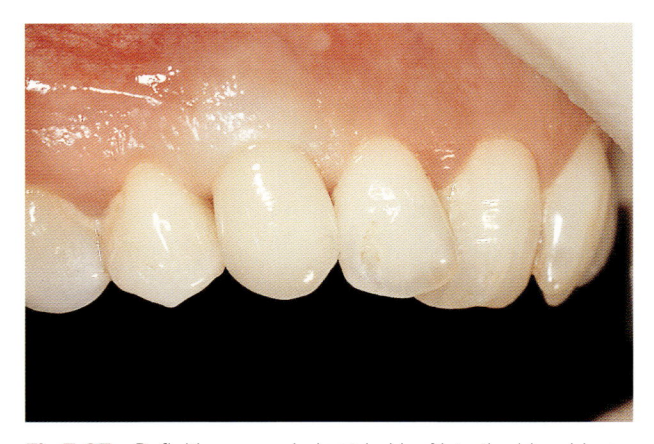

**Fig 7-87**  Definitive crown being tried in. Note the blanching, which is excessive and might lead to gingival recession.

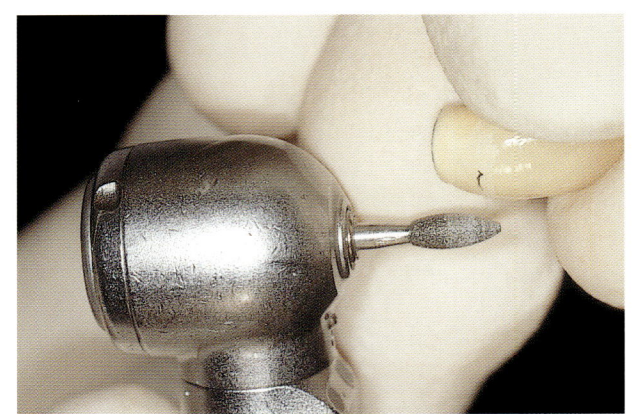

**Fig 7-88**  The crown is modified and polished to establish a form that does not exert pressure on the labial soft tissues on seating.

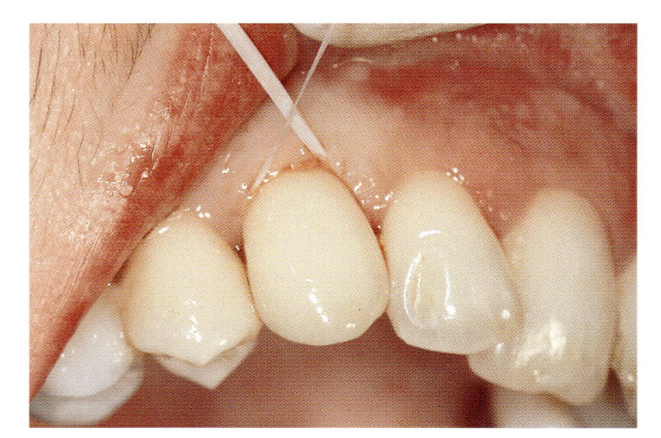

**Fig 7-89**  The crown is seated using a minimum amount of temporary cement avoiding excess material to be extruded subgingivally. Dental floss can be used to ensure that excess cement is removed.

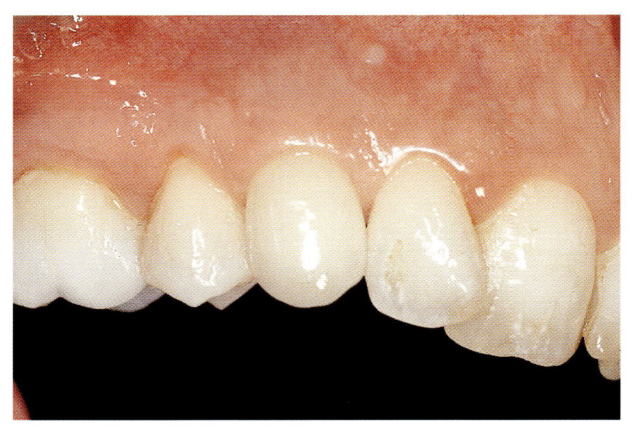

**Fig 7-90**  Labial view of definitive crown showing a natural appearance both in terms of tooth form and colour as well as gingival contours.

**Fig 7-91** Custom-made coping seated on an abutment prior to pick-up impression. This technique cannot be used if the abutment needs to be modified.

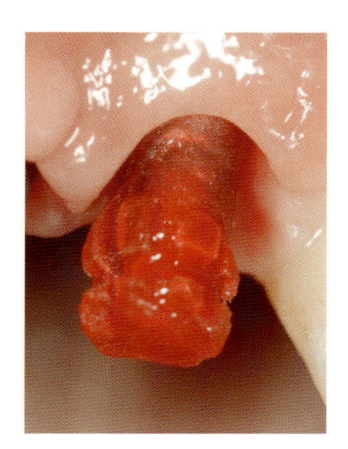

**Fig 7-92** Coping picked up in an impression. An abutment will be inserted into coping prior to casting providing a replica of the mouth.

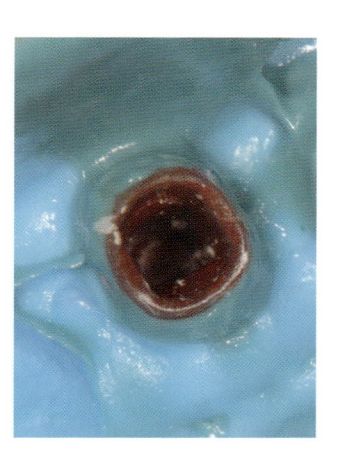

## Immediate Placement: Clinical Variations

Clinical variations will depend upon the anatomical region and the local conditions, as well as if multiple implants are being placed. The ideal situation for immediate implant placement is where the root form is such that the socket can be obliterated almost entirely by the implant. This is likely to produce the greatest amount of primary stability. Concerns relate to root morphology and local anatomy, particularly in the premolar and molar regions of both the maxilla and the mandible. With increasing gap size between implant and the socket, the amount of bone-to-implant contact will be reduced.[101,102]

In the aesthetically critical zone, the clinical protocol may need to be changed to minimise the post-operative hard and soft tissue changes.

There are, however, situations where immediate implant placement may be of benefit, but where the presence of multiple failing teeth does not support the conditions considered to be ideal. Situations where single teeth need to be replaced by means of an immediate implant depend on the adjacent teeth to sustain the level of bone. In situations where multiple teeth need to be extracted, legitimate concerns regarding the ability to sustain the level of bone may be raised. Loss of the bone between implants may result in the loss of the interdental papilla.[103,104] Treatment, therefore, needs to be planned and executed carefully.

CT scans provide essential preoperative information relating to the root morphology and the surrounding alveolar bone (Figs 7-9 and 7-10).

### Aesthetically Critical Zone

In situations where aesthetics are critical (e.g. high lip line) the technique should focus on preventing any hard or soft tissue changes to sustain a stable emergence profile. A number of steps can be taken; some of these are addressed here.

- **Implant position.** The implant should be positioned towards the palatal aspect of the socket.
- **Abutment.** It may be possible to use a ceramic abutment to minimise the risk of greying of the soft tissues. The ceramic abutment, which is biocompatible, will also offer better integration and support for the soft tissues. It further brings the crown margin closer to the gingival margin, thus facilitating cement removal (see the Treatment sequence; Figs 7-12–7-45).
- **Transitional restoration.** The soft tissue support that is essential to maintain the emergence profile is established, as described above, by means of a transitional restoration, which also seals the socket to protect the blood clot.
- **Biomaterials.** A biomaterial may be used to provide bulk should any remodelling of the labial plate take place (Figs 7-55–7-81). There are inherent risks of infection in implant dentistry, which may result in extensive bone loss. These are likely to be increased in the presence of biomaterials because of the

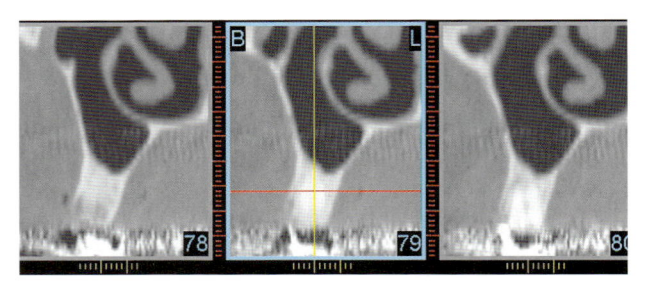

II Implant Placement: Surgery and Prosthodontics

**Fig 7-93** Cross-sectional CT image of a premolar requiring extraction. The root can be seen in close proximity to the maxillary sinus. Primary fixation, therefore, must be obtained from the socket walls. Additional height may be gained by means of manipulating the maxillary sinus floor.

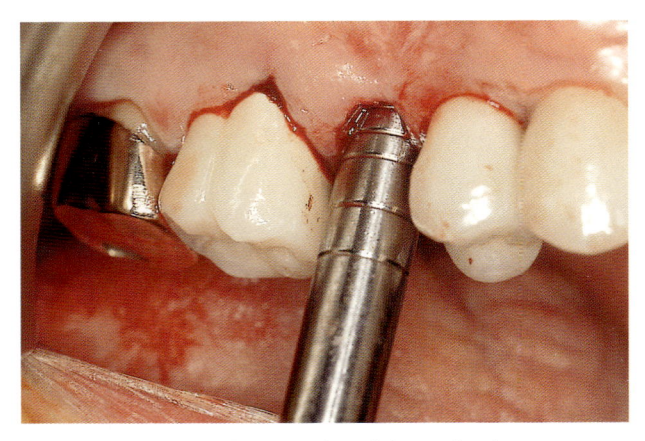

**Fig 7-94** Following the extraction of the tooth a bone condenser can be seen inserted in to the tooth socket to 8 mm.

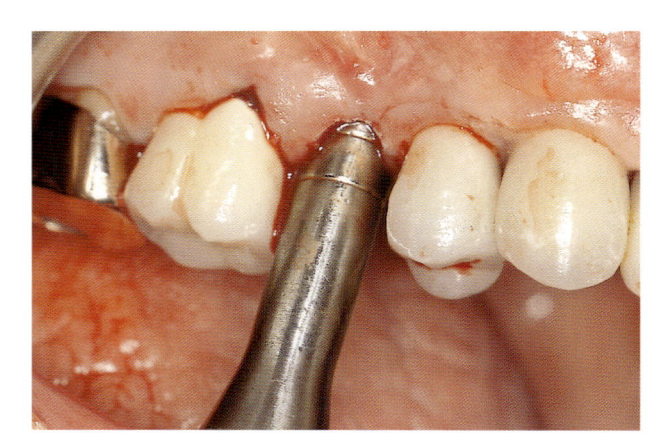

**Fig 7-95** Labial view showing the insertion of the bone condenser to 14 mm. Additional height has been gained by manipulating the floor of the maxillary sinus.

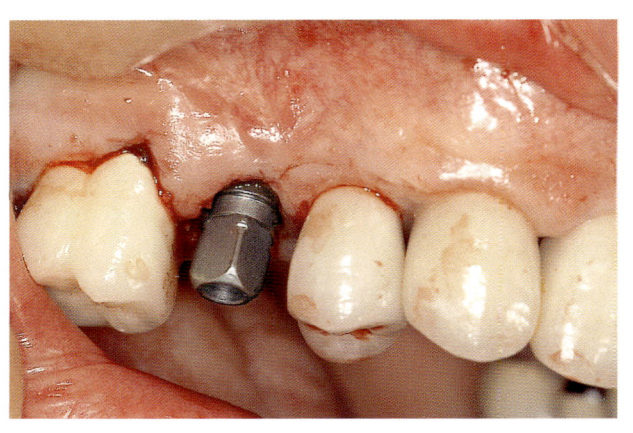

**Fig 7-96** The implant selected for placement into the socket can be seen inserted. An 11-mm implant has been inserted so that it is positioned 3 mm below the level of the labial gingival margin and 1.5 mm below the bony socket.

potential to develop biofilms. Antibiotic prophylaxis is recommended to reduce this risk.[105]

## Posterior Maxilla

In the posterior maxilla, the maxillary sinus may limit the amount of bone available (Fig 7-93). It then becomes necessary to obtain primary fixation from the walls of the socket and the labial and buccal cortical plates. In view of the poor quality of bone that normally exists in this region, it becomes necessary to manipulate the bone using bone condensers. These are used to increase the density of bone, the width of bone and possibly the height of bone by manipulation of the sinus floor (Figs 7-94–7-98). In the molar region, the root forms and separation need to be assessed preoperatively to ensure that primary stability can be achieved. Implant placement in any one of the sockets may result in the implant being placed away from the middle of the proposed crown. This can lead to an excessively large cantilever and hygiene maintenance problems. Consideration may be given to implant placement in the interradicular septum to overcome this problem. Use of 3D imaging and interactive planning is particularly valuable for preoperative decision making, including feasibility and component part selection (Figs 7-99–7-102).

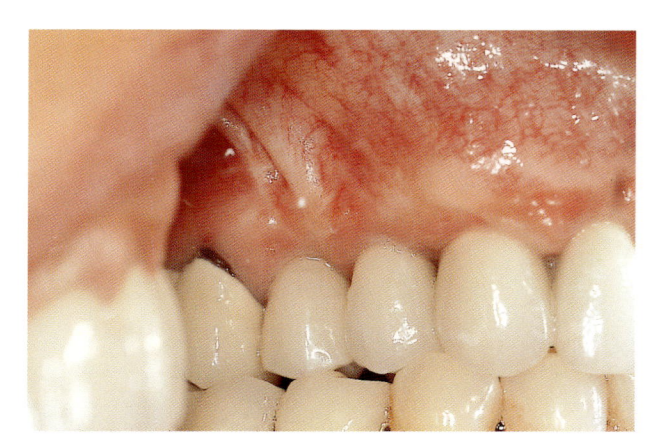

# 7  Immediate Placement and Computer-guided Surgery

**Fig 7-97** Labial view of the completed restoration replacing the second premolar.

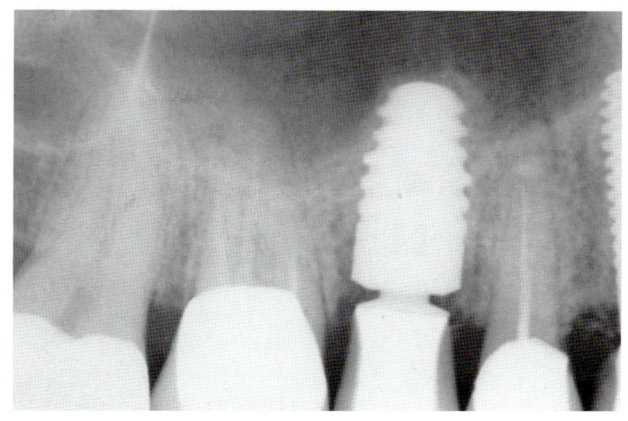

**Fig 7-98** Periapical radiograph of the restored implant. The amount of bone manipulated to gain additional height can be seen as can the close adaptation of the socket walls to the integrated and stable implant.

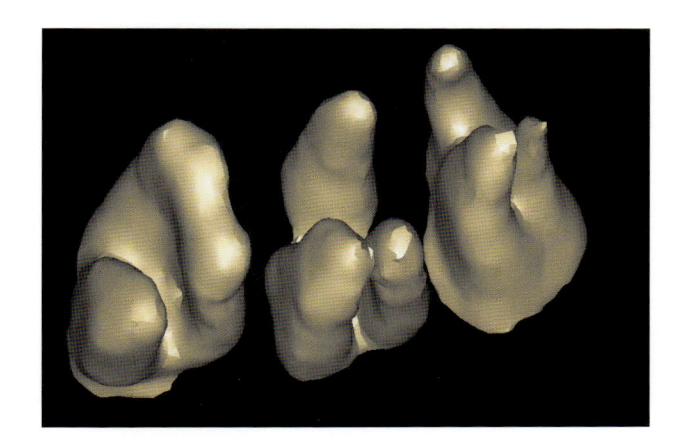

**Fig 7-99** CT reconstruction of maxillary molars showing divergent roots with adequate interradicular septae for implant placement.

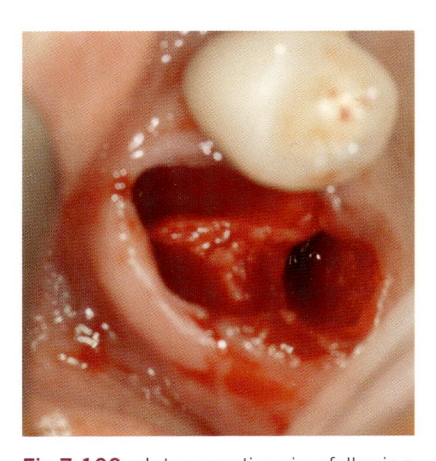

**Fig 7-100** Intraoperative view following tooth extraction showing adequate interradicular bone for implant placement. A larger implant is unlikely to gain primary stability due to the configuration and divergence of the roots.

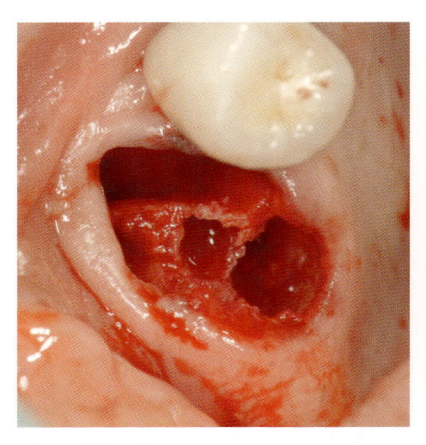

**Fig 7-101** Osteotomy commenced within the interradicular bone. Placing an implant using any of the root sockets would result in a malpositioned implant and abutment with excessive loads being transmitted via an exaggerated cantilever.

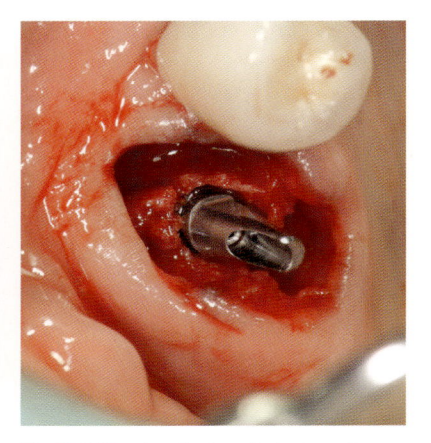

**Fig 7-102** Implant and abutment visible emerging from the interradicular septum. The abutment is positioned in the centre of the prosthetic envelope and will offer the most favourable load transmission on completion of healing.

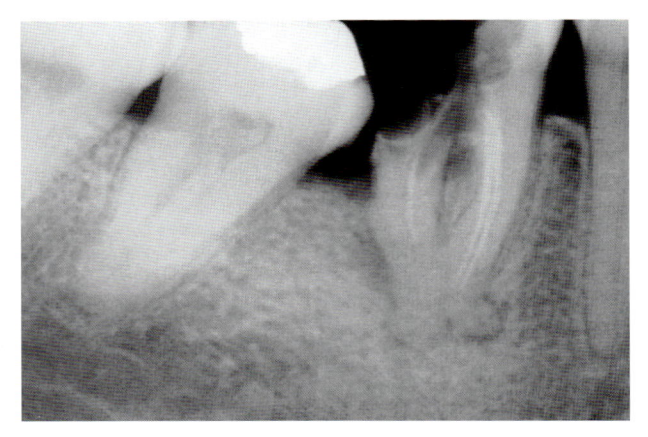

II  Implant Placement: Surgery and Prosthodontics

**Fig 7-103** Periapical radiograph of the failing first molar tooth. The root morphology and bone density is evident. The pathology evident is not considered to be acute as there are no symptoms.

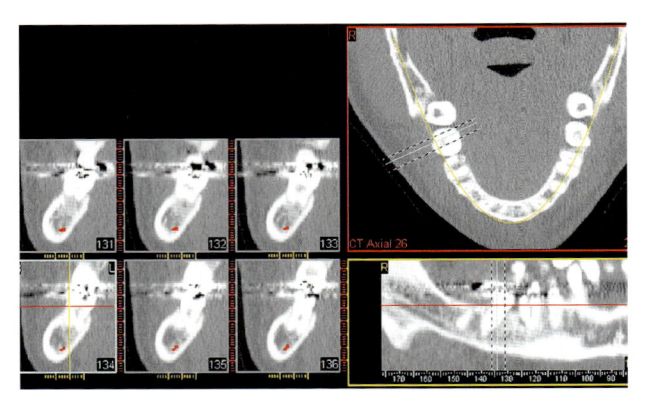

**Fig 7-104** Cross-sectional CT image of the molar tooth showing the density of bone and the width of bone available. The position of the inferior alveolar nerve has been marked interactively and can be seen clearly without confusion with other radiolucent areas in any one particular cross-section.

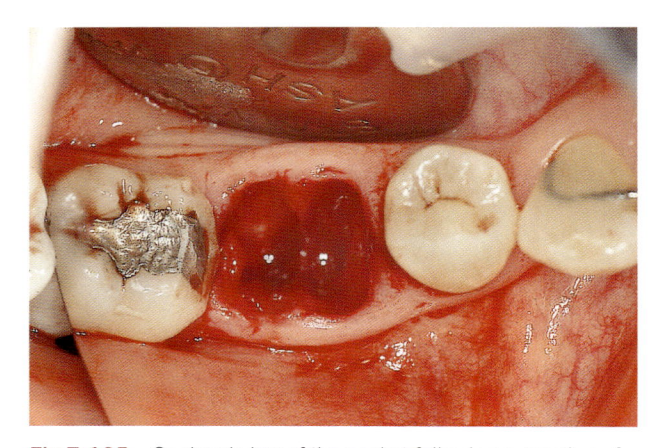

**Fig 7-105** Occlusal view of the socket following extraction of the molar tooth.

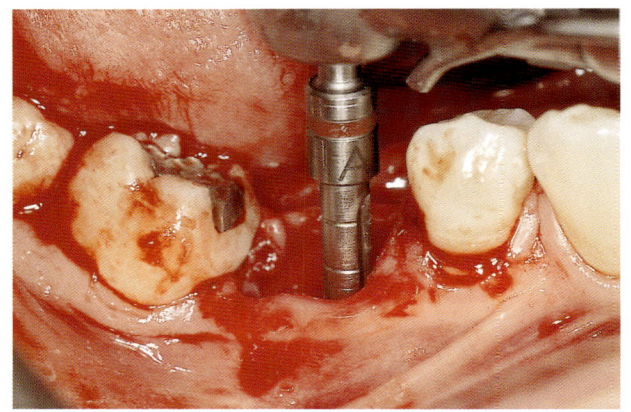

**Fig 7-106** Osteotomy bur being used to establish the osteotomy within the mesial aspect of the socket. The osteotomy bur is used to establish the direction and the precise depth to which the osteotomy will be prepared.

## Posterior Mandible

In the posterior mandible, the replacement of a molar tooth poses several problems (Fig 7-103). These relate to the limitations imposed by the inferior alveolar canal. This would typically restrict the amount of bone available beyond the socket for primary fixation. It, therefore, becomes necessary to establish primary fixation from the socket walls. In view of the complex morphology of the molar roots and the relatively large socket that results from extraction, a larger-diameter implant becomes necessary. Furthermore, a more accurate idea of the morphology of the mandible with respect to width and angulation becomes more important; CT scans, therefore, offer very critical information regarding feasibility as well as for components and types of instrument that might be required (Fig 7-104). The high density of the cortical bone plates in the mandible often requires careful osteotomy preparation using rotary instruments. Careful consideration must be given to the use of bone-tapping instruments to tap threads into dense labial and lingual cortical plates in order to ensure a precise fit and adequate primary stability (Fig 7-105–7-117).

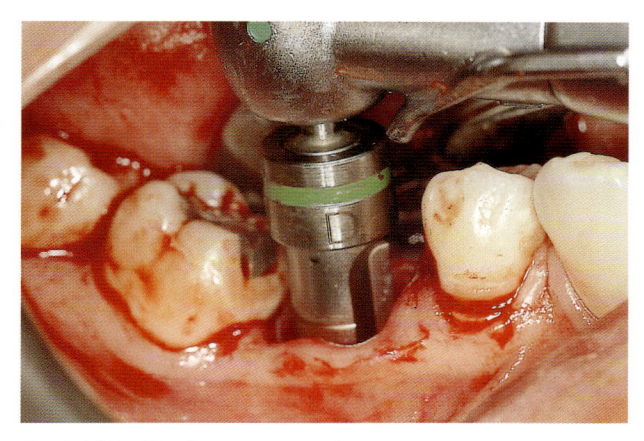

# 7  Immediate Placement and Computer-guided Surgery

**Fig 7-107** The final osteotomy bur being used, having enlarged the recipient site to receive an implant of 7 mm in diameter and 11 mm in length. An osteotomy extending 14 mm below the buccal gingival margin will enable the implant to be placed 3 mm below the level of the gingival margin.

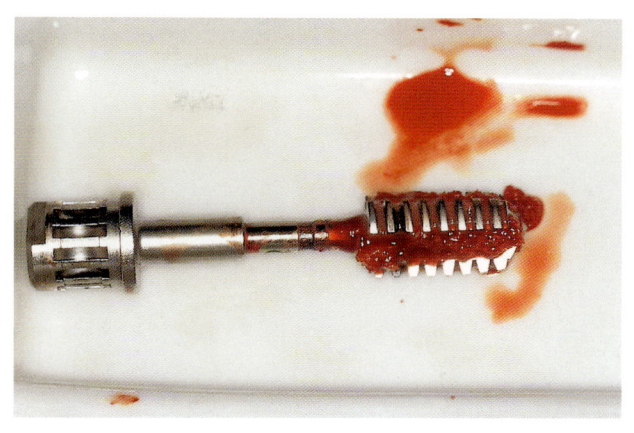

**Fig 7-108** A bone tap is used to prepare the threads within the dense cortical bone surrounding the socket. This will enable the implant to be seated precisely.

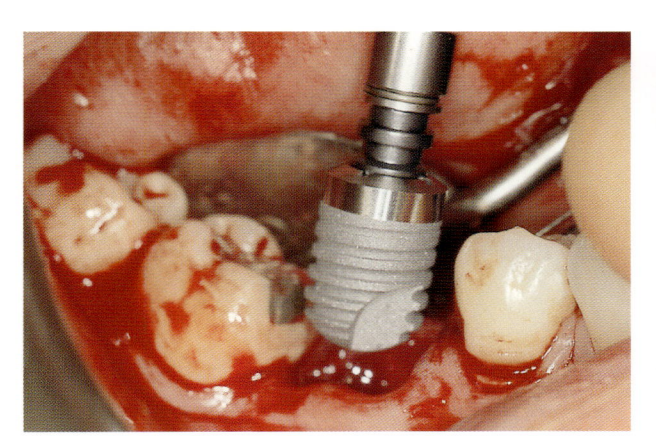

**Fig 7-109** A 7-mm diameter implant being inserted.

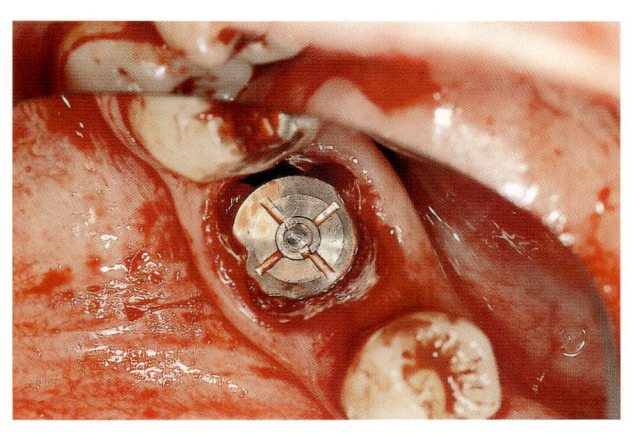

**Fig 7-110** Occlusal view of the implant in situ showing the obliteration of the socket with the wide diameter implant.

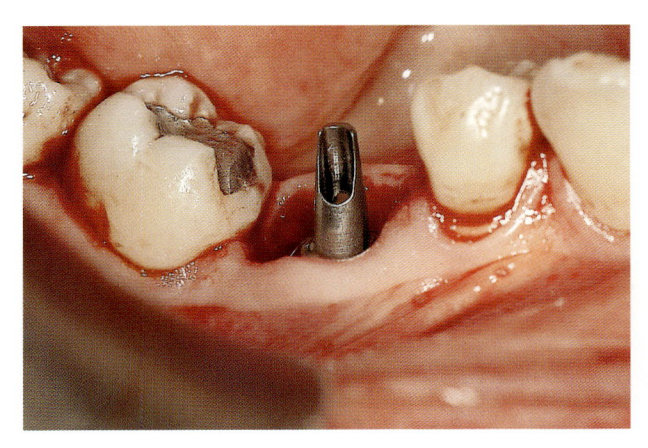

**Fig 7-111** The abutment (7.5-degree angulation) measured and attached to the implant after cover screw removal.

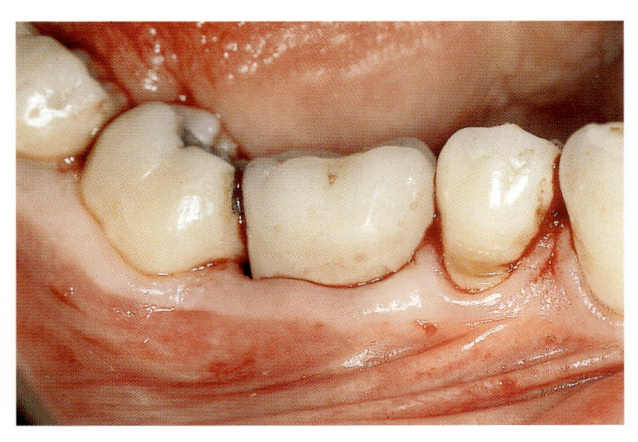

**Fig 7-112** Transitional restoration seated onto the abutment.

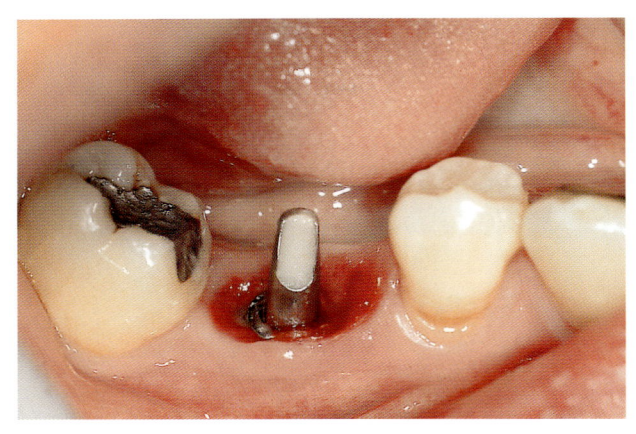

**II** Implant Placement: Surgery and Prosthodontics

**Fig 7-113** Labial view of the implant on completion of healing. The soft tissue contours developed by the transitional restoration can be seen.

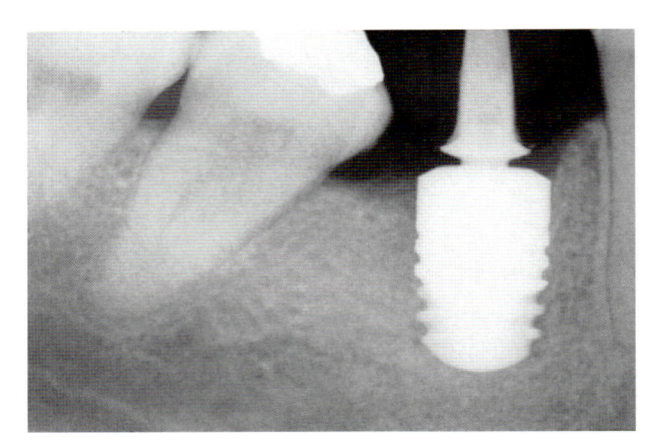

**Fig 7-114** Periapical radiograph showing the implant and abutment in situ at three months after insertion prior to restoration.

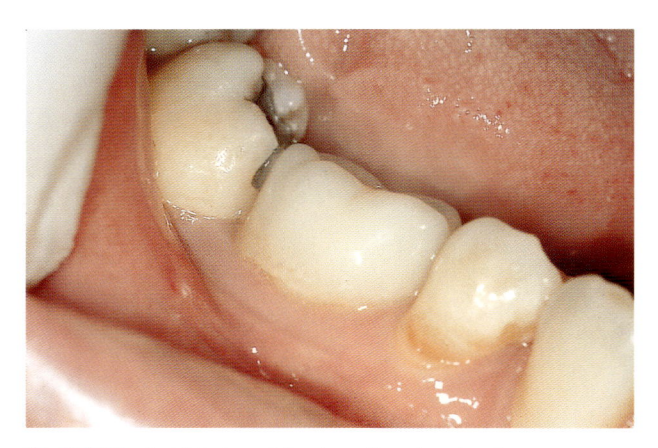

**Fig 7-115** Labial view of the transitional restoration on completion of healing at three months after insertion prior to restoration.

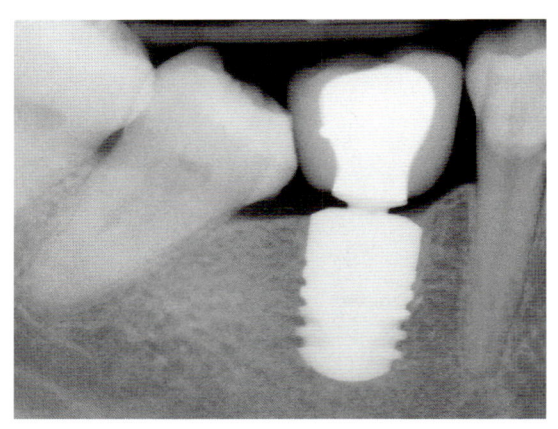

**Fig 7-116** Periapical radiograph one year after insertion. Note bone healing that has taken place.

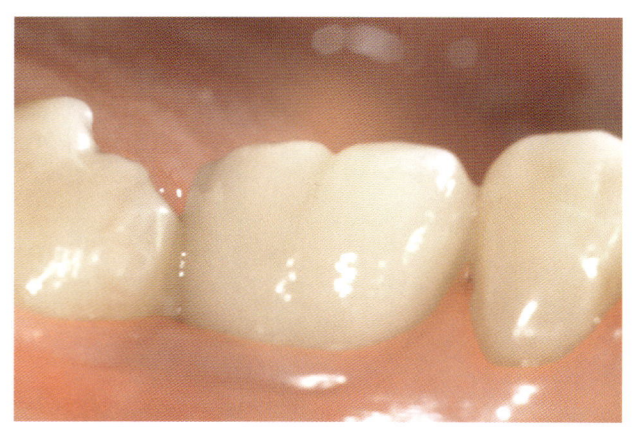

**Fig 7-117** Definitive restoration one year after implant insertion, showing a natural emergence profile, which prevents the collection of food that may otherwise occur.

Rough surfaces enable bone contact to be established even in the presence of large spaces between the socket and the implant, as seen in the radiographs of adjacent implants placed into molar sockets (Figs 7-118 and 7-119).[106]

It is sometimes necessary to place implants in either the mesial or distal root socket. For single teeth, this may result in a cantilevered crown. Placement of implants within the interradicular septum is possible in those situations where there is adequate separation. For multiple teeth, the positioning of implants within root sockets may be considered favourable in view of the reduction of effective cantilevers (Figs 7-120–7-129).

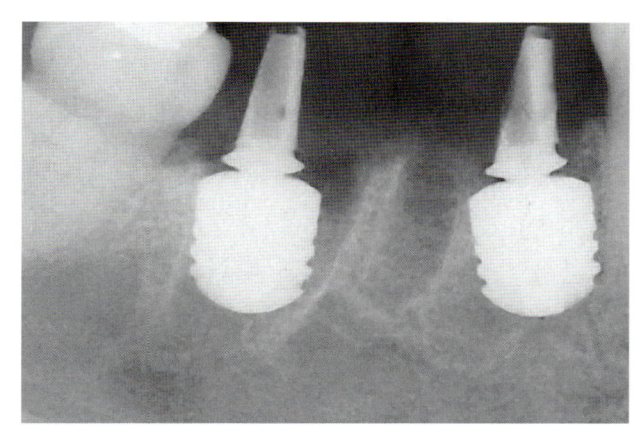

# 7 Immediate Placement and Computer-guided Surgery

**Fig 7-118** Periapical radiograph of two immediately placed 7-mm diameter implants in the posterior mandible, gaining primary stability from buccal and lingual aspects of the mandible. Note the distance between alveolar socket and the implant.

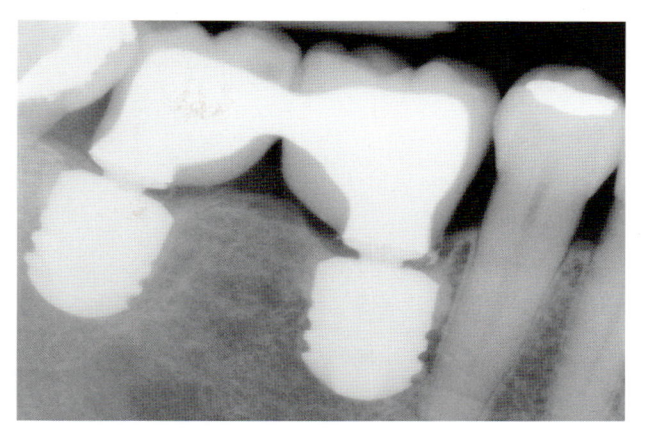

**Fig 7-119** Periapical radiograph of the patient shown in Fig 7-118. The radiograph was taken five years after insertion, following a recementation of the splinted restoration prior to cement removal. Note the bone healing and stability.

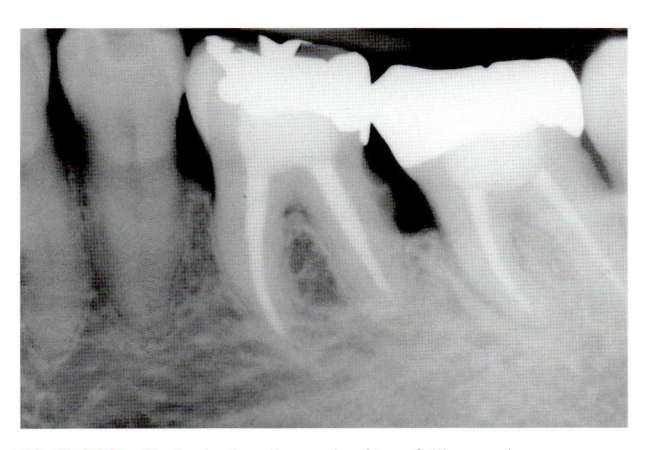

**Fig 7-120** Periapical radiograph of two failing molars.

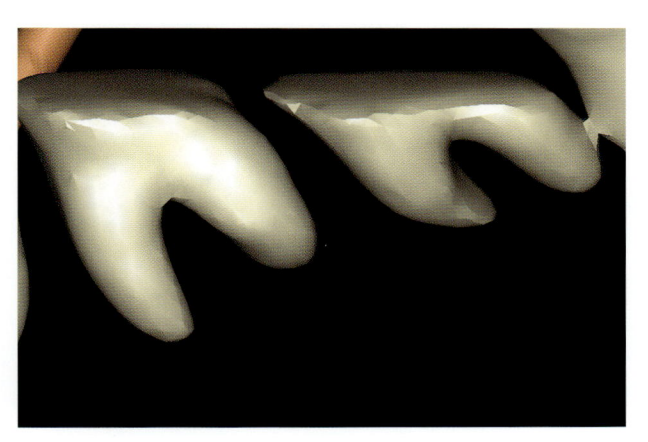

**Fig 7-121** Three-dimensional CT reconstruction of the roots of the failing molars showing the divergent roots.

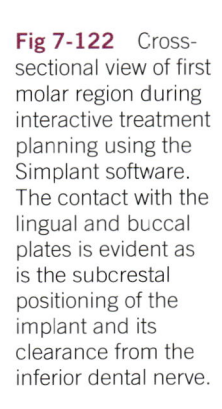

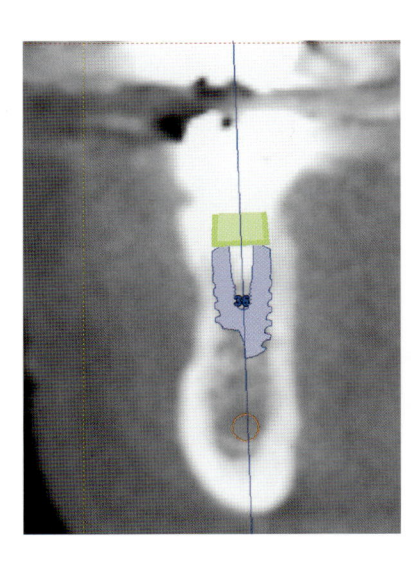

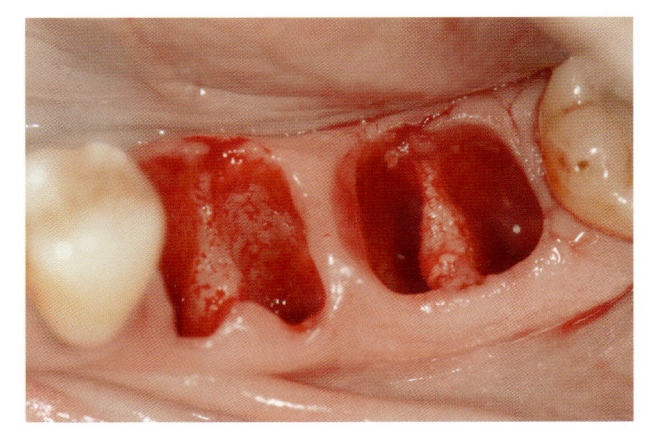

**Fig 7-122** Cross-sectional view of first molar region during interactive treatment planning using the Simplant software. The contact with the lingual and buccal plates is evident as is the subcrestal positioning of the implant and its clearance from the inferior dental nerve.

**Fig 7-123** Postextraction view of two sockets showing mesial and distal root sockets for each tooth and the interradicular septae.

81

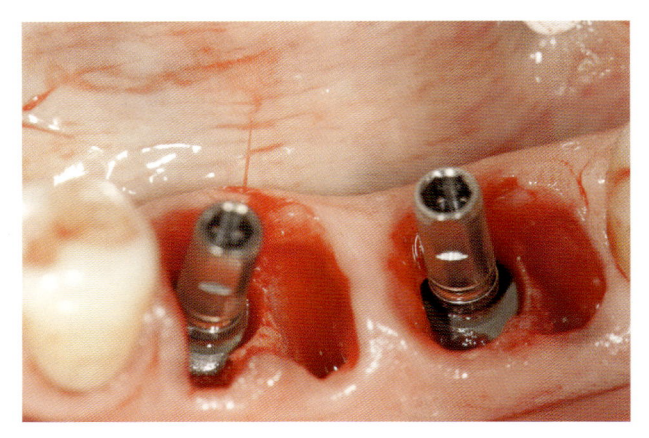

## II Implant Placement: Surgery and Prosthodontics

**Fig 7-124** Implants inserted in the mesial root socket of each tooth. Note the alignment and positioning in relation to the interdental septum.

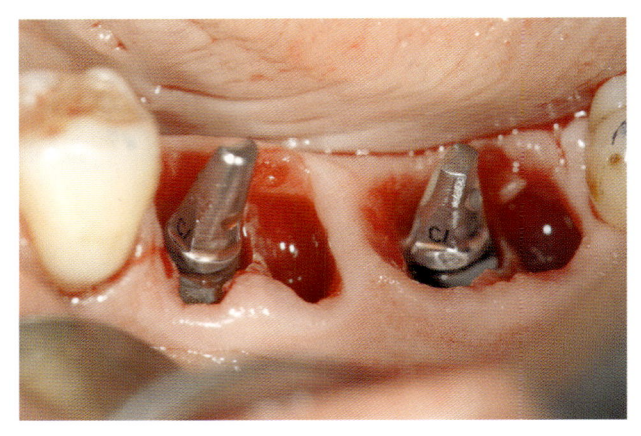

**Fig 7-125** Labial view of the angled abutments selected to correct the implant alignment and achieve parallelism.

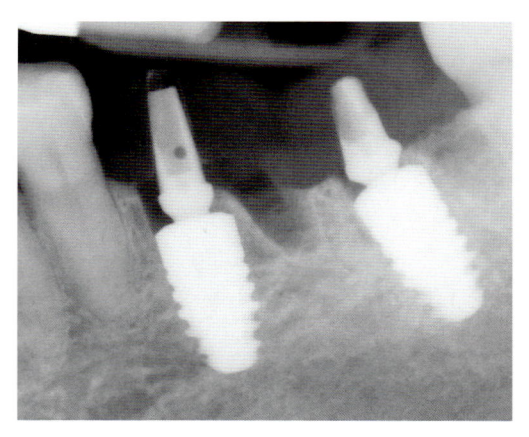

**Fig 7-126** Post-operative periapical radiograph showing positioning of implants and alignment of abutments.

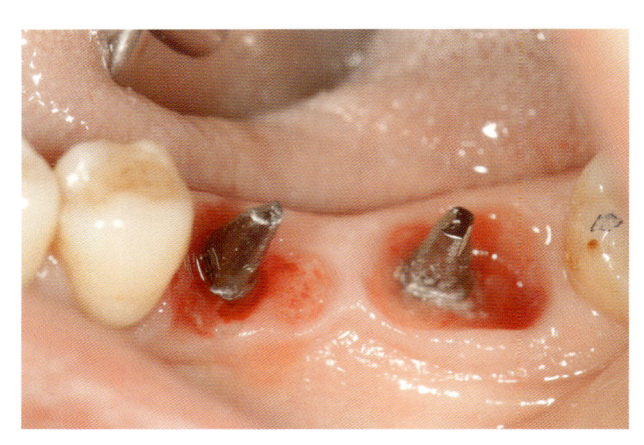

**Fig 7-127** Post-operative view at three months showing the healing sockets and the emergence contours developed by the transitional restorations.

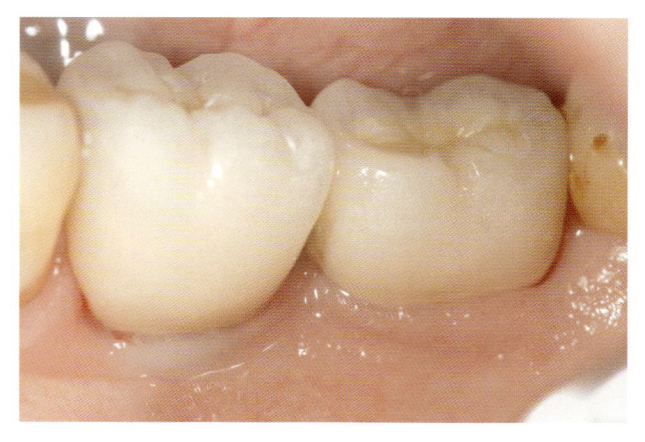

**Fig 7-128** The definitive restoration at the time of fitting, showing good emergence profile and surrounding tissues which will mature.

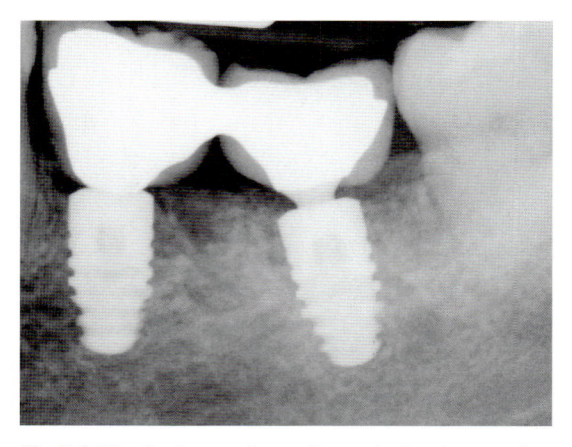

**Fig 7-129** Post-operative radiograph showing excellent bony healing at four months.

# 7  Immediate Placement and Computer-guided Surgery

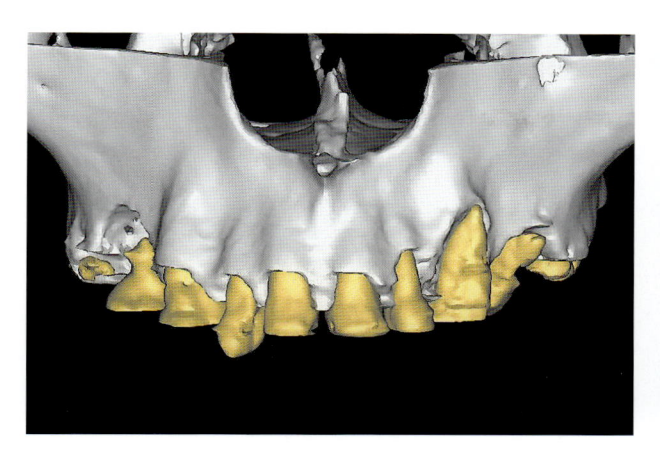

**Fig 7-130** Three-dimensional reconstruction of a maxilla, showing prominent alveolar bone with interdental depressions indicating thin bone overlying the roots. Such situations are susceptible to remodelling and recession.

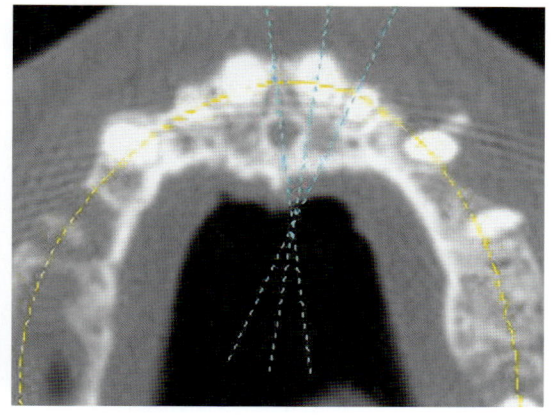

**Fig 7-131** Axial view of the patient shown in Fig 7-130. Thin labial bone and deep interradicular depressions are clearly visible and indicative of susceptibility to recession.

## Multiple Adjacent Implants

The challenge that faces a clinician is dependent upon the reason for tooth failure and the status of the alveolar ridge and remaining tooth structure.

- **Periodontal disease where bone has been lost.** Extraction is less likely to result in damage to the alveolar bone but poses the problem of hard and soft tissue replacement coupled with crown–implant ratio. Typically, further resorption is less likely to be a problem but susceptibility to peri-implant disease needs to be considered.
- **Endodontically compromised teeth.** If these have previously been restored with post-crowns and are supported by good alveolar structure, they can pose a number of problems. The fragility of a tooth with a compromised structure poses challenges for the maintenance of the surrounding bone during extraction of the tooth. Radiographically dense metal posts in roots will result in beam hardening and artefacts, which will make preoperative assessment more challenging.
- **Interradicular distance and thickness of labial and palatal bone.** These also need to be considered if the interdental septum is to be preserved.
- **Skeletal type.** High maxillary arch forms, where the available bone is present above the apices, need to be treated differently to low arch forms, where the available bone is on the palatal aspect. This also has a consequence for remodelling.

In the aesthetic zone, the remodelling of the very fine architecture has a consequence on the outcome and long-term stability of the tissues. Assessment of the hard and soft tissue biotypes is based on clinical observation and 3D imaging (Figs 7-130–7-133).

Management of these cases depends upon selecting sites that are likely to produce sufficient primary stability for loading at the time of placement. This assessment needs to be rigorous as the patient will be toothless if treatment is not completed as planned. Contingency plans for this eventuality should also be considered.

Osteotomy preparation is challenging as the position of the implant head is critical. The use of osteotomes runs the risk of fracture of the interseptal bone owing to the brittle nature of the lamina dura.

Following implant placement, abutments need to be attached to secure the prosthesis. For cement-retained prostheses, angled prefabricated abutments are used. For screw-retained prostheses, issues about the emergence of the screw come to the fore and may compromise the primary stability of the implants if addressed by altering implant angulation.

Implant placement can be carried out having estimated the position and using morphological landmarks for the orientation of the osteotomy burs.

Planning of the transitional prostheses needs accurate transfer of information from the intraoral records to the laboratory. Prediction of the point of emergence

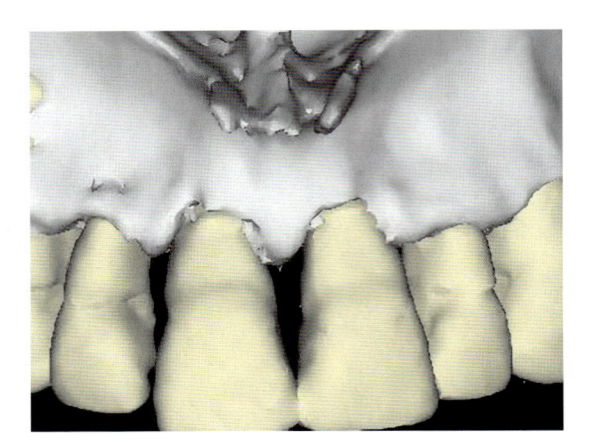

**Fig 7-132** Three-dimensional reconstruction of maxilla with minimal interradicular depressions unlikely to resorb.

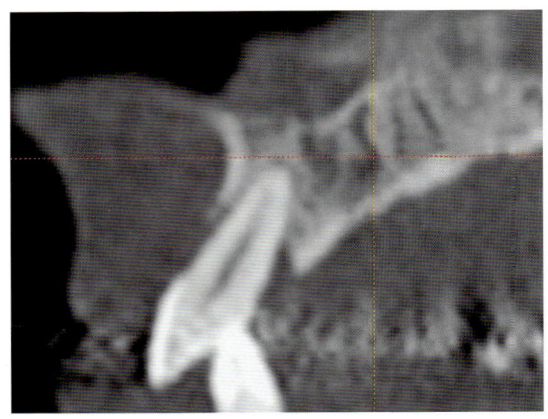

**Fig 7-133** Cross-sectional image of patient shown in Fig 7-132 showing thicker labial bone less susceptible to recession.

of the abutment is necessary so that the transitional restoration can be constructed to enclose the potential emergence site.

Execution of the treatment will, therefore, require extraction of the teeth, osteotomy preparation, abutment attachment and adaptation of the transitional restoration to the abuments. Consequently, planning is critical and requires experienced clinicians to be able to successfully complete such treatment.

An alternative approach is to use computer-guided surgery, which also should be carried out by experienced clinicians who can visualise the outcome.

# Immediate Loading: Principles of Primary Stability

For the implant to integrate, there can be no excess movement between the implant and the bone during the healing phase.[64,65] The primary stability of the implant at placement will depend on several factors, such as the quality and quantity of bone present, the design of the implant and the occlusal loads to which the transitional restoration will be subjected.[107]

A success rate equivalent to that with delayed loading can be achieved with immediately loaded implants.[108] This applies either when an implant is placed into an extraction socket, or following the completion of bone healing.

## Occlusal Load

The potential for overloading the implant will depend on the force that the patient is able and likely to exert. This will be influenced by whether treatment is for one tooth in a stable occlusion or for an edentulous jaw. The opposing dentition will also influence load. Reducing occlusal load may be achieved in two ways.

- The transitional crown can be left out of occlusion, ensuring that there are no interferences during excursions. Where aesthetics are not important, the implant may be left with the abutment attached and without a restoration, when an implant is placed into a healed site. This may then be considered as transmucosal healing.
- Several implants can be splinted with a passively fitting transitional restoration that is rigid.[109]

## Bone Quality

Bone quality can be manipulated by altering the method of osteotomy preparation and the judicious selection of instruments for this purpose:

- **Use of bone condensers**. Trabeculae within cancellous bone may be condensed using a series of osteotomes of increasing diameter to increase the density of bone surrounding the osteotomy[78,79]
- **Use of bone taps.** The use of bone taps may be partly or wholly omitted, allowing the implant to tap its own thread, resulting in a better-fitting implant with increased primary stability

- **Cortical engagement.** Increasing the diameter or length of an implant to engage cortical bone will invariably result in a more stable implant.

### Implant Design

The shape of the implant and its surface greatly influence primary stability and thus the precondition for osseointegration.[110–112]

- **Macro-design.** A screw-shaped implant with large, deeply cut threads will provide better stability than a tapered push-fit implant because of the greater surface area and the configuration of the threads, which will provide anchorage to resist movement that may be caused by multidirectional forces. Poorer success rates have been reported with non-threaded cylindrical implants when used for immediate placement and immediate loading.[113]
- **Precision of osteotomy.** The screw form enables vital bone to come into immediate contact with the entire surface of the implant, including the apex and the base of each thread. This is in contrast to a finned implant where the bone is only in contact with the edge of the fin.
- **Surface.** It is also clear that a rough surface provides higher frictional resistance to movement than a smooth surface. A blasted surface may, therefore, be preferred in view of the controversies that surround coated implants.

### Abutment Connection

Platform switching has demonstrated preservation of soft as well as hard tissues in immediately loaded implants. This is reported to result from changes in the positioning of the micro-gap.[114]

However, in this study, a micro-gap was present between the abutment and the implant. When a tight implant abutment connection is used, there is no micro-gap and, therefore, no potential for bacterial contamination. This may be assumed to offer further advantages.[92]

A conical connection that is sufficiently tight to prevent bacterial leakage is ideal, as the implant is often placed below the crest of the bone to compensate for potential resorption of the socket margins, as discussed above. This is particularly relevant for immediate placement of implants, where implants often have to be inserted below the crest of the bony socket.

For immediate loading, an abutment needs to be connected at the time of the implant insertion; consequently, a broad range and stock of angled abutments is needed.[7] The abutment should fit within the prosthetic envelope to avoid major modifications. This avoids the need for temporary abutments and, therefore, the replacement of the abutment at a subsequent visit. An abutment of the correct shape is required to ensure that the ideal soft tissue emergence profile can be established. The same considerations regarding soft tissue management, including the use of transitional restorations, apply in situations where the implant has been placed in a healed site (see Chapter 9).

The forces necessary to secure the abutment should be in such a range that the implant position is not altered and no precautions are necessary to prevent this (e.g. use of counter-torque). With the above-mentioned conical connection (Ankylos) a torque of 15 Ncm is needed to engage the conical connection of the abutment.

## Computer-guided Surgery

Computer-guided surgery may be used:
- to manufacture surgical drill guides to prepare the osteotomy
- to insert the implants
- to fabricate a transitional restoration as well as select the abutments for immediate loading in conjunction with a stereolithographic model.

Surgical guides may be constructed to be supported by:
- **Soft tissues.** This will require additional fixation to stabilise the drill guide, which reduces the discrepancy between the relative implant positions but does not eliminate the overall displacement caused by the resilience of the soft tissues.
- **Bone.** This will require flap reflection, which can be extensive. The 3D image and, therefore, the stereolithographic model has to be based on a careful determination of the threshold used to outline the bony surface.

- **Teeth.** Large dense metal restorations will cause artefacts and beam hardening, which introduces inaccuracies in seating. Study casts of the mouth need to be sent for scanning so that the distortions can be minimised. This will, however, introduce inaccuracies in the positioning of implants and, therefore, of abutments attached to these implants.
- **Supplementary implants/reference points.** It has been proposed that three reference points (mini-implants) may be used to support a radiopaque template during fabrication; these are worn during CT data acquisition, as well as providing location points for the drill guide during surgery.[115,116]

Computer-guided surgery will incur additional costs for the construction of the guide, the stereolithographic models and additional laboratory costs for the abutment selection and fabrication of the transitional restoration. Treatment of patients requires more detailed planning. The clinician needs to be experienced to visualise the outcome. Once the plan has been transmitted for the construction of the guide, no changes can be made to the positioning of the implants. Furthermore, there are some restrictions regarding the use of techniques to increase bone density (e.g. use of osteotomes).

There are inherent inaccuracies in the process, typically reported to be an angular deviation of 2 degrees or more and an implant head discrepancy of approximately 1 mm in the horizontal and vertical planes. These arise from the CT data, discrepancies in the stereolithographic process, subsequent positioning errors of the surgical guide on the cast and in the mouth, as well as discrepancies caused by the drill guide and osteotomy bur tolerances.[117,118]

## Planning
Planning has to be meticulous and follows a series of steps as outlined below.

### Clinical Observation and Preliminary Radiographic Examination
Careful clinical examination is required. Observations regarding the presence of infection and in particular acute infection need to be made. The hard and soft tissue biotypes need to be classified. The state of restoration of teeth that are present, with particular reference to heavy metal root canal posts, needs to be noted in order to maximise the CT data. The quality and quantity of soft tissue should be assessed. Many procedures will require a change in the intermaxillary relations. In view of this, careful assessment of the patient's ability to adapt to any proposed changes needs to be made.

### Laboratory Stage
Mounted study casts with intermaxillary records and proposed changes are required. Study casts may also need to be sent for scanning to verify accuracy of stereolithographic models.

A diagnostic preview (waxup) is required at this stage and construction of a template with radiopaque markers to identify proposed tooth positions.

### Computed Tomography
Acquisition of accurate 3D data is critical. Planning requires a sophisticated software program such as Simplant (Materialise Dental NV, Leuven, Belgium). Planning should be carried out using the cross-sectional image for simulated implant placement with a realistic representation of the implant system intended for use. Mesio-distal corrections may be carried out in the panoral view.

Final refinements are carried out in the 3D view, which enables the clinician to verify the position and visualize the emergence of the implant at the selected site, which is determined by the proposed prosthetic tooth.

### Drill Guide
The type of drill guide required needs to be decided and if required drill diameters selected. Guides may be selected specific to the diameters of the osteotomy burs to be used. Alternatively drill guides with replaceable sleeves may be ordered, which offer the benefit of not having to change the guide, thus enabling additional fixation (e.g. ExpertEase system, Dentsply Friadent). Responsibility for the drill guide and, therefore, implant position lies with the treating dentist.

### Stereolithographic Models and Laboratory Process
The stereolithographic models should have the planned osteotomy sites of the correct diameters and

depths for the insertion of implant analogues. Subsequently, selection of the abutments can be carried out once the models have been mounted on the articulator in the correct intermaxillary relationship. A matrix of the proposed teeth permits the selection of the correct abutment.

Acrylic sleeves are fabricated directly onto the abutments to allow accurate adaptation of the transitional restoration to the abutment. This technique allows for the inaccuracies that are inherent in the planning process as well as the surgical and prosthetic procedures.

## Surgery

### Seating of Surgical Guide and Osteotomy Preparation

Seating of the surgical guide will depend upon the type of support that was chosen. Flap reflection will be required for bone-supported guides. Additional fixation for soft tissue-supported guides is often achieved using the opposing dentition to assist positioning. Tooth-supported guides, when appropriate, offer stable support and may or may not require flap elevation depending upon the nature of the case.

Osteotomies should be prepared to the correct depth. Ideally the implant should be inserted to the planned depth using a guide such as the ExpertEase. In cases where a surgical drill guide has been used for osteotomy preparation only, the implants are placed to a depth estimated from adjacent landmarks.

Internal irrigation is of particular value as the drill guide prevents any external sprays from reaching the osteotomy site.

### Abutment Attachment

The abutments are removed from the stereolithographic model one at a time and transferred to the appropriate implant and loosely attached. On placement of all the abutments, alignment can be carried out using an index. The index offers only a rough guide because of the discrepancies described above.

Acrylic sleeves are transferred and seated on the abutments after the abutments have been secured in the correct position.

### Transitional Restoration

The loose-fitting transitional restoration is tried in and its position determined by the opposing dentition. Once its fit has been confirmed, it is filled with self-polymerising resin and seated connecting to the sleeve. In this way, inaccuracies in placement of implants can be compensated, providing a functional restoration accurately seated using the opposing dentition. The sleeves prevent the need to use excessive amounts of resin, which would otherwise pose a grave risk of being extruded beyond the abutment into the extraction socket around the implant. Any discrepancies between the transitional restoration and the sleeve can be rectified extraorally. The transitional restoration is seated using a minimum amount of temporary cement in order to avoid having any excess cement.

### Restorative Phase

The restorative phase can be carried out three months after insertion of the implants once integration has taken place. In view of the fact that definitive abutments have been attached to the implant, conventional impressions provide the most efficient way of transferring data to the laboratory. Typically, the preliminary registration is carried out at the time of impressions, followed by registration using a wax replica of the transitional restoration to permit minute changes to be made. A try-in of teeth, metal try-in, the try-in of porcelain and the fit of the definitive restoration is carried out as described in Chapter 10.

## Clinical Cases Using Computer-guided Surgery

### Case 1: Full Arch (Maxilla) Immediate Placement and Loading

A patient of long standing who suffered from progressive periodontal disease with very sensitive teeth required treatment. Preliminary assessment followed by 3D imaging confirmed the ongoing disease process and the possibility of replacing the failing teeth immediately with implants.

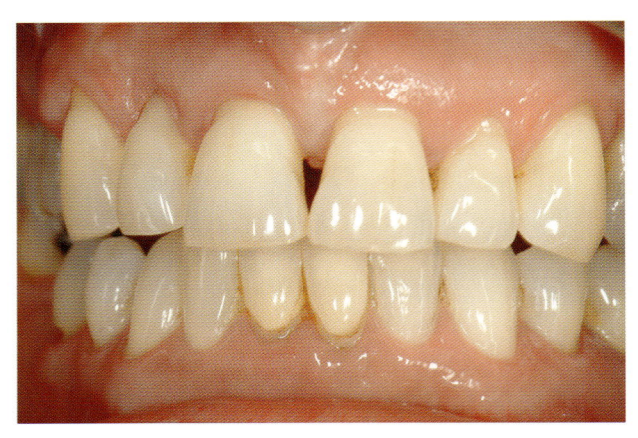

II Implant Placement: Surgery and Prosthodontics

**Fig 7-134** Intraoral labial view of patient with failing maxillary teeth.

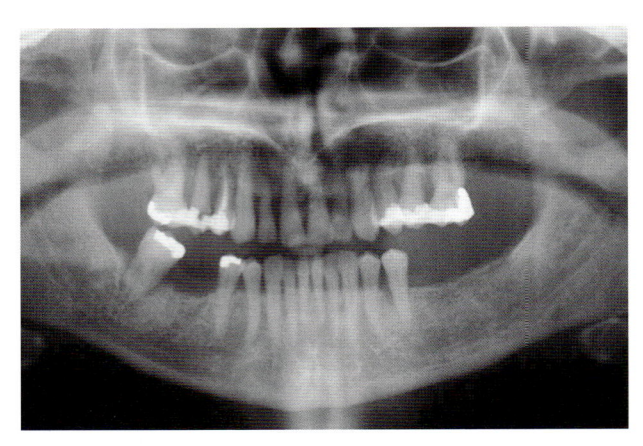

**Fig 7-135** Dental panoramic tomograph showing the overall status of teeth. In addition to the failing maxillary teeth, the missing molars in the mandible as well as the failing mandibular right second molar can be seen.

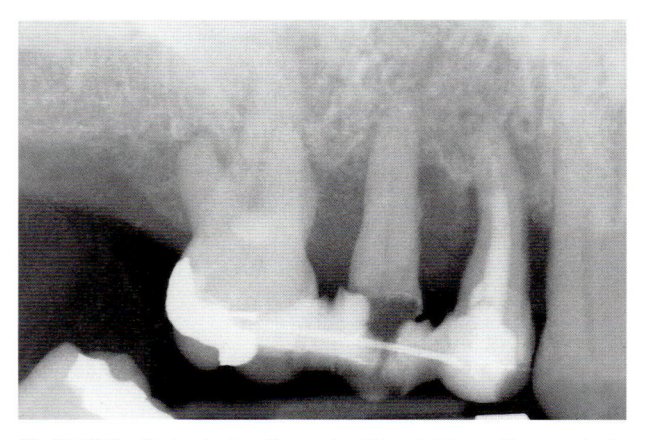

**Fig 7-136** Periapical radiograph of the right maxillary sextant showing severely compromised teeth.

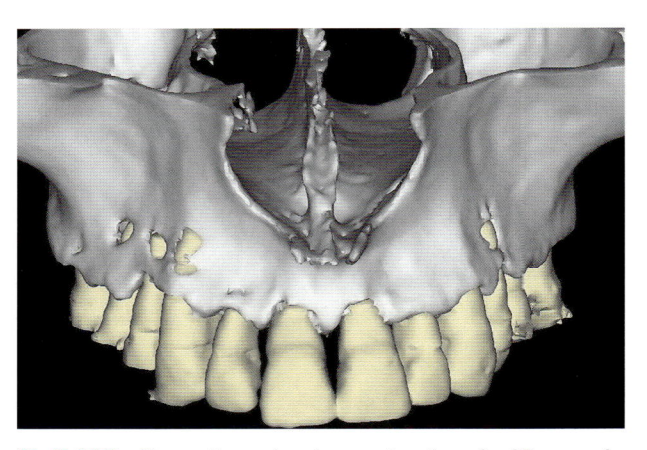

**Fig 7-137** Three-dimensional reconstruction of a CT scan of the maxilla, showing the overall status.

Computer-guided surgery was used to plan treatment so that failing teeth could be replaced without any loss of function. The case describes the location of bone with 3D imaging that would not have been clearly evident from conventional imaging. Use of 3D imaging also enabled the prediction of a biotype less susceptible to ongoing resorption. Tooth-supported surgical guides were planned, being supported by teeth where implants did not need to be positioned. The treatment was carried out uneventfully using conventional surgical guides, which did not allow for implant positioning to the correct depth. The depth to which the implants were placed was estimated using the thickness of soft tissues and adding 2 mm, thus positioning the implants 2 mm subcrestally. Abutment attachment was carried out methodically and the transitional restorations adapted simultaneously to the soft tissues and the abutments using acrylic resin sleeves and cold-curing acrylic resin.

Three months later, the definitive restorations were constructed and have subsequently been monitored using photography and radiography, which have demonstrated a stable outcome. Key to the successful outcome has been the ability to obtain good primary stability based on accurate bone density assessment and the use of an implant design that generates a high degree of primary stability. The ongoing stability of the tissues seems to be attributable to the tight implant–abutment connection. The case is outlined in Figs 7-134–7-170.

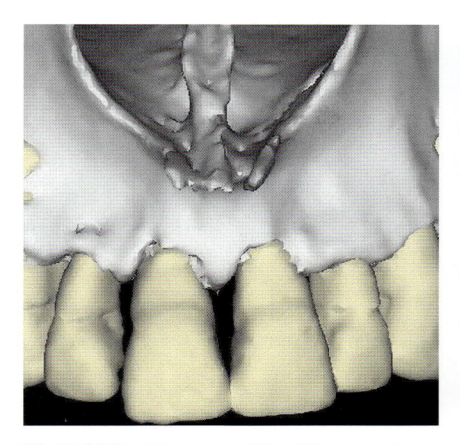

7   Immediate Placement and Computer-guided Surgery

**Fig 7-138**   Close-up of the 3D reconstruction of the CT scan of the anterior region showing the very limited amount of bone available under the nasal floor.

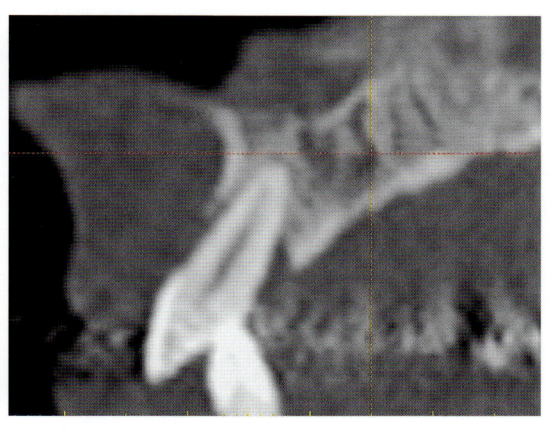

**Fig 7-139**   Cross-sectional image of the central incisor tooth confirming minimum bone for implant placement below the floor of the nose. However, considerable amount of bone is available towards the palatal aspect of the root.

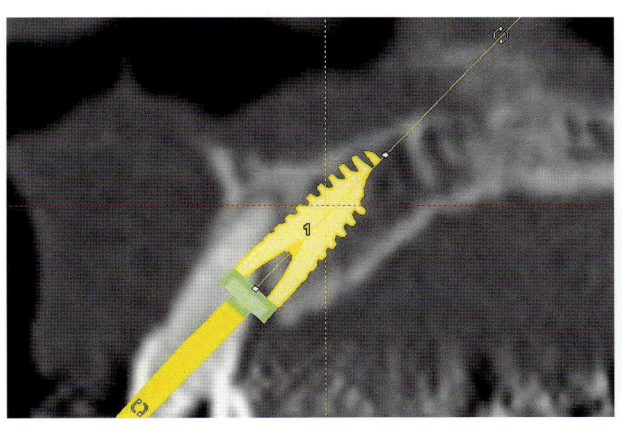

**Fig 7-140**   Interactive planning using the Simplant software. The implant is positioned into the available bone palatal to the root.

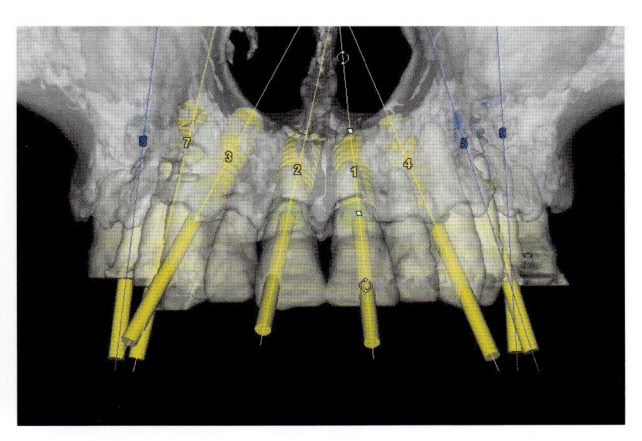

**Fig 7-141**   Three-dimensional view with all the implants positioned permits the clinician to assess the clinical outcome and facilitates refinement of implant positions if required.

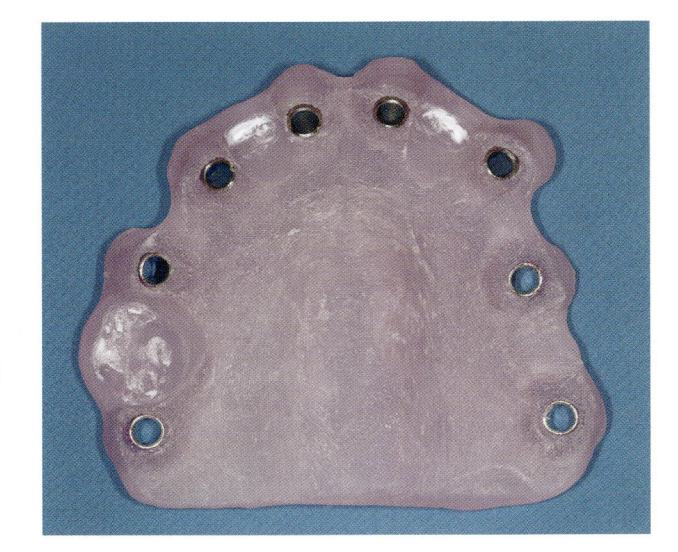

**Fig 7-142**   Once the clinician is satisfied with the implant positions in terms of angulation, siting and depth, the data can be transmitted for the construction of a surgical guide based on the planning data. A surgical guide for the preparation of the osteotomies can be seen. A tooth-supported guide, to be supported by the two lateral incisors and maxillary left first molar has been returned. The drilling tubes are matched to each diameter of the osteotomy bur to be used. Three guides were obtained for the pilot, 3-mm and 4-mm drills.

89

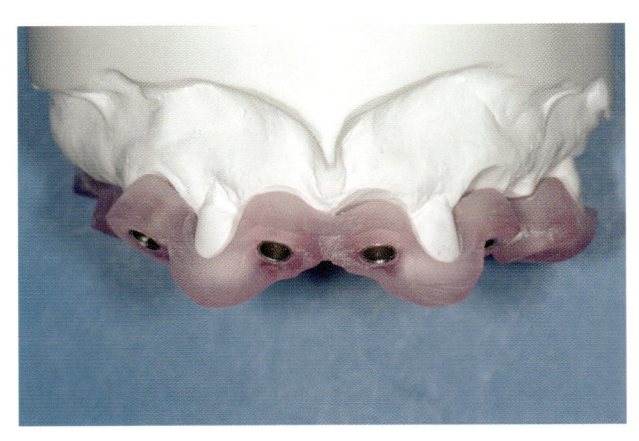

## II Implant Placement: Surgery and Prosthodontics

**Fig 7-143** The surgical guide being tried on a study cast to ensure accurate seating.

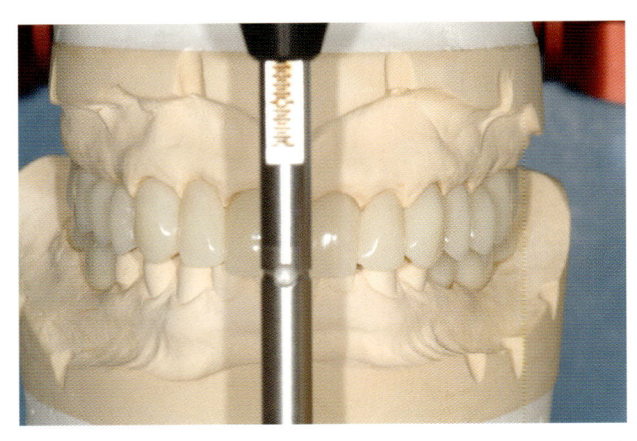

**Fig 7-144** Mounted study casts with the maxillary transitional restoration constructed.

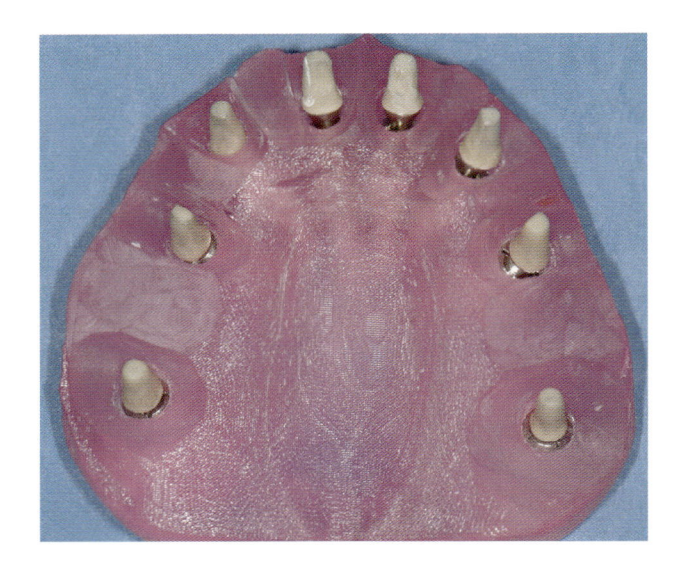

**Fig 7-145** Stereolithographic models are returned with osteotomy preformed to the correct depth for the insertion of implant analogues. Pre-angled abutments have been inserted ensuring parallelism. Thin acrylic resin sleeves have subsequently been constructed on the abutments for connection to the transitional bridge at the time of surgery.

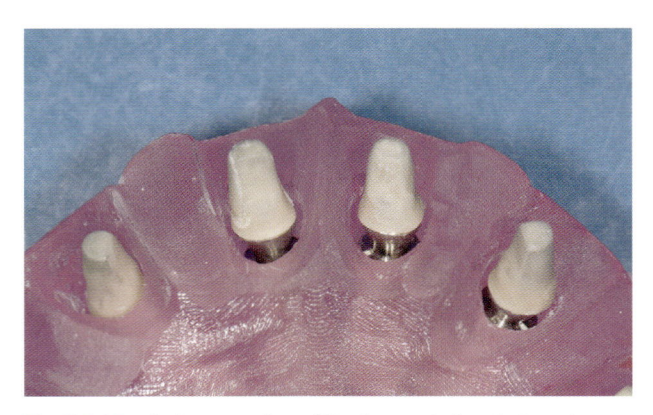

**Fig 7-146** A close-up view of the four anterior abutments showing details of the acrylic resin sleeves.

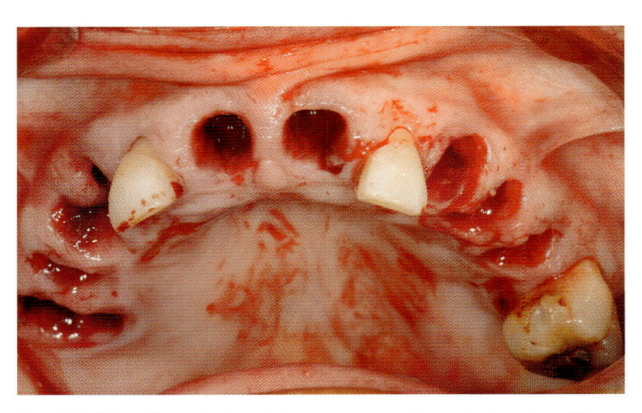

**Fig 7-147** Clinical view following extraction of all teeth with the exception of the lateral incisors and the maxillary eft first molar prior to seating the drill guide.

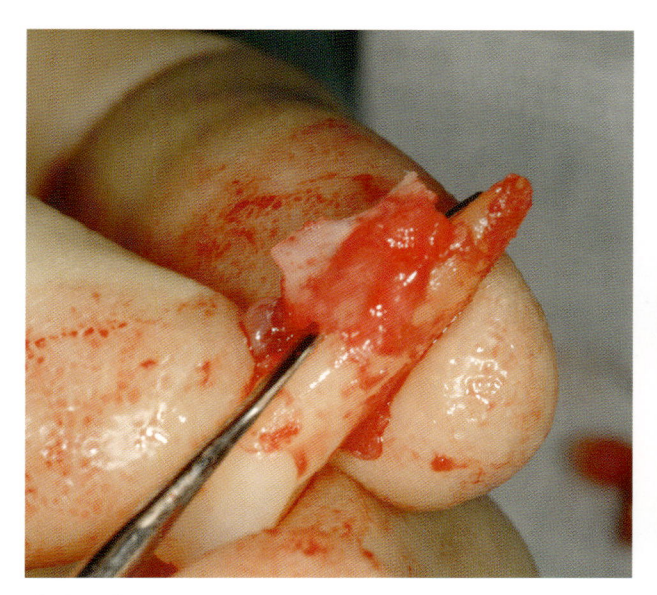

# 7 Immediate Placement and Computer-guided Surgery

**Fig 7-148** The labial plate fractured during extraction of the maxillary right canine. Fortunately sufficient bone was available on the palatal aspect to permit insertion of the implant as planned. The impact of bone loss can be seen in the image of the definitive restoration.

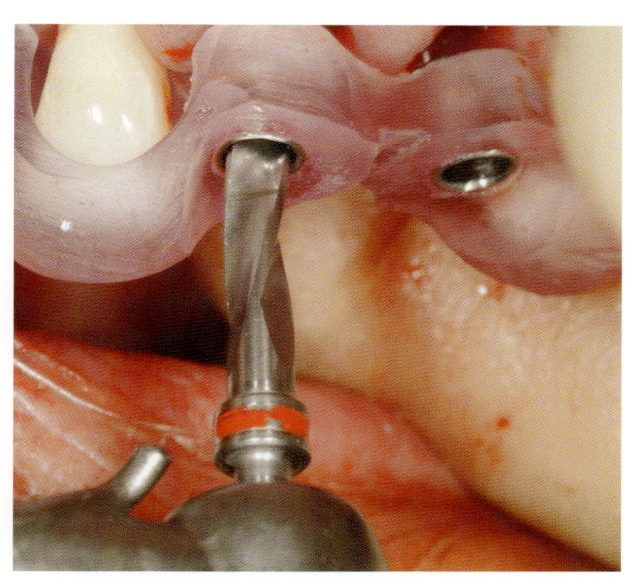

**Fig 7-149** Intraoperative view of the surgical guide in situ supported by the selected teeth with an internally irrigated osteotomy bur (3 mm diameter) being used to prepare the osteotomy in the selected position and at the right angle.

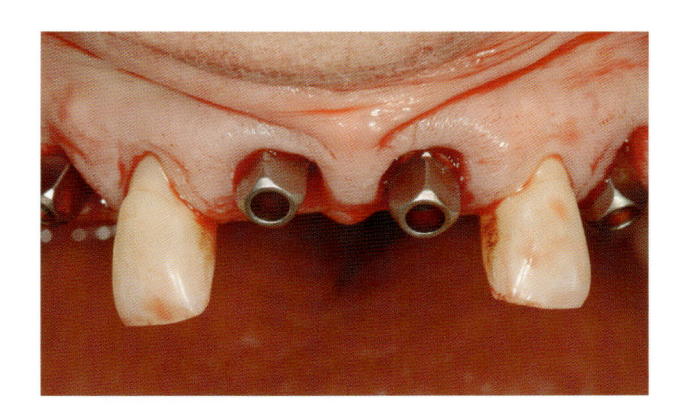

**Fig 7-150** The implants have been inserted to the depth estimated from soft tissue thickness measurements. The carriers of the anterior implants are visible as are the lateral incisors, which were used for supporting the surgical drill guide.

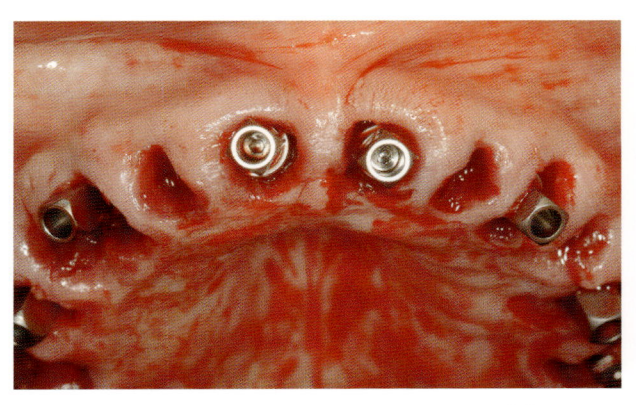

**Fig 7-151** Intraoral view of the maxillary implants following extraction of the remaining teeth. The angulation of the implants can be seen and related to the 3D CT image.

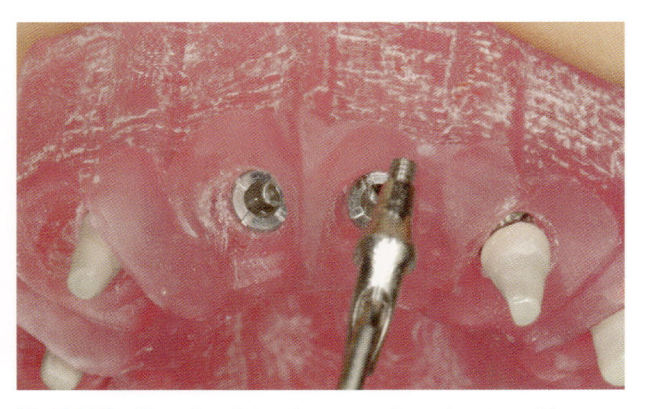

**Fig 7-152** Transfer of the abutments from the stereolithographic model is carried out one at a time to ensure an accurate transfer.

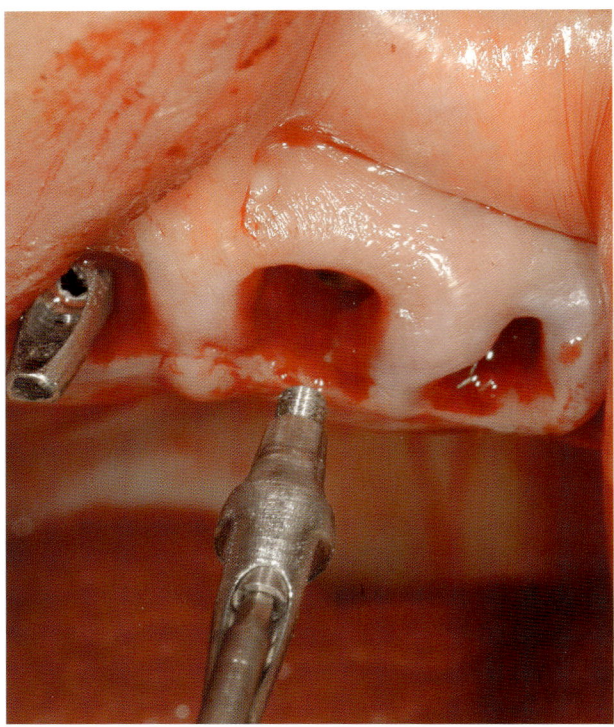

II  Implant Placement: Surgery and Prosthodontics

**Fig 7-153**  Abutment being transferred to the mouth for connection to the implant.

**Fig 7-154**  Labial view of all the abutments following sealing of the screw access holes.

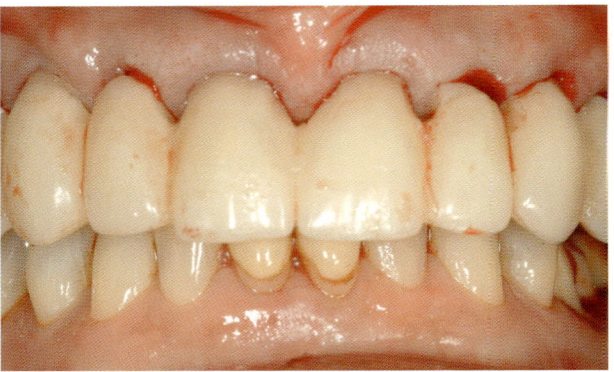

**Fig 7-155**  The transitional restoration fitted following its connection to the closely adapted acrylic resin sleeves. Note the relationship of the transitional restoration to the surrounding soft tissues.

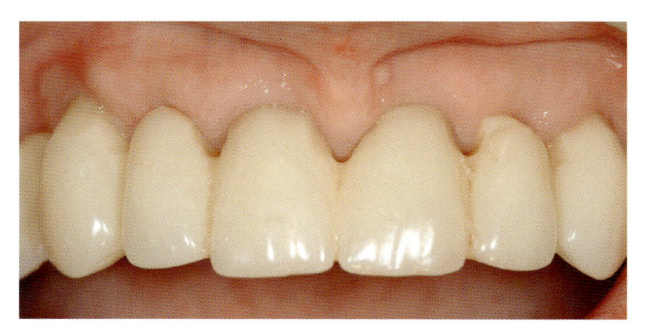

**Fig 7-156**  The transitional restoration three months after insertion. Note the stability of the soft tissues.

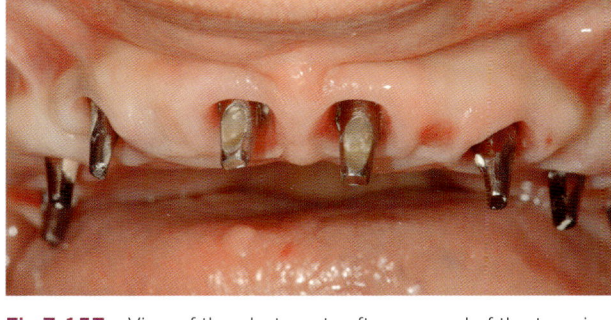

**Fig 7-157**  View of the abutments after removal of the transitional restoration, showing the emergence profile created and the healed healthy tissues.

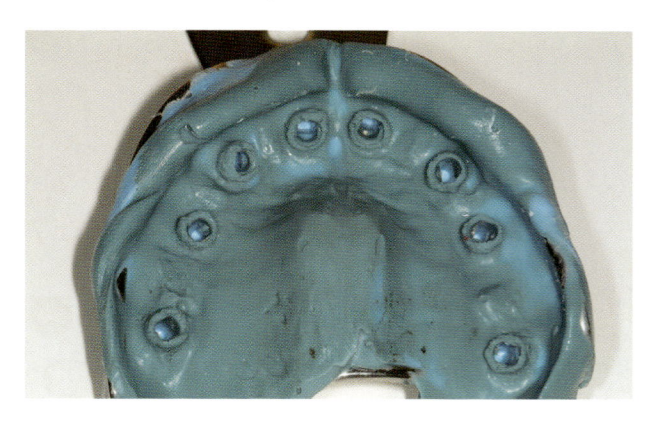

**Fig 7-158**  Conventional impression taken using addition-cured silicone in a rimmed metal tray. Retraction cord has been used to identify the margins of the abutment. The soft tissue contours have also been recorded.

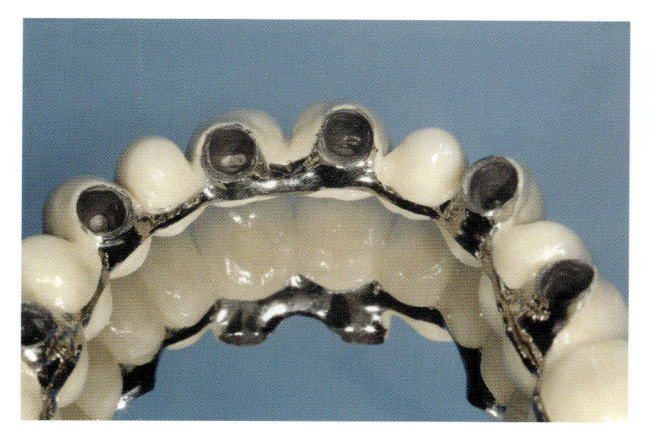

# 7 Immediate Placement and Computer-guided Surgery

**Fig 7-159** View of the fit surface of the definitive cement-retained full arch bridge.

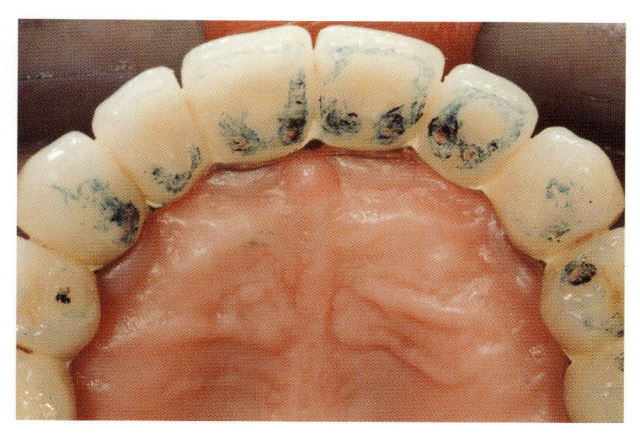

**Fig 7-160** Occlusal view of the cemented restoration showing contacts in centric relation and during excursive movements.

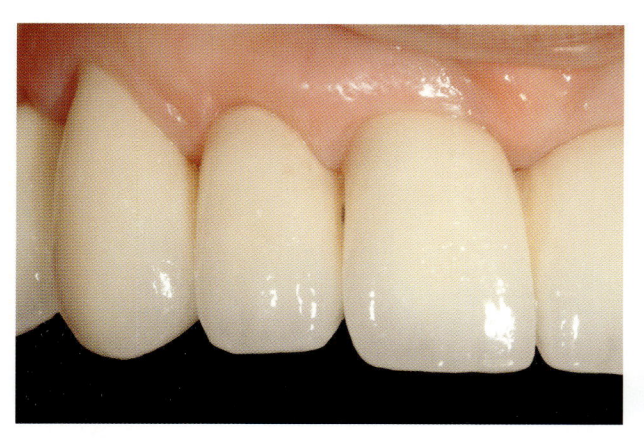

**Fig 7-161** Labial view of the right side showing a more apically positioned gingival margin in the area of the canine.

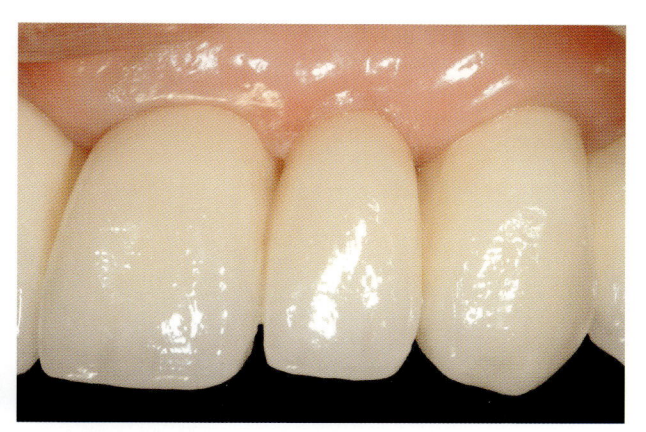

**Fig 7-162** Labial view of the left side showing soft tissue contours in relation to the porcelain bridge. Note gingival margin levels.

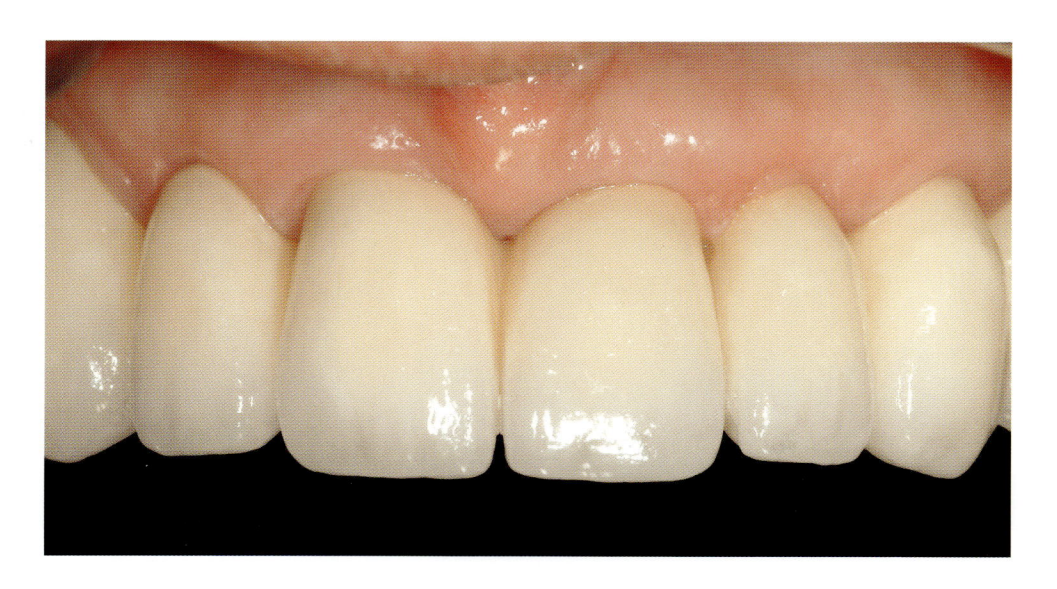

**Fig 7-163** Anterior view providing an overview of the soft tissue contours and relative gingival margin levels.

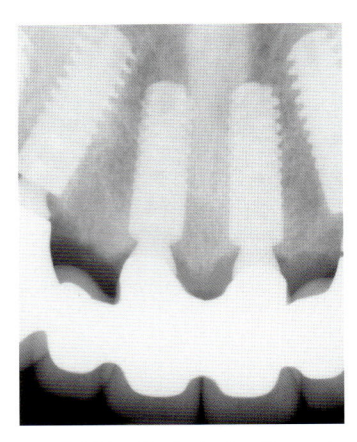

II   Implant Placement: Surgery and Prosthodontics

**Fig 7-164**   Periapical radiograph taken one year after surgery showing bone levels. Note the interdental peaks of bone being sustained above the implant shoulder level. These are dependent upon the absence of micro-leakage between abutments and implants and are responsible for maintenance of the papillary form.

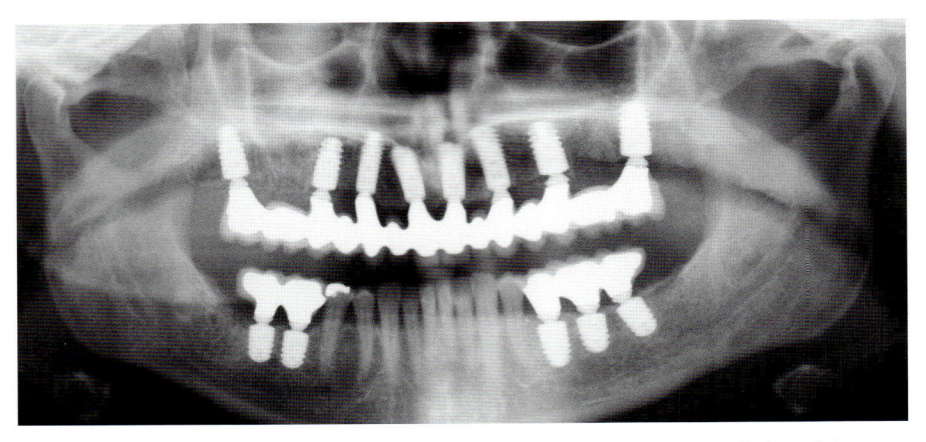

**Fig 7-165**   Post-operative dental panoramic tomograph providing an overall view of the status of the mouth.

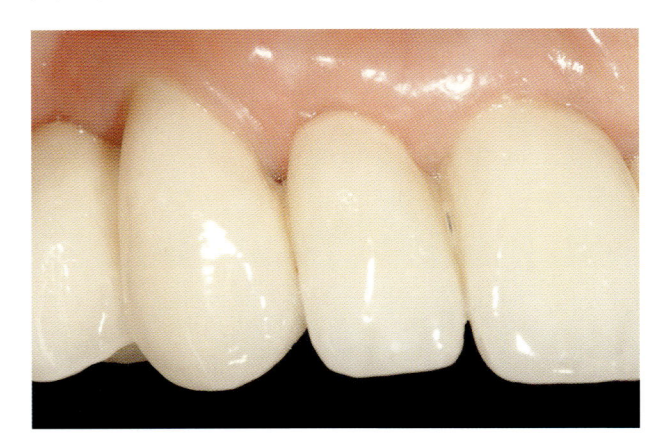

**Fig 7-166**   Clinical view of the right anterior region showing stability of the tissues two years after the procedure.

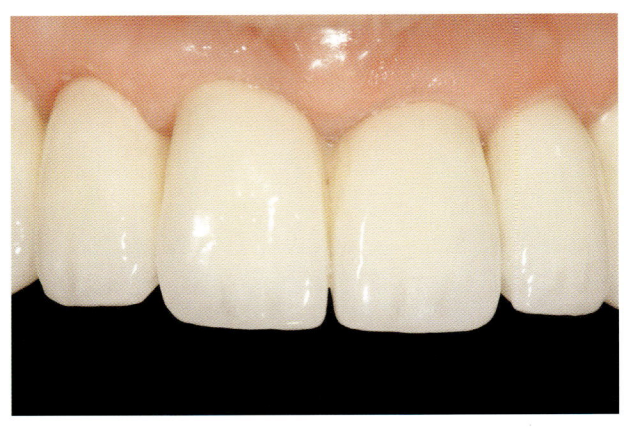

**Fig 7-167**   Clinical view of the anterior region showing stability of the tissues two years after the procedure.

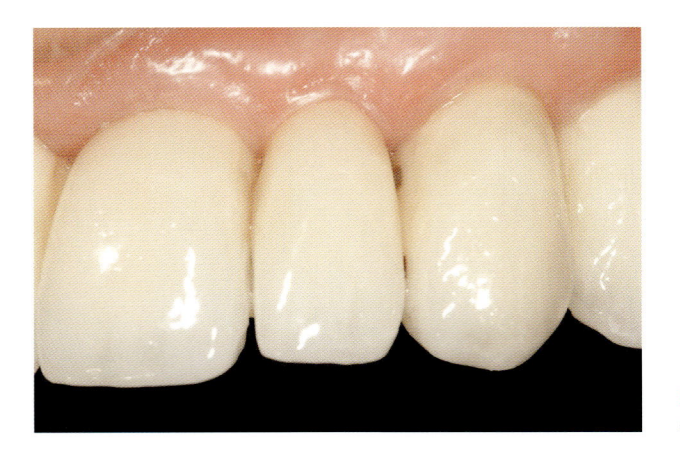

**Fig 7-168**   Clinical view of the left anterior region showing stability of the tissues two years after the procedure.

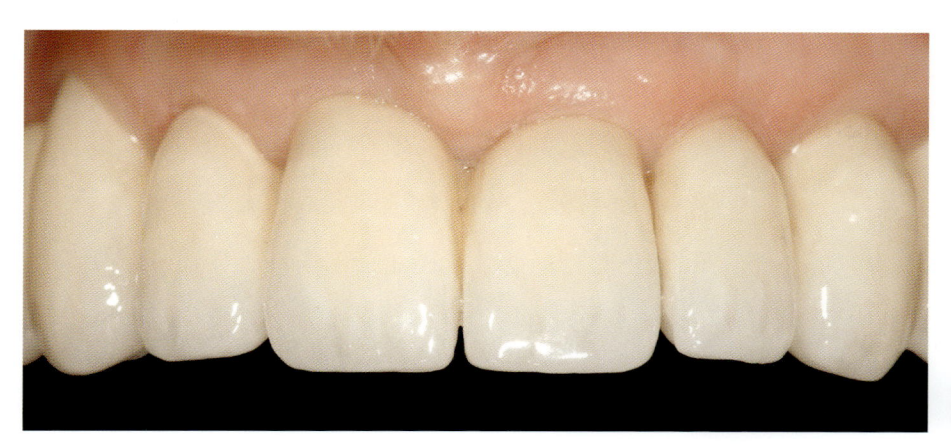

**7** Immediate Placement and Computer-guided Surgery

**Fig 7-169** Overall view of the anterior region two years after the procedure.

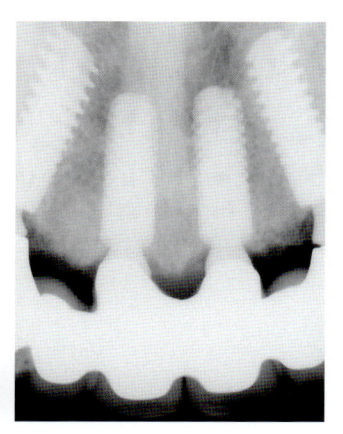

**Fig 7-170** Periapical radiograph two years after the procedure showing stable hard tissues.

### Case 2: Management of a Complex Restorative Case

Tooth-supported guides were used for this patient, with implants being placed into healed sites via a transmucosal approach. This was a complex case that required a change in the intermaxillary relations to correct overclosure caused by bruxism-induced tooth wear.

The treatment formed part of the overall management of the patient, which required multiple restorations. Acceptance of the change in the intermaxillary relation was established in stages using provisional restorations followed by implant-supported transitional restorations, prior to proceeding to the definitive restorations (Figs 7-171–7-186).

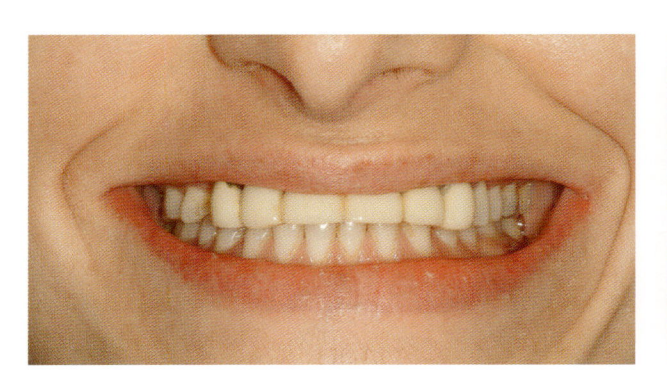

**Fig 7-171** Preoperative view of patient smiling.

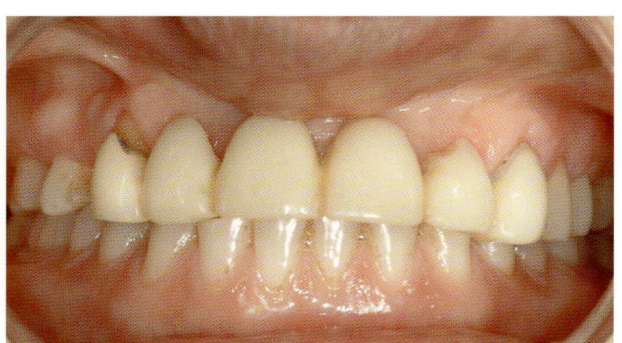

**Fig 7-172** Intraoral view of failing bridge.

95

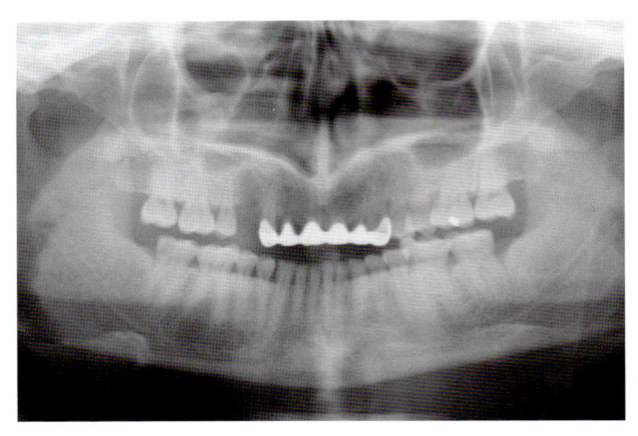

## II Implant Placement: Surgery and Prosthodontics

**Fig 7-173** Preoperative panoral radiograph showing the failing bridge and minimally restored but worn teeth.

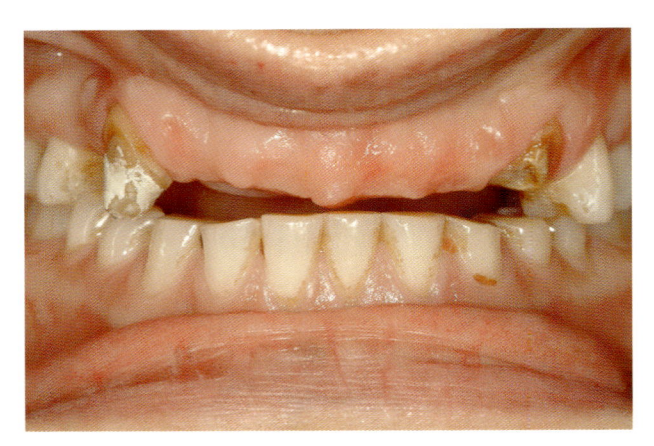

**Fig 7-174** Intraoral view showing reduced occlusal clearance and overclosure resulting from excessive tooth wear.

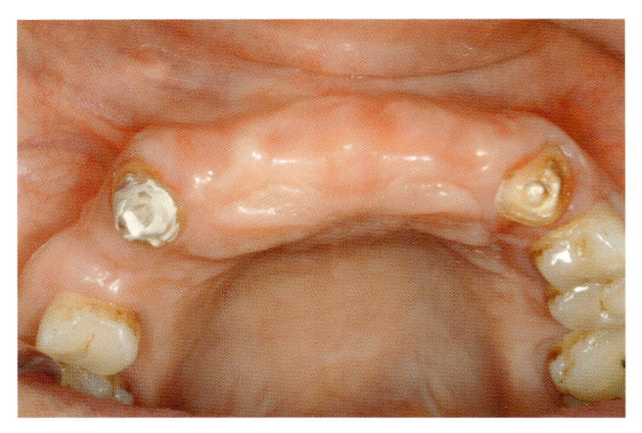

**Fig 7-175** Occlusal view of the ridge showing ample keratinised soft tissues suitable for transmucosal implant placement. Bone volume would need to be estimated prior to implant placement.

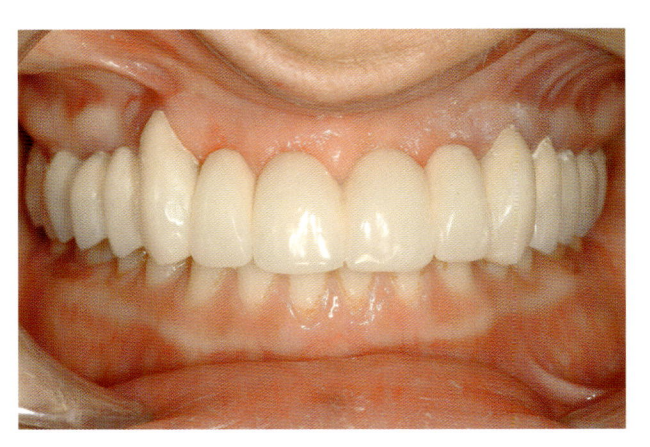

**Fig 7-176** Provisional restoration constructed to permit the correct intermaxillary relationship to be established. No treatment of the mandible is proposed at present.

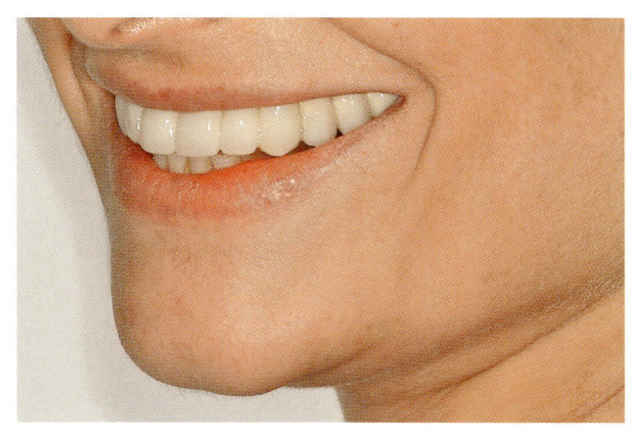

**Fig 7-177** Assessment of facial form following fitting of provisional restoration.

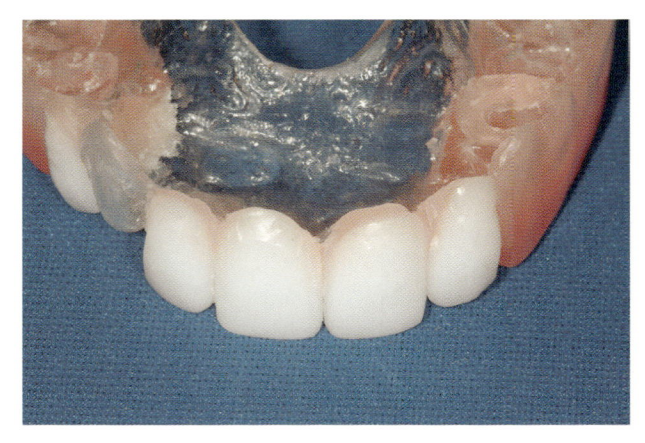

**Fig 7-178** Radiopaque teeth for use during CT scanning to identify proposed tooth position.

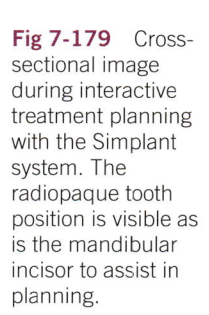

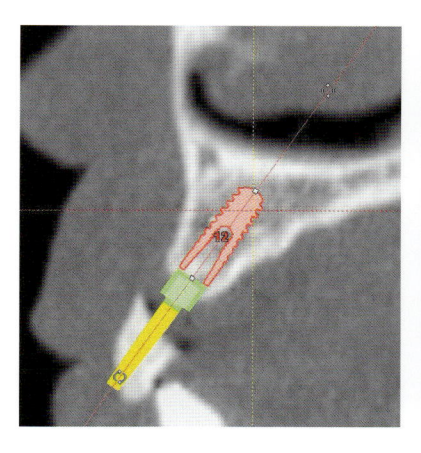

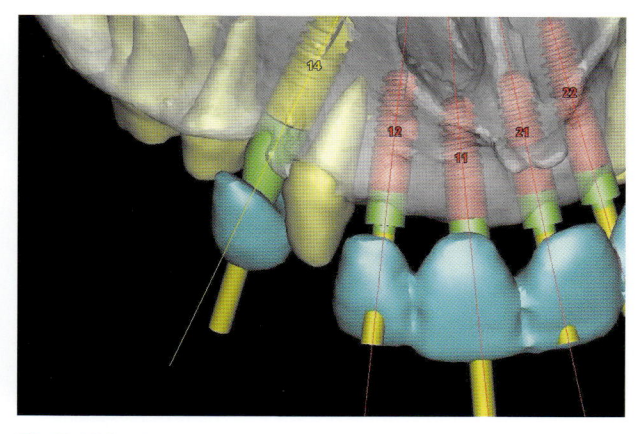

**7** Immediate Placement and Computer-guided Surgery

**Fig 7-179** Cross-sectional image during interactive treatment planning with the Simplant system. The radiopaque tooth position is visible as is the mandibular incisor to assist in planning.

**Fig 7-180** Three-dimensional reconstruction based on CT data being used to assess and refine implant position during treatment planning.

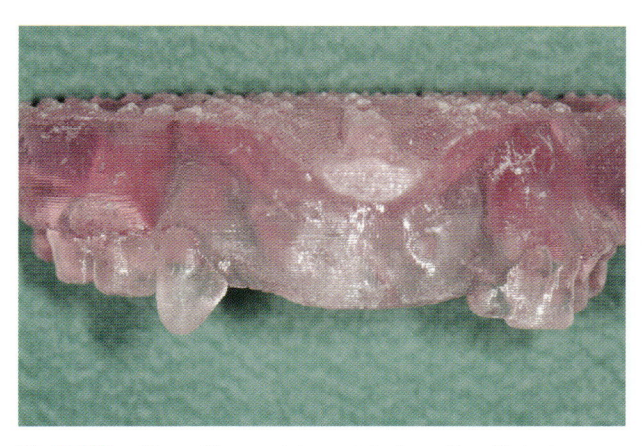

**Fig 7-181** Stereolithographic model of maxilla with holes prepared based on treatment planning data to receive implant analogues.

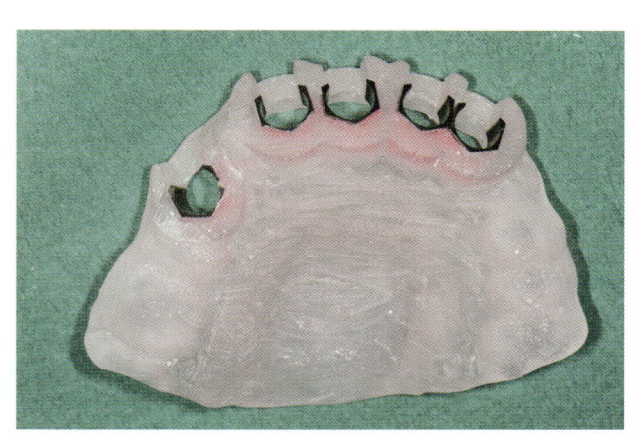

**Fig 7-182** ExpertEase surgical guide (Dentsply Friadent) with open titanium sleeves (prototypes) to enable the entire range of instruments to be used without the need to remove the guide. This is made possible by sleeves that fit on the internally irrigated drills.

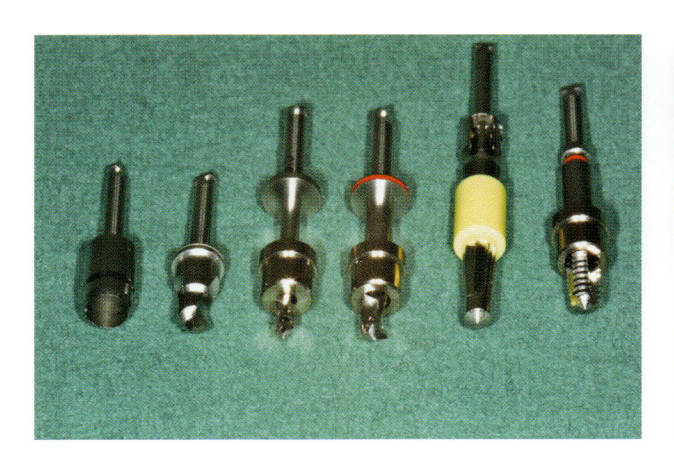

**Fig 7-183** Range of instruments designed for osteotomy preparation using the ExpertEase surgical guide to predetermined depths.

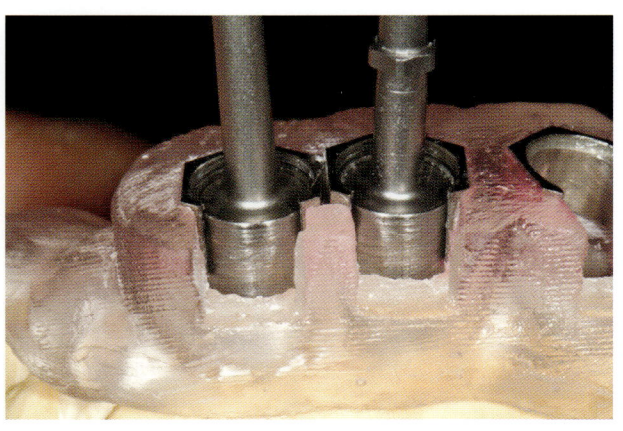

**Fig 7-184** Image demonstrating use of guide and instruments on a study cast.

97

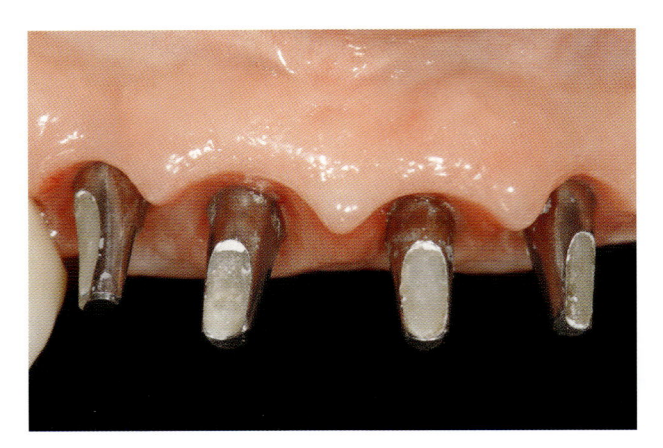

**Fig 7-185** Intraoral view of abutments emerging from contoured soft tissues.

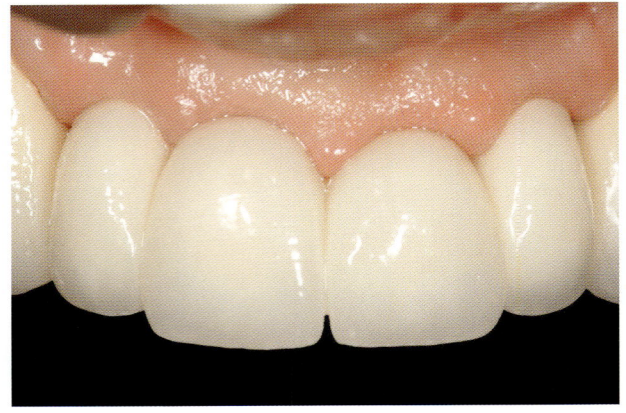

**Fig 7-186** Definitive restorations in situ showing excellent aesthetic outcome.

## Case 3: Immediate Full Mouth Rehabilitation with Substantial Changes in the Intermaxillary Relationship

This case describes the management of a patient with failing teeth and non-functional occlusion. The patient's medical condition required general anaesthesia for treatment and, consequently, treatment of both jaws was carried out simultaneously to minimise the number of anaesthetics. Extraction of all failing teeth with simultaneous implant placement in conjunction with implants placed into healed sites with immediate loading was planned to provide the patient with functional restorations in both jaws at the same time.

Changes to the occlusion were planned by careful observation of the speech patterns to predict the adaptation to the change in the occlusal scheme. Guided surgery provided an ideal mechanism for producing a predictable outcome with minimum risk of failure of implants or restorations.

Considerable planning is required with close collaboration between dental surgeon, dental technician and the imaging and rapid prototyping company.

This case depicts effective treatment carried out in one session that provided the patient with immediate improvement in the quality of life (Figs 7-187–7-210).

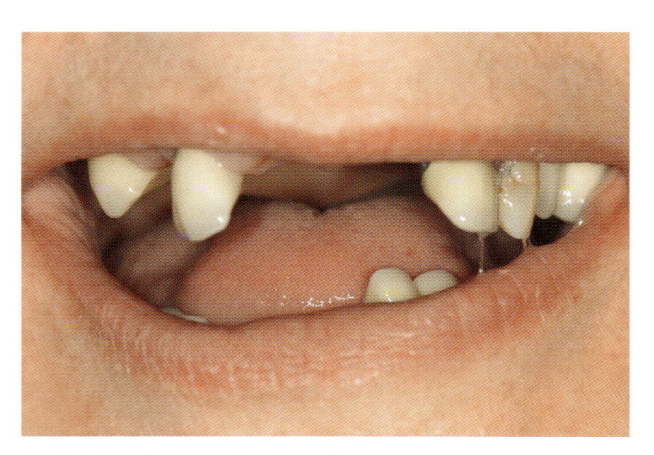

**Fig 7-187** Preoperative view of patient.

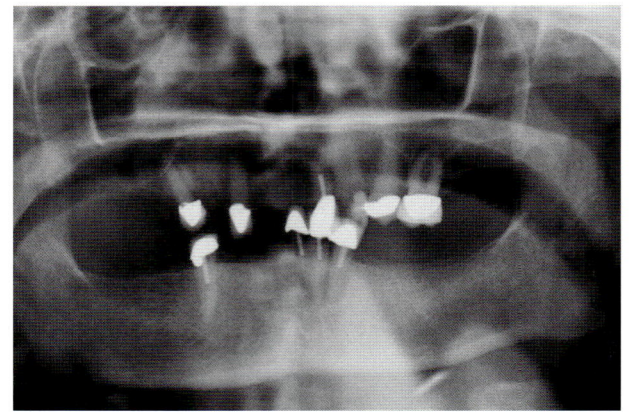

**Fig 7-188** Preoperative panoral radiograph showing the oral status.

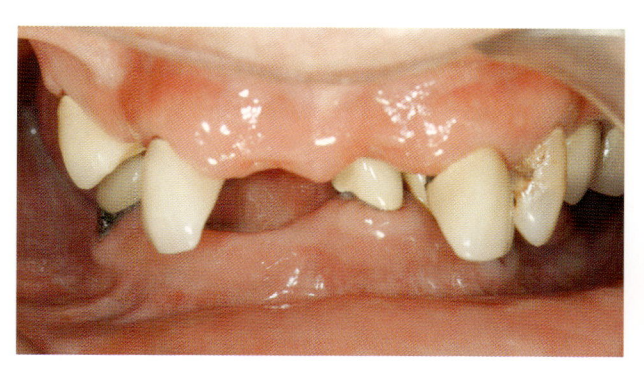

# 7 Immediate Placement and Computer-guided Surgery

**Fig 7-189** Labial view showing non functional occlusion with mandibular remaining teeth biting directly into the palatal soft tissues.

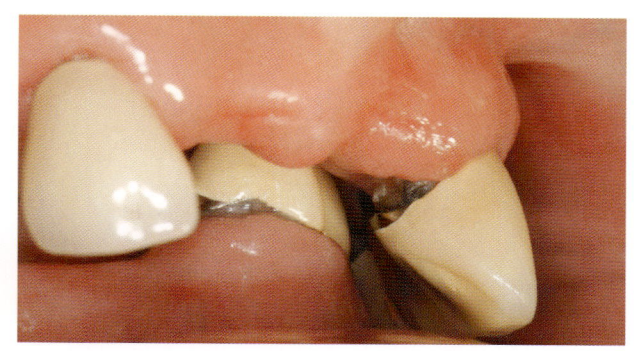

**Fig 7-190** Lateral view depicting the occlusal relationship.

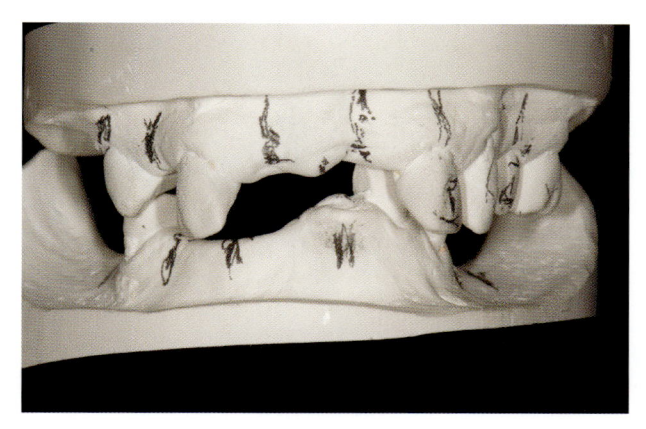

**Fig 7-191** Study casts mounted on a semi-adjustable articulator for assessment and planning of transitional restoration.

**Fig 7-192** Interactive planning ensuring that the position, depth and angulation of the implant will translate effectively to the clinical situation. Artefacts caused by heavy metal restorations can be seen at the level of the clinical crowns (sporadic black and white areas which are indicative of loss of image). Therefore, accurate representation of the tooth form for stereolithographic reconstruction would not be possible and a tooth-supported guide is contraindicated.

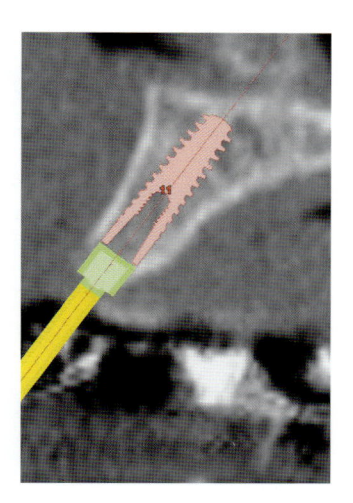

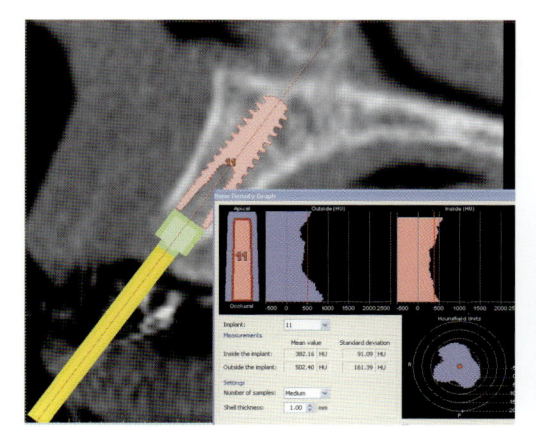

**Fig 7-193** Bone density assessment of each proposed implant site to evaluate the clinical procedures required to ensure adequate primary stability.

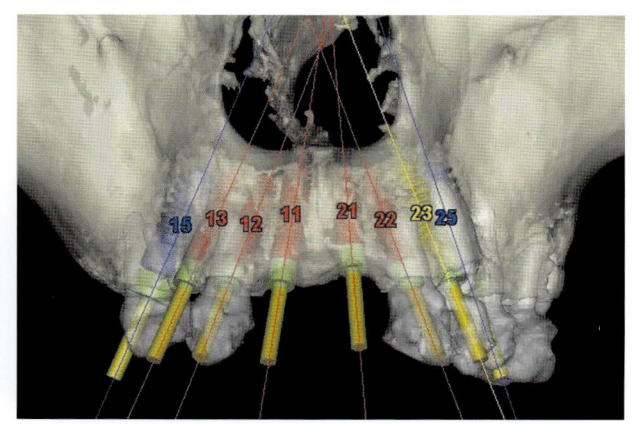

**Fig 7-194** Three-dimensional reconstruction of the maxilla with proposed implants in situ, which is critical to ensure translation to the clinical treatment phase to ensure an aesthetic result. All refinements of implant positions are made here.

99

II   Implant Placement: Surgery and Prosthodontics

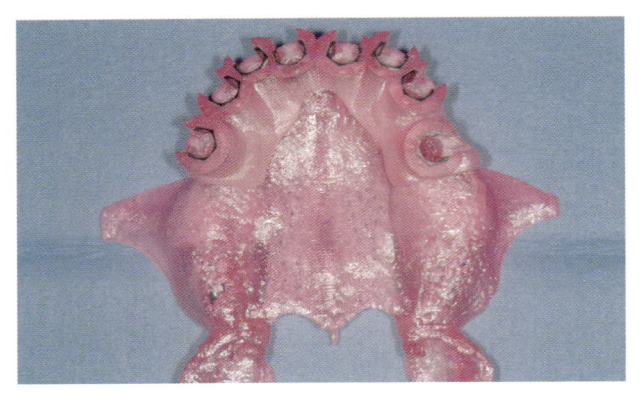

**Fig 7-195**   Interactive planning data is sent to Materialise, Leuven, Belgium for the construction of stereolithographic models and an ExpertEase drill guide to be used for osteotomy preparation as well as implant placement. Implant position data without abutment selection constitutes the information required for the fabrication of the drill guide.

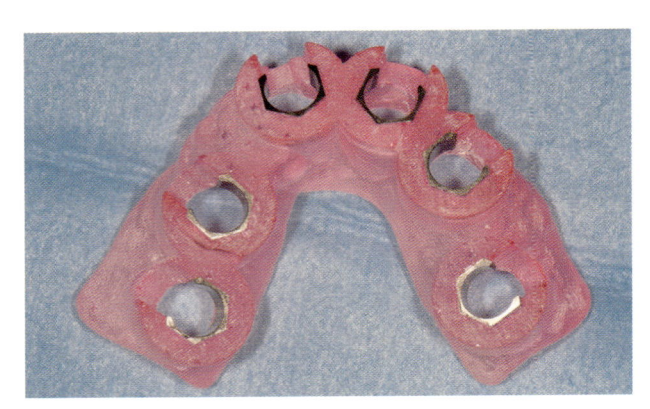

**Fig 7-196**   Drill guide for the mandible.

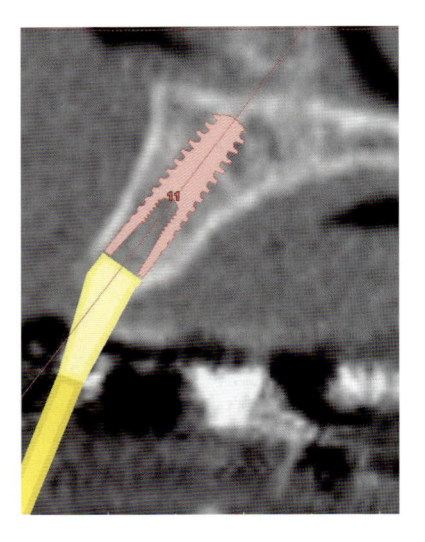

**Fig 7-197**   Interactive selection of abutments will provide an indication to the technician regarding the abutment that might be required. Data gathered here may also be used to alter implant position and orientation prior to sending data for surgical guide construction.

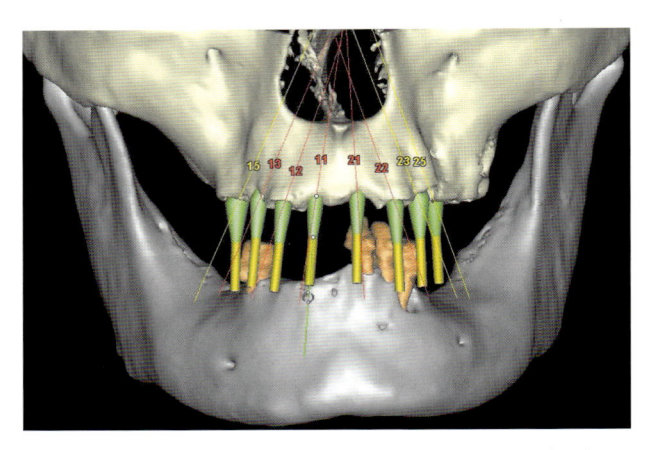

**Fig 7-198**   Three-dimensional image with abutments for the arbitrary assessment of abutment alignment as well as the relationship to the opposing jaw.

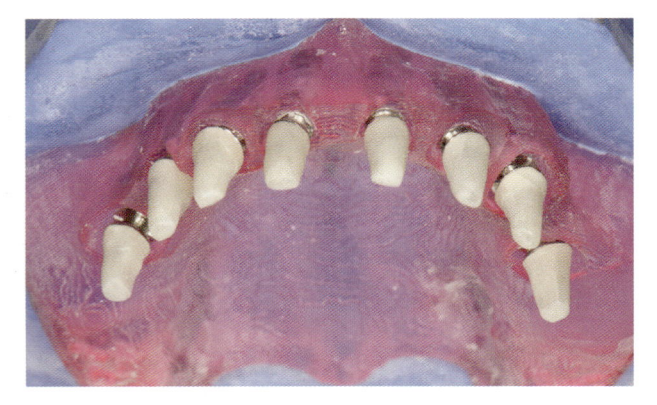

**Fig 7-199**   Prefabricated abutments selected by the technician to ensure alignment and parallelism. Acrylic sleeves have been constructed for connection to the transitional restoration.

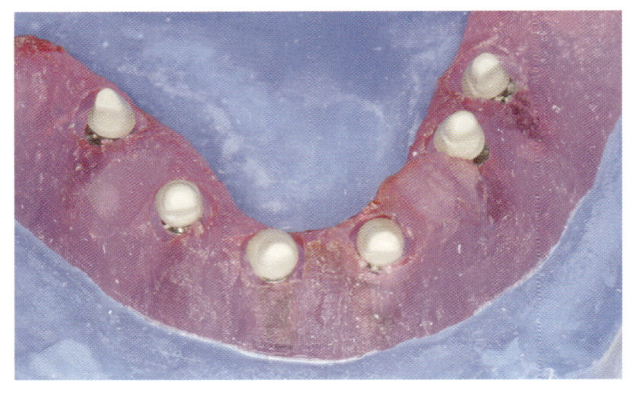

**Fig 7-200**   Abutments and sleeves for the mandible. Note the proclination of the abutments to allow function between the maxillary and mandibular teeth.

100

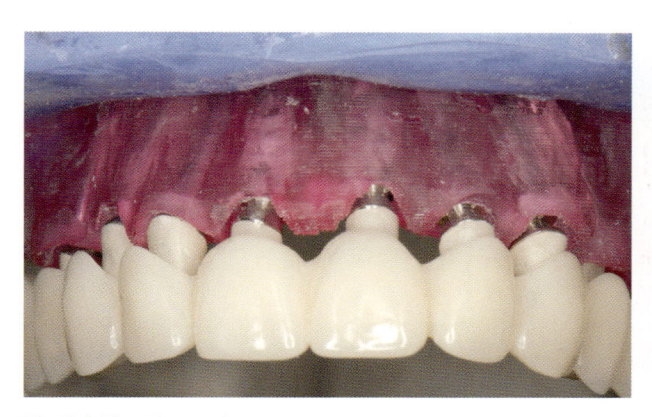

# 7 Immediate Placement and Computer-guided Surgery

**Fig 7-201** The prefabricated abutments and sleeves in relationship to the transitional restoration. Information transfer from mounted study casts to the stereolithographic model with teeth present and a further stereolithographic model with prepared osteotomy replicas.

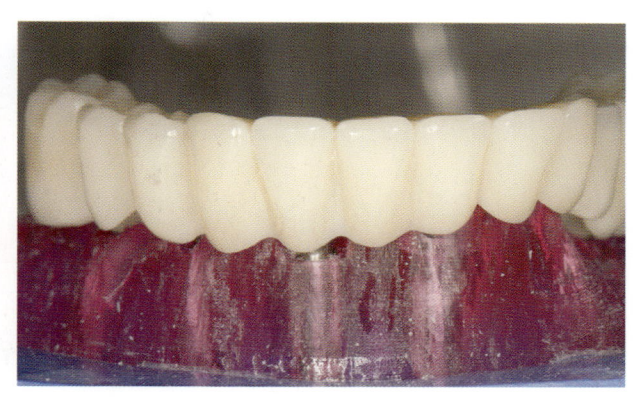

**Fig 7-202** Mandibular transitional restoration on the abutments and sleeves. It has been designed to occlude against the maxillary teeth.

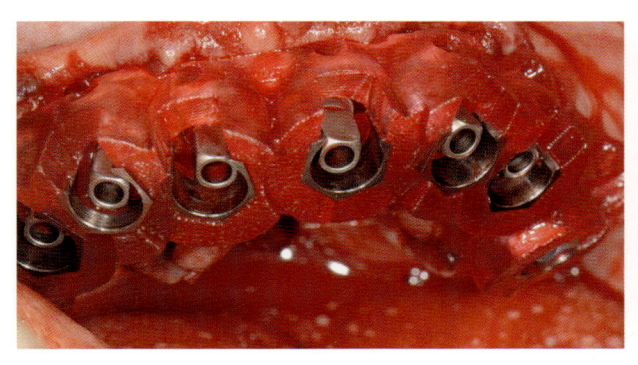

**Fig 7-203** Intraoperative view of the bone-supported surgical guide with the implants inserted to the prescribed position and depth.

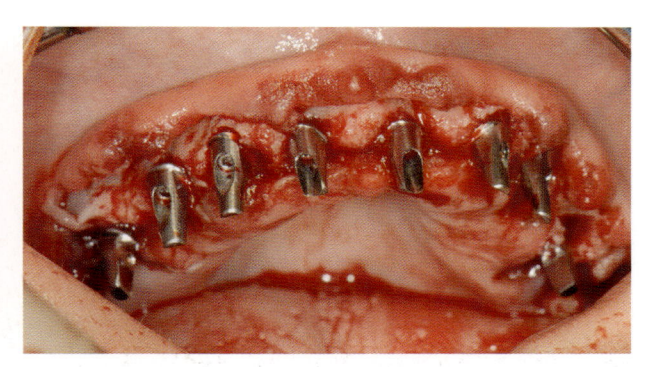

**Fig 7-204** The abutments transferred to the mouth from the stereolithographic model prior to sealing of the access holes, seating of the sleeves for connection to the transitional restoration. Any compensation for the discrepancies during surgery is made by the tolerances allowed for within the hollow acrylic resin transitionals. Guidance for positioning of the upper transitional is provided by the lower transitionals and vice versa.

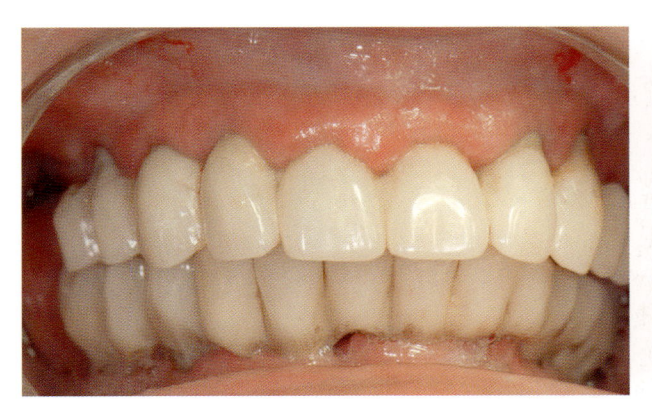

**Fig 7-205** Upper and lower transitional restorations can be seen in function with the mandibular teeth proclined and the maxillary teeth marginally retroclined. The image describes the clinical situation approximately two weeks post-operatively.

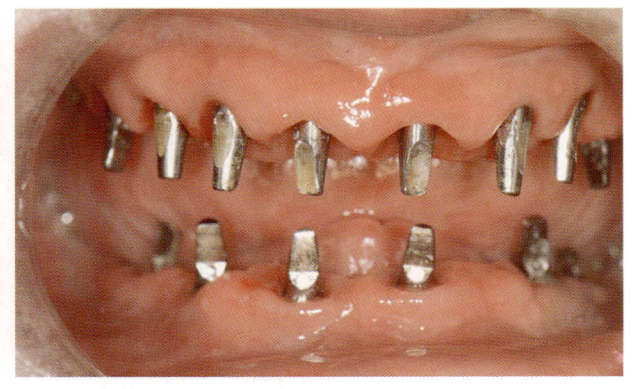

**Fig 7-206** The abutments emerging from the soft tissues three months after implant insertion. The soft tissue healing is evident and the relationship of the upper and lower abutments as planned can be seen.

II Implant Placement: Surgery and Prosthodontics

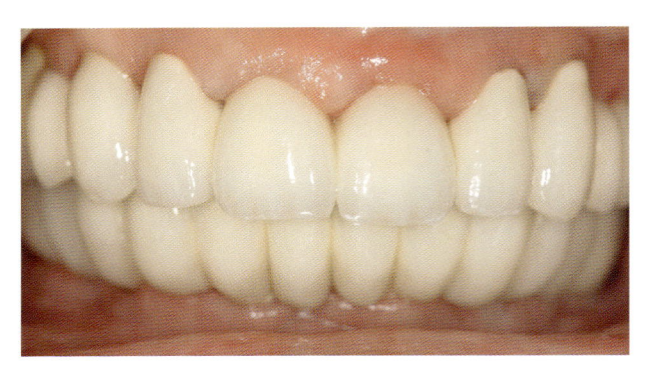

**Fig 7-207** Definitive restoration showing functional occlusal scheme with the teeth in contact.

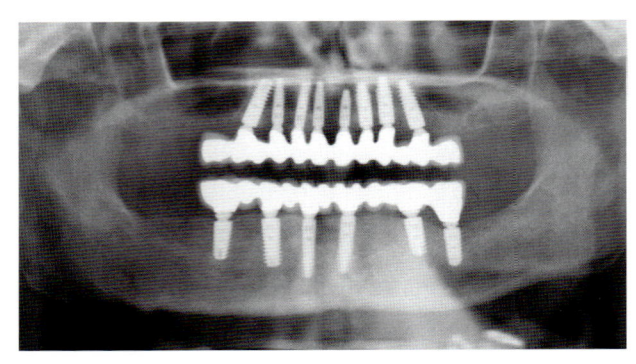

**Fig 7-208** Post-operative panoral radiograph showing the positioning of the implants to avoid anatomical structures and make maximum use of the available bone.

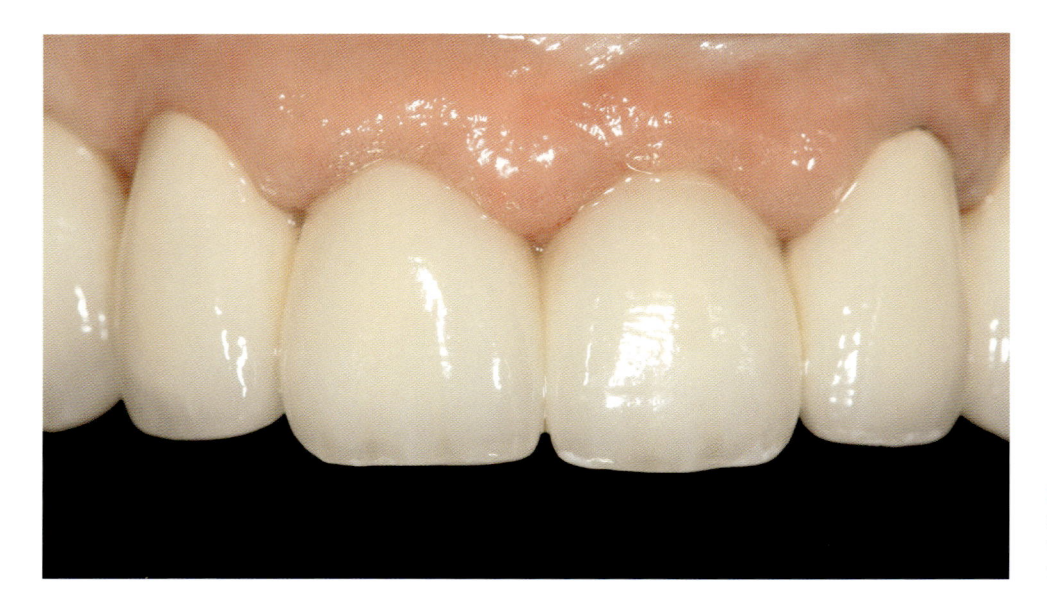

**Fig 7-209** Natural appearance of definitive restoration and soft tissues.

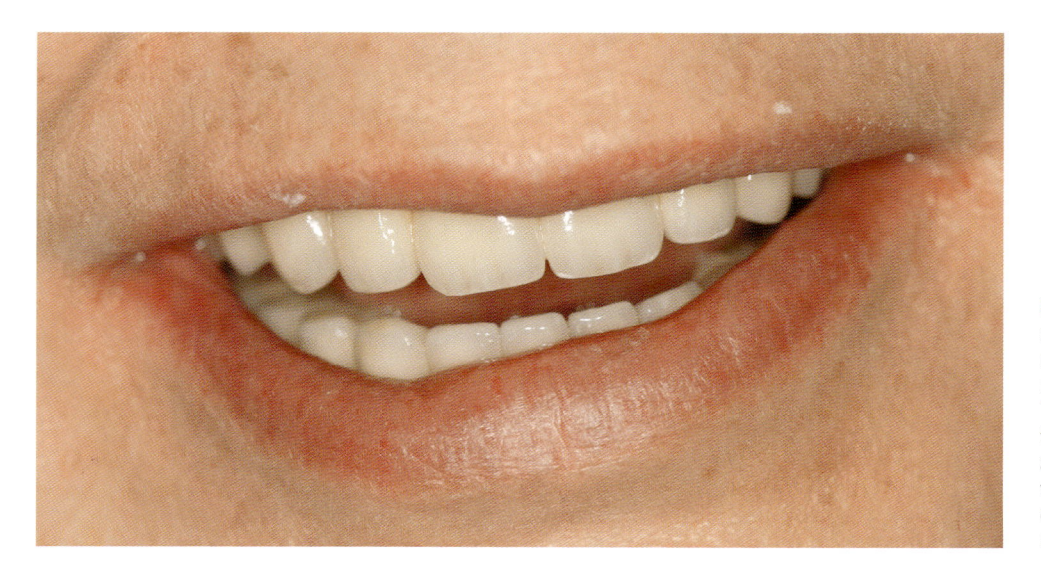

**Fig 7-210** Patient smiling naturally. A considerable improvement has been achieved. The occlusal and aesthetic improvement was accomplished in one day with the aid of modern diagnostic technology and rapid prototyping

# Chapter 8

# Delayed Placement in Adequate Bone with Mature Ridge

## Introduction

Delayed insertion of implants into mature bone of adequate width and height is a very safe and predictable technique with which to achieve osseointegration. It enables the clinician to select the implant site with precision and to be assured of the attachment of bone to the implant.

An extraction socket matures at approximately six months, confirmed by radiographic assessment. This provides a healed bony site where an osteotomy can be prepared. This can be predicted by proper assessment of the bony biotype. Other techniques have been described to commence treatment at completion of soft tissue healing and often require advanced surgical techniques using membranes and biomaterials to correct any deficiency that naturally would be present. These techniques are described elsewhere.

Typically in situations where malpositioned teeth need to be replaced, allowing the extraction site to heal will permit implant site selection to match the proposed ideal tooth position as predicted based on bone biotype (see Case 4, below). Carrying out treatment in stages also permits bone deficiencies caused by infection to be repaired naturally. This in specific biotypes permits implant placement without the need for augmentation. In other cases staged treatment allows the clinician to confirm the need for augmentation based on a visual assessment of the provisional restoration and a radiographic assessment of the bone volume (Case 4 in Chapter 14).

Furthermore, the bone level on the completion of healing and remodelling can be predicted specific to the implant system used. For example, for an externally hexed system, the minimum interimplant distance has been specified as 3 mm.[103] This was based on the expected remodelling of bone resulting from microleakage at the implant–abutment interface. Other systems that have an implant–abutment junction with no micro-gap are beginning to redefine the minimum interimplant distance.[119]

For a 3.5-mm implant, a minimum ridge height of 12 mm and a minimum width of 6 mm is considered necessary (Figs 8-1 and 8-2). This will leave more than 1 mm of residual bone on the buccal and lingual aspect of the ridge. The length of the ridge for a single tooth should ideally be 8 mm and 14 mm for two implants of the above diameter (Figs 8-2 and 8-3; Flowchart 8-1).

Delayed placement in mature bone offers the opportunity to load an implant immediately at the time of placement. Assessment for this is carried out in the preoperative phase, as the requirements in terms of the surgical approach, component parts and the transitional restorations will differ (Flowchart 8-2).

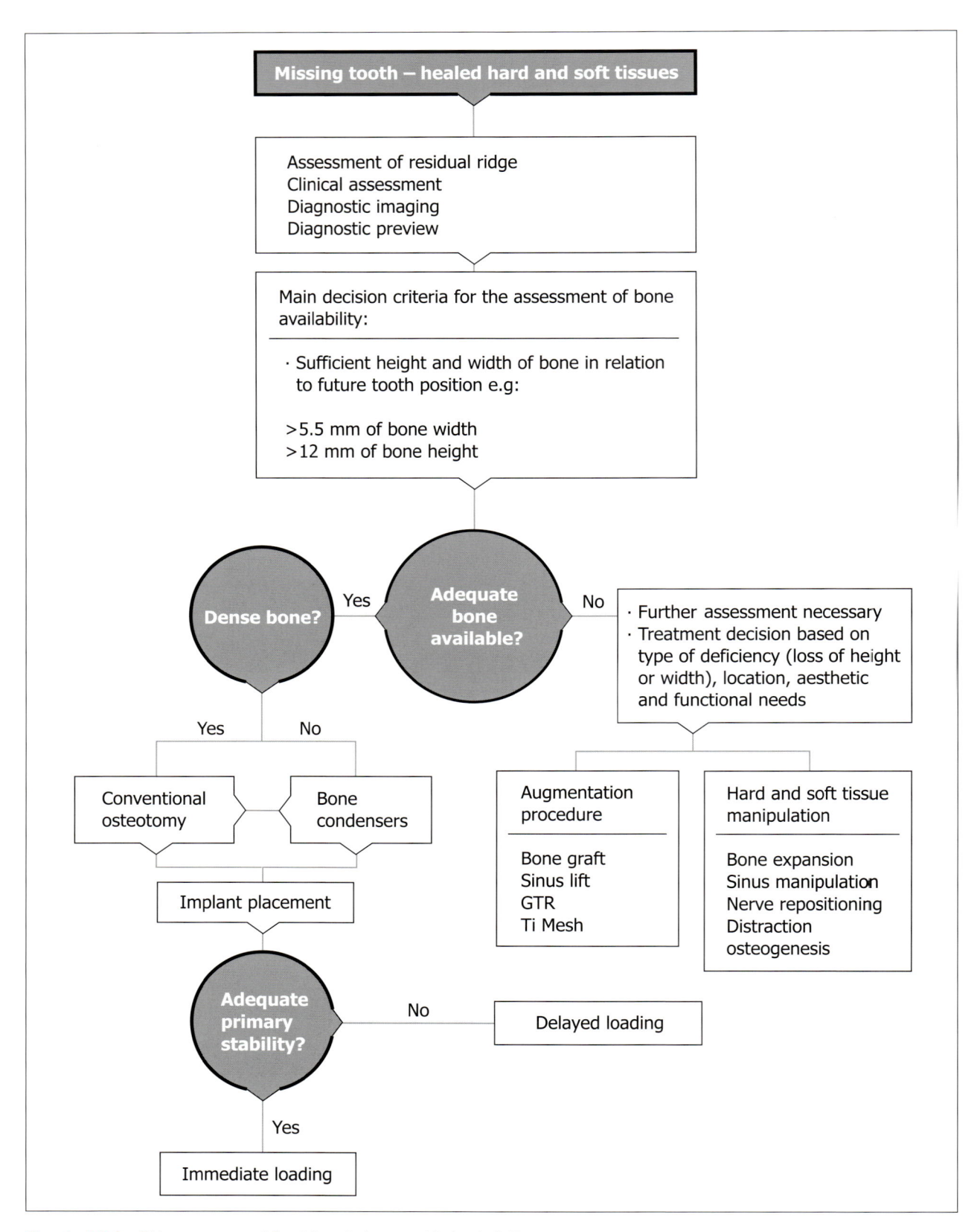

## II  Implant Placement: Surgery and Prosthodontics

**Missing tooth – healed hard and soft tissues**

Assessment of residual ridge
Clinical assessment
Diagnostic imaging
Diagnostic preview

Main decision criteria for the assessment of bone availability:

- Sufficient height and width of bone in relation to future tooth position e.g:

>5.5 mm of bone width
>12 mm of bone height

**Adequate bone available?**

- Yes → **Dense bone?**
  - Yes → Conventional osteotomy
  - No → Bone condensers
  
  → Implant placement → **Adequate primary stability?**
  - No → Delayed loading
  - Yes → Immediate loading

- No →
  - Further assessment necessary
  - Treatment decision based on type of deficiency (loss of height or width), location, aesthetic and functional needs
  
  → Augmentation procedure
  - Bone graft
  - Sinus lift
  - GTR
  - Ti Mesh
  
  → Hard and soft tissue manipulation
  - Bone expansion
  - Sinus manipulation
  - Nerve repositioning
  - Distraction osteogenesis

**Flowchart 8-1**  Ridge assessment for delayed placement in healed site.

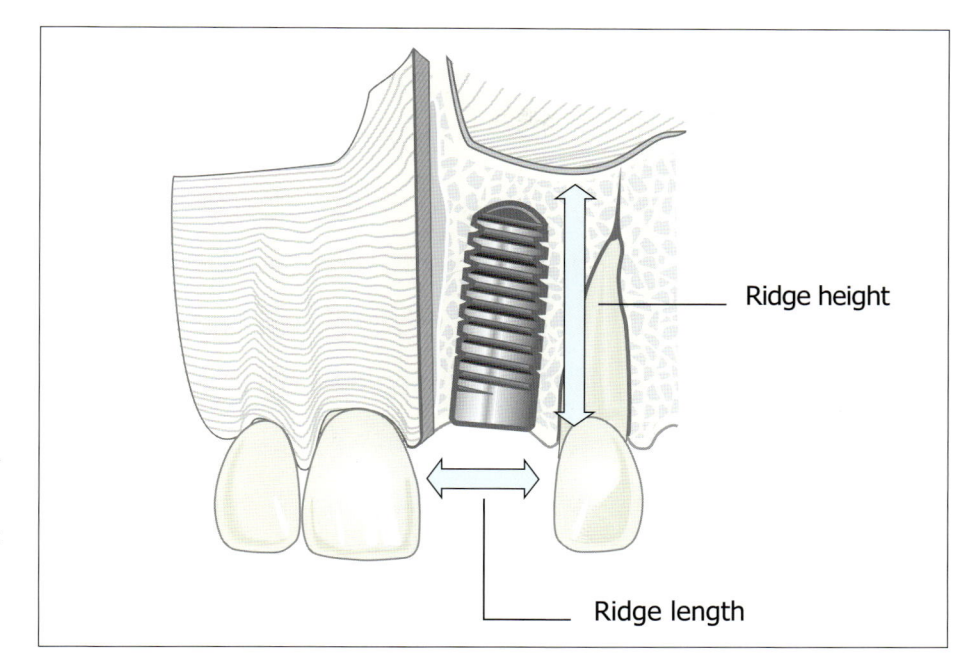

# 8  Delayed Placement in Adequate Bone with Mature Ridge

**Fig 8-1** Schematic representation of an implant placed to replace the maxillary left central incisor. The ridge length (L) represents the distance between the adjacent teeth. The ridge height (H) represents the height of alveolar ridge available for an implant and corresponds to the length of an implant that could be used.

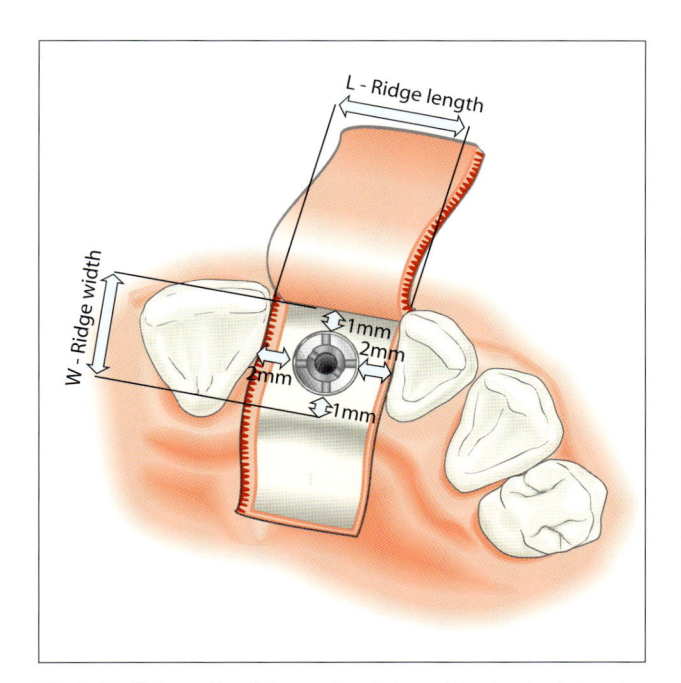

**Fig 8-2** Schematic of the occlusal view of the implant showing the ridge length (L), which has an impact on the implant diameter. The width of the ridge (W) determines the diameter of the implant that can be used. The ideal ridge length and width have been estimated based on the most common implant diameter (approximately 3.5 mm). The estimated ridge length allows for up to 2-mm clearance from adjacent teeth and the minimum ridge width allows for 1-mm thickness of bone on both the buccal and palatal sides of the implant.

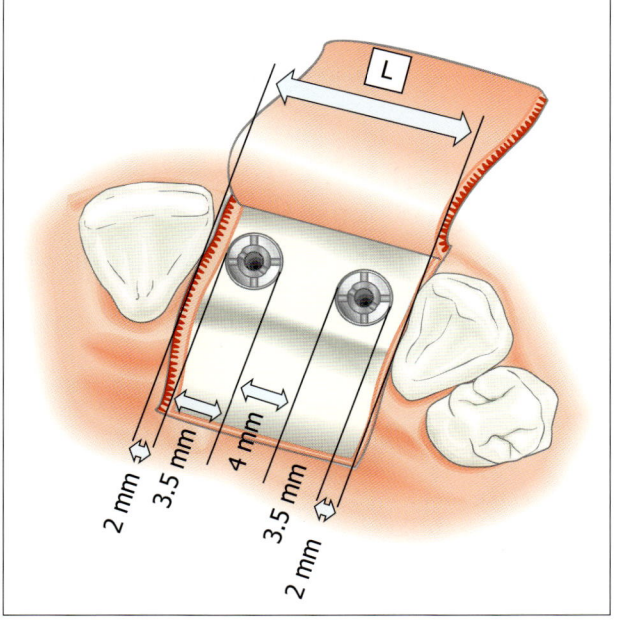

**Fig 8-3** The estimated minimum ridge length for two implants placed interdentally. A space of 15 mm is considered suitable allowing 2-mm clearance between the adjacent teeth and implants and a 4-mm clearance between the two implants.

105

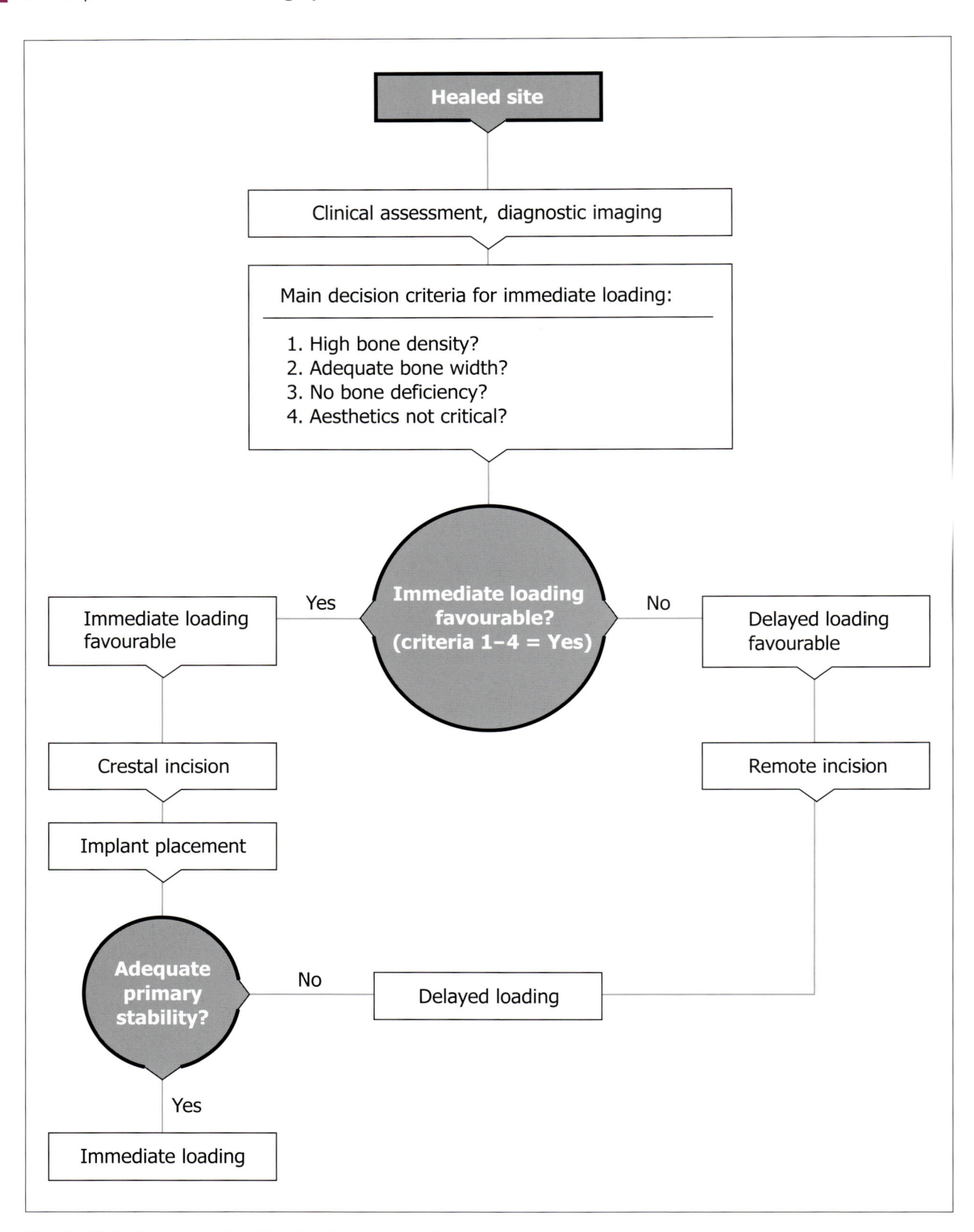

II Implant Placement: Surgery and Prosthodontics

```
                    ┌─────────────┐
                    │ Healed site │
                    └──────┬──────┘
                           │
           ┌───────────────┴───────────────┐
           │ Clinical assessment, diagnostic imaging │
           └───────────────┬───────────────┘
                           │
      ┌────────────────────┴────────────────────┐
      │ Main decision criteria for immediate loading: │
      │                                               │
      │   1. High bone density?                       │
      │   2. Adequate bone width?                     │
      │   3. No bone deficiency?                      │
      │   4. Aesthetics not critical?                 │
      └────────────────────┬────────────────────┘
                           │
                           ▼
                 ┌─────────────────────┐
       Yes       │ Immediate loading   │       No
    ┌────────────│ favourable?         │────────────┐
    │            │ (criteria 1–4 = Yes)│            │
    │            └─────────────────────┘            │
    ▼                                               ▼
┌──────────────┐                            ┌──────────────┐
│ Immediate    │                            │ Delayed      │
│ loading      │                            │ loading      │
│ favourable   │                            │ favourable   │
└──────┬───────┘                            └──────┬───────┘
       │                                           │
       ▼                                           ▼
┌──────────────┐                            ┌──────────────┐
│ Crestal      │                            │ Remote       │
│ incision     │                            │ incision     │
└──────┬───────┘                            └──────────────┘
       │
       ▼
┌──────────────┐
│ Implant      │
│ placement    │
└──────┬───────┘
       │
       ▼
  ┌─────────┐     No      ┌──────────────────┐
  │Adequate │─────────────│ Delayed loading  │
  │primary  │             └──────────────────┘
  │stability│
  └────┬────┘
       │ Yes
       ▼
┌──────────────┐
│ Immediate    │
│ loading      │
└──────────────┘
```

**Flowchart 8-2** Assessment for delayed or immediate loading.

**8** Delayed Placement in Adequate Bone with Mature Ridge

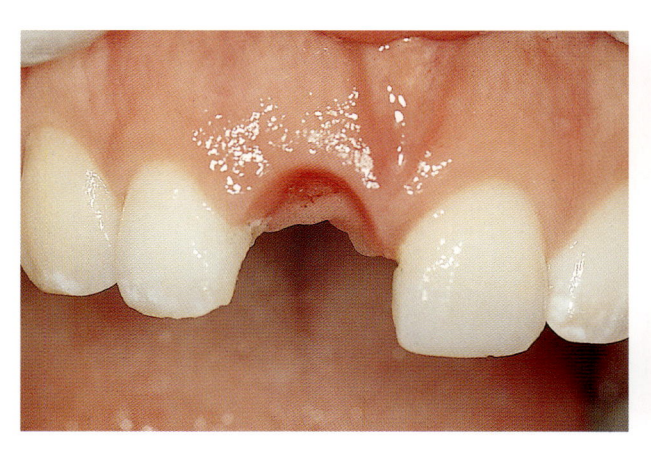

**Fig 8-4** Preoperative labial view: the gingival contours can be seen following the removal of the provisional restoration.

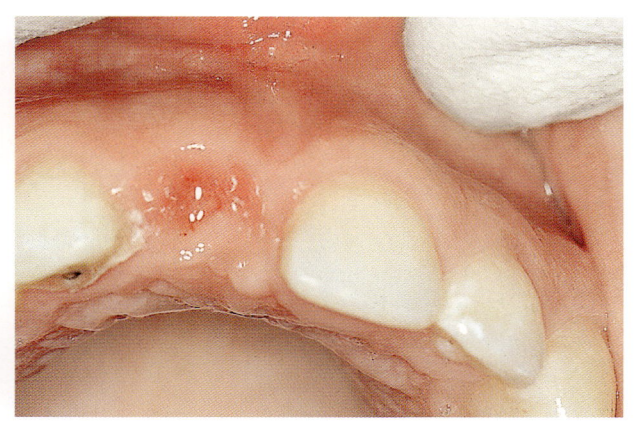

**Fig 8-5** Occlusal view showing adequate width of the residual ridge.

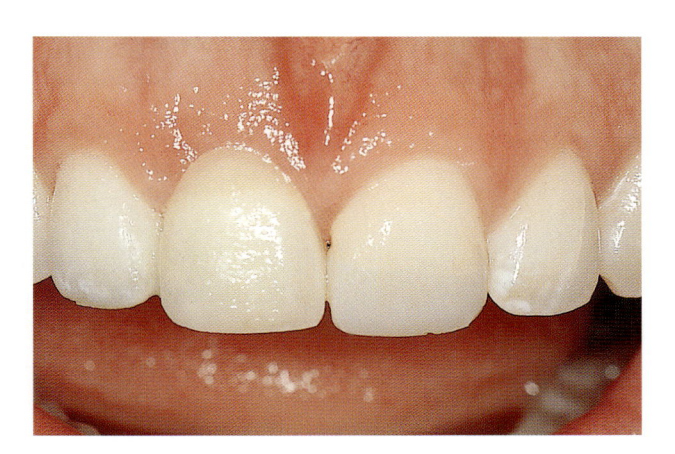

**Fig 8-6** Metal-acrylic resin Rochette bridge replacing the maxillary right central incisor demonstrating excessive tooth length.

## Assessment

### Clinical Assessment

The clinical appearance of the ridge height and width should be assessed (Figs 8-4 and 8-5). The ridge height should be compared with the papillary height of the adjacent teeth. The width should be assessed in relation to the labial contour around the adjacent teeth. The gingival margin and the height of the papillae should be noted, because scalloped thin papillae are more difficult to reproduce than flat and thick papillae (see Figs 6-6 and 6-7, p. 34).

Although the height and width of bone can be assessed using radiographic means (CT) or ridge mapping, the relationship of the ridge to the future tooth requires assessment. This can be achieved accurately by positioning a tooth in the desired position and noting the projected gingival contours (Fig 8-6).

The number of missing teeth will also have a bearing on the treatment outcome; consequently the length of the ridge (e.g. mesiodistal space) in relationship to the number and size of the teeth will influence the treatment plan. The precise location of the implant site will influence the emergence profile, the interdental bone height and the soft tissue contours.

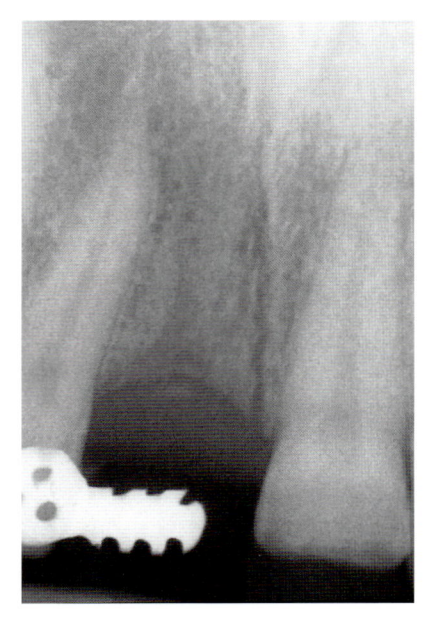

## Implant Placement: Surgery and Prosthodontics

**Fig 8-7** Preoperative periapical radiograph demonstrating adequate bone and local anatomy such as naso-palatine canal and proximity of roots.

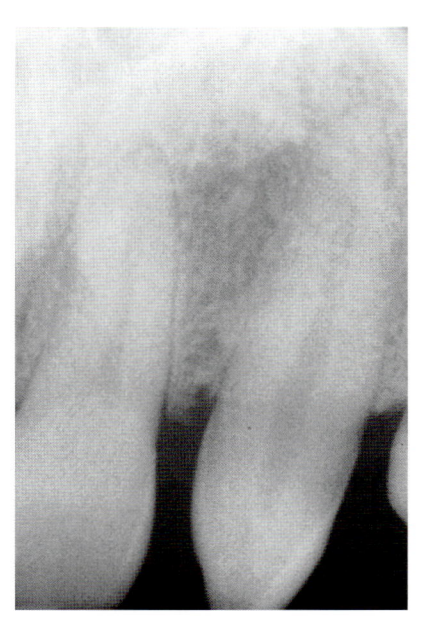

**Fig 8-8** Preoperative periapical radiograph of the region requiring restoration, showing inadequate space for implant placement.

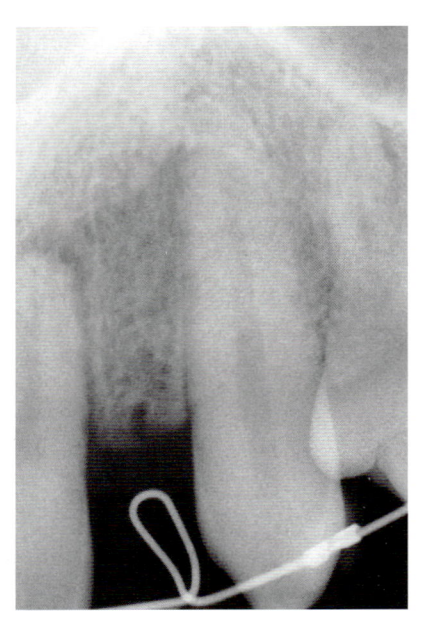

**Fig 8-9** Periapical radiograph on completion of the orthodontic treatment, showing sufficient interdental space. (Orthodontics carried out by Dr Peter Gascoigne, London, UK.)

### Radiographic Assessment
#### Periapical Radiograph

Periapical radiographs are valuable for establishing the status of healing following tooth loss and for the elimination of any pathology. Any residual roots or pathology can be identified on the radiograph. The interdental ridge height as well as the bone level at the proposed implant site can be measured in relation to the cementoenamel junction of the adjacent teeth.

An impression of the ridge width can be gained by trabecular density, although this cannot be relied on. Relevant anatomical structures (e.g. naso-palatine canal or the inferior alveolar canal) and their proximity to the implant site can be estimated from a periapical radiograph.

The height of the available bone can be accurately assessed using techniques where the distortion is known or minimal. The mesiodistal dimensions of the available bone and the space available between the adjacent roots and the orientation of the roots can also be determined using this type of radiograph (Figs 8-7–8-9).

#### Dental Panoramic Tomography (Orthopantomography)

DPTs provide an excellent overview of the jaws, confirming the information obtained from periapical radiographs.

#### Computed Tomography

CT provides very useful 3D information regarding the spatial orientation of the ridge when the tooth position has been identified with markers of distinct radiopacity. Additional information relating to bone density measurements will facilitate the decision whether to load immediately or not. Furthermore, CT will provide guidance regarding techniques to be employed during surgery.

### Preoperative Stage

Where there will be delayed insertion of an implant in a mature ridge, the following preoperative stages are considered pertinent to accurate assessment. Impressions of the mandible and maxilla, coupled with a facebow when required, can be used to provide the diagnostic and treatment aids described below.

## Diagnostic Preview

The arrangement of acrylic resin denture teeth of the correct form on a baseplate in the ideal aesthetic and functional position can be used to assess the possible treatment outcome by transferring the preview to the patient's mouth. Pink wax should not be used on the labial aspect, and flanges are contraindicated. An assessment of the tooth length can only be made when the tooth or tooth-coloured wax is used in contact with the soft tissues, providing a contrast to facilitate assessment.

The relationship of the ideal tooth form to the residual ridge can be used to establish the need for augmentation. A decision regarding the use of maxillary bone expansion or autogenous onlay graft to achieve the ideal ridge contour can be made in conjunction with appropriate diagnostic imaging techniques. Patients' involvement in this assessment process is fundamental to informed consent. More effective feedback can be obtained by transferring this information into a fixed provisional restoration.

## Diagnostic Template

On completion of the assessment, the information gathered can be transferred to a template constructed from the diagnostic preview.

The concept of a hollow prosthetic envelope to transfer the validated aesthetic and functional parameters to the surgical site is considered to be the most effective means of guidance during surgical phases.[120] The diagnostic template may be used for a number of purposes:
- positioning a bone graft to ensure insertion of an implant in the ideal position
- confirming the implant site selected using established guidelines that take into account local anatomical parameters
- selecting and confirming the abutment and its position within the prosthetic envelope to permit the proposed restoration
- indicating any requirement for manipulation of the soft tissues to establish the desired contour.

Templates designed in the laboratory to guide the surgeon in the positioning of the implant are considered inappropriate and liable to cause surgical error, since anatomical details are not available to the laboratory. Furthermore, directional drilling guides built into templates by the laboratory without accurate guidance from 3D imaging are considered to be equally dangerous.

## Drill Guides Based on CT Data

Guides may be fabricated based on accurate planning using interactive CT data-based computer software. The clinician is, therefore, responsible for selecting the precise implant position and angulation, using appropriate software. This is limited by the accuracy of the technology used. The ideal tooth position must also be transferred and visualised on the CT scan in order to accurately coincide implant and tooth position. The template should then be fabricated by direct and accurate means, such as stereolithography, using the data provided by the clinician. The template must be supported by a rigid structure, such as bone or teeth. If soft tissue support for the template is planned, additional fixation is recommended. However, the prerequisites for transmucosal (flapless) surgery are adequate keratinised non-mobile soft tissue in addition to adequate hard tissue. Artefacts from restorations might prevent accurate planning and further limit the use of this approach (see Fig 7-192, p. 99).

## Provisional Restoration

Provisional restorations may be used to replace missing teeth during the phases of treatment. They serve the valuable purpose of providing verification for the established aesthetic design and occlusal scheme. Varying benefit can be gained depending on the type of restoration used.

### Removable Dentures

Removable dentures should be made of acrylic resin to allow modifications to be easily made in situations where the ridge contour is altered. Limited diagnostic information is available for aesthetic assessment, particularly if flanges are used (Figs 8-10 and 8-11).

Furthermore, dentures are inherently unstable and provide little information with respect to function. They pose an increased risk when used during augmentation procedures.

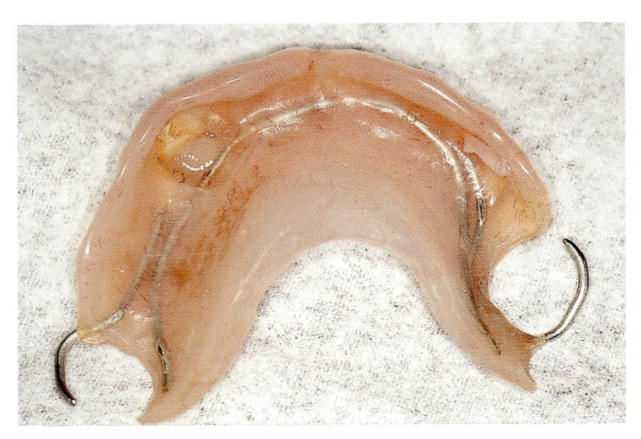

## II  Implant Placement: Surgery and Prosthodontics

**Fig 8-10** Partial acrylic resin denture with flange that requires replacement.

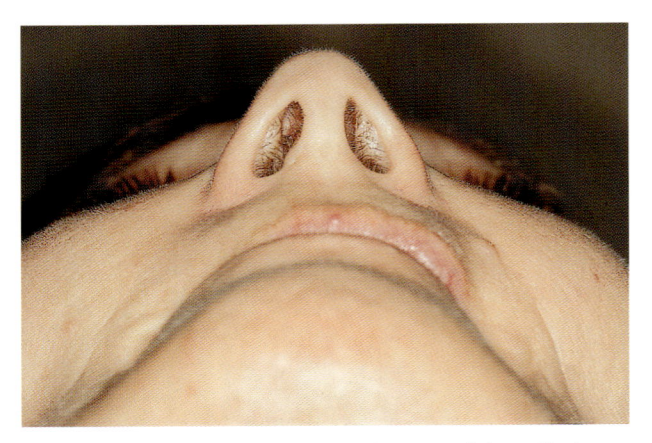

**Fig 8-11** Extraoral view from caudal aspect of the patient without the denture demonstrating the loss of lip support.

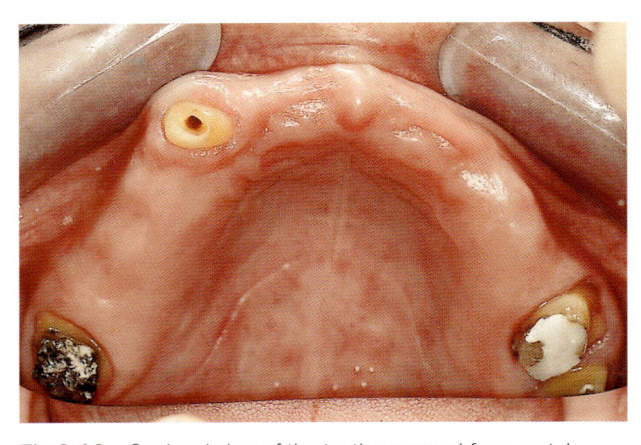

**Fig 8-12** Occlusal view of the teeth prepared for a metal-acrylic bridge to provide the patient with a fixed restoration throughout the treatment time. The treatment of this patient has been described in Chapter 10.

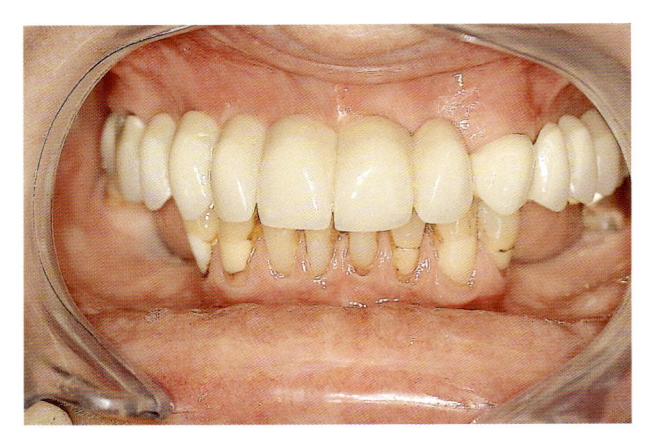

**Fig 8-13** Labial view of the metal-acrylic bridge in place. The bridge will provide functional and aesthetic feedback during the course of the treatment, which requires augmentation and implant placement.

### Conventional Bridgework

Bridgework is indicated when the crowning of adjacent teeth is necessary or justified. Changes in occlusal scheme can be effected when necessary. Bridges should be constructed from metal and acrylic resin and designed to allow for changes in ridge contours. They provide an excellent diagnostic aid to assess aesthetics as well as function in terms of masticatory and phonetic performance (Figs 8-12 and 8-13).

### Fixed Resin-bonded Bridges

The preferred type of resin-bonded bridge is the Rochette constructed from metal and acrylic.[121] The design of the retainer with retention holes allows for predictable removal and re-cementation at the time of surgery (Figs 8-14–8-17). The acrylic resin allows the pontic to be bonded directly to the tooth, when required, for additional stability. Furthermore, alteration, both in terms of reduction and addition, is facilitated. The design of the metalwork should allow modifications of the acrylic resin without interference with the metal (Figs 8-18–8-20). The choice of material should be such that it has sufficient strength in thin sections. The preferred material for bonding the Rochette retainer is a powder- and liquid-based composite (New super C; Amco, Fremont, CA, USA). This bonds

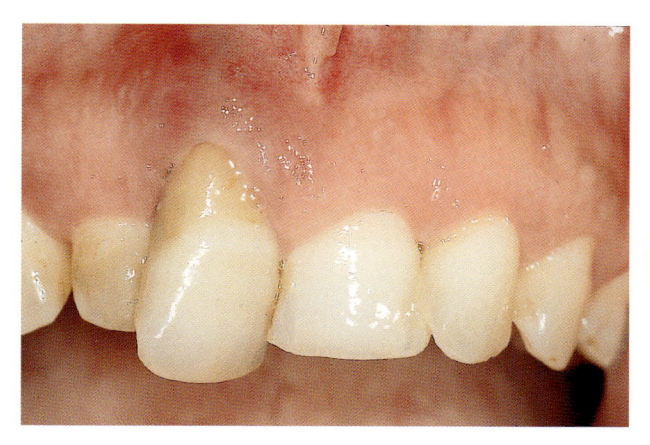

**8** Delayed Placement in Adequate Bone with Mature Ridge

**Fig 8-14** Labial view of a periodontally involved central incisor. The extrusion of the tooth as well as the associated bone loss is apparent.

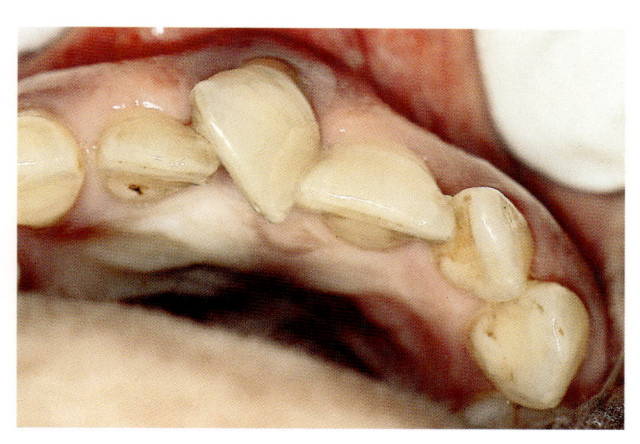

**Fig 8-15** Occlusal view of the same patient showing a limited amount of space available for the rotated central incisor between the adjacent teeth.

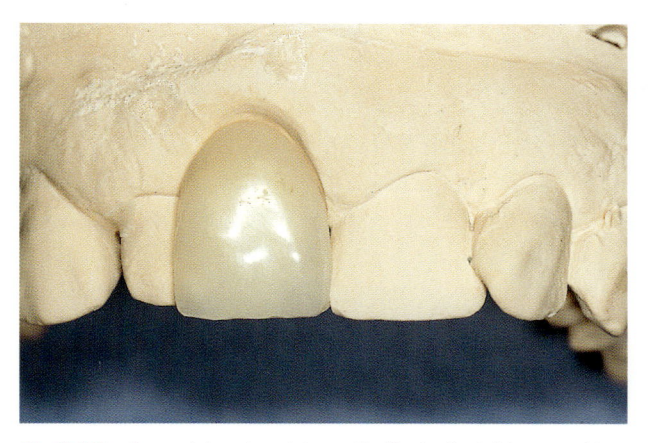

**Fig 8-16** A provisional metal-acrylic Rochette bridge provides an excellent opportunity to assess the manner in which the reduced space can be managed. The clinician and patient are able to assess the appearance that can be achieved by overlapping the lateral incisor with a tooth matching the left central incisor in width.

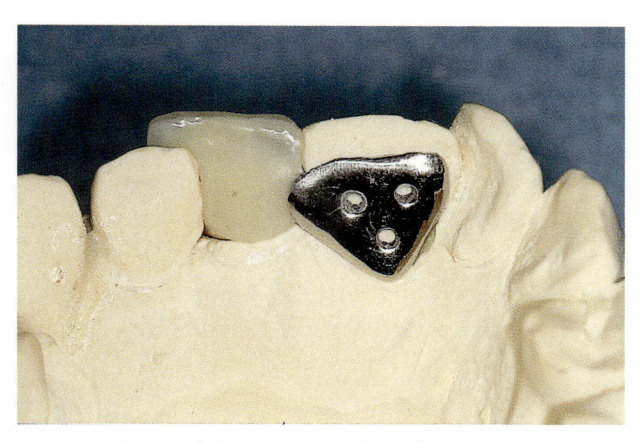

**Fig 8-17** Occlusal view of the metal-acrylic Rochette bridge showing the use of a single retainer on the palatal aspect of the central incisor. The design of the Rochette bridge using three holes to provide mechanical retention for the bridge to the tooth greatly facilitates the removal and replacement of the bridge. The single retainer provides very predictable retention during the treatment period. The manner in which the reduced amount of space available is used for the broader incisor is also apparent.

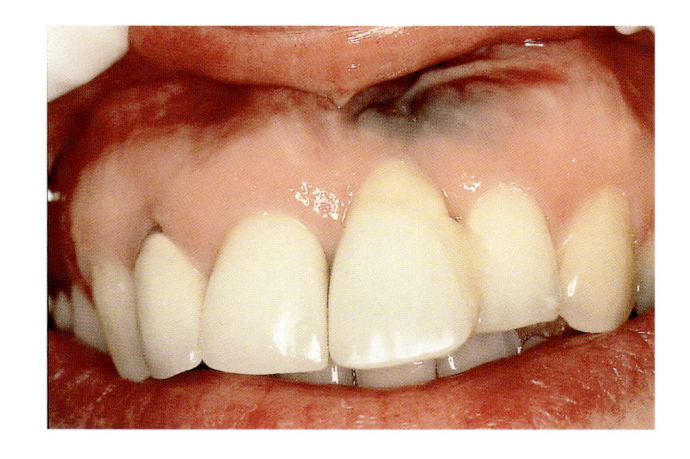

**Fig 8-18** Labial view of metal-acrylic Rochette bridge showing the increased cervical length of tooth caused by the loss of bone in the left central incisor region. This Rochette pontic is diagnostic of the need to increase the amount of bone by means of a bone graft.

111

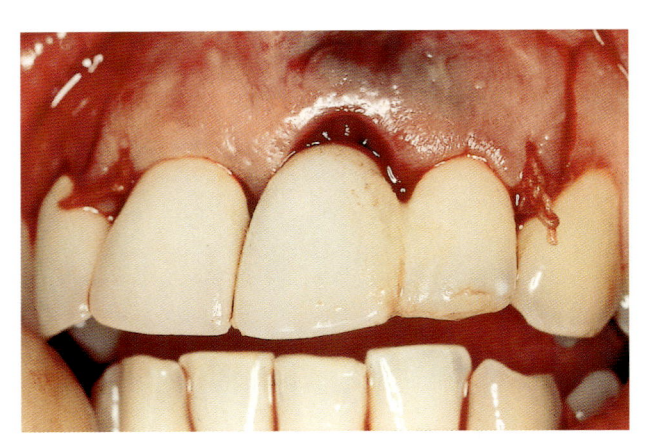

**Fig 8-19** The Rochette bridge fitted following the bone grafting procedure to reconstruct the deficiency. The Rochette pontic has been reduced to permit seating and is indicative of adequate reconstruction. The amalgam tattoo has been displaced coronally as the soft tissue is advanced to cover the graft.

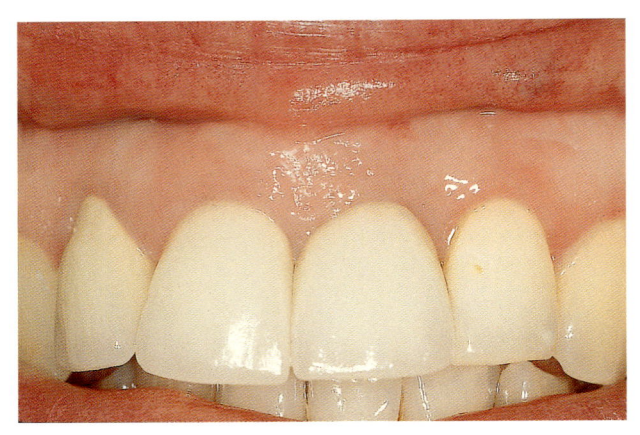

**Fig 8-20** The completed definitive restoration supported by an implant following soft tissue corrective surgery. (Restorative phase completed by Dr Russ Ladwa, London, UK.)

directly to the acrylic tooth, any residual composite on the tooth surface and the etched surface of the tooth. Consequently, re-cementation after completion of surgical procedures is greatly facilitated. The clinical evaluation of the Rochette bridge demonstrates its usefulness as a means of temporarily replacing missing teeth during implant treatment.[122]

The design of the Rochette will depend on the clinical situation as follows.

- **Tooth surface.** The ideal surface for bonding is enamel, which can be etched for adhesion of the composite cement. Porcelain surfaces need to be blasted, etched with hydrofluoric acid and treated with a silane-coupling agent before bonding with composite. Dentine-bonding agents do not offer the same bond strength as those bonding to enamel. Metal surfaces are unsuitable for bonding within the mouth if they are not silicoated (e.g. tribochemical coating with CoJet, 3M-ESPE; St Paul, MN, USA) and prepared with a silane-coupling agent.[123–125] Enamel remains the most predictable surface, producing good bond strength. When an adequate surface area for bonding is available, single retainers offer the most predictable results for single anterior teeth (Figs 8-17 and 8-21).
- **Occlusal clearance.** Sufficient space is necessary for a stable retainer (minimum thickness of 0.5 mm). In the absence of adequate space, the retainer needs to be located at a distance from the pontic area (Figs 8-22–8-24). Alternatively, the Dahl principle can be applied, which involves incorporating a platform that will come into contact with the opposing teeth prematurely, thus adjusting the occlusal levels; alternatively the opposing dentition can be adjusted, but this may be met with resistance from the patient (Figs 8-25–8-30).[126]
- **Location of retainer and pontic.** When posterior teeth are being replaced, retention for the Rochette bridge can be gained from the buccal and palatal surfaces of the molar teeth. The ability to provide retention and occusal rests makes posterior Rochette bridges very stable, with a minimum risk of debonding.
- **Distance between pontic and retainer.** In the event that no suitable teeth are available to bond to, a retainer at a site distant to the pontic may be selected and connected by a spring cantilever.

Rochette bridges can be constructed to extend over long spans replacing many teeth with several retainers and offer the advantage of preserving tooth tissue, particularly where the abutment teeth are sound (Figs 8-31–8-44). However, only limited changes in the occlusal scheme are practicable with this modality.

**8** Delayed Placement in Adequate Bone with Mature Ridge

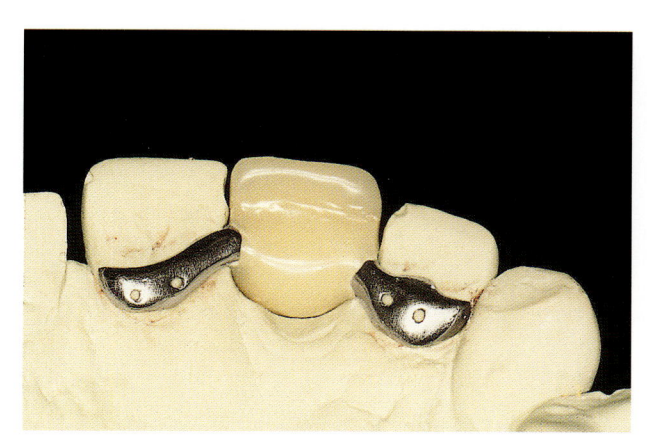

**Fig 8-21** The use of two wings may become necessary because of the amount of space available in patients where there is substantial contact with the teeth in the opposing jaw. Using bilateral retainers compensates for the reduction in the surface area for retention.

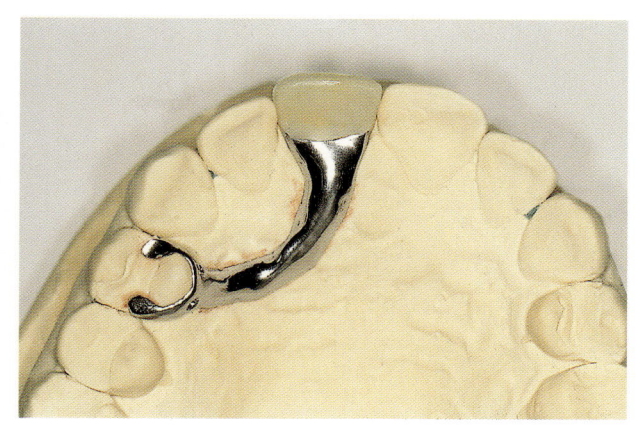

**Fig 8-22** Occlusal view of a spring cantilever metal-acrylic Rochette bridge that gains support and retention from a premolar tooth. The spring cantilever bridge becomes indicated in situations where the adjacent teeth have a surface that is difficult to bond to or when inadequate occlusal clearance is available. The use of occlusal rests facilitates seating. The extension of the retentive wing onto the buccal aspect would provide greater security but interferes with aesthetics.

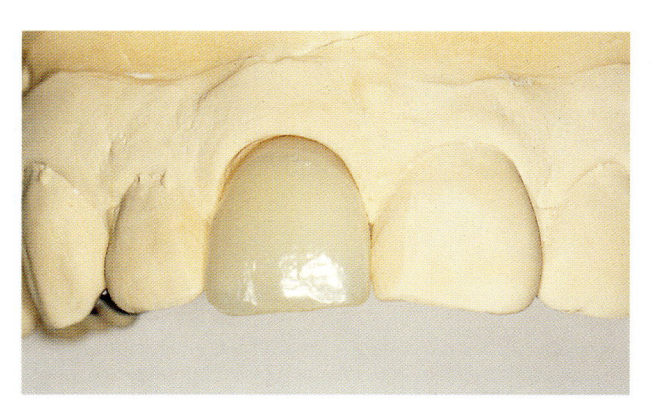

**Fig 8-23** Labial view of the spring cantilever Rochette bridge demonstrating its use as a diagnostic tool.

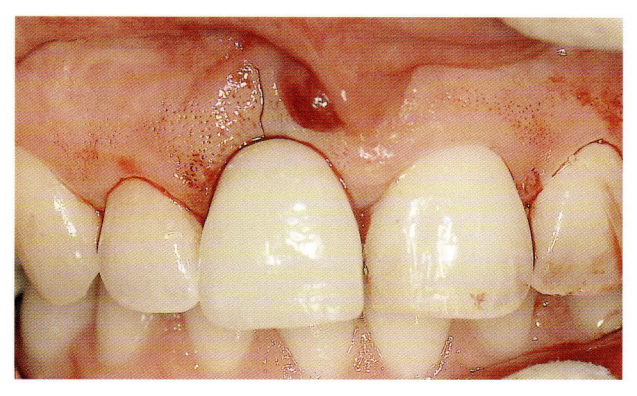

**Fig 8-24** Clinical view of the Rochette bridge described above on cementation immediately after the extraction of the maxillary right central incisor.

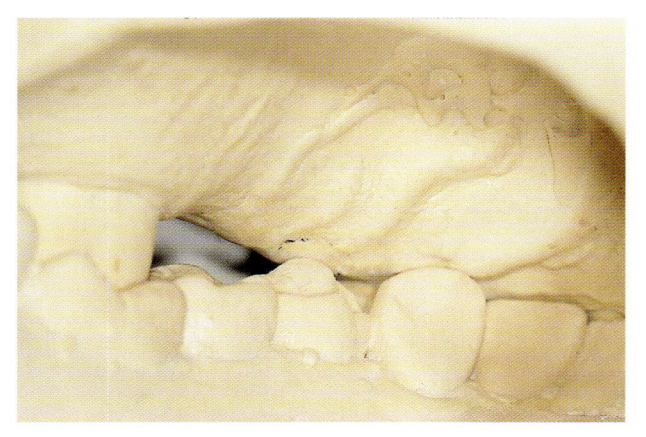

**Fig 8-25** Palatal view of diagnostic study casts in occlusion showing inadequate occlusal clearance. The mandibular premolar can be seen in contact with the upper mucosa.

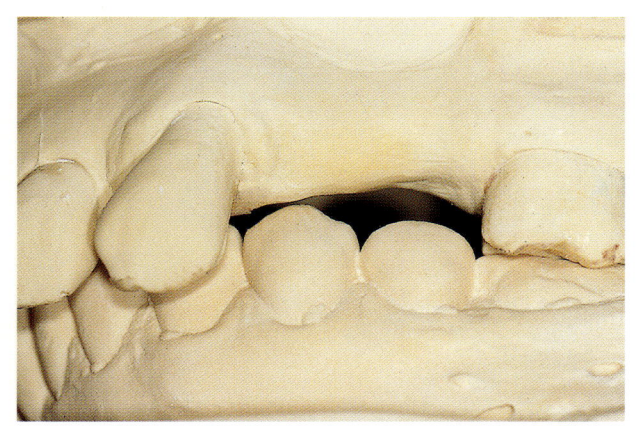

**Fig 8-26** Labial view of the study casts showing the buccolingual relationship of the teeth and the opposing alveolar ridge.

113

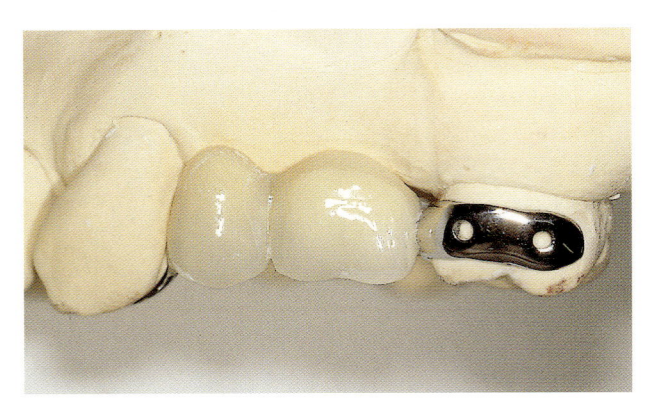

II  Implant Placement: Surgery and Prosthodontics

**Fig 8-27** Labial view of metal-acrylic resin Rochette bridge, which utilises a buccal wing on the second molar for support and retention.

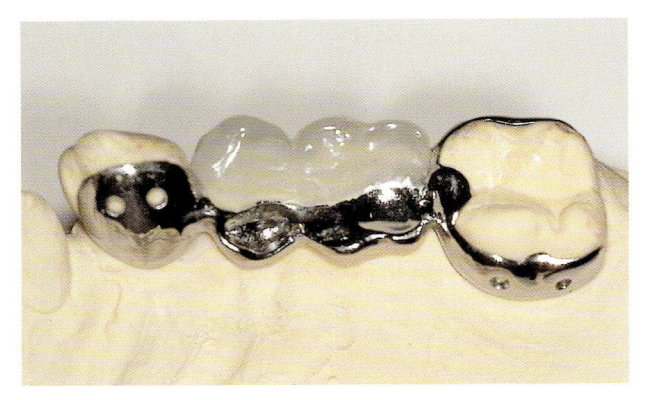

**Fig 8-28** Occlusal view of Rochette bridge showing a palatal wing on the canine and the second molar. In addition the occlusal rest on the molar is visible. The occlusal surfaces of the premolar and molar teeth have been designed out of metal to intercuspate with the overerupted mandibular premolars, utilising the Dahl principle for the creation of interdental space.

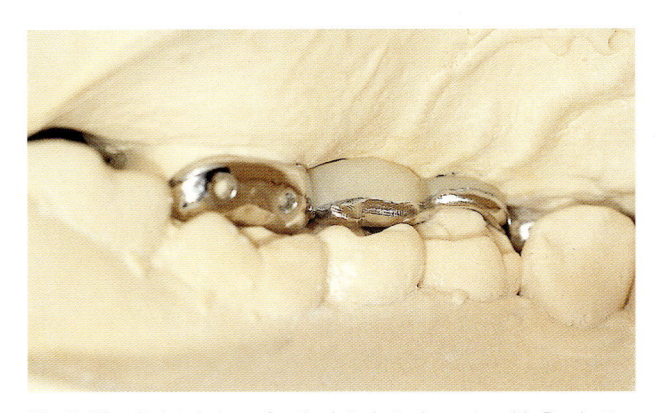

**Fig 8-29** Palatal view of articulated study casts with Rochette bridge in situ.

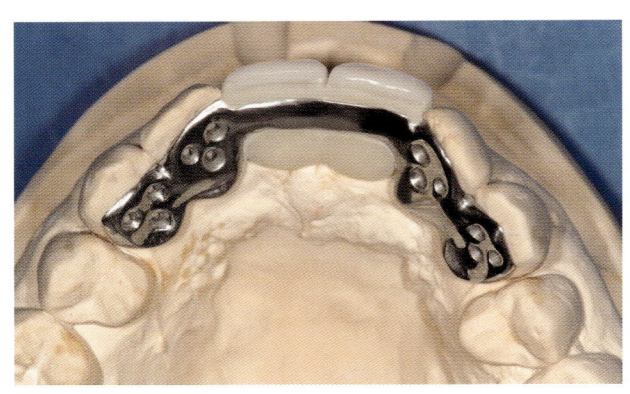

**Fig 8-30** Occlusal view of a Dahl appliance/Rochette bridge, designed to intrude the mandibular incisors to create space for bone graft and implants in a patient with a traumatic bite directly into the palatal soft tissues. The use of retainers on the lateral incisors and canines was designed to provide stability to the maxillary provisional restoration.

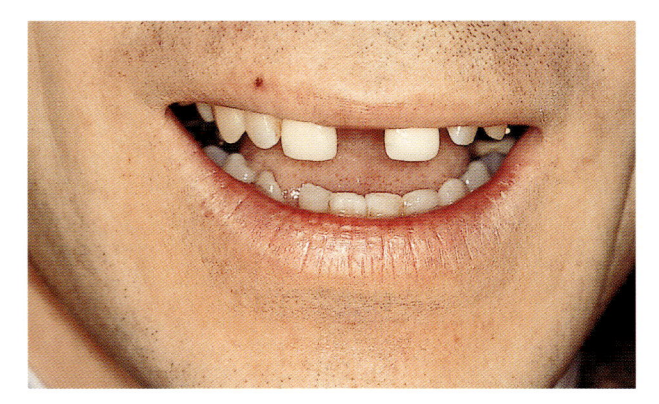

**Fig 8-31** Preoperative photograph of a patient with a large central diastema posing a difficult restorative problem which requires accurate diagnostic resolution prior to embarking on surgical procedures to replace the two central incisors with implants.

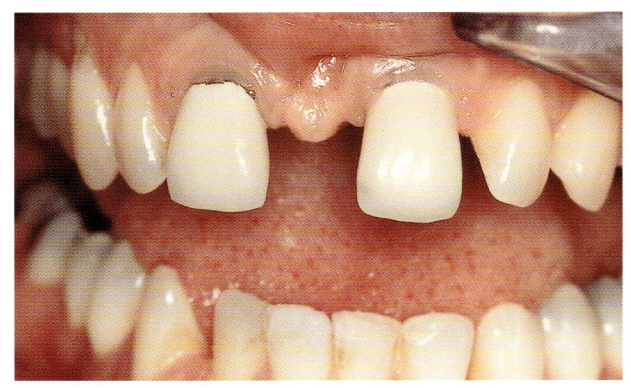

**Fig 8-32** Intraoral labial view of failing crowns providing an idea of the dimensions of the diastema that need to be addressed.

**8** Delayed Placement in Adequate Bone with Mature Ridge

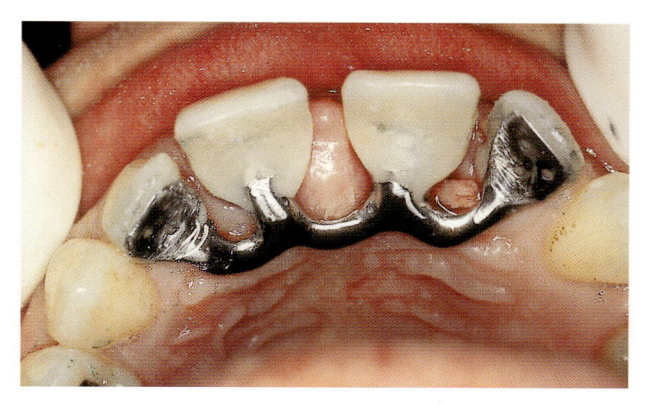

**Fig 8-33** Palatal view of spring cantilever metal-acrylic Rochette bridge retained by the two lateral incisors.

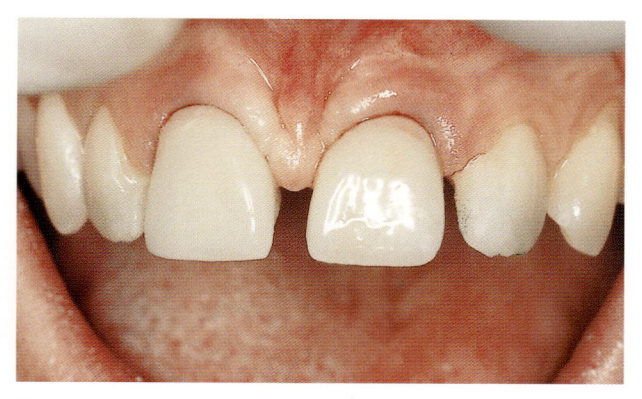

**Fig 8-34** Labial view of the metal-acrylic Rochette bridge in situ. The bridge will provide both the clinician and the patient with an opportunity to assess the appearance before proceeding with the surgical treatment. The position of the bone graft and implants is determined by the tooth position, which must first be approved.

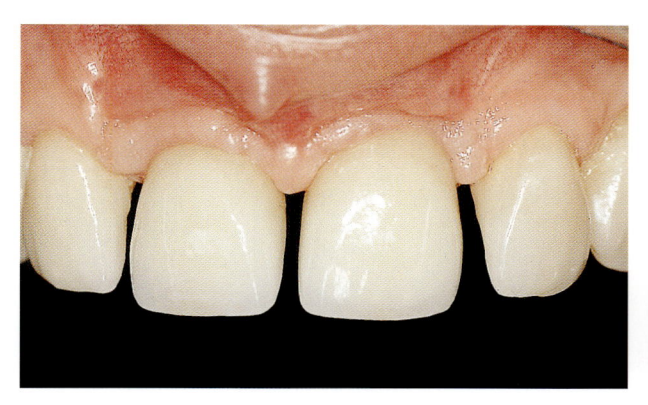

**Fig 8-35** Labial view of the definitive restorations consisting of two implant-supported crowns replacing the central incisors and porcelain veneers on the lateral incisors reducing diastemas between the central and lateral incisors.

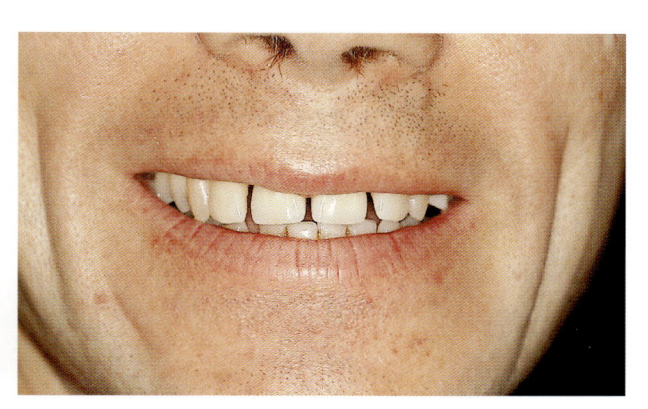

**Fig 8-36** Frontal view of the patient smiling with the definitive restorations.

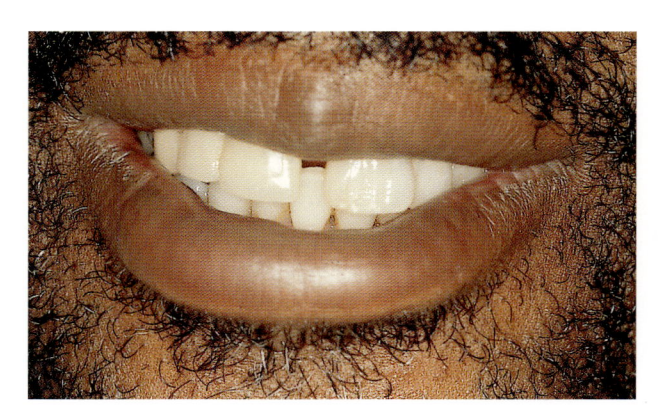

**Fig 8-37** Anterior view of patient with advanced periodontal disease exhibiting a large diastema caused by the drifting of the anterior teeth. (Same patient as in Fig 14-42.)

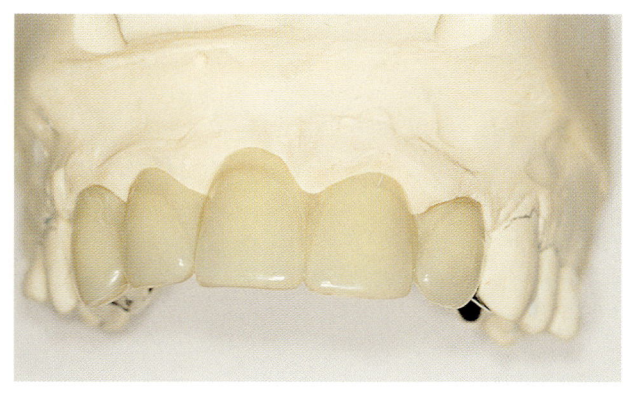

**Fig 8-38** Labial view of the metal-acrylic Rochette bridge designed to replace five anterior teeth. Note that the diastema has been eliminated and the size and position of the replacement teeth needs to be verified functionally and aesthetically.

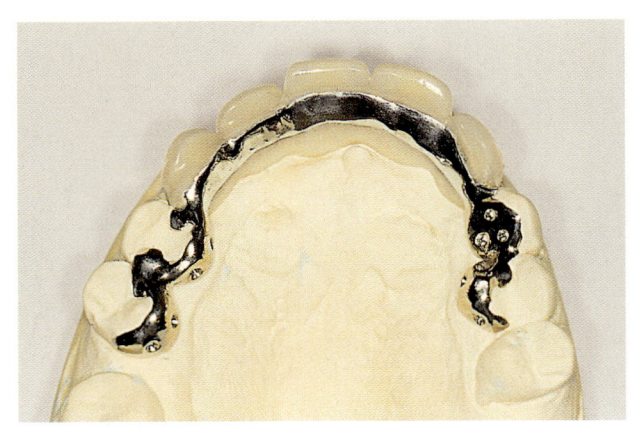

II Implant Placement: Surgery and Prosthodontics

**Fig 8-39** Occlusal view of the Rochette bridge showing the wings, which will provide retention for the bridge.

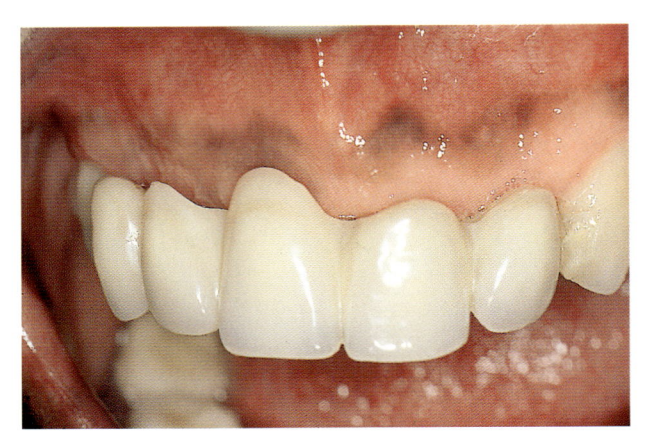

**Fig 8-40** Rochette bridge in situ showing the appearance that has been achieved.

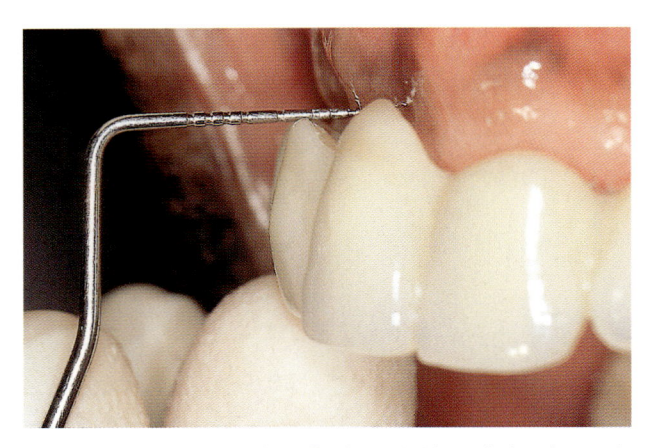

**Fig 8-41** Lateral view of the Rochette bridge relating the tooth position, which has been selected for functional and aesthetic outcome, to the healed residual alveolar ridge.

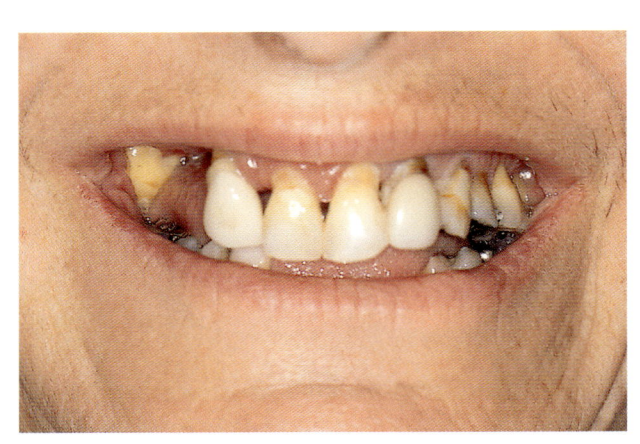

**Fig 8-42** Preoperative anterior view of a patient with failing dentition.

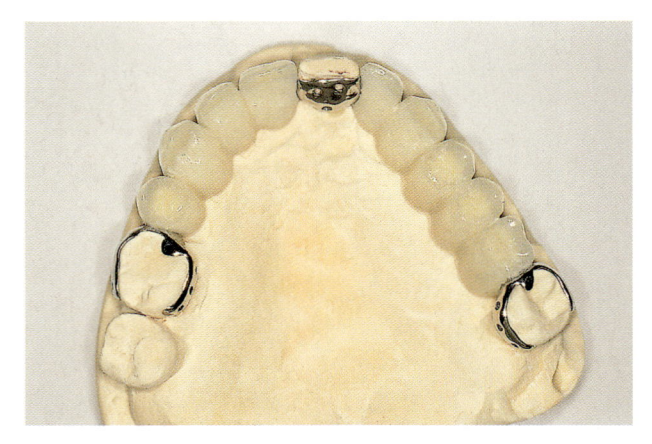

**Fig 8-43** Occlusal view of the laboratory cast with large-span metal-acrylic Rochette bridge.

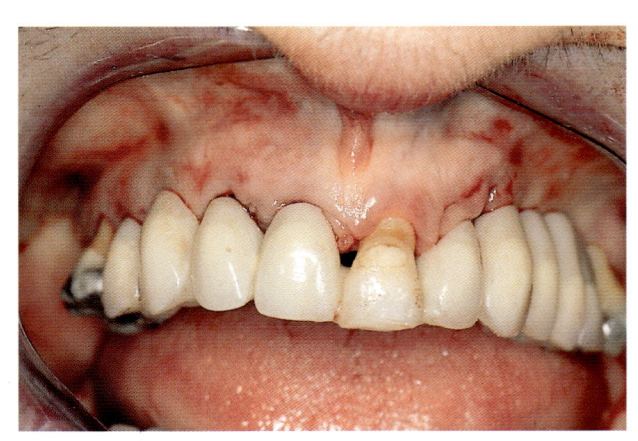

**Fig 8-44** Labial view of the same Rochette bridge cemented into place immediately on extraction of the failing teeth.

## 8 Delayed Placement in Adequate Bone with Mature Ridge

### Hybrid Bridges

Rochette retainers and full-preparation retainers can be combined wherever appropriate, resulting in a hybrid bridge. Such a structure is typically used when there is a large space bounded at one end by a tooth that needs crowning and at the other by a tooth that would be inappropriate to crown (Figs 8-45–8-50).

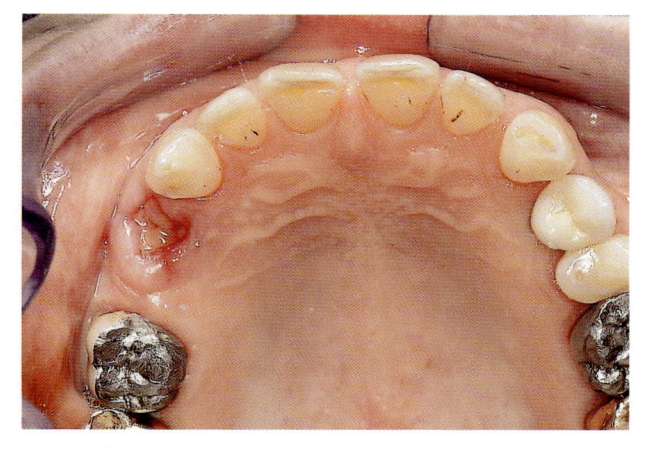

**Fig 8-45** Occlusal view of patient requiring restoration of the maxillary premolars with implants. The molar is restored with a crown that requires replacement, the canine is unrestored. (Same patient as Fig 10-18.)

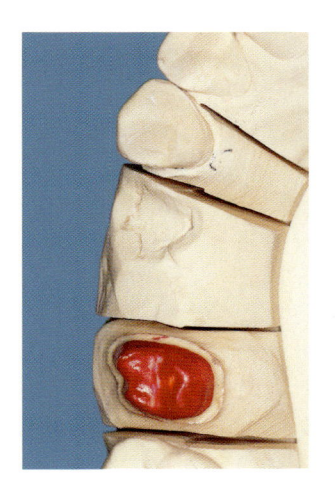

**Fig 8-46** Occlusal view of the working cast with the prepared die of the first molar.

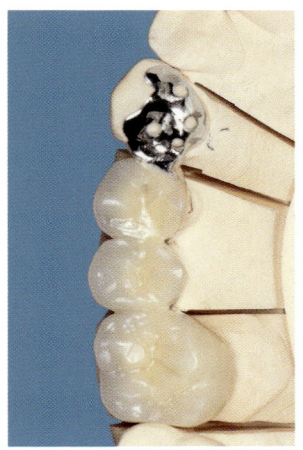

**Fig 8-47** The completed metal-acrylic bridge with full coverage retainer on the first molar and a metal Rochette wing on the canine.

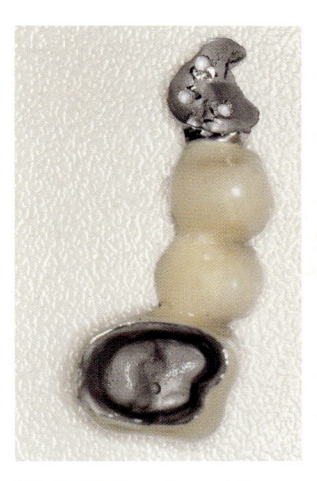

**Fig 8-48** Fit surface of the hybrid metal-acrylic Rochette bridge.

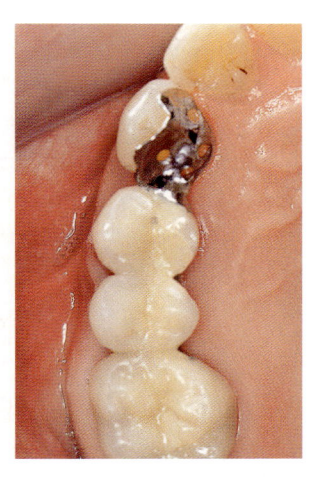

**Fig 8-49** Occlusal view of the fitted metal-acrylic hybrid Rochette bridge.

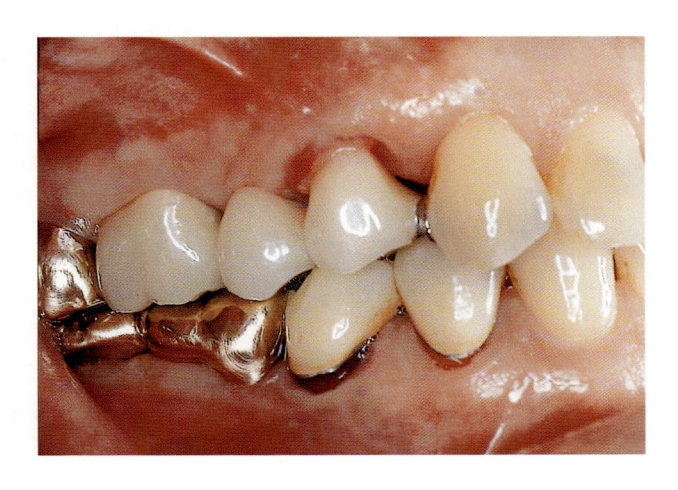

**Fig 8-50** Labial view of the same fixed partial denture as shown in Fig 8-49.

II  Implant Placement: Surgery and Prosthodontics

## Considerations Specific To Immediate Loading

When deciding whether immediate loading is possible, the main criteria to be considered are as follows (see also Chapter 7):

- Adequate bone density to allow primary stability to be achieved.
- There should be adequate bone width as it may not be appropriate for an implant to be loaded immediately following the manipulation of the labial plate, which may well, in turn, result in compromised primary stability.
- The absence of any minor bone deficiencies that may require the use of a membrane for guided bone regeneration.
- Aesthetics are of prime importance for consideration in the anterior maxillary region. The protocol for delayed loading offers more opportunities to position the implant precisely and to re-contour the soft tissues during implant placement. It also provides a second opportunity to create the required emergence profile by positioning the incision for implant exposure based on the contours established on completion of integration. Furthermore, impressions at first-stage surgery can be taken. This provides the opportunity to have the abutment and transitional restoration available at the time of implant exposure to create the desired soft tissue profile.

**Table 8-1** Assessment checklist of a future implant site for delayed placement

| | |
|---|---|
| Degree of healing | |
| Pathology | |
| Amount of bone | |
| • height | |
| • width | |
| • length of ridge | |
| Soft tissue check | |
| Gingival margin | |
| Papillae | |
| Bone density | |
| Diagnostic preview | |
| Provisional restoration | |

If immediate loading is planned, its execution will be dependent on the achievement of adequate primary stability at implant placement, as introduced in the chapter on immediate placement (Chapter 7).

Therefore, additional component parts and laboratory work must be planned (see below under immediate loading). The steps prior to delayed placement of an implant in a healed site are summarised in Table 8-1.

## Implant Placement

Access to the bony ridge depends on the preoperative criteria, which would determine whether immediate or delayed loading is planned. The clinical stages for delayed placement of implants with intended immediate loading are summarised in Flowchart 8-3 (see pp. 120–121). Where delayed loading is planned, two-stage surgery is intended using a remote incision for stage one and a suitable incision for exposure of the implant at the second stage, as outlined in Chapter 9.

### Incision for Delayed Loading

Access to the bony ridge should be made using remote incisions to reduce the risk of early implant exposure. Remote palatal incisions are used in the maxilla (Figs 8-51 and 8-52) and remote buccal incisions in the mandible. Crestal incisions may also be used, particularly in the mandible. Closure of a crestal incision should be carried out using a suturing technique that ensures tight wound closure.

### Incision for Immediate Loading or for Transgingival Healing

A crestal incision is necessary to be able to attach the abutment or sulcus former following implant placement. The precise location of the incision should be designed to create the soft tissue contours required. In the maxilla, the incision is made towards the palatal aspect of the crest, which provides a surplus of tissue on the labial aspect and thus the option of manipulating it to create the gingival margin and papillae (Figs 8-53 and 8-54). Alternatively, a broad 'H'-shaped incision may be used where the procedure can be carried out with minimum exposure of the bony ridge. Attached

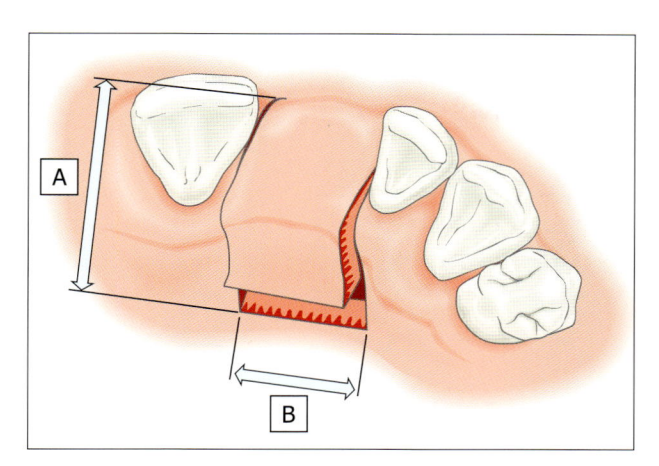

**8**  Delayed Placement in Adequate Bone with Mature Ridge

**Fig 8-51**  Diagram of a palatal incision for delayed loading. Little or no exposure of the labial cortical plate is necessary. The incision consists of two separate components: (A) incisions perpendicular to the ridge extending 10 mm into the palate on either side of the gap; (B) a bevelled component, which is executed parallel to the ridge and joins the two incisions made perpendicular to the ridge. This is normally carried out by means of a Blake's knife. This produces a buccally based flap, the incision remaining distant from the site where the implant and any augmentation material might be positioned.

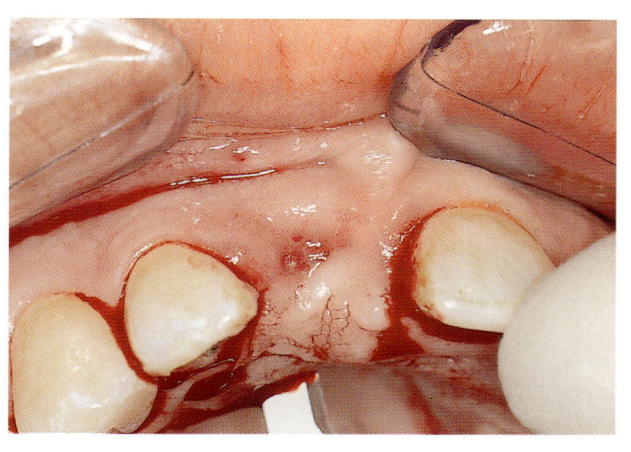

**Fig 8-52**  Occlusal view of the ridge showing the palatal component of the incision for the remote buccally based flap made using a Blake's knife. The flap design is depicted in Fig 8-51.

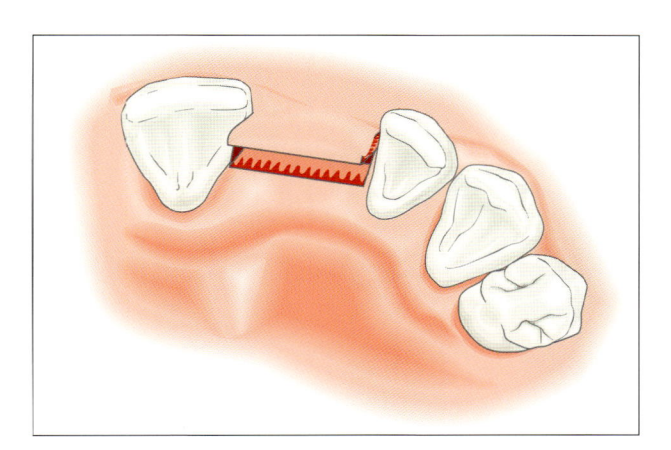

**Fig 8-53**  Incision for immediate loading. A crestal incision positioned on the palatal aspect of a ridge crest is considered ideal. It will permit the manipulation of the soft tissues to close the wound around the abutment and create papillae, as outlined in Chapter 9 on implant exposure. Alternatively, an 'H'-shaped incision may be used as long as adequate access to the ridge can be gained.

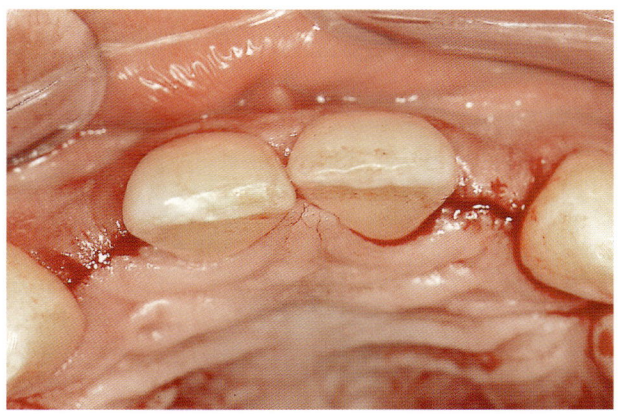

**Fig 8-54**  Full-thickness incision on the palatal aspect of the ridge, as shown in Fig 8-51.

keratinised tissues are sparse in the mandible and it therefore becomes necessary to bisect the available tissue. Certainly the incision should not be made towards the lingual aspect because of the very friable nature of the mucosa and the risk of damage to anatomical structures.

## Site Selection

Selection of the proper implant site is crucial for the successful clinical outcome of prosthetic restoration and must be confirmed by use of the diagnostic template, which outlines the planned position of the tooth.

II  Implant Placement: Surgery and Prosthodontics

**Laboratory**

- Study casts
- Set up teeth for preview
- Fabricate provisional restoration if required

Fabricate diagnostic template

Fabricate hollow acrylic transitional restoration

U/L & jaw relations

**Clinical**

Impressions

Clinical and radiographic assessment
Healed adequate hard and soft tissues

Implant placement

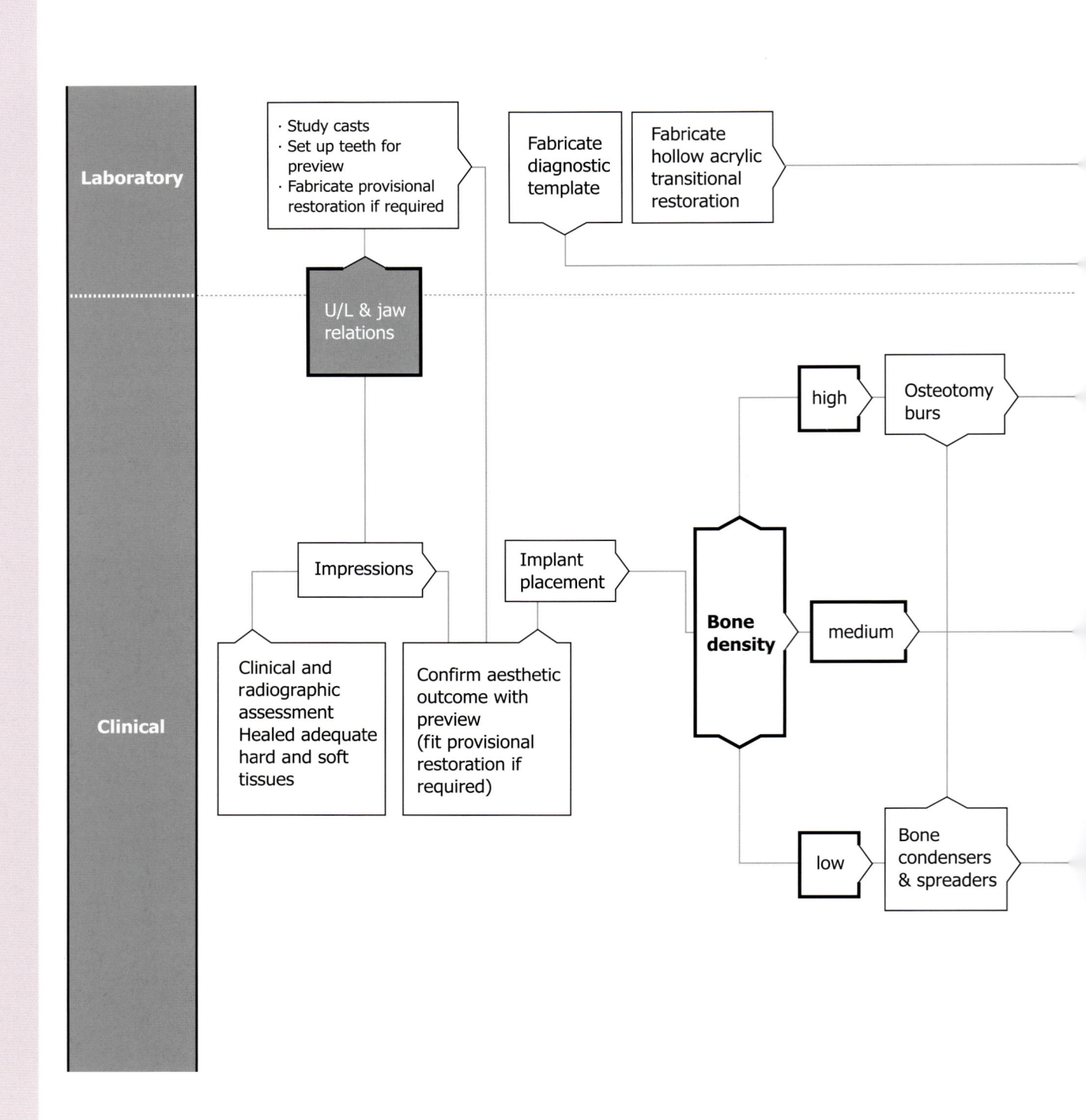

Confirm aesthetic outcome with preview (fit provisional restoration if required)

**Bone density**

high — Osteotomy burs

medium

low — Bone condensers & spreaders

**Flowchart 8-3**  Clinical stages for delayed placement of implants with intended immediate loading.

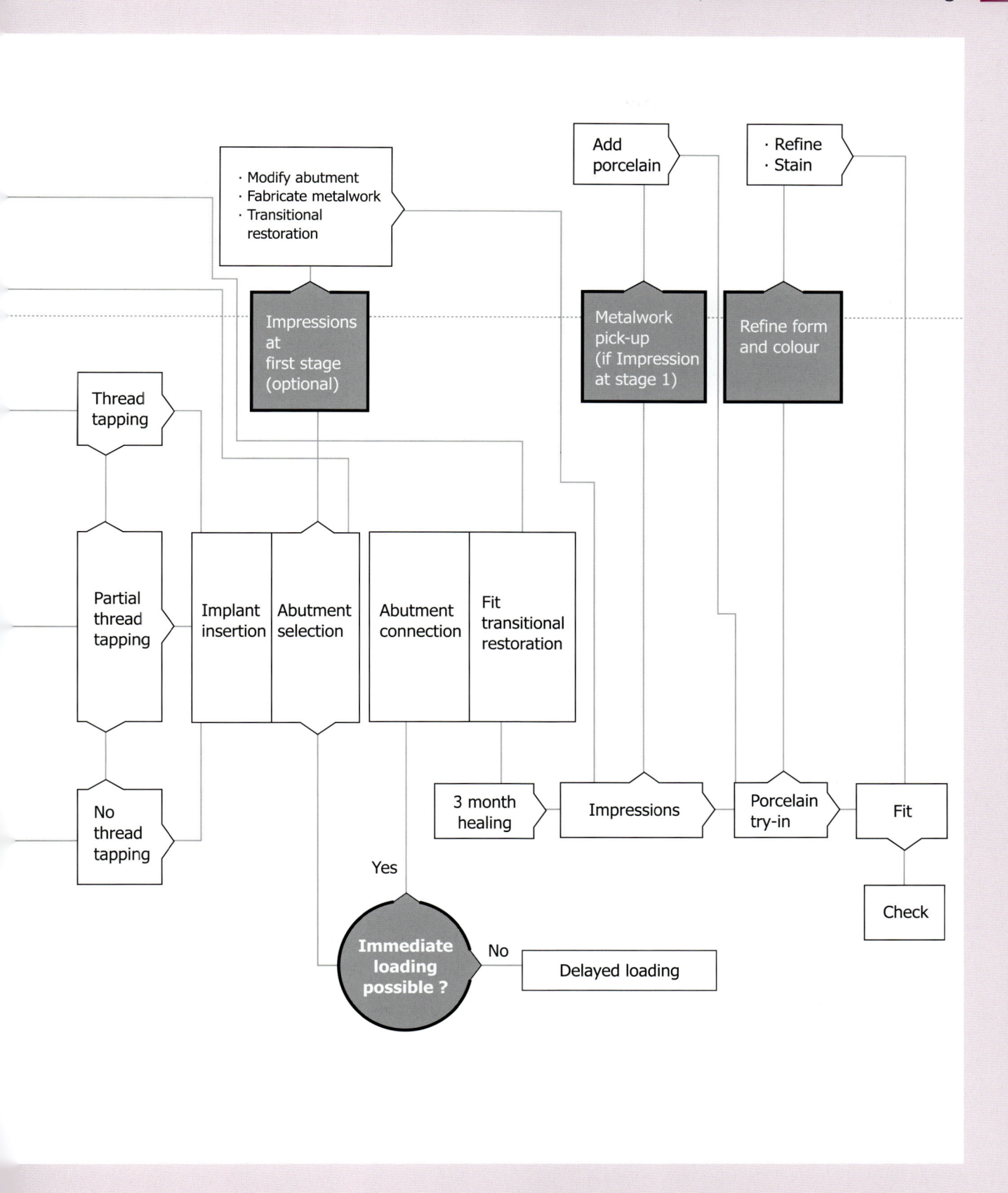

# 8 Delayed Placement in Adequate Bone with Mature Ridge

- Modify abutment
- Fabricate metalwork
- Transitional restoration

Add porcelain

- Refine
- Stain

Impressions at first stage (optional)

Metalwork pick-up (if Impression at stage 1)

Refine form and colour

Thread tapping

Partial thread tapping

Implant insertion

Abutment selection

Abutment connection

Fit transitional restoration

No thread tapping

3 month healing

Impressions

Porcelain try-in

Fit

Check

Yes

**Immediate loading possible ?**

No

Delayed loading

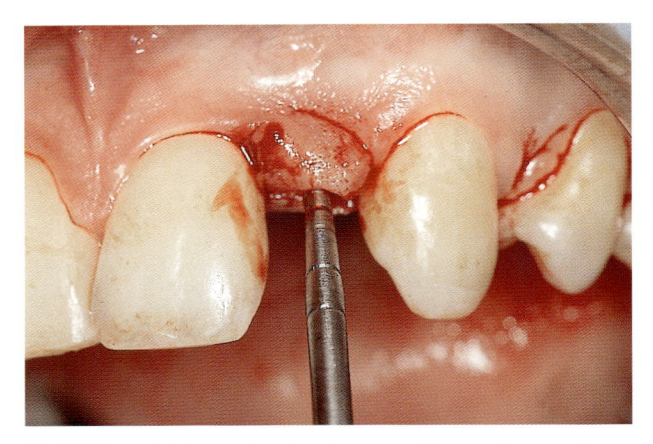

**II** Implant Placement: Surgery and Prosthodontics

Fig 8-55 Labial view showing the use of the position marker.

The osteotomy site is selected using a small round bur or a position marker (Fig 8-55) to determine the centre of the osteotomy. For a single implant, this should be positioned equidistant from the adjacent teeth and sufficiently distant from any critical anatomical structures to avoid any damage on completion of the osteotomy to the correct diameter. The osteotomy site should be positioned in the middle of the crest, and this position is best assessed visually. Any minor alteration in the position can be carried out as the site is enlarged and the margin of the osteotomy comes close to any of the boundaries. The consequences of incorrect site selection may only become evident during the restorative phase. Implant placement too far labially may result in abutment and implant dehiscence, thus compromising aesthetics. Palatal placement may result in interference with the occlusion or the need to use ridge-lapped crowns, with their inherent disadvantages.

For multiple implants the site must be selected to be in the middle of the ridge and centre of the prosthetic tooth as determined by the diagnostic template. The marked sites should be verified by direct measurements. They should be no closer than 4 mm to an adjacent tooth and no less than 7 mm from an adjacent implant site. For example, a 3.5-mm diameter implant should be placed no less than 2 mm away from an adjacent tooth and more than 3 mm away from an adjacent implant.[103,104]

When the dimensions of a tooth dictates that adjacent implants should be placed closer than 3 mm, then either a narrower diameter implant should be selected (e.g. 3 mm) or an implant that has a conical connection that prevents micro-leakage.[119] In relation to teeth where the crown width is less than 6 mm (e.g. mandibular incisors) it may become necessary to use a pontic between implants not placed adjacent to each other or to accept the mechanical disadvantage of a cantilevered tooth.

**Osteotomy Preparation**

The aim of the osteotomy is to use the maximum amount of bone available at the selected implant site, following sound surgical principles. Therefore, the osteotomy should be prepared without any dehiscence. The direction of the osteotomy should be determined using the adjacent teeth and the alveolar cortical plates as direction guides.

The position marker or a pilot bur (Lindemann bur) can be used to establish the direction of the osteotomy to the predetermined depth based on radiographic measurements. This will also provide an indication of the bone density or confirm the bone density established by a previous CT scan (Fig 8-56). The diameter of the osteotomy is then sequentially enlarged until the diameter of the desired implant has been attained (Fig 8-57). This provides an opportunity with each increased bur size to confirm the site position and the diameter of the implant to be used. To avoid thermal trauma to the bone,[127] internal irrigation for the burs is recommended.[128–130] Delivery of the coolant to the cutting tips greatly facilitates surgery, as the clinician can be assured of adequate irrigation and can concentrate on the completion of the osteotomy in the desired position.

In bone of high density, the bed for the implant must be formed completely. This may involve the use of any hand reamers and bone taps required by the implant system that is being employed (Fig 8-58). This is frequently true for the mandible and occasionally for the maxilla, particularly when implants of wider diameter are used.

In bone of low density in the maxilla, bone condensers are the preferred instruments because they enable the osteotomy to be formed with a minimal risk of perforating the labial or lingual plates (Fig 8-59). Furthermore, they increase the density of the surrounding bone, thus improving the degree of primary fixation that can be achieved.

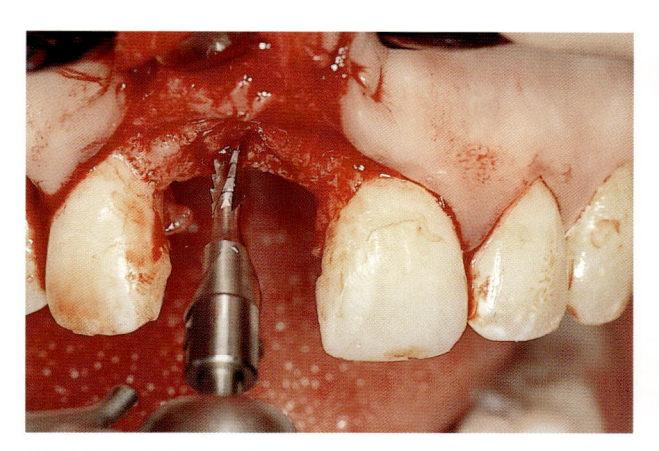

**8** Delayed Placement in Adequate Bone with Mature Ridge

**Fig 8-56** Lindemann bur being used to prepare pilot osteotomy establishing direction.

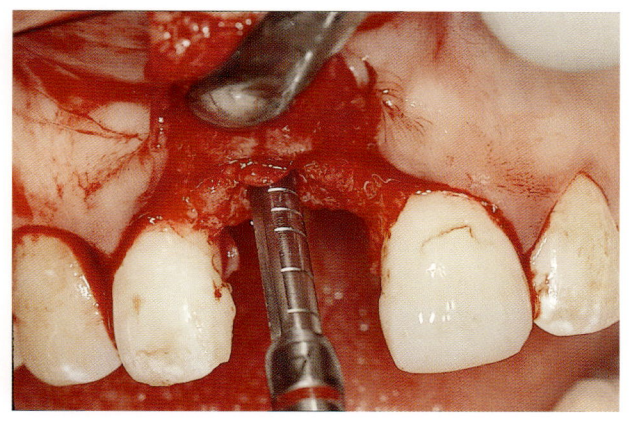

**Fig 8-57** Parallel drill (internally irrigated) being used to establish depth. In this case, the final diameter was established as well.

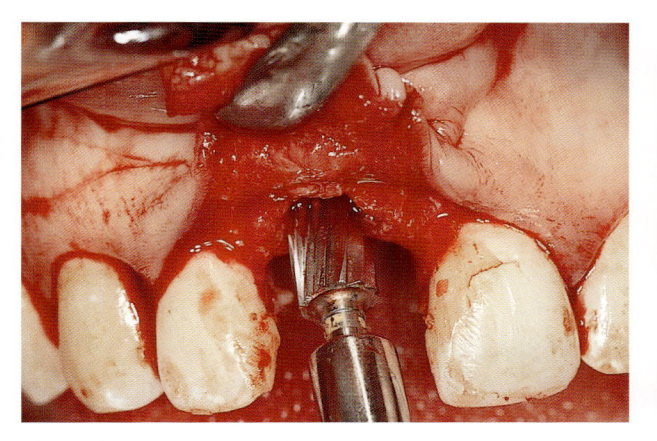

**Fig 8-58** Hand reamer being used to prepare osteotomy.

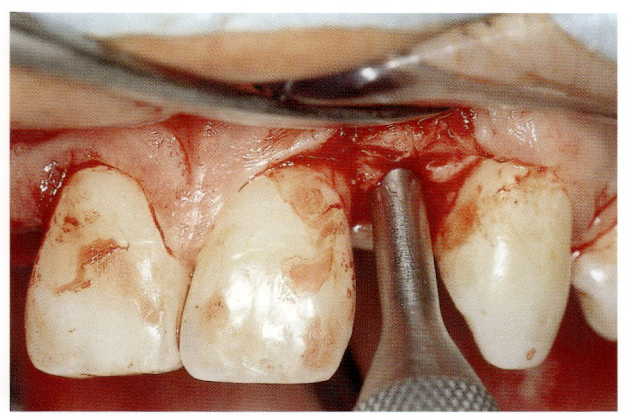

**Fig 8-59** Bone condenser being used to increase bone density.

In low-density bone, the implant may be inserted without any further development of the osteotomy. If excessive resistance is met during the insertion of the implant, the implant should be unscrewed by one to two turns and reinserted using the implant as a tap. Where there is greater resistance to insertion than met previously, the implant should be removed, the thread tapped and the implant reinserted.

In bone of moderate density, a hand reamer may be used and the osteotomy partly threaded with a bone tap before insertion of the implant. This variation in osteotomy preparation will ensure that adequate primary stability for the implant can be achieved, particularly where immediate loading is intended.

The depth of the osteotomy should be measured from the point on the crest of the ridge, which is used for the radiographic assessment of depth. The osteotomy should be planned so that it is 1 mm deeper than the selected implant length. It is imperative, of course, that the depth to which the osteotomy is going to be prepared is the depth that is used to establish clearance from vital structures. It is a wise clinician who always measures his osteotomy bur directly prior to drilling.

This provides some flexibility regarding the depth to which the implant is inserted without having to remove it to deepen the osteotomy when the implant needs to be inserted deeper. The need to increase the insertion depth of the implant may arise where a rounded ridge is present and the implant may be level with the crest of the ridge but prominent on the labial and lingual aspects. The labio-palatal position of the abutment will also be affected where the ridge is at an angle to the longitudinal axis of the proposed restoration. This is discussed in a later section. It should be borne in mind that cylindrical threaded implants are best suited for precise seating.

## Osteotomy Preparation Based on CT Data

Based on bone density measured from a CT scan, the following guidelines may be used. This is particularly critical when immediate loading is intended, where the clinician needs to ensure that he can complete the planned treatment. This is to bring the implant into function, which, in turn, is dependent on achieving adequate primary stability. The implant site, whether in the maxilla or the mandible, will have an influence on the management.

- **Low-density bone** (less than 300 HU). Immediate loading in low-density bone requires considerable skill and judgement during site preparation. Managing occlusal load becomes critical and full benefit should be gained from splinting of implants with multiple implant insertions. Most importantly the clinician should recognise those clinical situations where immediate loading of the implant should not be carried out.
  – *Maxilla.* Low-density bone is most commonly found in the posterior maxilla, particularly the tuberosity, which may be even as low as 0 HU (Fig 8-60). In these situations, there is no reason to use osteotomy burs, except perhaps to perforate the crest. Osteotomes are the primary means of preparing the implant bed. Bone taps are contraindicated. Manipulation of the sinus floor may also be carried out simultaneously.
  – *Mandible.* Low trabecular density in the mandible (most commonly the posterior mandible) is often combined with a denser cortical plate, which would need to be prepared using rotary instruments penetrating the crest. However, minimum preparation of the trabecular bone is required beyond the pilot bur unless the lingual and labial cortical plates are going to be engaged. Subcrestal placement would in this situation compromise the stability of the implant and a staged approach may be required.

- **Medium-density bone** (300–700 HU). This is the most favourable range of densities, where osteotomy preparation to gain good primary stability for the implant can be achieved (Fig 8-61).
  – *Maxilla.* The use of a pilot bur followed by bone condensers is indicated in the maxilla when minimum resistance to bone manipulation is met. This quality of bone is most commonly found in the anterior region. Osteotomy burs may be used in conjunction with tapered reamers when there is excessive resistance. If during insertion of the implant a torque greater than 30 Ncm is required, consideration needs to be given to either using the implant as a bone tap, by unscrewing and reinserting, or using a bone tap. The maximum force for insertion should not exceed 50 Ncm.
  – *Mandible.* Osteotomy burs and tapered reamers are invariably indicated in this quality of bone, which is found both in the anterior and posterior regions. Bone tapping can be commenced and stopped if no resistance is met. Caution should be exercised where labial and lingual plates are likely to be engaged.

- **High-density bone** (more than 700 HU). Preparing an osteotomy site in high-density bone is challenging, as adequate primary stability is required, but care needs to be taken not to underprepare the site and thus exceed the optimum insertion torque (Fig 8-62).
  – *Anterior maxilla and mandible.* This density of bone is most commonly found in the anterior regions and less commonly in the maxilla. Osteotomy burs, tapered reamers and bone taps are indicated. Where less resistance is met during the bone-tapping procedure, partial tapping of the site will ensure adequate primary stability.

The precise protocol used will vary depending on the design of the implantable device. The above guidelines apply to the numerous implants now available that incorporate a tapered core combined with a progressive deep thread. The use of excessive insertion forces, although likely to produce high primary stability, runs the risk of damage to the implant site and the insertion device. Forces in excess of 50 Ncm are not considered to be suitable.

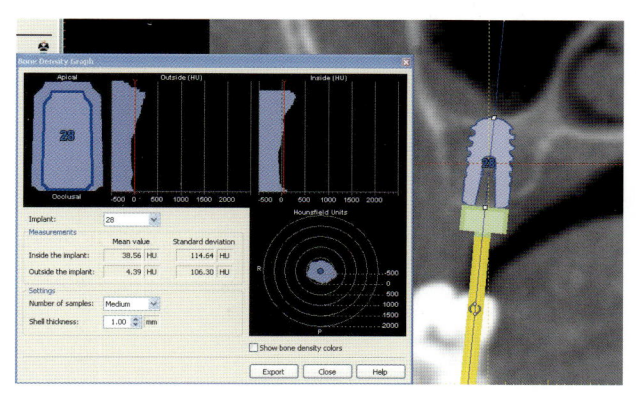

**8  Delayed Placement in Adequate Bone with Mature Ridge**

**Fig 8-60** Cross-sectional CT image with implant placed interactively for the assessment of bone density. A bone density of < 0 HU demonstrates the presence of fatty tissue. Such a case is not normally suitable for immediate loading. To achieve primary stability even for staged treatment would require judicious osteotomy preparation.

**Fig 8-61** Cross-sectional CT image with implant interactively inserted into anterior maxilla with a density of 500–700 HU. This is ideally suited for immediate loading. Site preparation must be carried out with assessment at the time of osteotomy preparation as to whether bone tapping would be necessary.

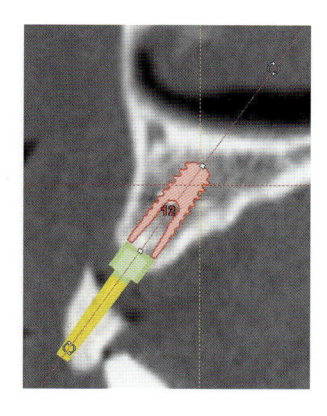

**Fig 8-62** Typically bone density of more than 700 HU is found in the anterior mandible and requires osteotomy preparation, including the partial or complete preparation of threads using a bone tap.

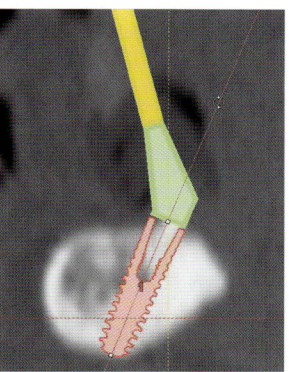

## Implant Insertion

The implant is inserted using established protocols which ensure that neither the implant nor the insertion device is damaged by the use of excessive force, but that the implant is stable for whichever mode of loading is chosen. The clinician will already be aware of the orientation of the ridge from the preoperative assessment. If the angle is likely to be less than 15 degrees, the primary concern will be developing an emergence profile. The margin of the clinical crown will need to be below the gingival margin to create a natural emergence profile. Placing the implant level with the bone normally provides an approximately 3-mm thickness of attached tissue with which to create this profile. Subcrestal placement of implants is recommended by those systems (e.g. Ankylos) that have a conical connection which does not permit micro-leakage. In this case, the depth and the sulcus height of the abutment needs to be appropriately compensated.

Care should be taken to ensure that the implant is also approximately 3 mm below the gingival margin of the corresponding contralateral natural tooth. The positioning of the implant must always take into account the shape of the abutment that will be attached to the implant, as this will significantly affect the contours that are produced (Fig 8-63).

With implants that require an abutment angle greater than 15 degrees, the depth to which the implant is inserted will have an effect on the labio-palatal position of the abutment. Increasing the depth to which the implant is inserted in the maxilla will move the abutment towards the palate and may interfere with the occlusion. Conversely, decreasing the depth will move the abutment in the labial direction, which will cause gingival recession and compromise the aesthetics because there will not be adequate space available for the prosthetic reconstruction (Figs 8-64 and 8-65). It is, therefore, appropriate that the abutment be tried in at this stage, particularly as the pivot point of the angle is set at a variable height from the implant surface for different abutments.

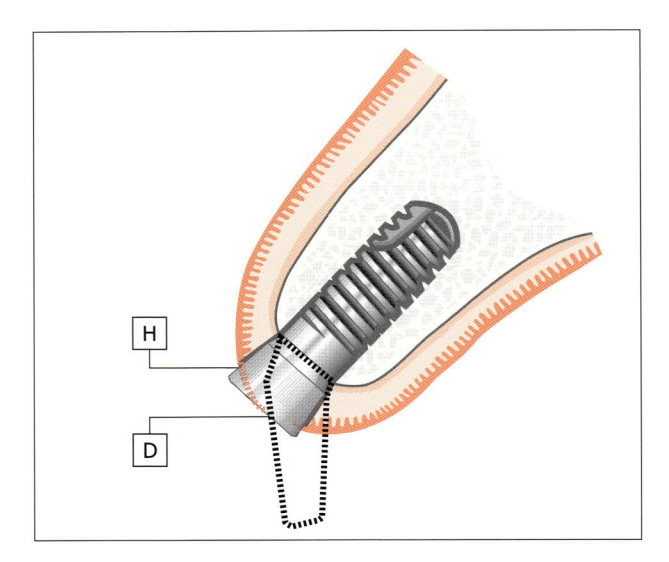

II   Implant Placement: Surgery and Prosthodontics

**Fig 8-63**   The influence of the abutment on the emergence profile. A wider abutment or a healing abutment, which does not compensate for the angle or the emergence profile, may result in the soft tissues healing in a more apical position, exposing a greater proportion of the crown or abutment. Similarly one-piece implants or implants with a transgingival healing collar invariably face this problem and should be considered carefully when an implant needs to placed in a ridge inclined to the tooth axis. The line H represents the level at which the gingiva may heal if a bulky healing abutment is attached. The line D represents the level of gingiva that results from a properly contoured or angled abutment. The pivot point of an angled abutment will also have a similar effect. Trying in an abutment, therefore, enables the clinician to refine the implant position.

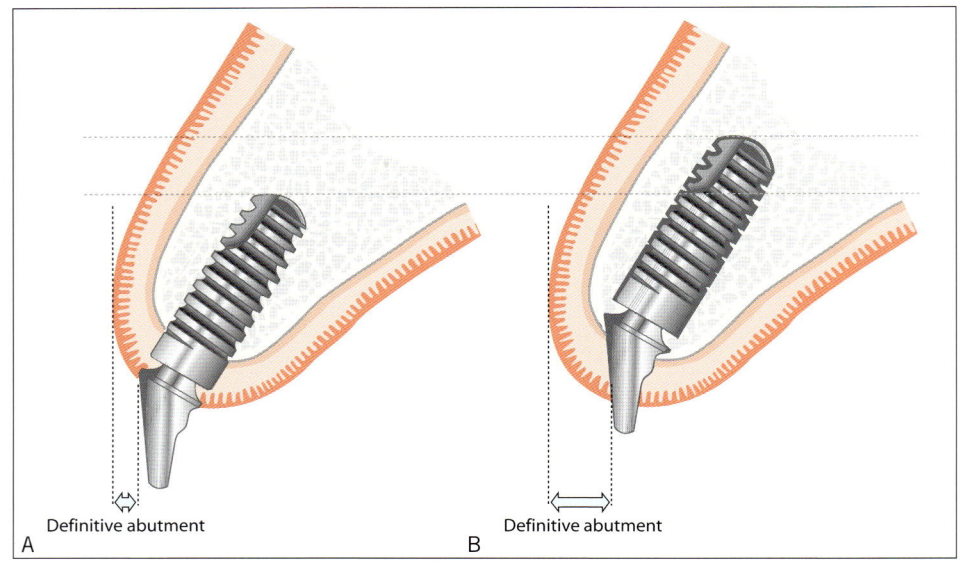

**Fig 8-64**   The impact of the depth of an implant placed at an angle upon the position of the abutment. Abutment position A reflects the position when the implant is positioned superficially and position B represents an implant placed at a greater depth. The position of the abutment will clearly have an effect on the emergence profile and the point at which the gingival tissues mature.

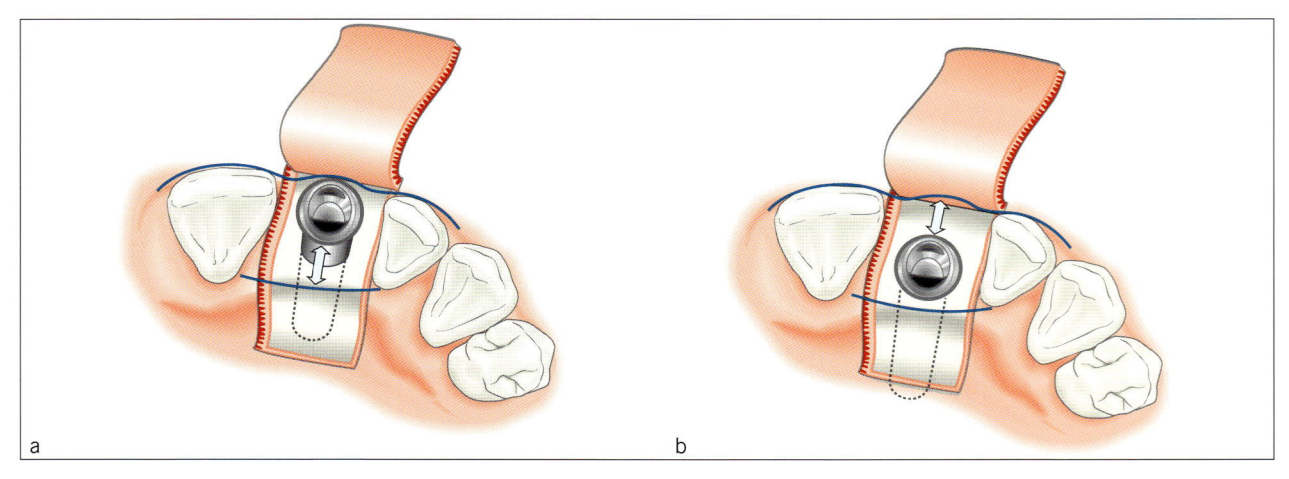

**Fig 8-65**   (a) The occlusal view of an abutment positioned labially in relation to the teeth, reflecting a more superficial positioning of the implant. (b) The position of an abutment in relation to the teeth when an implant is positioned to a greater depth.

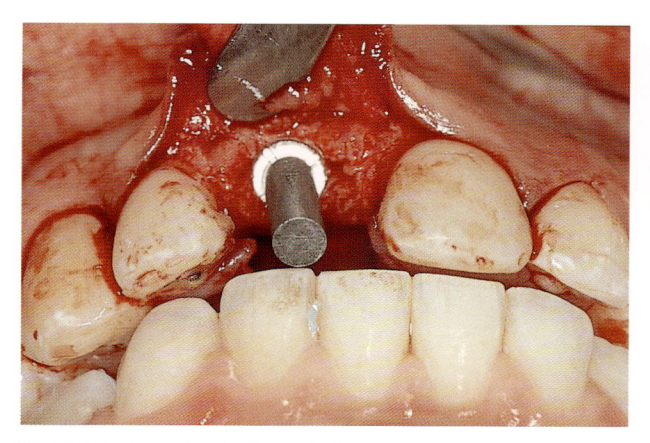

**8** Delayed Placement in Adequate Bone with Mature Ridge

**Fig 8-66** Direction indicator being used to establish occlusal clearance.

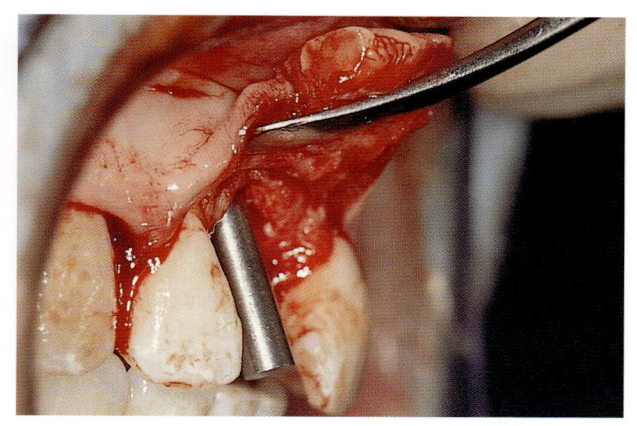

**Fig 8-67** Lateral view of the direction indicator in situ.

## Abutment Selection

Once the implant has been seated to the desired depth, the implant carrier may be removed and an abutment analogue (trial abutment or direction indicator) may be tried in (Figs 8-66 and 8-67). The abutment analogue is inserted and its position confirmed using a diagnostic template. If it falls in the desired position, the angle of the abutment is recorded. If the abutment is not in the centre, a different angle is tried in. In the event that the abutment body is placed too far in the labial or lingual direction, the depth of the implant is altered to move the abutment bodily into the right position.

With an implant system that uses a tapered connection as a means of mating with an abutment, the appropriate abutment can be selected using trial abutments after the removal of the implant carrier. For example, the Ankylos implant system uses a range of trial abutments (direction indicators) to measure the abutment angle and confirm implant position in combination with the diagnostic template outlining the future tooth position. Rotating an implant with an internal hex (or any other type of indexed connection) might be necessary in order to align the abutment in the middle of the future tooth position and parallel to the adjacent teeth or abutments. With an internal conical connection, rotational positioning is not necessary since the conical connection allows the abutment to be attached to the implant at an infinite number of rotational points. This eliminates the need to rotate the implant in order to orientate the abutment into the correct plane.[7] The ability to use an angled abutment enables the clinician to make full use of the available bone when inserting the implant, thus increasing the success rate as well as the aesthetic and functional outcome.[6,7,131–134]

## Impressions at First-stage Surgery: Special Considerations During Surgery

Different techniques have been described for the transfer of the implant position to the laboratory directly following insertion of the implant.[135–139] These consist of the use of open and closed tray techniques with impression material or the use of acrylic resin splints (Flowchart 8-4). A variety of component parts can be used to transfer the implant position, including the implant carrier, abutment transfer coping and the implant transfer coping for either the closed or open tray techniques.

The impression can be taken before the removal of the implant carrier by using a perforated stock tray that has been modified for use as an open tray with access to the implant carrier, using a pre-inserted hex driver. This enables the implant position to be transferred to the laboratory. However, we find the use of the implant carrier in combination with the open tray technique the most cost-effective and time-efficient method in the majority of cases (Figs 8-68 and 8-69). This technique is described in further detail below.

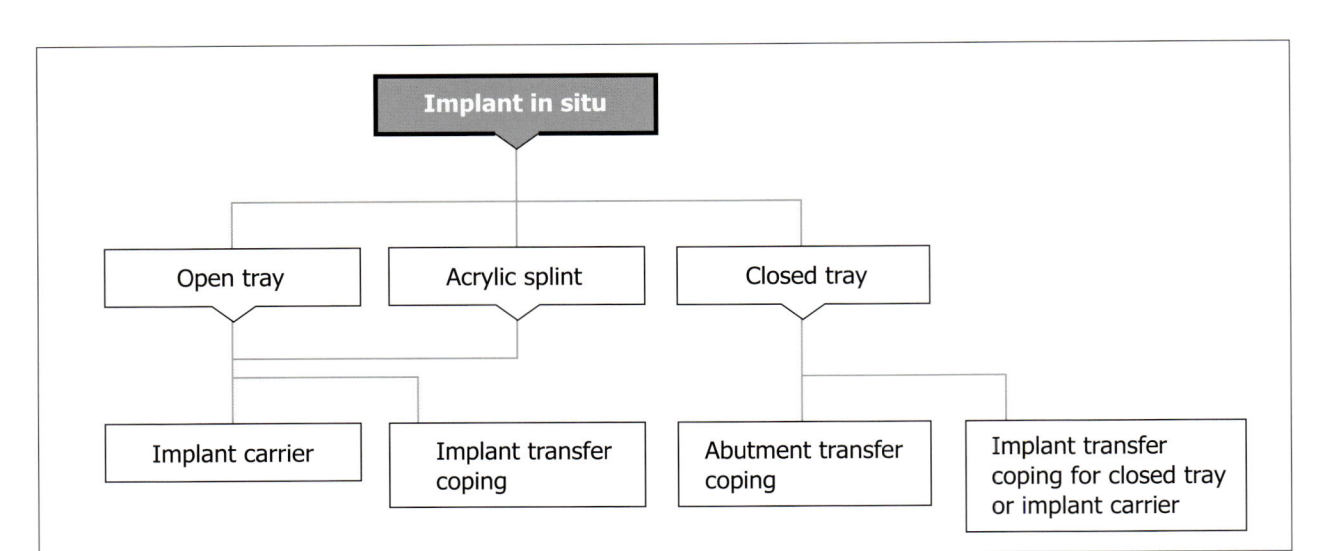

Flowchart 8-4  First-stage surgery impression.

## Impression Tray

A sterile, rigid stock tray needs to be prepared prior to impression taking, with an opening for access to the implant carrier for detachment. Either a plastic tray can be customised or a prefabricated metal tray with detachable sections (Fig 8-70) may be used.

Alternatively, special trays may be constructed beforehand in the laboratory, with the estimated position of the access hole being based on the study cast. This offers the advantage of obtaining accurate impressions without the use of excessive impression material. The hex driver for removal of the implant carrier is inserted into the carrier. The open tray is tried in with the finger over the opening to allow the hex driver to be located during seating of the impression tray. The tray is now removed in readiness for the impression.

## Impression Material

A medium-bodied vinyl polysiloxane elastomeric impression material is used, which is not toxic, does not support bacterial growth and is of a viscosity that ensures that it does not entangle within the surgical field.[140–143] In order to maintain asepsis, the nozzle of the mixing gun should also be sterilised (e.g. with gamma irradiation).

## Impression Technique

The tray is loaded with the impression material while the opening is occluded with a finger. Some impression material is also extruded around the implant carrier to ensure good adaptation. The impression tray is then carefully offered until the hex driver contacts the finger to orientate the tray, which is then seated into a stable position.

## Tray Removal

On completion of polymerisation, excess material around the hex driver is removed to gain access to the driver in order to detach the carrier. Once the fixing screw of the carrier has been completely disengaged, the tray can be removed.

The impression is removed from the mouth and disinfected. The implant analogue is then mounted onto the implant carrier. The stability of the implant carrier within the impression is confirmed and the impression is then sent to the laboratory for casting.

## Wound Closure
## Delayed Loading

Prior to closure, the contours of the ridge should be assessed. It is possible to increase the labial and vertical dimension of the soft tissue. This can be carried out using hydroxyapatite particles for increasing the labial bulk. A cover-screw extension may be used to increase the height in conjunction with hydroxyapatite (e.g. OsteoGraf D-300 or D-700; CeraMed Dental, Dentsply Friadent) (Figs 8-71–8-73).

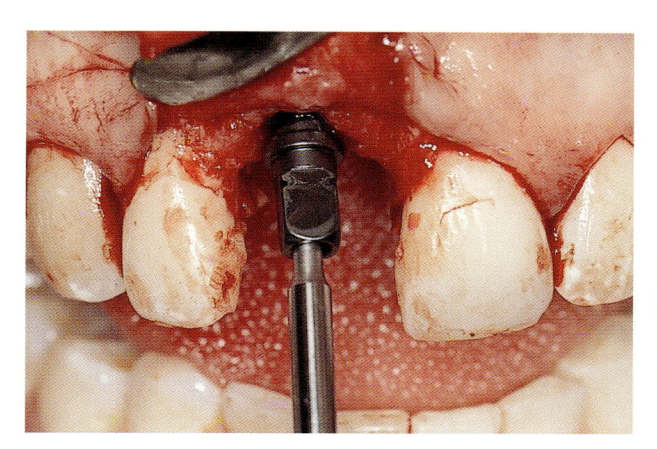

**8** Delayed Placement in Adequate Bone with Mature Ridge

**Fig 8-68** Labial view of the implant carrier with hex driver inserted prior to impression at first-stage surgery.

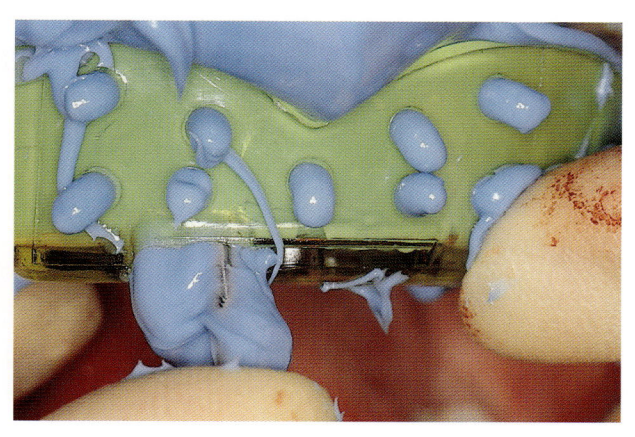

**Fig 8-69** A perforated stock tray being used to record the implant position (addition-cured silicone impression material: Provil Monophase; Heraeus Kulzer, Hanau, Germany). The hex driver can be seen emerging through the perforation in the tray.

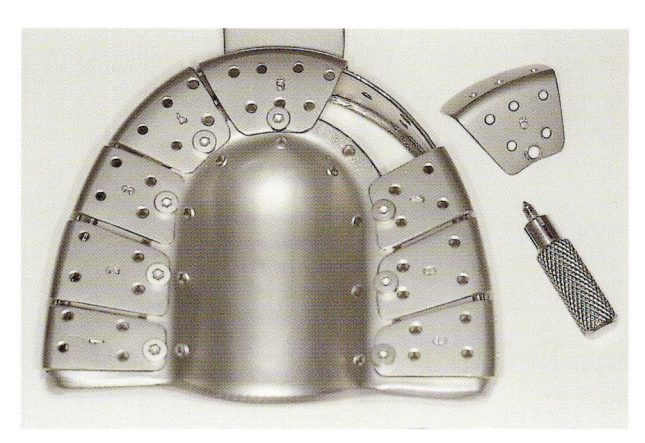

**Fig 8-70** Metal tray designed with removable segments to enable impressions to be taken using the open tray technique. This type of tray is well suited to impressions that are planned to be taken at first-stage surgery.

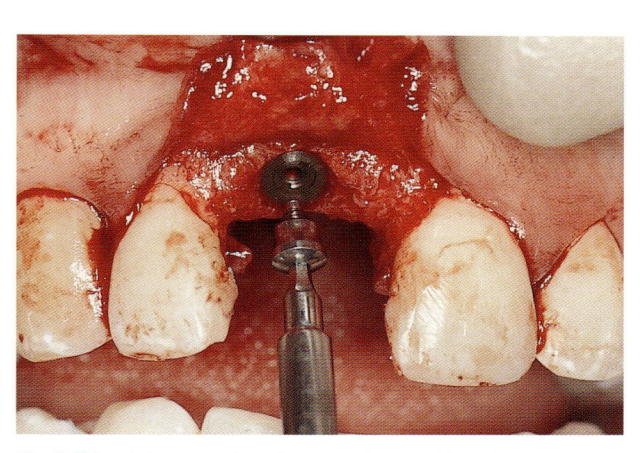

**Fig 8-71** A 3-mm sulcus former is inserted into the cover screw to provide support for the increased thickness of soft tissue that is required for the aesthetic outcome.

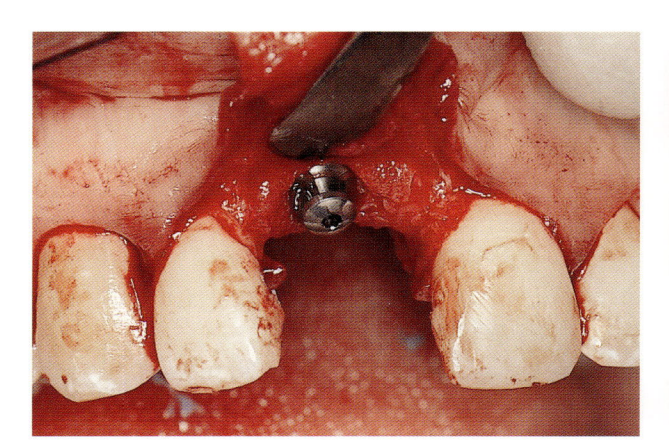

**Fig 8-72** Sulcus former in situ showing the increase in height that is planned.

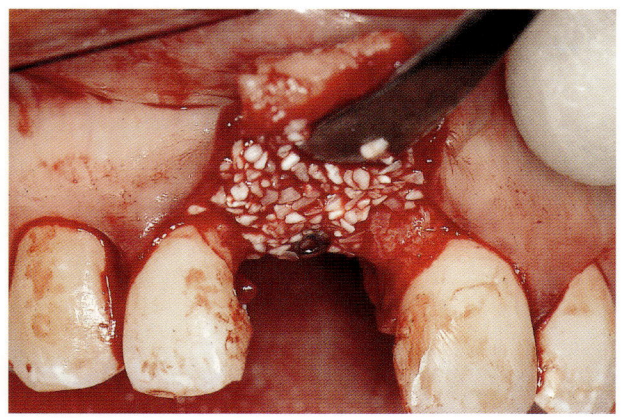

**Fig 8-73** Non-resorbable hydroxyapatite of 700 μm particle size placed around the sulcus former to increase soft tissue height (Osteograf, CeraMed Dental, Dentsply Friadent).

129

II  Implant Placement: Surgery and Prosthodontics

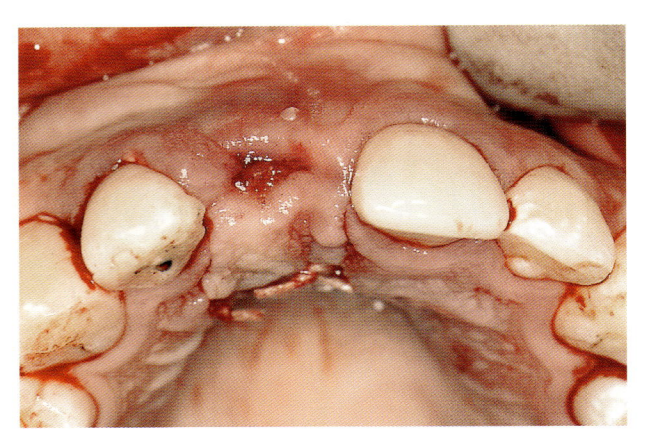

**Fig 8-74** Wound closure ensuring complete closure over implant site.

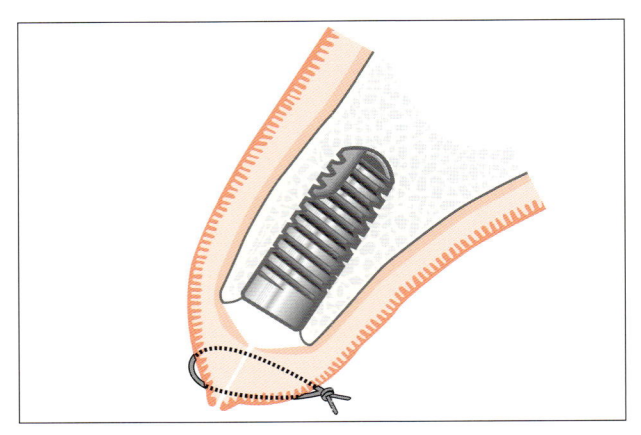

**Fig 8-75** Closure of a crestal incision over an implant using a vertical mattress suture.

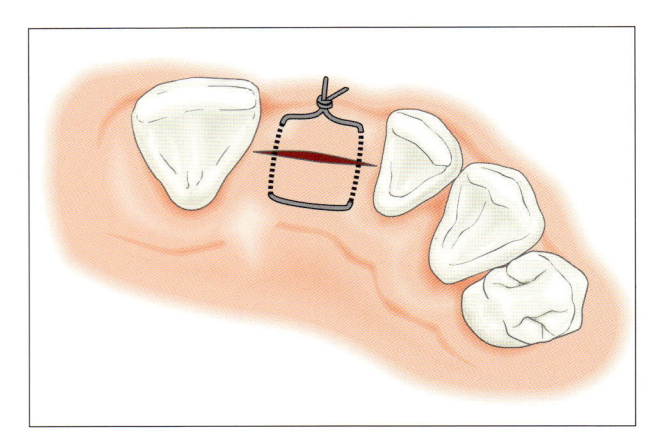

**Fig 8-76** The use of a horizontal mattress suture to close an incision placed over an implant. Additional interrupted sutures may be required to ensure a good seal.

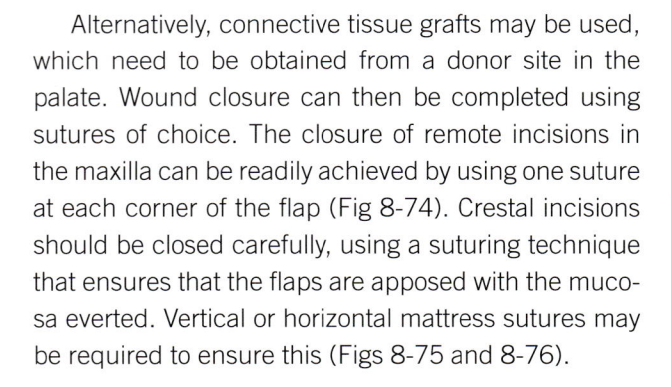

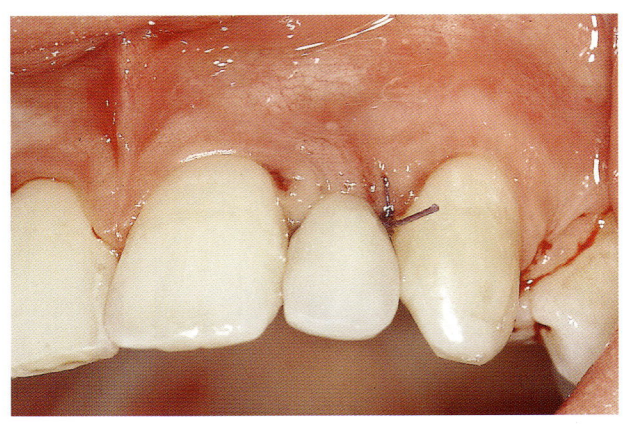

**Fig 8-77** 'S'-shaped incision has been used to close around the transitional restoration, creating papillae.

Alternatively, connective tissue grafts may be used, which need to be obtained from a donor site in the palate. Wound closure can then be completed using sutures of choice. The closure of remote incisions in the maxilla can be readily achieved by using one suture at each corner of the flap (Fig 8-74). Crestal incisions should be closed carefully, using a suturing technique that ensures that the flaps are apposed with the mucosa everted. Vertical or horizontal mattress sutures may be required to ensure this (Figs 8-75 and 8-76).

### Immediate Loading
Where the implant is to be loaded immediately, the soft tissue needs to be closed around the abutment and the transitional restoration (Fig 8-77). Typically, the soft tissue needs to be manipulated to ensure that the gingival margin is at the desired level and that primary closure in the interdental regions takes place. These techniques are described in greater detail in Chapter 9, as the objective is the same.

### Transgingival Healing
There may be many instances where the patient could benefit from the attachment of a sulcus former at the time of implant placement. This is particularly true in areas where aesthetics are not critical, such as the posterior quadrants (Figs 8-78 and 8-79).

In fact, attachment of a sulcus former may become necessary where immediate loading was intended but the primary stability of the implant was not considered to be adequate for the anticipated loads. Attachment of a sulcus former prevents the need for second-stage

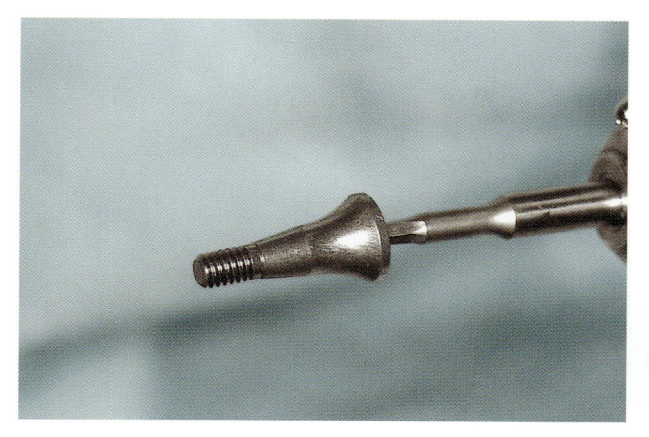

**8** Delayed Placement in Adequate Bone with Mature Ridge

**Fig 8-78** The sulcus former can be seen with the tapered profile, which will engage the conical connection within the implant.

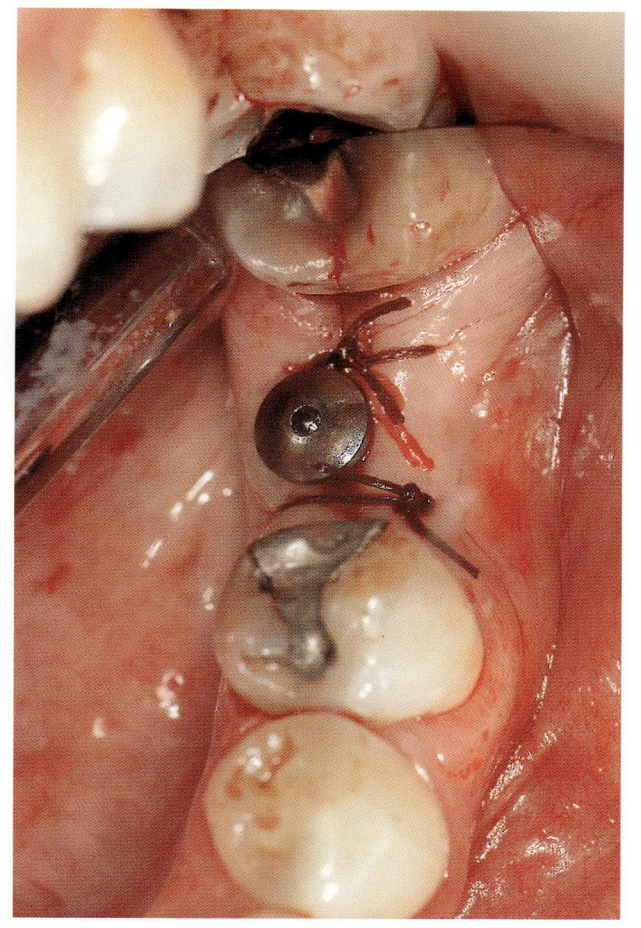

**Fig 8-79** Sulcus former in situ after implant placement.

surgery and allows the abutment to be seated after integration has taken place.

In these cases, a sulcus former may be attached to maintain access to the implant to enable loading to be instituted at the appropriate time. The impression technique suitable for the restorative phase is implant transfer using either the open or closed tray technique.

Alternatively, an abutment may be selected and fitted with an acrylic sleeve to maintain access to the abutment for conventional impressions or abutment transfer impressions at the desired time. In both cases, the cover screw would require removal before fitting the component. The wound may be sutured to achieve closure around the component part, using sutures of choice. Minor incisions to advance the flap around the component part may be necessary.

## Restorative Phase

After a healing phase of approximately one month, the restorative phase is started on the basis that soft tissue levels have stabilised. This is confirmed by observing the gingival margin and papillary levels, using the transitional restoration as a reference. Continuing soft tissue changes indicate that the restorative phase should be delayed.

Informaton may be transferred to the laboratory for the fabrication of the definitive restoration using one of the following impression techniques:
- pick-up impressions after first-stage impression
- conventional impressions
- implant transfer (open or closed tray)
- abutment transfer.

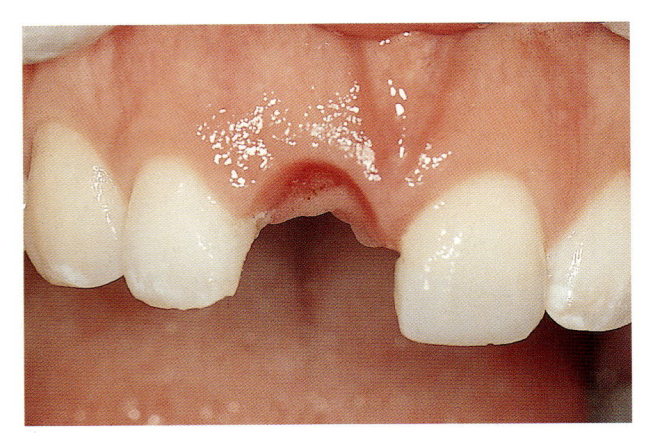

**Fig 8-80** Preoperative labial view; the gingival contours can be seen following the removal of the provisional restoration.

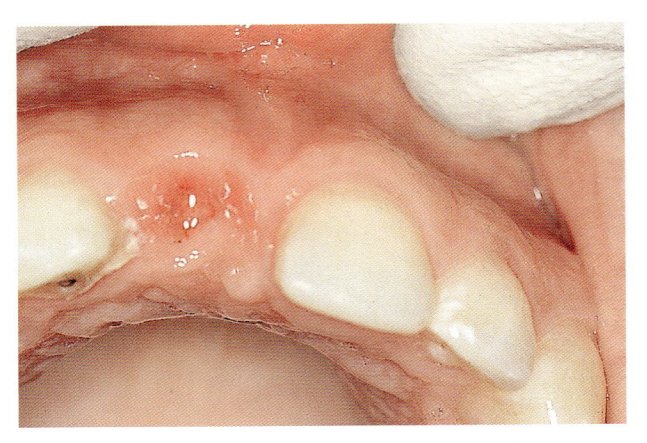

**Fig 8-81** Occlusal view showing adequate width of the residual ridge.

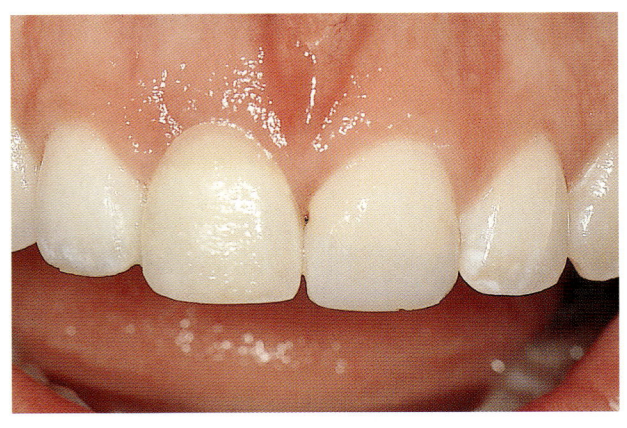

**Fig 8-82** Labial view of provisional Rochette bridge showing the gingival margin established following the extraction of the central incisor. It is evident that the tooth length of the maxillary right central incisor is greater than that of the natural left central incisor. This minor deficiency will require correction.

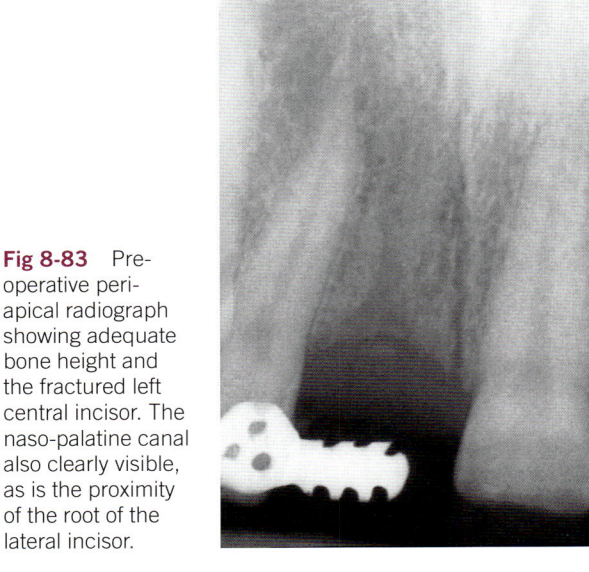

**Fig 8-83** Preoperative peri-apical radiograph showing adequate bone height and the fractured left central incisor. The naso-palatine canal also clearly visible, as is the proximity of the root of the lateral incisor.

## Delayed Placement of Implants: Clinical Cases

### Case 1: Delayed Placement with Delayed Loading

A 25-year-old woman was referred for the replacement of the maxillary right central incisor following an accident that had resulted in the fracture of both central incisors. The left central incisor was fractured, involving the dentine, and an oblique fracture of the maxillary right central incisor involved the upper-third of the root and extended subgingivally. The right central incisor was removed and the patient was provided with a metal-acrylic resin Rochette bridge so that the healing of the hard and soft tissues could be monitored.

The decision was made not to replace the tooth with an immediate implant because of the high lip-line and the risk of producing a less than satisfactory aesthetic result. A decision was also made not to load the implant immediately on insertion in order to maximise the opportunity of increasing the thickness of the soft tissue by using a delayed loading protocol, as described above (Figs 8-80–8-134).

# 8 Delayed Placement in Adequate Bone with Mature Ridge

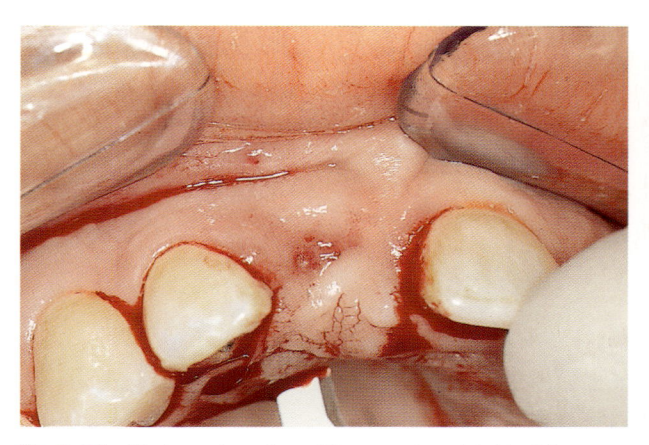

**Fig 8-84** Horizontal portion of the remote palatal incision being made by a Blake's knife as shown in Fig 8-51.

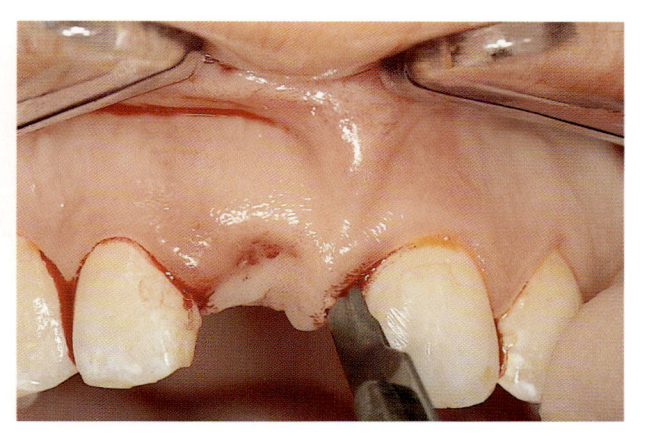

**Fig 8-85** Labial view showing the incision being extended within the sulcus around the cervical margin of the central incisor.

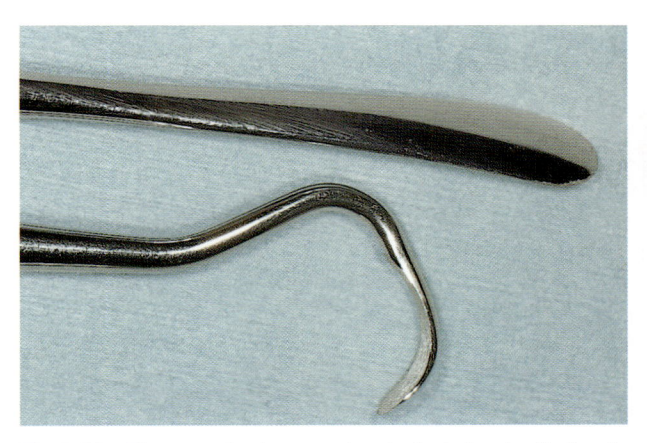

**Fig 8-86** Photograph of a curved periosteal elevator (bottom), which can be used to elevate the flap from the palatal aspect of the ridge. A conventional periosteal elevator (top) is used to elevate the flap over the crest of the ridge.

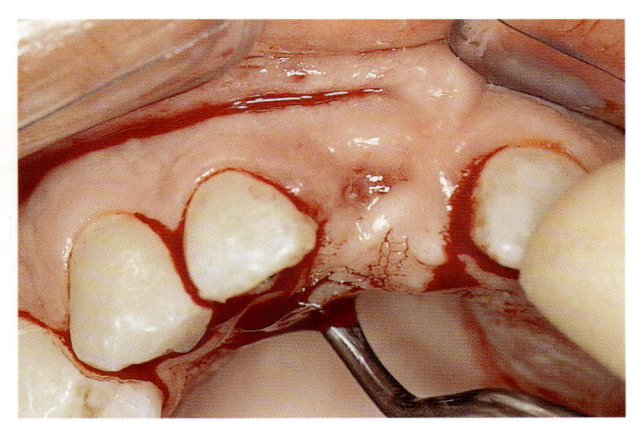

**Fig 8-87** Curved periosteal elevator being used to elevate the palatal portion of the flap.

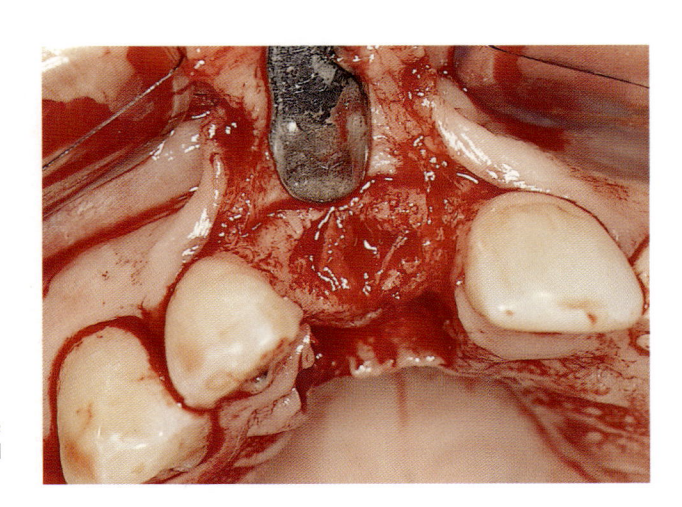

**Fig 8-88** Occlusal view of the flap elevated showing adequate ridge width present. The flap is not elevated to expose the labial cortical plate to minimise trauma.

133

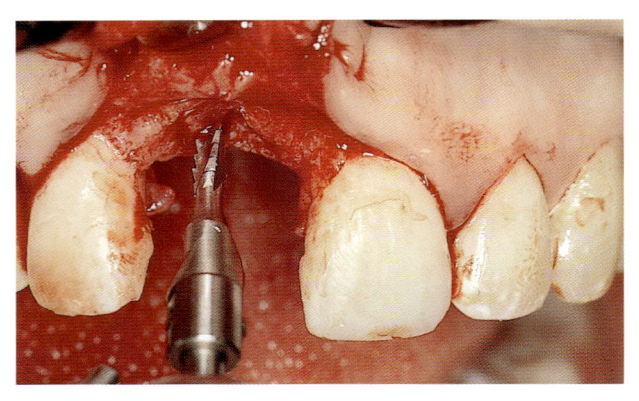

II  Implant Placement: Surgery and Prosthodontics

**Fig 8-89**  The pilot (Lindemann) bur can be seen being used to commence the osteotomy establishing the precise site in the base of the residual socket as well as the direction. The direction is established obtaining guidance from the adjacent teeth and the palatal cortical plate of the exposed ridge. Note that the osteotomy site has been selected towards the distal aspect of the exposed ridge in order to avoid the naso-palatine foramen.

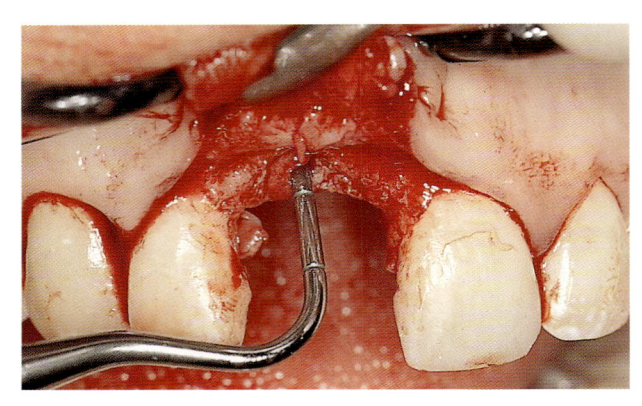

**Fig 8-90**  An osteotomy probe being used to ensure that no perforations on the apical, labial or palatal aspect have inadvertently been made. The direction can also be confirmed.

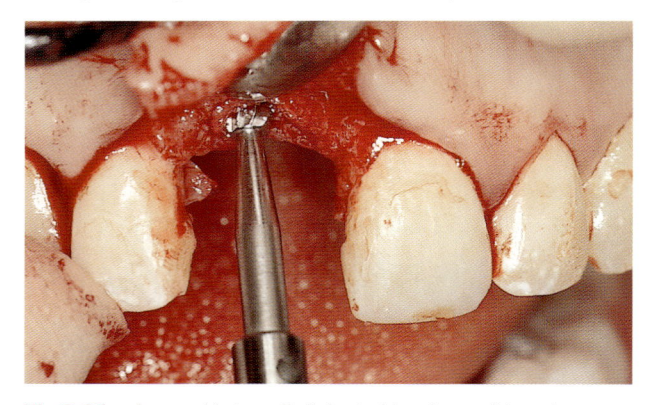

**Fig 8-91**  A round internally irrigated bur is used to enlarge the osteotomy. Any minor corrections in the site that has been selected can be made at this stage.

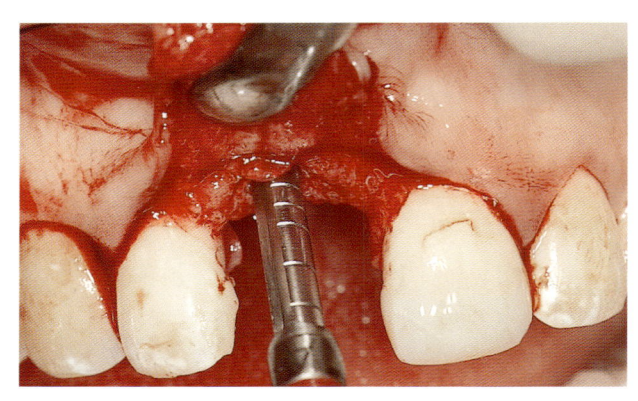

**Fig 8-92**  A parallel-sided osteotomy bur (parallel drill 'A', representing a diameter of 3.5 mm) can be seen being used to establish the depth to which the implant will be placed. The diameter of the implant that is to be inserted is selected by the final osteotomy bur that is used. In this case a 4.5-mm diameter implant was planned because adequate width was present.

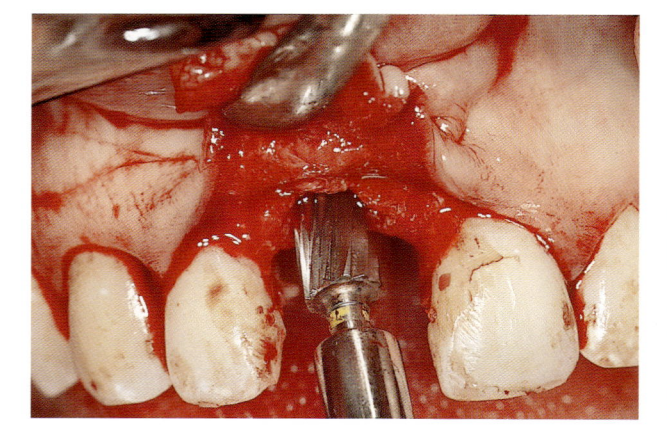

**Fig 8-93**  Reamer for the 4.5-mm implant being used to create the shape for the tapered implant body.

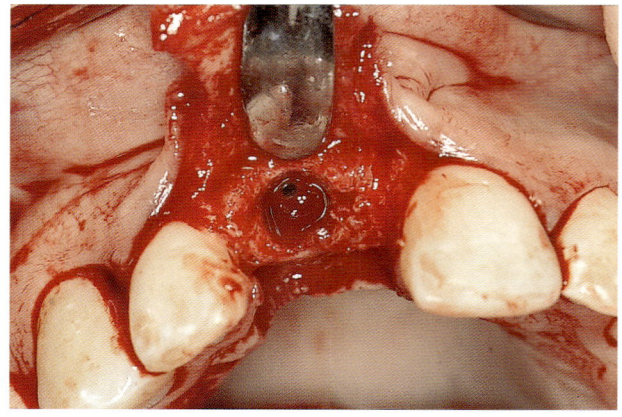

**Fig 8-94**  Occlusal view of the completed osteotomy. At least 1 mm of labial and palatal bone remain and at least 2 mm between the osteotomy and the adjacent teeth can be seen.

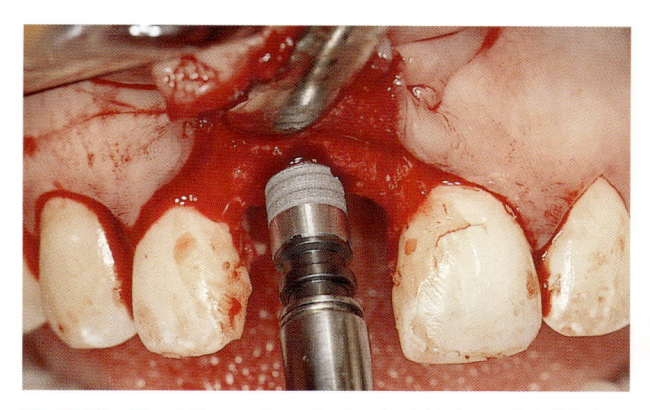

**8** Delayed Placement in Adequate Bone with Mature Ridge

**Fig 8-95** The 4.5-mm diameter implant (Ankylos B 14) being inserted.

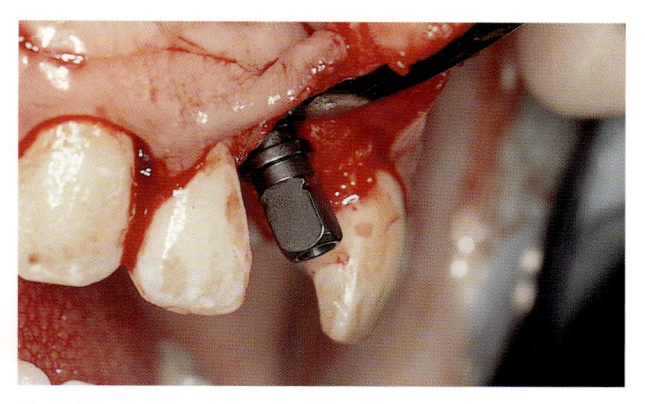

**Fig 8-96** The implant seated to a level approximately 1 mm below the bony margin. The implant carrier shows the angle at which the implant has been placed.

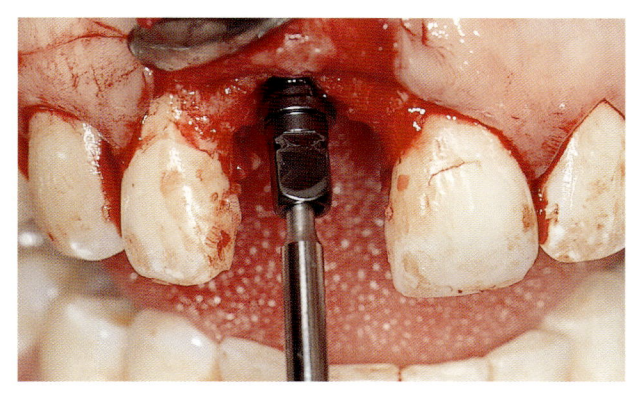

**Fig 8-97** Labial view of the implant carrier with hex driver inserted prior to impression at first-stage surgery.

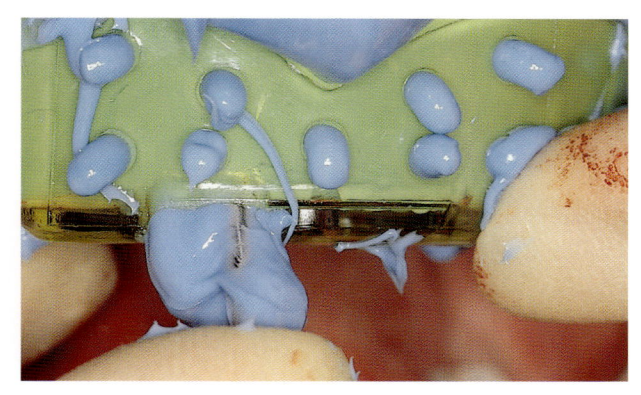

**Fig 8-98** A perforated stock tray being used to record the implant position (addition-cured silicone impression material: Provil Monophase). The hex driver can be seen emerging through the perforation in the tray.

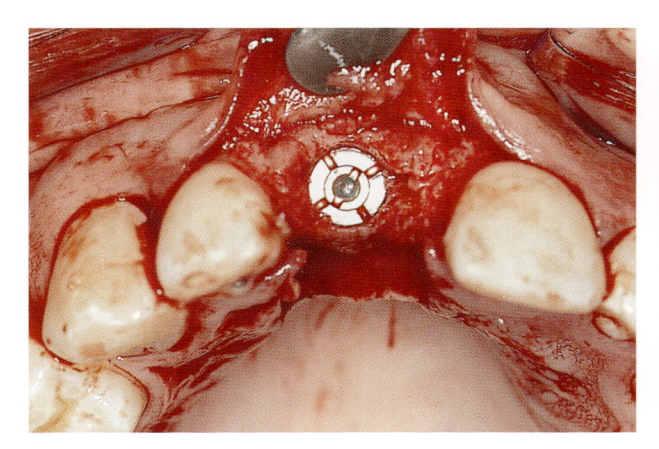

**Fig 8-99** Occlusal view of the implant after removal of the impression tray. The cover screw can be seen attached.

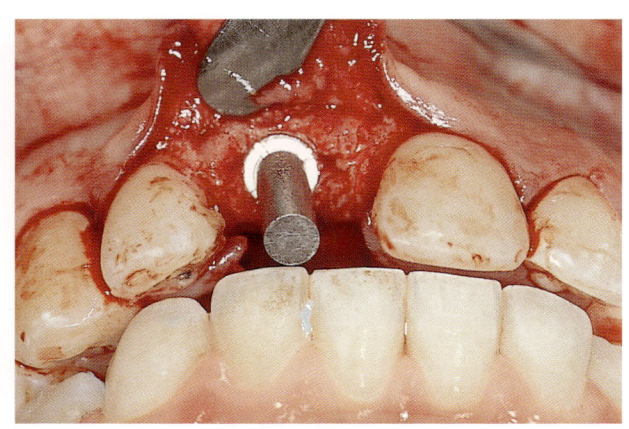

**Fig 8-100** Occlusal view of the prototype direction indicator being used to select the abutment angle. The relationship of the direction indicator (15 degrees) to the opposing dentition can be seen.

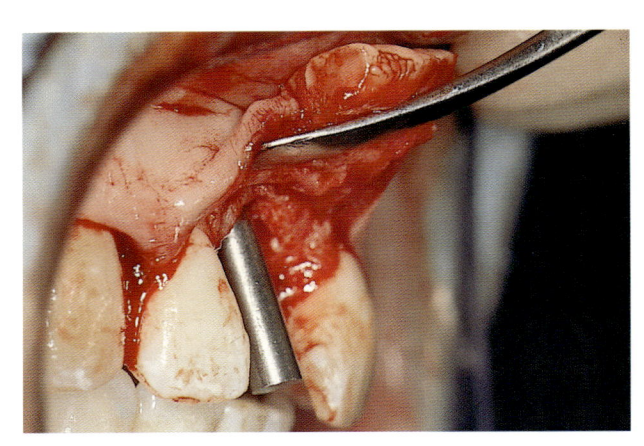

II   Implant Placement: Surgery and Prosthodontics

**Fig 8-101**   Lateral view of the direction indicator in situ.

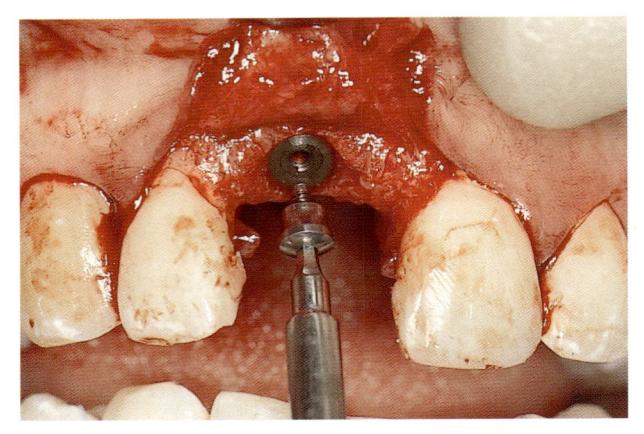

**Fig 8-102**   A 3-mm sulcus former is inserted into the cover screw to provide support for the increased thickness of soft tissue that is required for the aesthetic outcome.

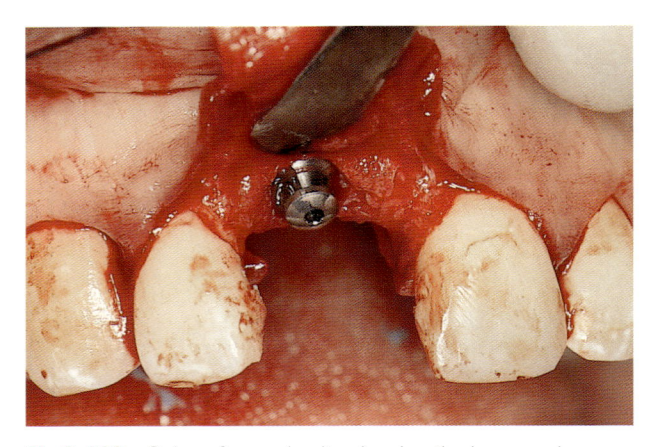

**Fig 8-103**   Sulcus former in situ showing the increase in height that is planned.

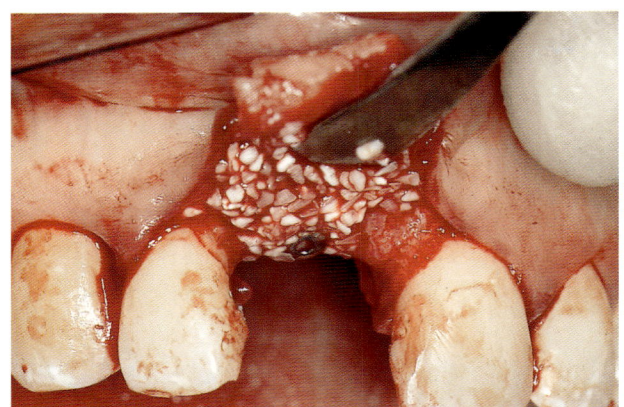

**Fig 8-104**   Non-resorbable hydroxyapatite of 700 µm-particle size placed around the sulcus former to increase soft tissue height (Osteograf).

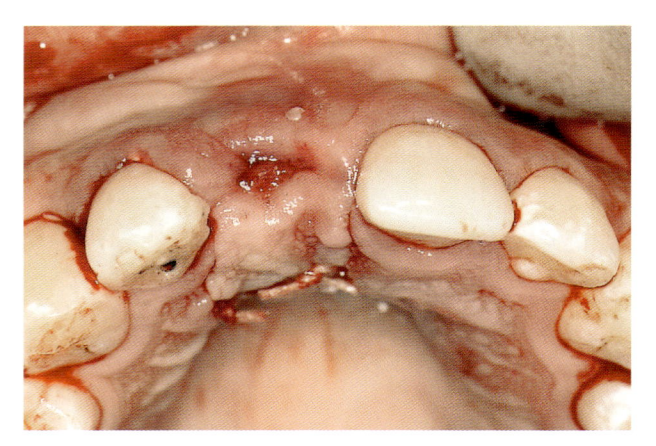

**Fig 8-105**   Wound closure effected by two sutures placed in the palate.

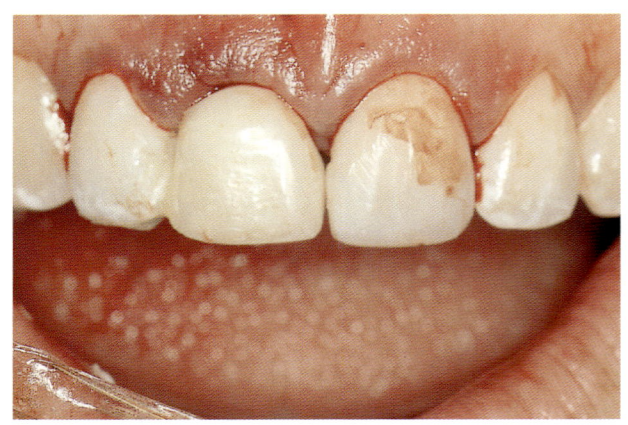

**Fig 8-106**   Labial view of the provisional metal-acrylic Rochette bridge demonstrating the reduced size of the tooth length resulting from the increased soft tissue dimensions.

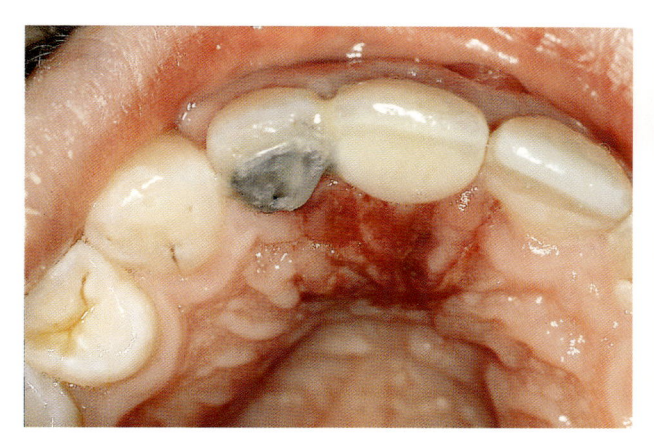

**8** Delayed Placement in Adequate Bone with Mature Ridge

**Fig 8-107** Occlusal view of the Rochette bridge in situ one week after surgery showing adequate healing of the flap.

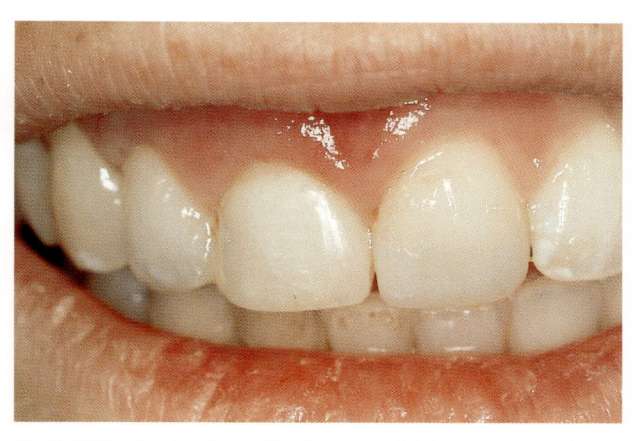

**Fig 8-108** Labial view of the Rochette bridge at one week showing the adaptation of the soft tissues to the pontic.

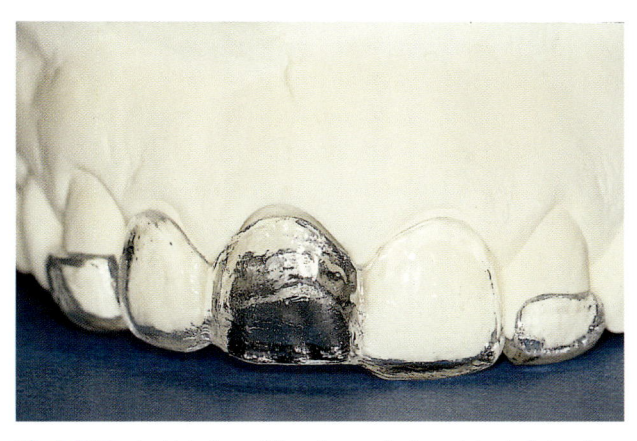

**Fig 8-109** Labial view of the diagnostic template defining the tooth length.

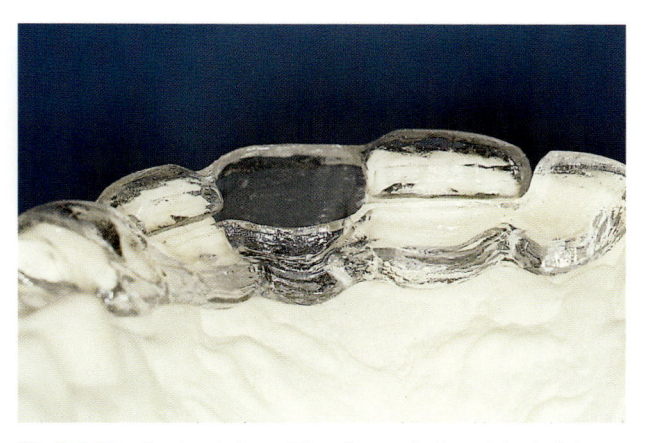

**Fig 8-110** Occlusal view of the diagnostic template defining the prosthetic envelope within which the abutment must fit. The template is used during surgery for the selection of the abutment and can also be used in the laboratory for the same purpose.

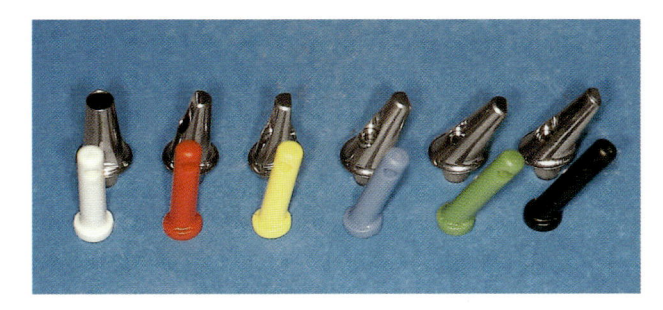

**Fig 8-111** Range of direction indicators with matching abutments. These are graduated at 7.5-degree increments and are colour coded corresponding to the abutments. The colour codes represent the angles in degrees as follows: white, 0; red, 7.5; yellow, 15; blue, 22.5; green, 30; and black, 37.5. The sequence of colours may be memorised as they correspond to the sequence of colour codes used for the implant diameters (Ankylos system).

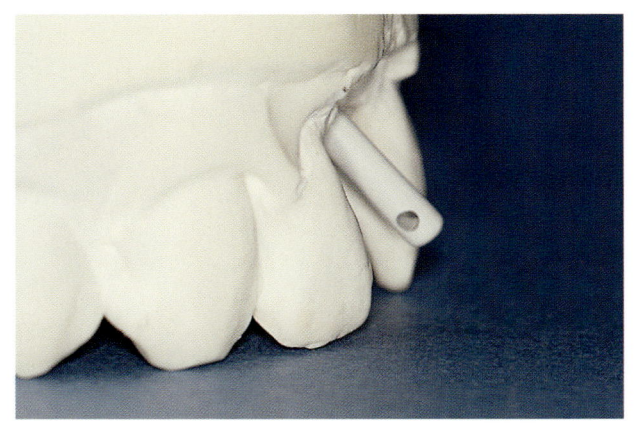

**Fig 8-112** A 0-degree direction indicator being tried in on the laboratory cast with the cover screw in situ. Note the angle at which the implant has been placed corresponds to the clinical images of the implant carrier (see Fig 8-96).

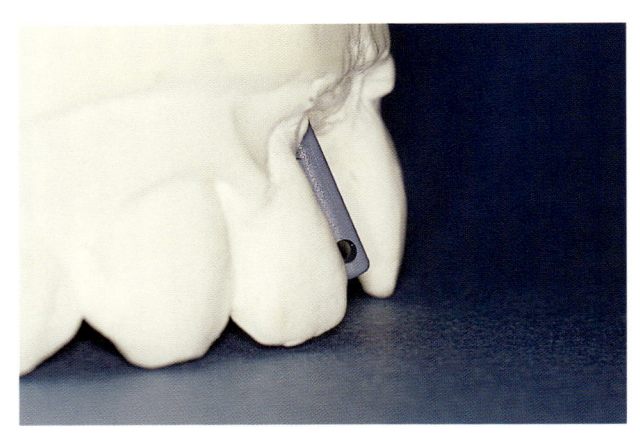

II Implant Placement: Surgery and Prosthodontics

**Fig 8-113** The use of a 22.5-degree direction indicator showing the correction that can be obtained. This corresponds to the clinical picture of the prototype direction indicator (Fig 8-101).

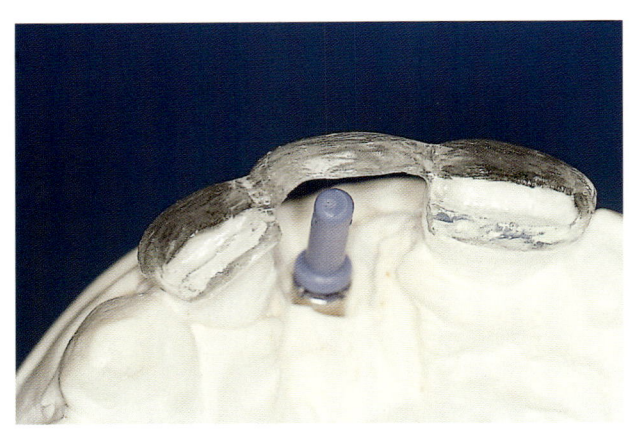

**Fig 8-114** The direction indicator with the labial part of the sectional template showing adequate clearance for aesthetics.

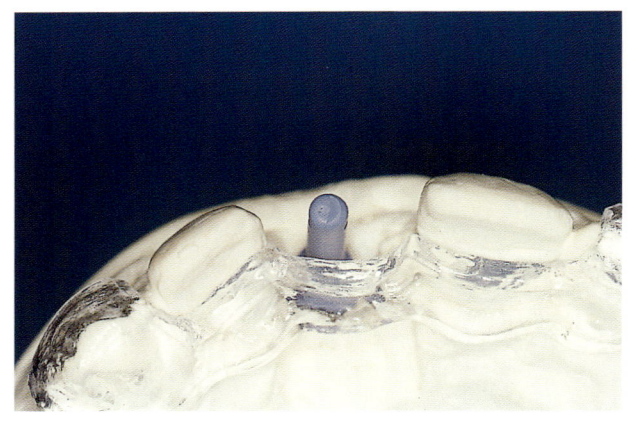

**Fig 8-115** The direction indicator with the palatal part of the sectional template showing adequate clearance for occlusion.

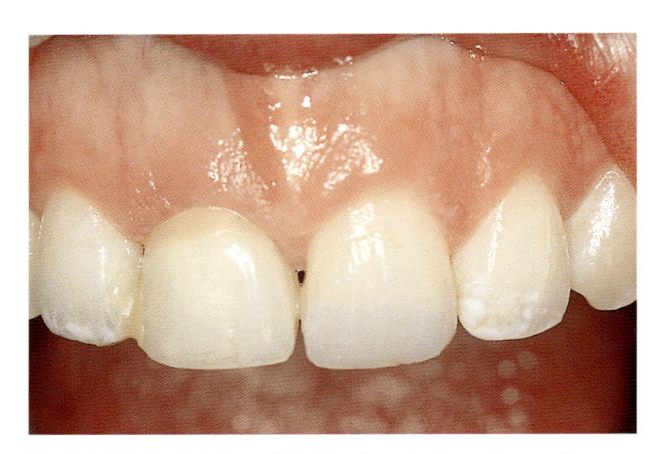

**Fig 8-116** Labial view of the Rochette bridge, six months post-operatively and prior to implant exposure.

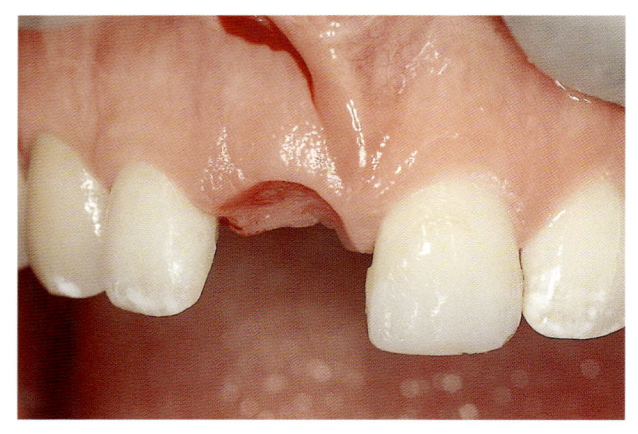

**Fig 8-117** Labial view of the soft tissue contours created by the Rochette bridge.

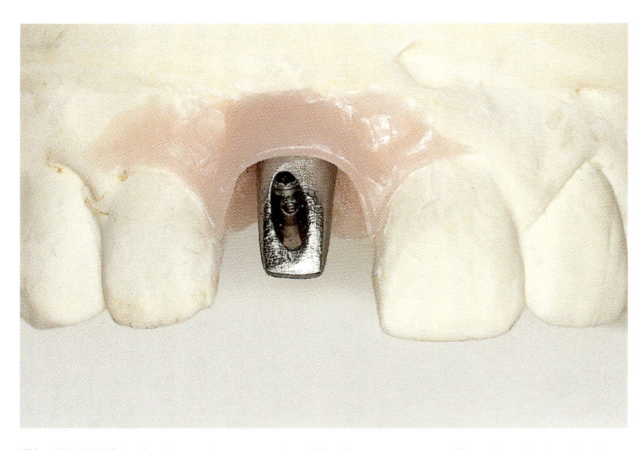

**Fig 8-118** Laboratory cast with the prepared, selected abutment in situ. The cast has been fabricated from the impression taken at first-stage surgery, which transferred the implant position.

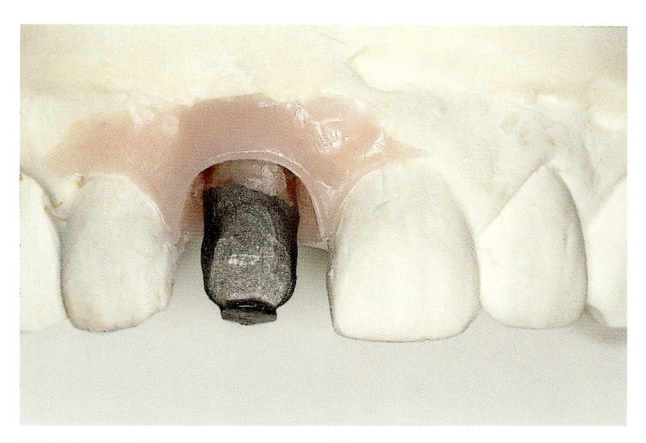

**8** Delayed Placement in Adequate Bone with Mature Ridge

**Fig 8-119** The metalwork was fabricated directly on the abutment, providing a very accurate fit.

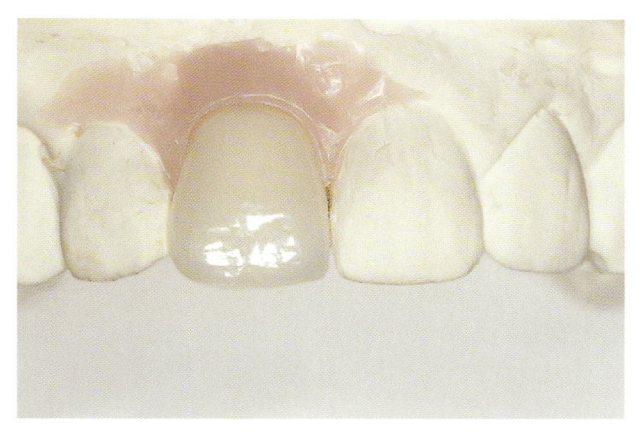

**Fig 8-120** The transitional restoration constructed on the abutment with the soft tissues depicted in pink wax. The transitional restoration will be used to develop the emergence profile.

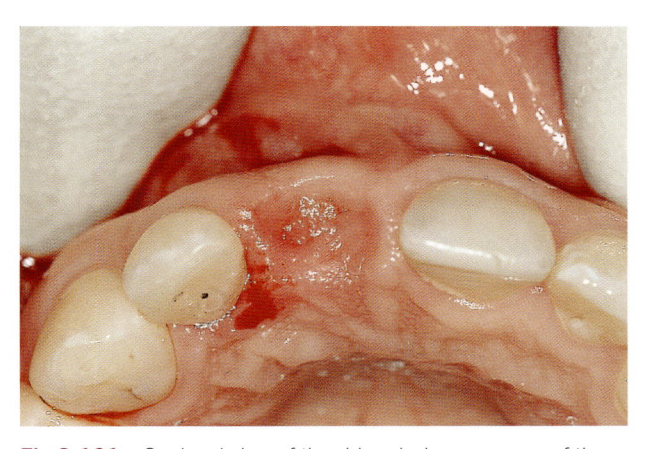

**Fig 8-121** Occlusal view of the ridge during exposure of the implant using an 'H'-shaped incision.

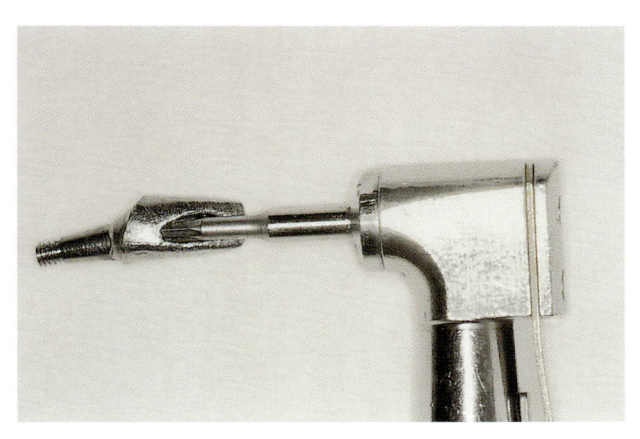

**Fig 8-122** The abutment prior to seating. Note the abutment has been modified by the dental technician to compensate for the distal placement of the implant to avoid the naso-palatine canal.

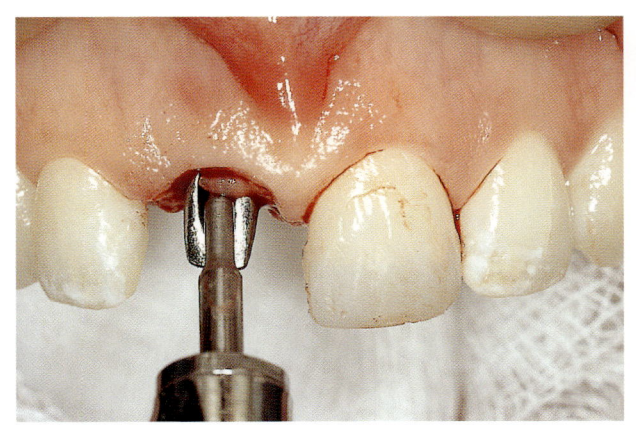

**Fig 8-123** Labial view showing the abutment being seated through the 'H'-shaped incision. The abutment is tightened to 15 Ncm to engage the conical connection.

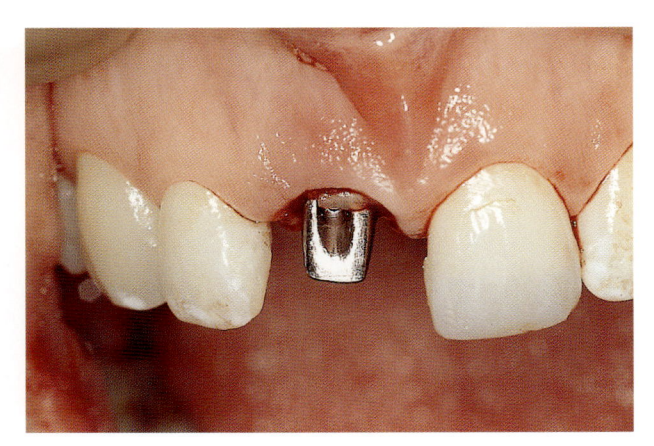

**Fig 8-124** Labial view of the abutment.

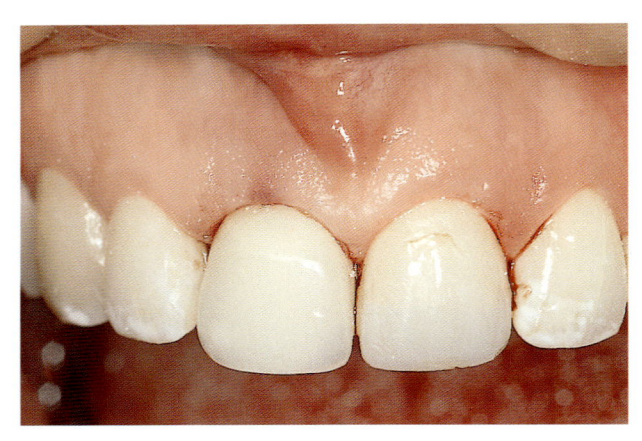

II Implant Placement: Surgery and Prosthodontics

**Fig 8-125** Labial view of the transitional crown seated on the abutment.

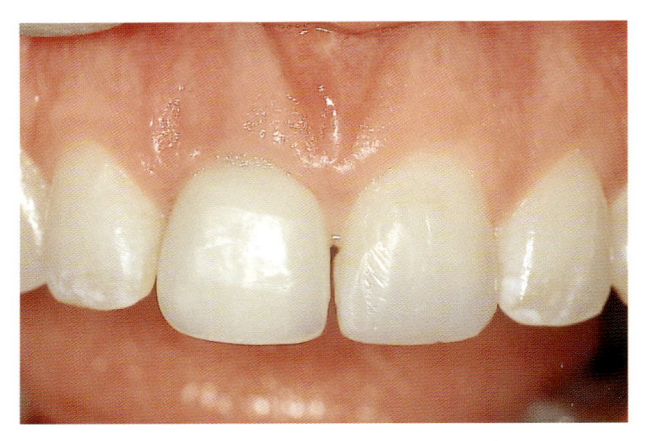

**Fig 8-126** Labial view of the transitional restoration one month after exposure, showing the mature soft tissue contours.

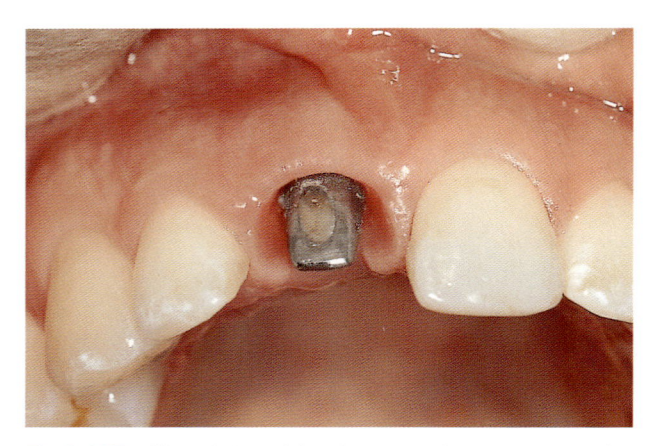

**Fig 8-127** Clinical view of the abutment after the removal of the transitional restoration showing the contours created by the transitional restoration.

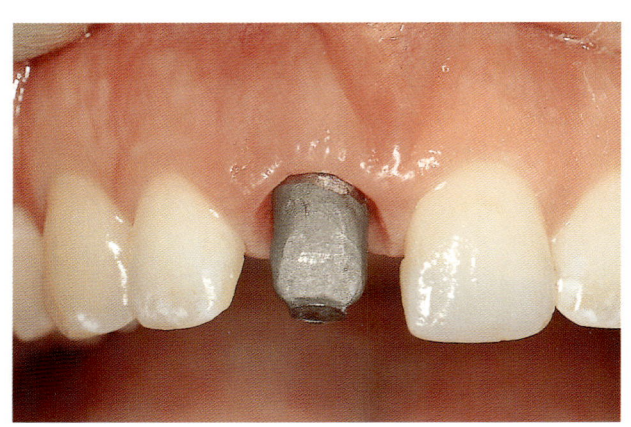

**Fig 8-128** Metalwork seated on the abutment prior to pick-up impression.

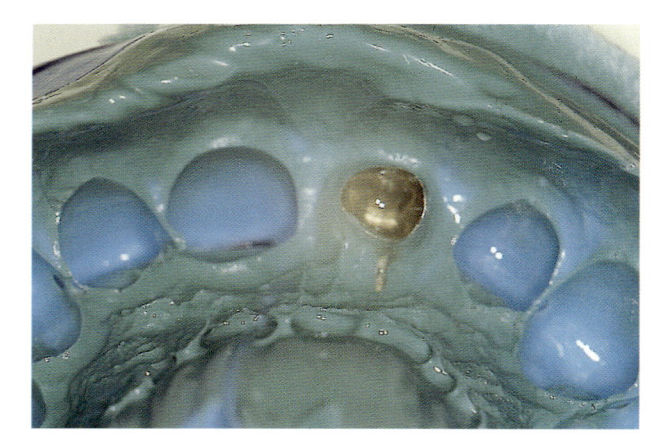

**Fig 8-129** Close-up of the pick-up impression with the metalwork and the relationship of the surrounding soft tissues ready for transfer to the laboratory.

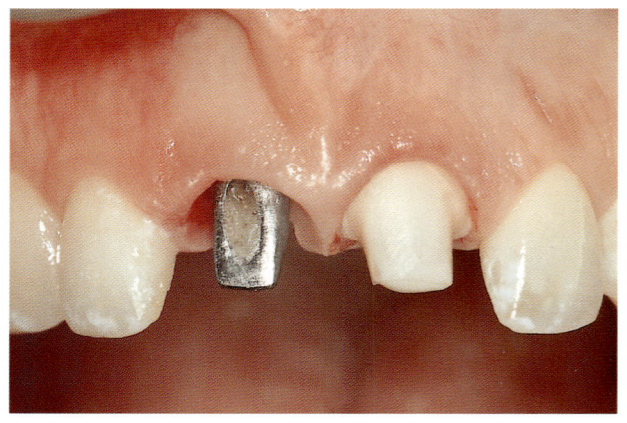

**Fig 8-130** Following dislodgement of the composite repair of the adjacent central incisor, a decision was made to construct a metal-ceramic crown. The prepared tooth can be seen adjacent to the implant abutment.

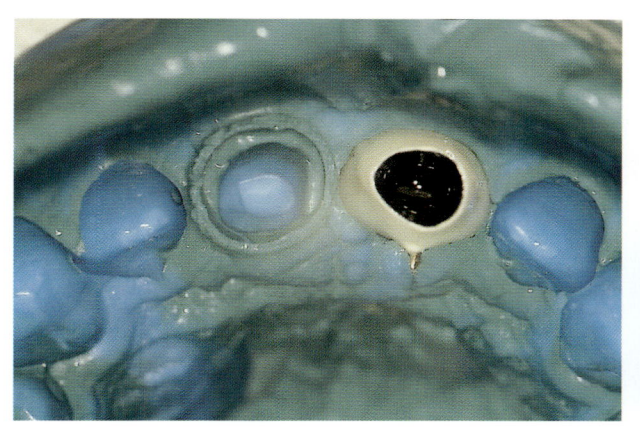

**8** Delayed Placement in Adequate Bone with Mature Ridge

**Fig 8-131** Impression of the prepared tooth with a combined pick-up of the unglazed restoration refined to the soft tissues.

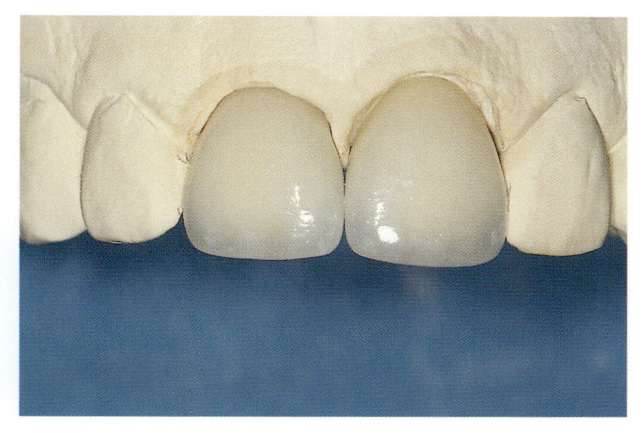

**Fig 8-132** Final restorations before cementation.

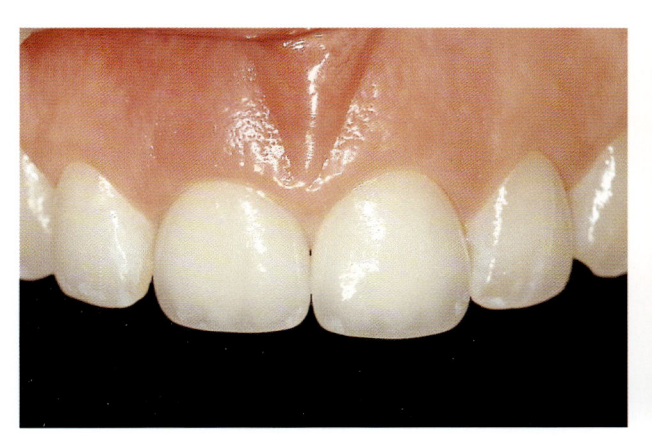

**Fig 8-133** Final restorations in situ showing acceptable aesthetic outcome.

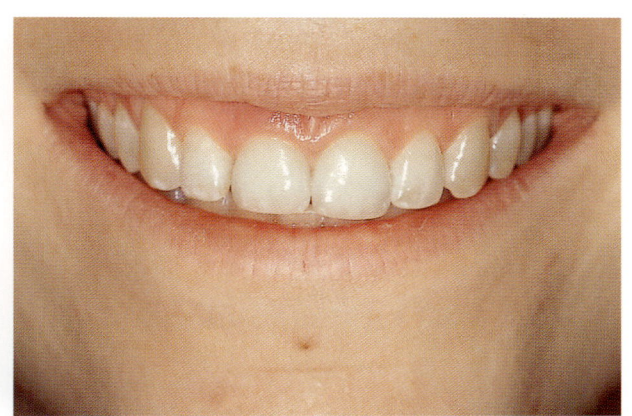

**Fig 8-134** Labial view of patient with high smile line after cementation of definitive restorations.

## Case 2: Delayed Placement with Immediate Loading

A 28-year-old man who had lost the lateral incisor eight months previously attended for its replacement with an implant. Conventional radiographs demonstrated adequate height; ridge width was assessed using ridge mapping to ensure adequate width in spite of the labial depression. Visual assessment of soft tissue height indicated the possibility of manipulating it to bulk out the deficiency caused by disuse atrophy. An implant for immediate loading was planned, with surgical access designed to develop soft tissues. The incision was similar to that carried out for implant exposure when staged treatment is carried out. Implant placement was carried out with simultaneous abutment attachment and fitting of the transitional restoration. Restorative treatment was completed three months later using conventional impressions (Figs 8-135–8-148).

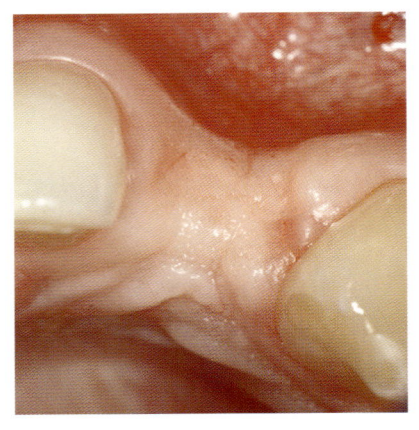

II  Implant Placement: Surgery and Prosthodontics

**Fig 8-135** Occlusal view of an edentulous lateral incisor region showing the labial depression following natural postextraction atrophy.

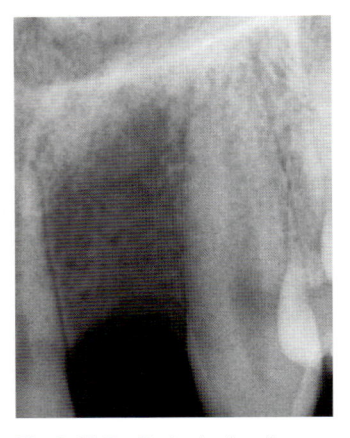

**Fig 8-136** Periapical radiograph showing adequate bone height. The radiolucent appearance is indicative of low-density bone in view of the adequate width as measured by ridge mapping.

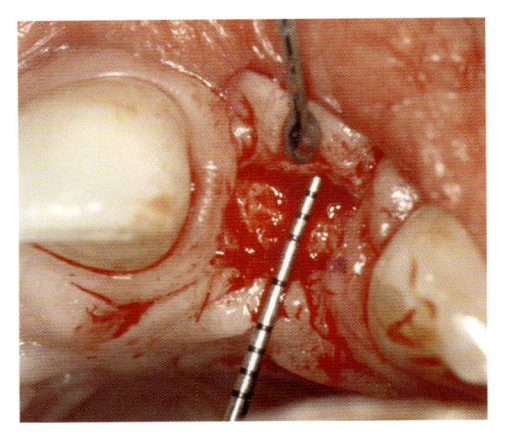

**Fig 8-137** Access to the bony ridge is obtained by means of an 'H'-shaped incision and designed towards the palatal aspect of the ridge, with the deflection of the tissues labially to increase the bulk in order to compensate for the atrophy.

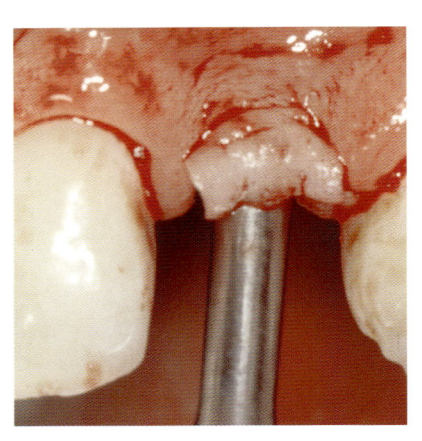

**Fig 8-138** The osteotomy was prepared using a pilot bur, followed by a round bur to penetrate the crest and a bone condenser to complete the osteotomy to the depth and diameter required.

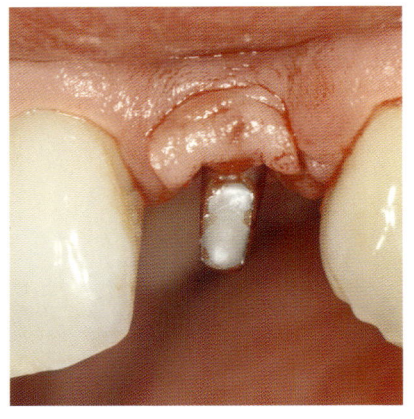

**Fig 8-139** The implant was inserted, the angle of the abutment selected as described above using direction indicators and the definitive abutment inserted and attached to the implant. The abutment is visible with the access hole for the fixation screw sealed with wax and glass-ionomer cement.

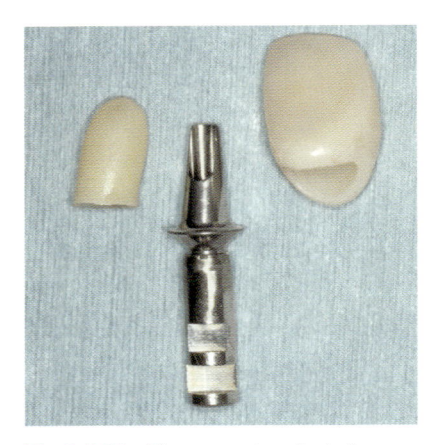

**Fig 8-140** The accurate adaptation of the transitional restoration is carried out by connecting the hollow acrylic transitional restoration (seen to the right of the abutment) to the acrylic sleeve (seen left of the abutment), which has been constructed to fit accurately onto the abutment. This is done using self-curing resin.

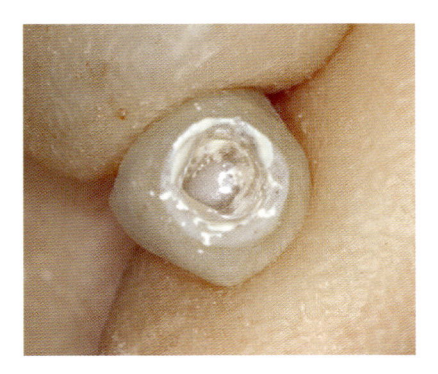

**Fig 8-141** The fit surface of the transitional restoration loaded with a thin smear of temporary cement prior to cementation. A prudent amount of temporary cement prevents any excess and, therefore, any adverse soft or hard tissue response.

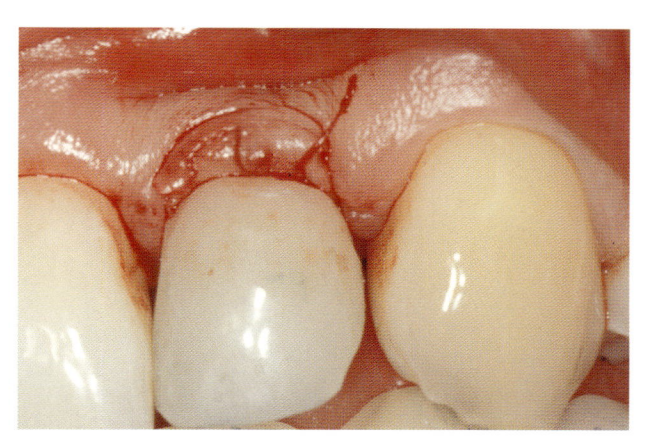

**8** Delayed Placement in Adequate Bone with Mature Ridge

**Fig 8-142** The transitional restoration fitted on the abutment. The deflected tissues are visible and have been sutured using a fine (6-0 Vicryl; Ethicon, Somerville, NJ, USA) suture.

**Fig 8-143** Post-operative radiograph showing the implant and abutment relationship.

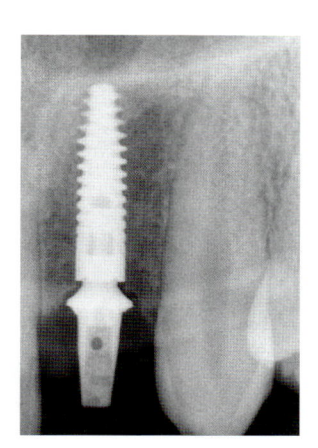

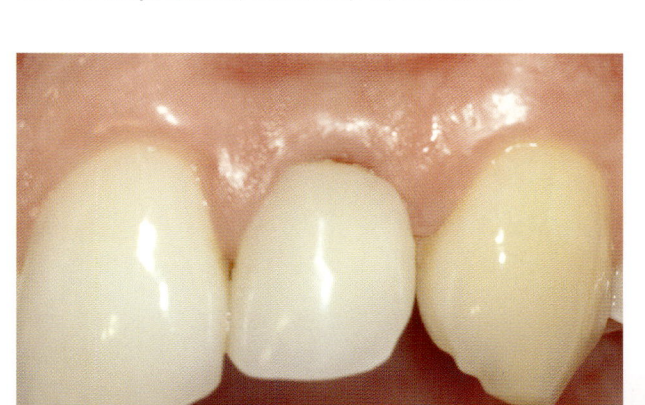

**Fig 8-144** Healing of the soft tissues at one week.

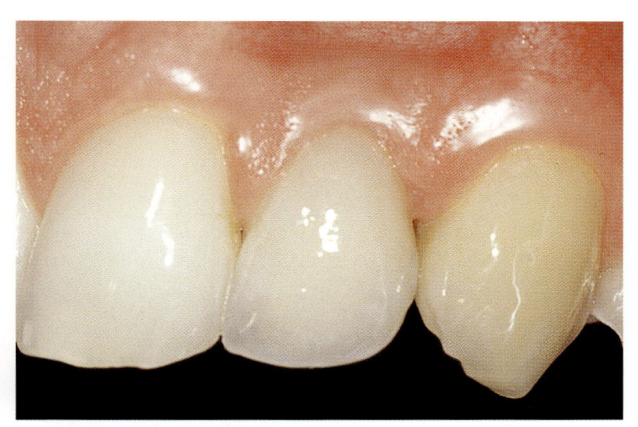

**Fig 8-145** Definitive restoration in situ, constructed three months after implant insertion.

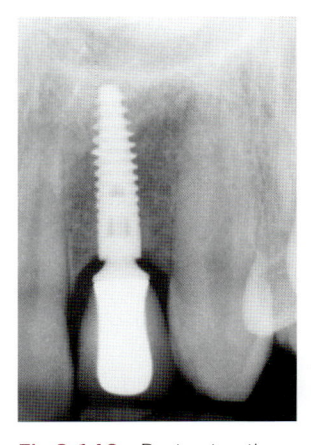

**Fig 8-146** Postrestorative radiograph showing the level of bone in relationship to the implant.

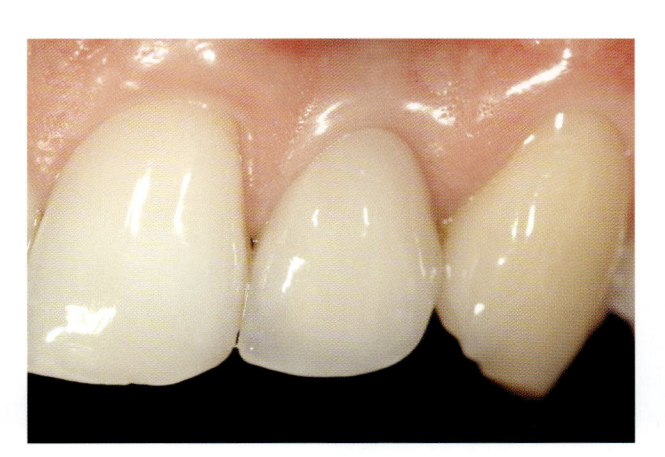

**Fig 8-147** Labial view of the definitive restoration seven years after the procedure. Stable gingival contours are evident.

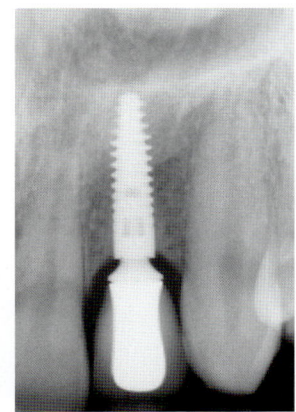

**Fig 8-148** Periapical radiograph taken seven years after the procedure showing stable bone levels compared with the postrestorative radiograph.

143

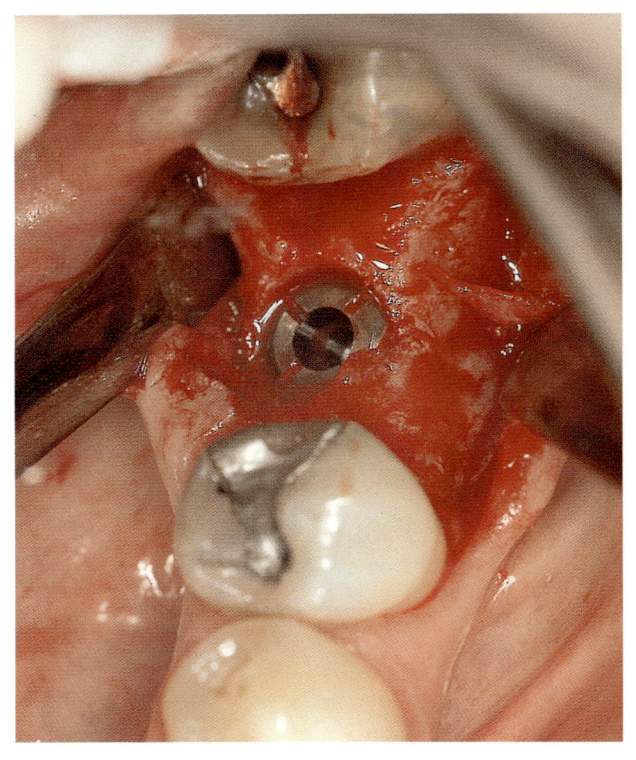

II | Implant Placement: Surgery and Prosthodontics

**Fig 8-149** Occlusal view of the implant replacing the mandibular first molar. The cover screw has been removed to receive the sulcus former.

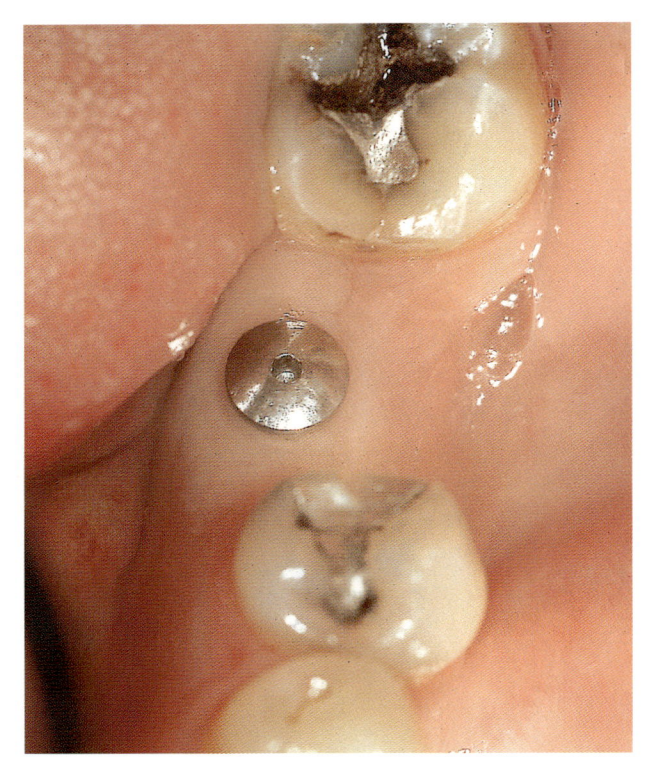

**Fig 8-150** The sulcus former prior to attachment of the abutment and restorative phase.

### Case 3: Delayed Placement with Transgingival Healing

This case demonstrates the use of a sulcus former to enable transgingival healing to take place. When a posterior tooth is replaced by a single implant, transmucosal healing is favoured where a prosthesis is not worn and where aesthetics are not critical (Figs 8-149 and 8-150).

### Case 4: Delayed Placement with Immediate Loading

This 50-year-old woman returned for treatment several years after treatment of the left mandible. A history of advanced periodontal disease and a need to retain her natural teeth resulted in disease progression, both in terms of caries and bone loss. Her final decision to proceed with the treatment was based on the success of the previous treatment and a need to improve the appearance of her anterior teeth.

The decision to carry out the treatment on the completion of healing was based on a number of factors:

- the poor position of her present teeth and, therefore, the impossibility of locating the implants in the desired tooth position
- the need for augmentation in the posterior quadrants
- the need to ensure that the patient would tolerate a change in the occlusal scheme
- the need for the patient to approve the aesthetic changes proposed.

Treatment involved a diagnostic preview subsequently translated into a provisional restoration. Augmentation under the sinuses and manipulation of the inferior alveolar neurovascular bundle was implemented. Subsequent placement of implants in the correct position with immediate loading and their eventual restoration was undertaken (Figs 8-151–8-201).

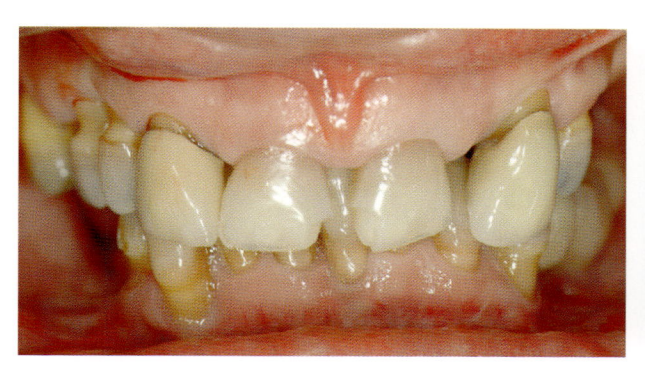

**8** Delayed Placement in Adequate Bone with Mature Ridge

**Fig 8-151** Labial view of patient showing intraoral status with respect to spacing of teeth as well as the relationship between the maxillary and mandibular teeth. A complete traumatic and increased overbite is evident.

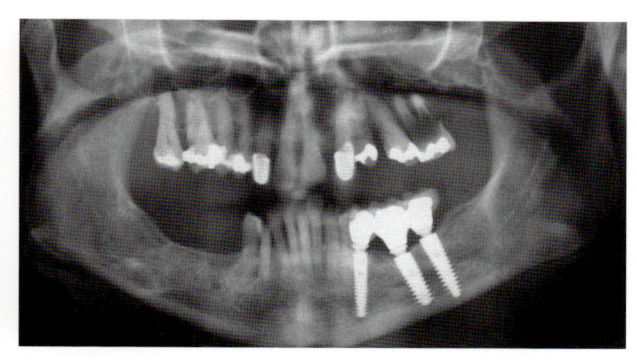

**Fig 8-152** Dental panoramic tomograph showing considerable pathology with respect to caries and periodontal bone loss. Previous treatment carried out on the lower left-hand side is visible.

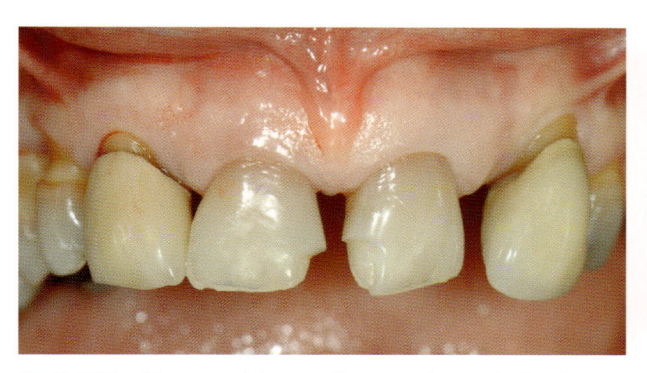

**Fig 8-153** Close-up of the maxillary anterior teeth showing the spacing, discolouration and positioning.

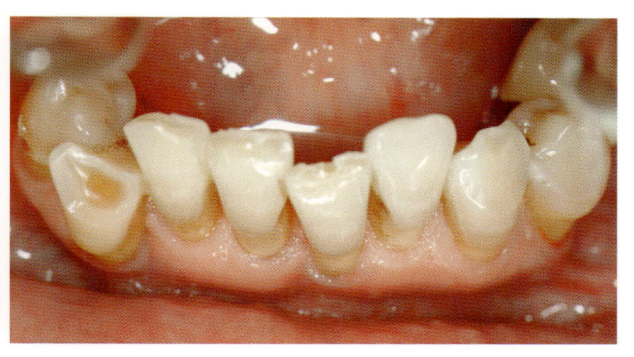

**Fig 8-154** Close-up of the mandibular anterior teeth showing the overcrowding, imbrication and the wear indicative of parafunctional activity.

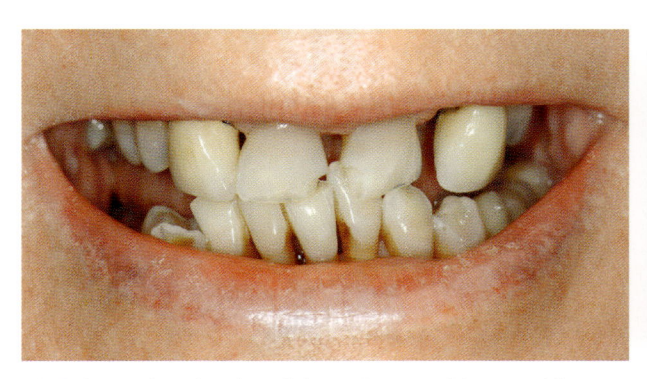

**Fig 8-155** Anterior view of the patient speaking, providing valuable information relating to normal functional intermaxillary distance. This information can be used to predict tolerance to planned changes in the occlusal scheme.

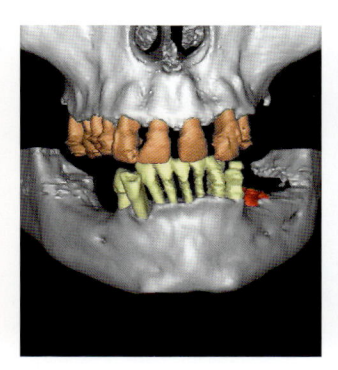

**Fig 8-156** CT scan of the maxilla and mandible taken parallel to the occlusal plane and providing an image of both the jaws. The interrelationship of the jaws can be seen.

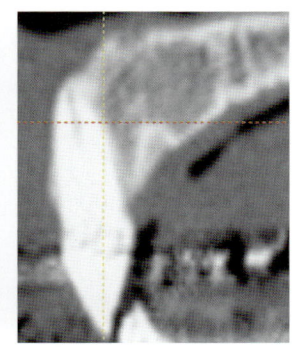

**Fig 8-157** Cross-sectional CT image of the central incisor providing valuable information about the bone biotype and, therefore, predicting postextraction resorption.

145

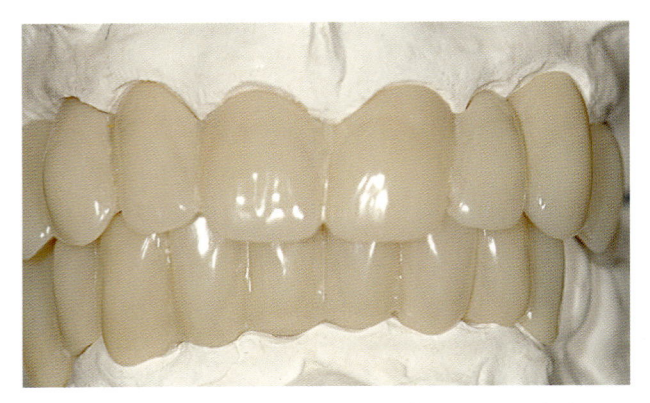

## II  Implant Placement: Surgery and Prosthodontics

**Fig 8-158**  A diagnostic preview on study casts mounted on a semi-adjustable articulator. The proposed change in the intermaxillary distance was based on interdental speaking distance.

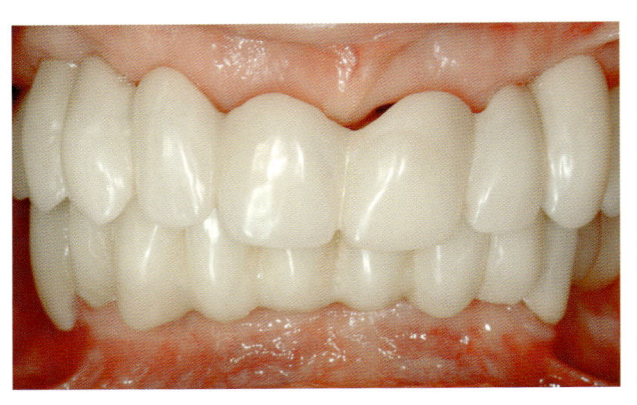

**Fig 8-159**  Information gathered during the diagnostic preview is translated to metal-acrylic provisional restorations and transferred to the mouth for assessment of aesthetics and function.

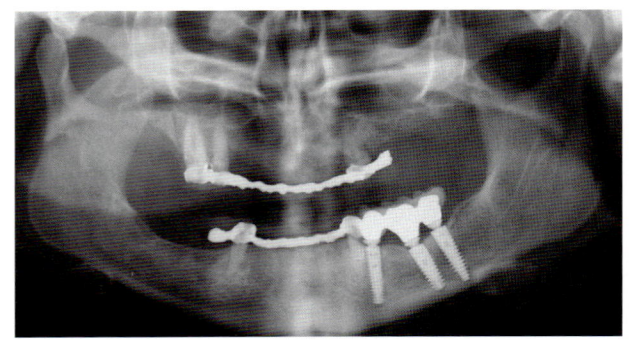

**Fig 8-160**  A panoramic tomograph showing the positioning of the teeth selected for the support of the metal-acrylic provisional restoration.

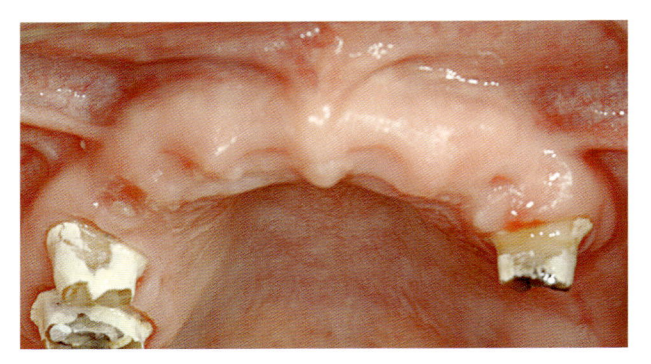

**Fig 8-161**  Intraoral view of the healed ridge three months following extraction. The position of the implants can now be selected as dictated by tooth position following the complete healing of the tooth sockets.

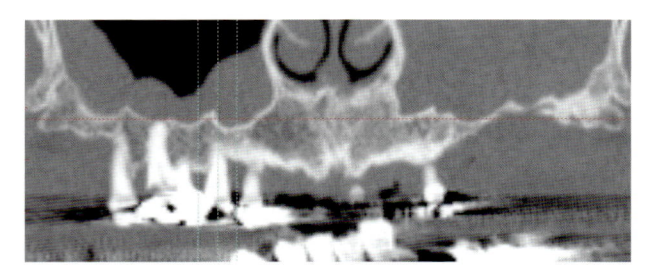

**Fig 8-162**  CT panoral view showing a thickened sinus lining. The occluded sinus on the left-hand side may be attributable to the pathology associated with the recently extracted molar teeth, which had breached the floor of the sinus.

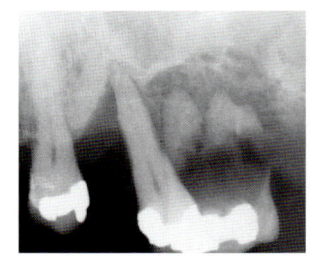

**Fig 8-163**  The radiograph showing the pathology associated with the failing left molar.

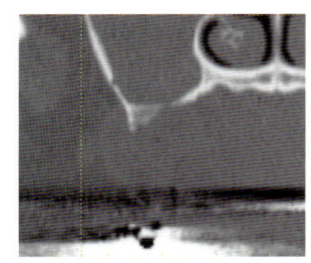

**Fig 8-164**  Cross-sectional CT image showing the residual bone thickness and the thickened sinus lining. A branch of the maxillary artery is visible in the lateral wall of the sinus.

8   Delayed Placement in Adequate Bone with Mature Ridge

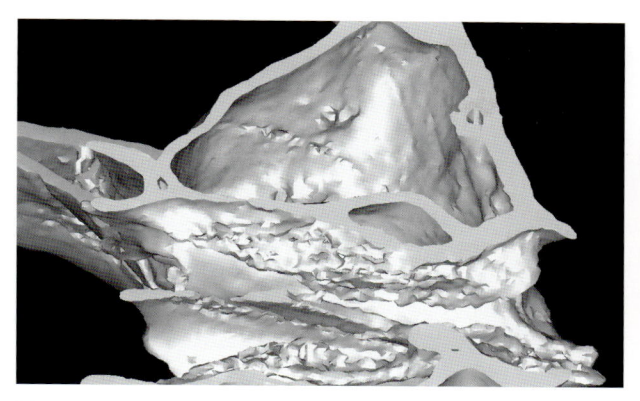

**Fig 8-165**   Three-dimensional CT view of the internal surface of the left maxillary sinus showing the scoring of the lateral wall by the branch of the maxillary artery.

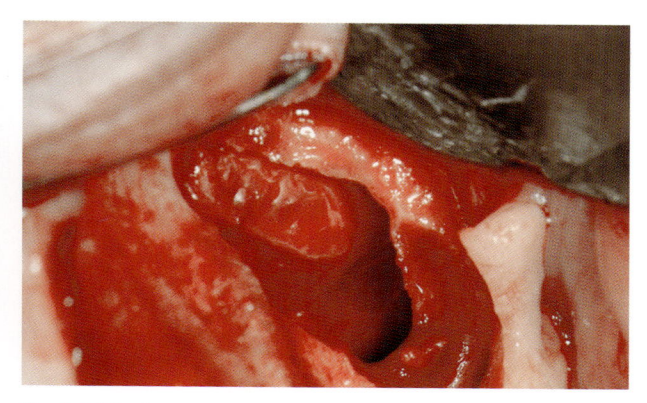

**Fig 8-166**   Lateral window approach for subantral augmentation. Inspiration by the patient results in the inward movement of the lining. This is indicative of an intact lining. In this case, it is also indicative of a resolution of the obliterated sinus following extraction of the teeth that were causing the pathological response of the lining.

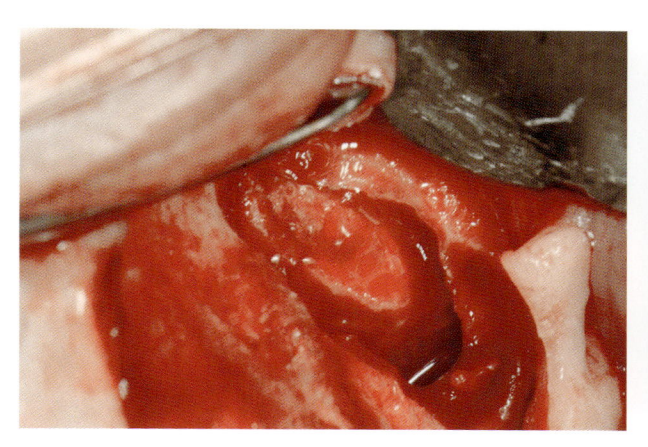

**Fig 8-167**   Exhalation by the patient results in the outward movement of the lining.

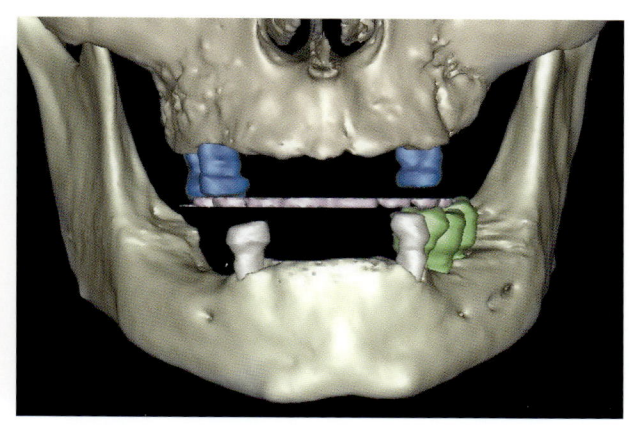

**Fig 8-168**   Three-dimensional CT view of maxilla and mandible showing complete healing of the sockets at six months after extraction. The second CT scan is used to plan implant placement in the healed sites as well as in the augmented sinuses.

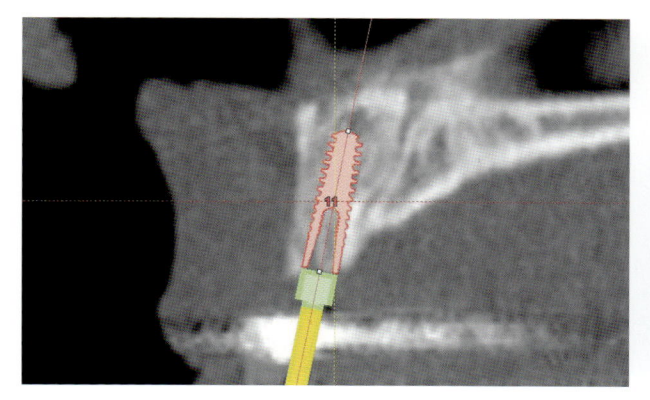

**Fig 8-169**   Cross-sectional CT image of the anterior maxilla showing interactive positioning of the implant in adequate bone, as predicted from bone biotype assessment.

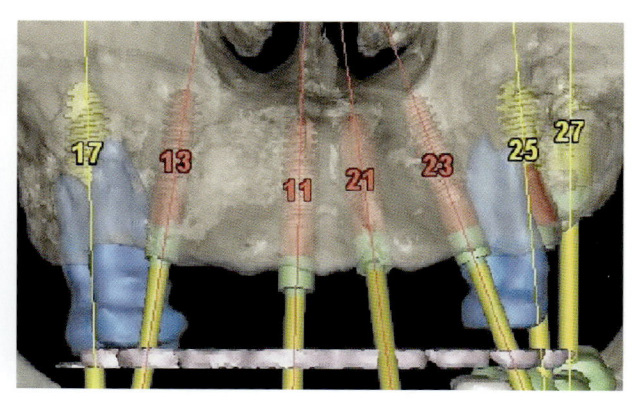

**Fig 8-170**   Interactive planning on the CT 3D view enables the assessment of the implant positions with respect to tooth position identified by the provisional restoration and adjacent teeth.

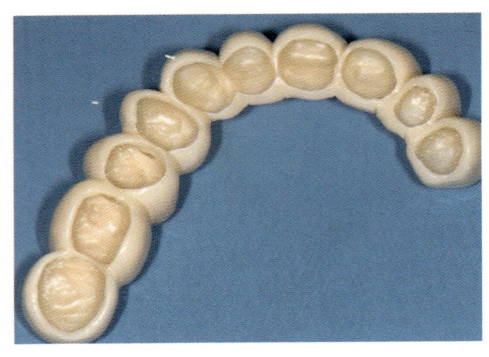

II  Implant Placement: Surgery and Prosthodontics

**Fig 8-171** Hollow acrylic transitional restoration fabricated from preliminary diagnostic information and provisional restorations. This is produced in readiness for the immediate loading of the implants that had been planned.

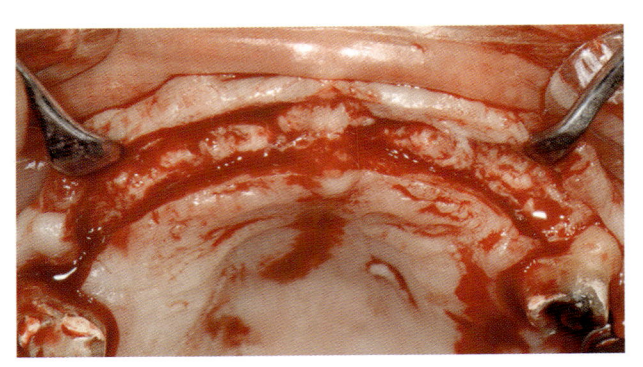

**Fig 8-172** An incision on the palatal aspect of the crest of the ridge is used to expose the crest for siting of implants.

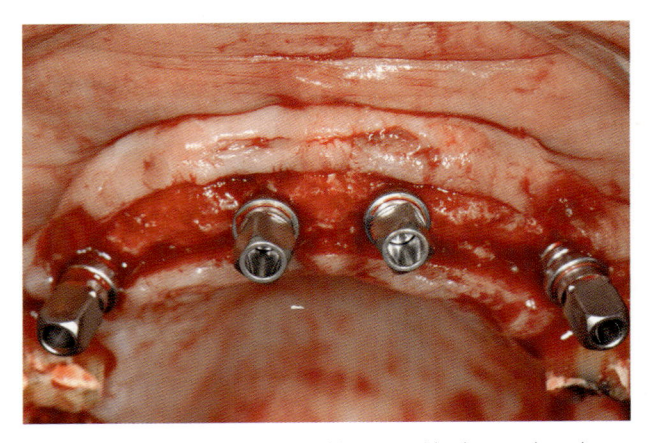

**Fig 8-173** Implants positioned in central incisor and canine positions according to interactive planning. Implant positions were estimated based on landmarks, namely the naso-palatine foramen and the retained first premolars.

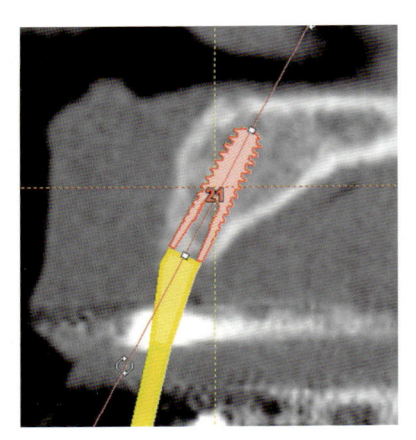

**Fig 8-174** Abutment selection using the interactive Simplant program.

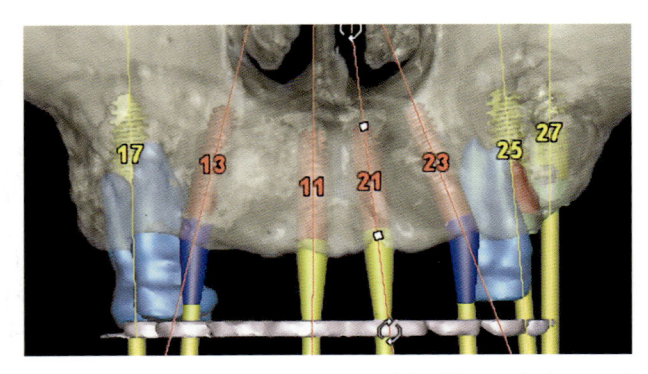

**Fig 8-175** Three-dimensional view of the CT scan being used to verify the abutment position in relation to the provisional restoration.

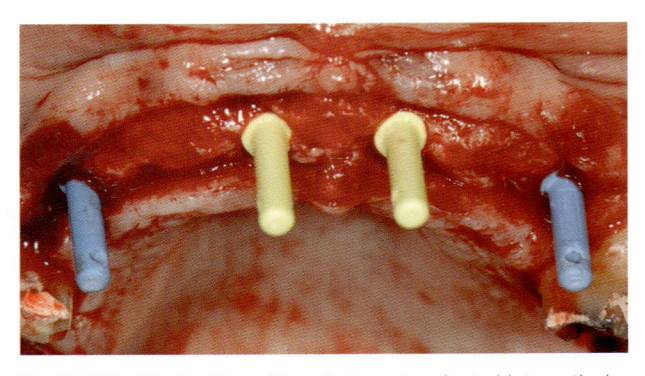

**Fig 8-176** Verification of the abutments selected interactively. This is done directly using the direction indicators placed into the cover screws of the implants.

8   Delayed Placement in Adequate Bone with Mature Ridge

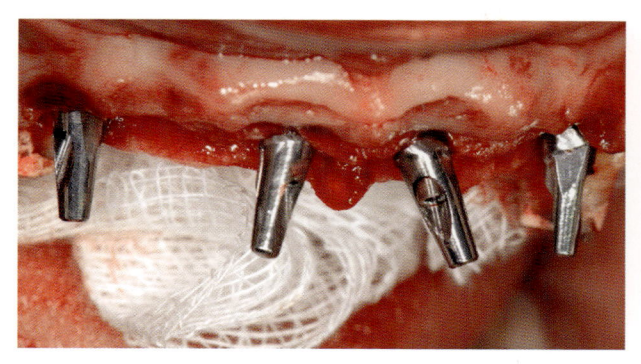

**Fig 8-177**   Pre-angled abutments inserted into the implants following cover screw removal. A non-indexed system depending upon a conical connection enables the abutment to be rotated into the correct alignment, as shown in Fig 8-178. An indexed system would require the rotation of the implant to satisfactorily align the abutments.

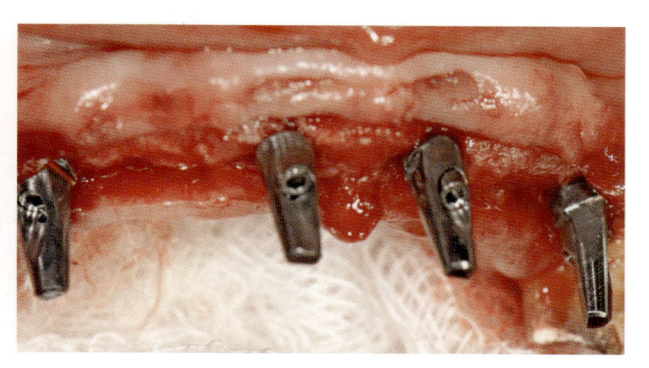

**Fig 8-178**   Correctly aligned abutments prior to engaging the conical connection with a screw tightened to 15 Ncm.

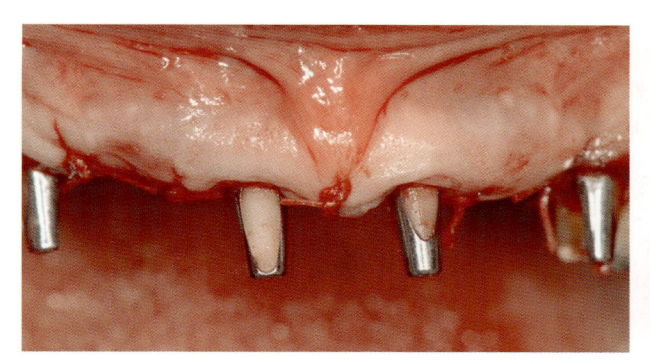

**Fig 8-179**   The wound sutured around the abutments. Note that the access holes have been sealed with the glass-ionomer cement to permit effective relining of the transitional restoration directly onto the abutments. The abutment in the central incisor region on the left-hand side has been changed to a 22.5-degree abutment to achieve better alignment.

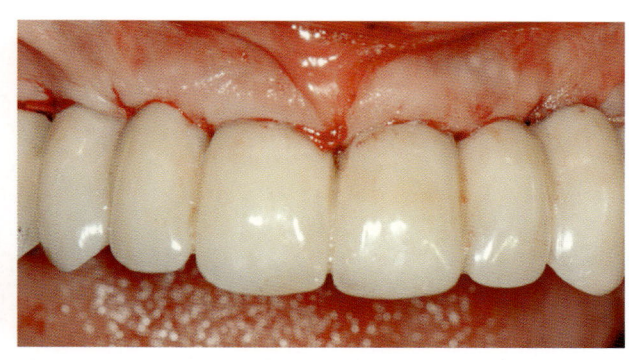

**Fig 8-180**   The relined transitional restoration seated over the abutments is used to establish gingival contours.

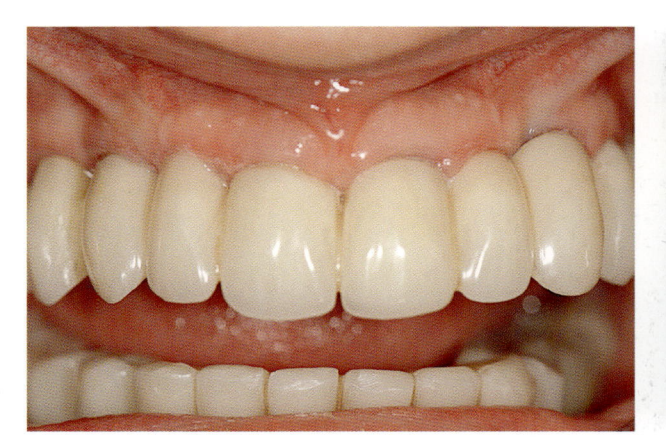

**Fig 8-181**   Healed and contoured soft tissues.

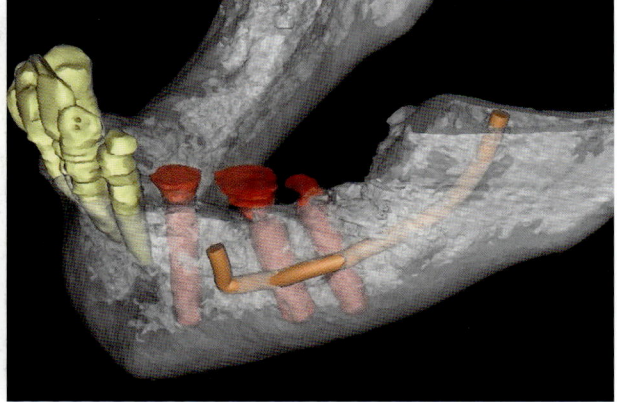

**Fig 8-182**   Three-dimensional CT view of left mandible showing previous treatment with implants in situ, which extend to the lower border. The inferior alveolar nerve has been repositioned and is visible on the surface.

## II  Implant Placement: Surgery and Prosthodontics

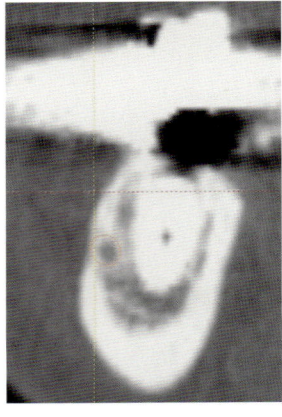

**Fig 8-183** Cross-sectional view showing one of the implants with the inferior alveolar nerve adjacent to it.

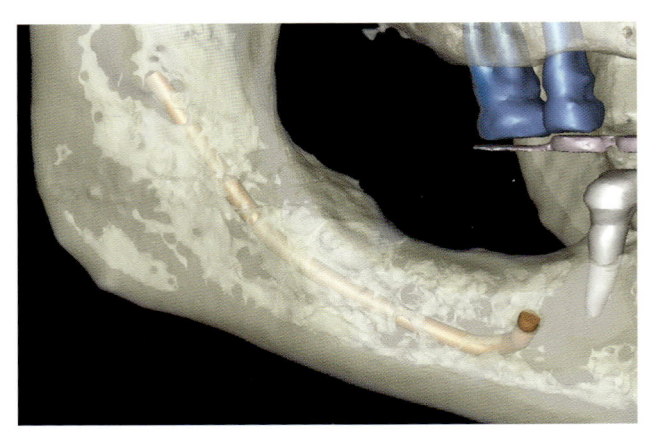

**Fig 8-184** Three-dimensional CT view of lower right-hand side with the inferior alveolar nerve outlined.

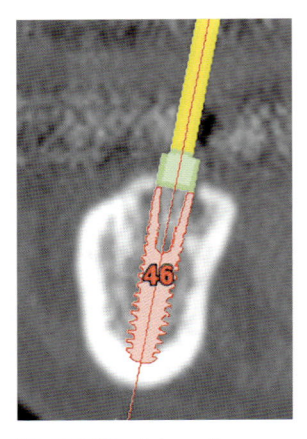

**Fig 8-186** Interactive planning showing a 17-mm implant with the nerve transpositioned towards the buccal.

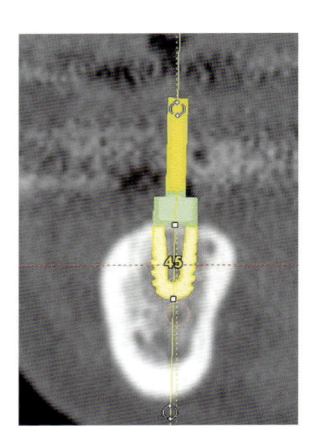

**Fig 8-185** Cross-sectional view with interactive placement of an implant. The shortest implant (8 mm) can be seen in contact with the inferior alveolar nerve. The placement of such an implant would be hazardous and would carry a high risk of damage to the nerve. The patient's predisposition to periodontal disease would also be of concern with respect to future bone loss around a short implant.

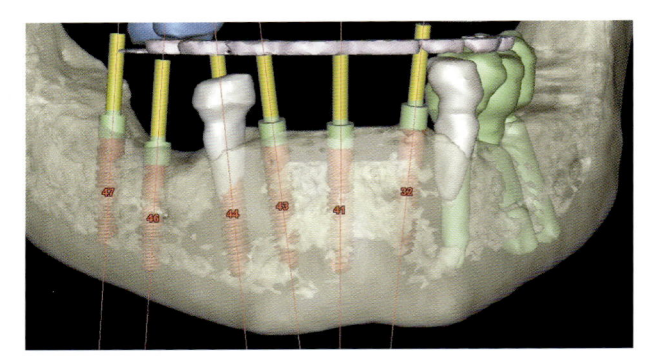

**Fig 8-187** Three-dimensional visualisation of the planning of implants.

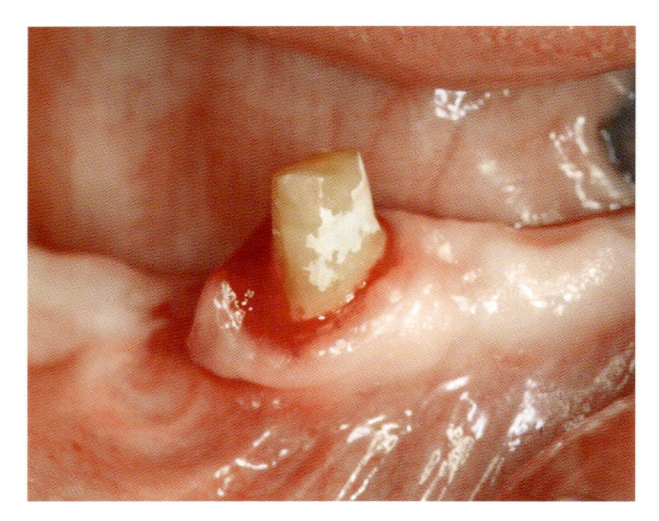

**Fig 8-188** Preoperative view of lower right side.

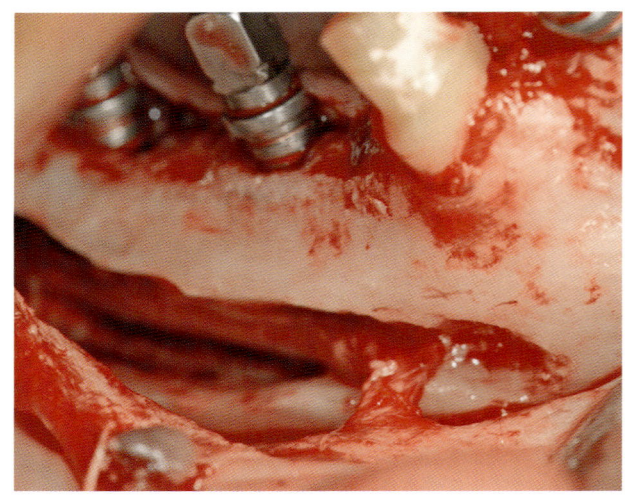

**Fig 8-189** Intraoperative image showing the intact repositioned nerve lying beside the implants. The mental and incisive branches are visible.

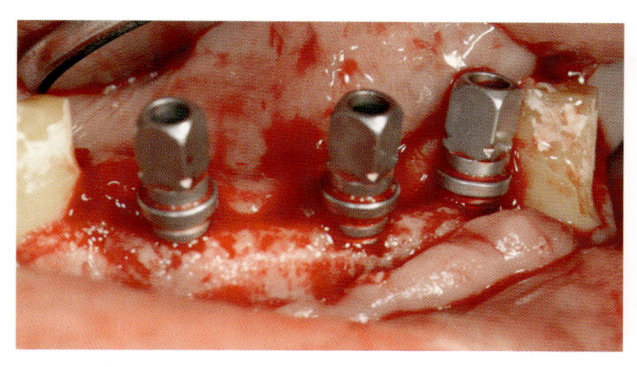

**8** Delayed Placement in Adequate Bone with Mature Ridge

**Fig 8-190** Anterior implants in situ as planned during the interactive CT scan planning session.

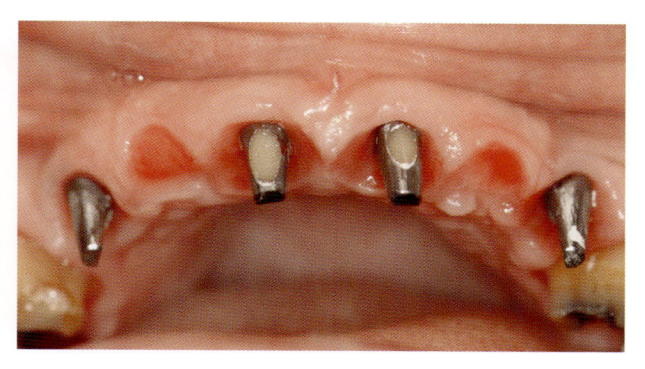

**Fig 8-191** Maxillary abutments emerging out of soft tissues contoured by the transitional restoration.

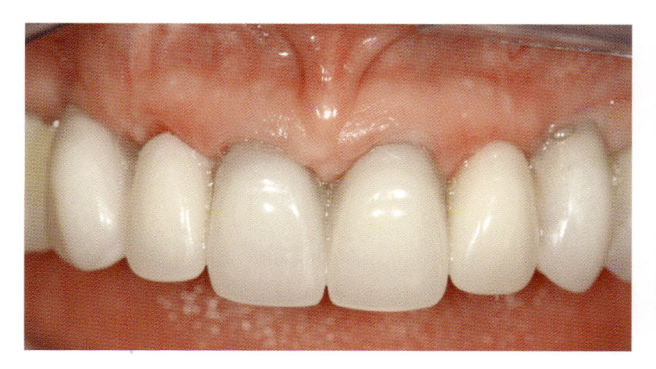

**Fig 8-192** A new diagnostic preview is fabricated from acrylic teeth and wax to enable the direct relationship between the abutments and the working casts to be accurately established. Any changes that are necessary should be made at this stage prior to the construction of the metalwork.

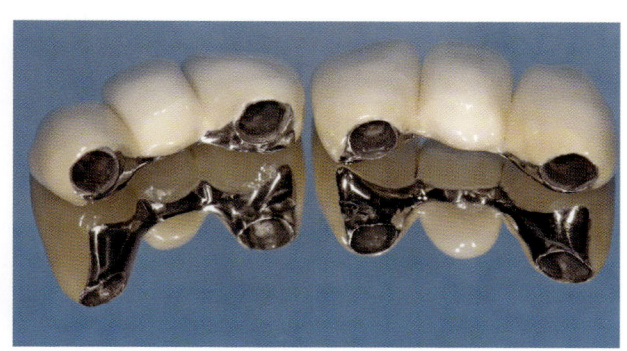

**Fig 8-193** The definitive restoration fabricated from porcelain fused to metal. Two separate bridges have been constructed for the six anterior teeth. Individual crowns for the remaining teeth and splinted crowns for the posteriors were also fabricated.

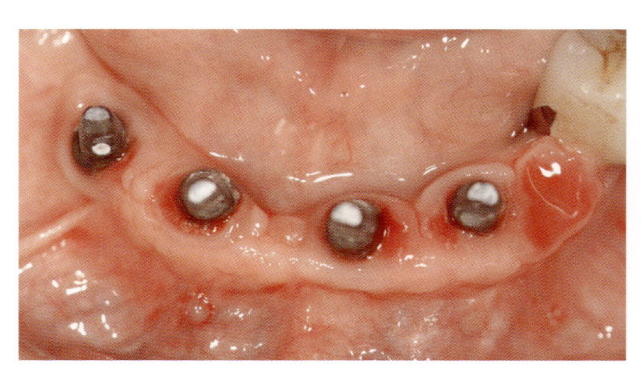

**Fig 8-194** Intraoral view of the mandibular abutments.

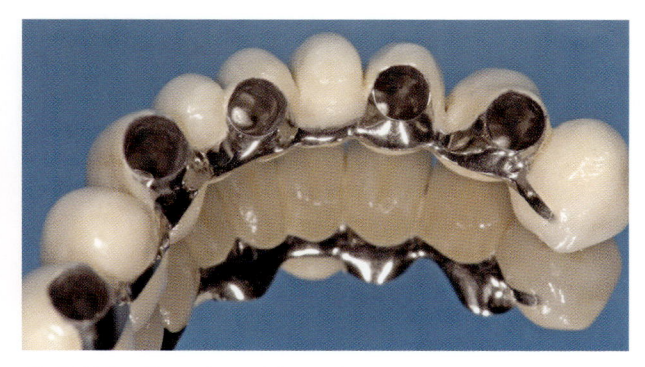

**Fig 8-195** Fit surface of the splinted bridge that has been constructed for the mandibular implants.

II    Implant Placement: Surgery and Prosthodontics

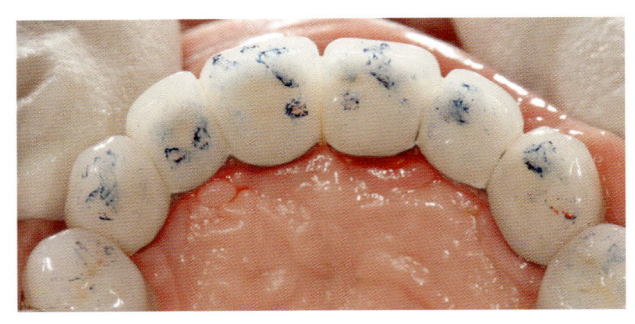

**Fig 8-196**  View of the occlusal surface of the maxillary restoration showing the established contact with the mandibular restoration. Anterior guidance with posterior disclusion was the preferred scheme.

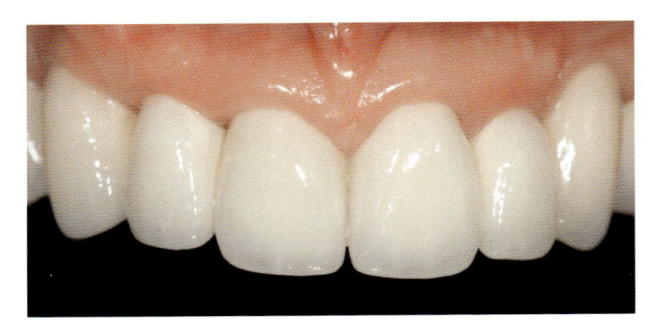

**Fig 8-197**  Labial view of the definitive restoration.

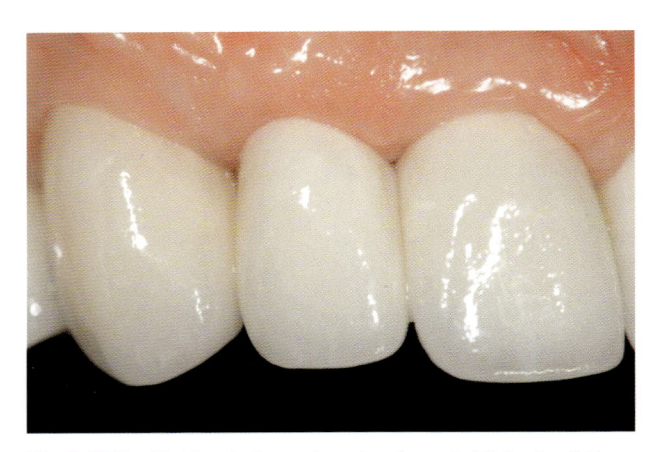

**Fig 8-198**  Right anterior region showing established soft tissue contours and emergence profile.

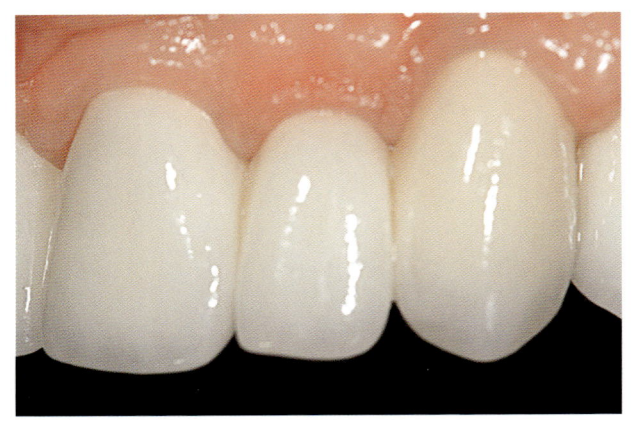

**Fig 8-199**  Left anterior region.

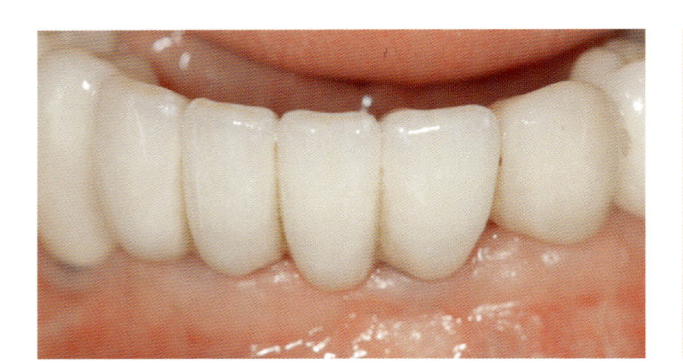

**Fig 8-200**  Labial view of mandibular restoration.

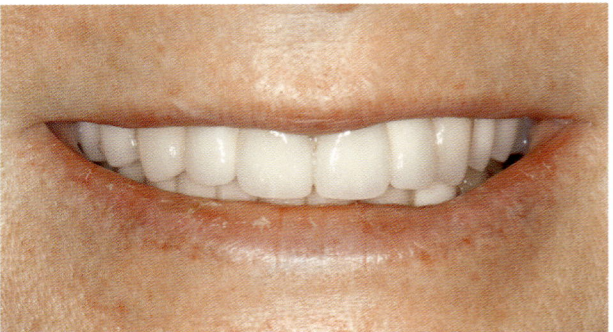

**Fig 8-201**  Anterior view of the patient showing the corrected position of the teeth as well as the relationship between the two jaws.

# Chapter 9

# Delayed Loading: Implant Exposure

## Introduction

The philosophy that has been described in the earlier chapters has as its main objectives the predictable achievement of osseointegration and the creation of an adequate hard tissue foundation to provide support for the soft tissues. It is intended that sufficient soft tissues in bulk and contour are present to facilitate the development of the desired harmonious emergence profile.

It is the shape of the component part, which is attached at the time of exposure, that influences the emergence profile. It is, therefore, obvious that the size and the shape of the component part used should closely match the final abutment and restoration. It is for this reason that the definitive abutment, selected at first-stage surgery, is considered to be ideal for attachment at this stage.

This enables the abutment that is ideally shaped for the proposed restoration to be connected at the time of implant exposure. Attachment of the definitive abutment at this stage of treatment prevents the repeated disconnection and reconnection of component parts. This has several benefits:

- it prevents excessive negative tissue reactions associated with repeated disconnection and reconnection[144]
- it avoids inaccuracies that are associated with repeated transfers of component parts between the surgery and laboratory[145–148]
- it reduces costs by avoiding the purchase of component parts required for transfer of information and additional laboratory procedures

Furthermore, a transitional restoration fabricated from impressions taken at first-stage surgery may also be contoured and fitted at this stage.

Healing abutments are, therefore, not considered ideal unless they can be shaped to prevent the soft tissues from being unacceptably deformed. Attention needs to be paid, in particular, to implants requiring restorations with abutment angles greater than 15 degrees. Re-contouring by healing abutments may result in unacceptable gingival recession (Fig 8-63, p. 126). Nevertheless, if the conditions are such that a healing abutment is used as a sulcus former, modification of the existing provisional restoration might be necessary in order to provide continuing function after implant exposure.

The incisions that are described to gain access to the implant are designed to allow the creation of a natural papillary and marginal contour consistent with the adjacent teeth. The aim of the protocol is

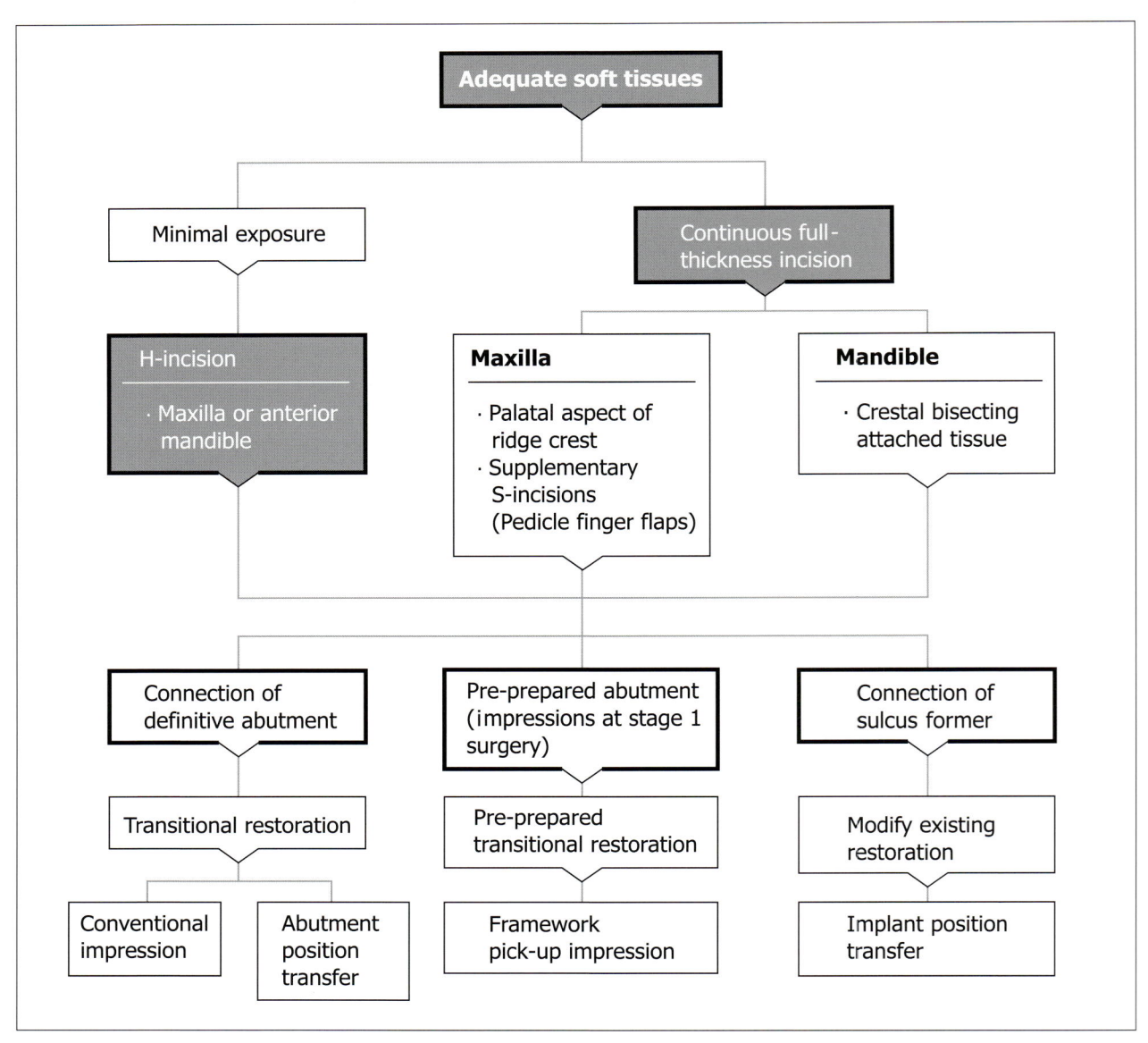

II Implant Placement: Surgery and Prosthodontics

**Flowchart 9-1** Surgical exposure of implant.

```
Adequate soft tissues
├── Minimal exposure
│   └── H-incision
│       · Maxilla or anterior mandible
│       └── Connection of definitive abutment
│           └── Transitional restoration
│               ├── Conventional impression
│               └── Abutment position transfer
└── Continuous full-thickness incision
    ├── Maxilla
    │   · Palatal aspect of ridge crest
    │   · Supplementary S-incisions (Pedicle finger flaps)
    │   └── Pre-prepared abutment (impressions at stage 1 surgery)
    │       └── Pre-prepared transitional restoration
    │           └── Framework pick-up impression
    └── Mandible
        · Crestal bisecting attached tissue
        └── Connection of sulcus former
            └── Modify existing restoration
                └── Implant position transfer
```

to simplify the treatment for the patient, clinician and dental technician.

## Preoperative Planning

A hollow acrylic resin transitional restoration should be fabricated based on the original diagnostic preview with respect to the tooth form and position. Additional impressions may be required to incorporate any changes made during the course of treatment to this stage.

## Implant Exposure

Sound surgical principles to minimise the surgical exposure based on the access required should be employed. A series of surgical approaches to achieve this are described in Flowchart 9–1.

### Minimal Exposure Incision

When adequate tissue is present, the purpose of this phase is to remove tissue for the insertion of

# 9 Delayed Loading: Implant Exposure

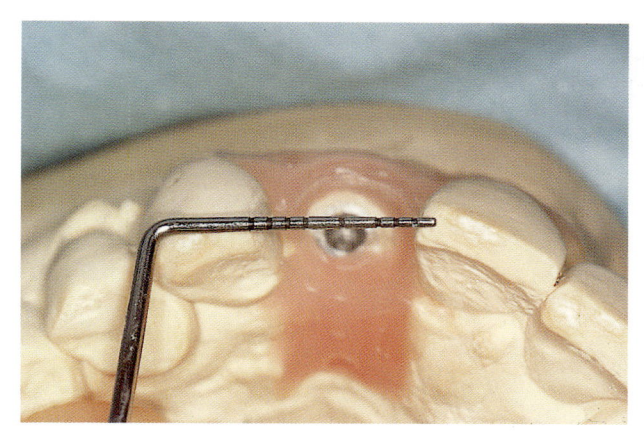

**Fig 9-1** Occlusal view of the stone cast constructed from impressions taken at first-stage surgery showing the position of the implant. This position can be transferred to the clinical situation. An abutment selected at first-stage surgery is modified based upon this cast containing an implant analogue. The transitional crown, as well as the metalwork, has been constructed.

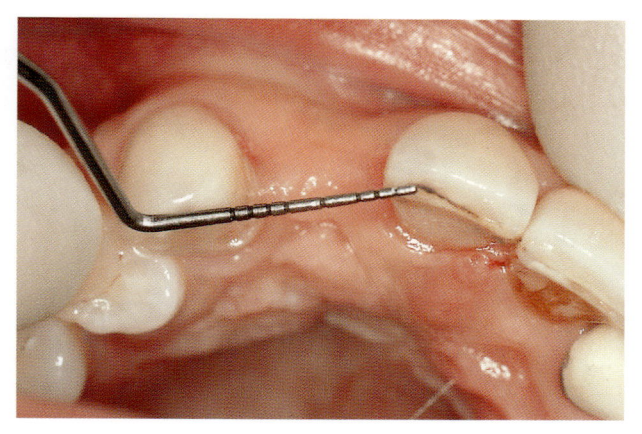

**Fig 9-2** Occlusal view of the healed ridge prior to exposure of the implant. The position of the implant can be accurately located in the mouth by transferring the information from the laboratory cast.

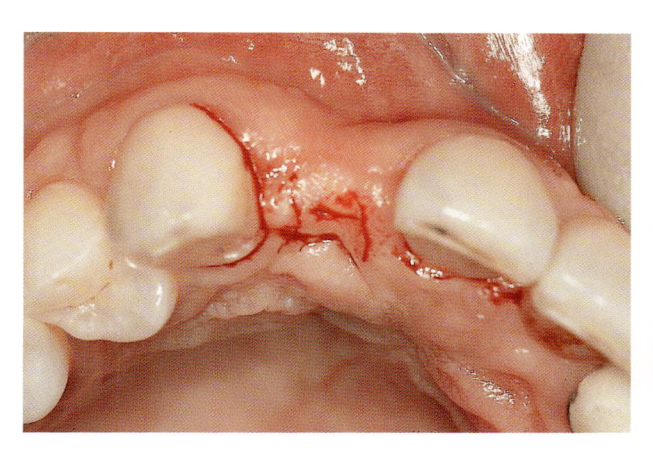

**Fig 9-3** The 'H'-shaped incision can be seen inscribed in the ridge. The crossbar of the 'H' is positioned towards the palatal aspect of the crest. This will enable soft tissues to be displaced towards the labial where the depression is visible in this view.

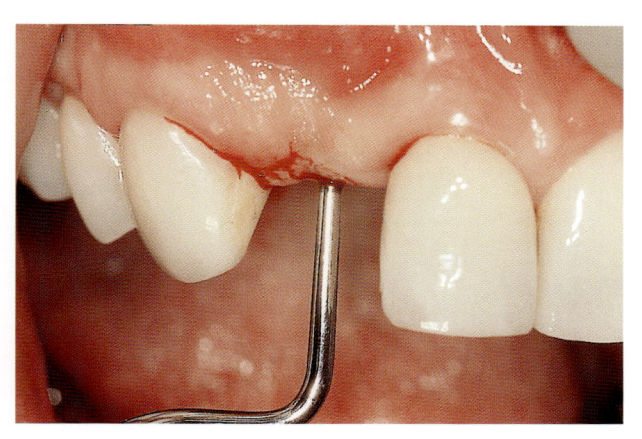

**Fig 9-4** Labial view showing a sharp probe (Ankylos exposure kit [available from Dentsply Frident, Mannheim, Germany]) being used to accurately locate the implant.

the abutment and a transitional restoration. However, excision of this tissue with a circular punch, for example, may not achieve the ideal position for the gingival margin. It is for this reason that the minimal incision ('H' shaped) was devised. This provides an opportunity to assess the contours and manipulate the tissues, if necessary, or to excise them, if more appropriate (Figs 9-1–9-14).

## 'H'-shaped Incision

This type of incision is especially useful for:
- the anterior maxilla or mandible
- accurately identified implant position
- exposure of a single implant
- multiple implants with adequate interimplant distance.

The incision is made directly over the implant, with the main incision over the palatal area of the implant

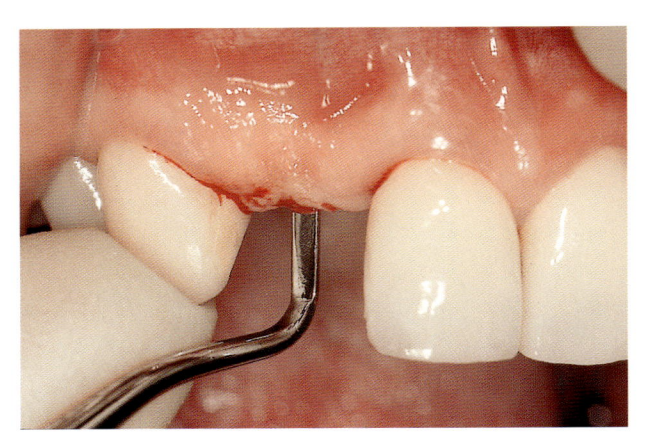

## II  Implant Placement: Surgery and Prosthodontics

**Fig 9-5**  Flat instrument (Ankylos exposure kit) can be seen being used to clear the soft tissues from the implant surface to gain access to the cover screw.

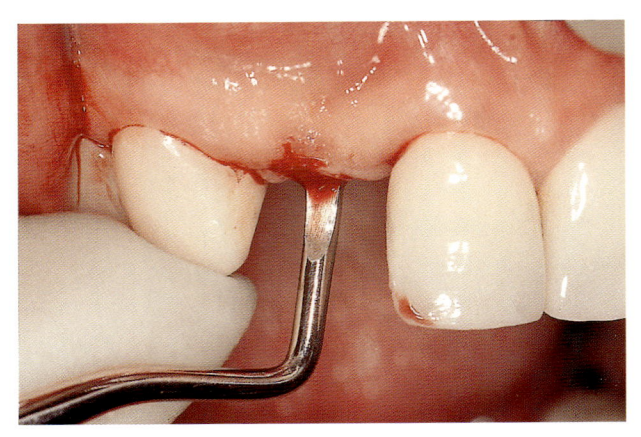

**Fig 9-6**  Excavator (Ankylos exposure kit) maybe used to undermine the soft tissues to allow their manipulation and for the removal of any bone that may have grown over the implant and may prevent access to the cover screw.

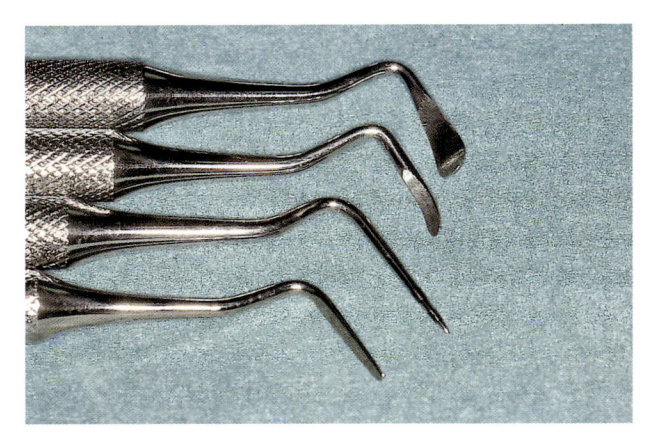

**Fig 9-7**  Ankylos exposure kit showing the four instruments that facilitate exposure of the implant and the clearance of hard and soft tissues particularly when a minimal incision is used.

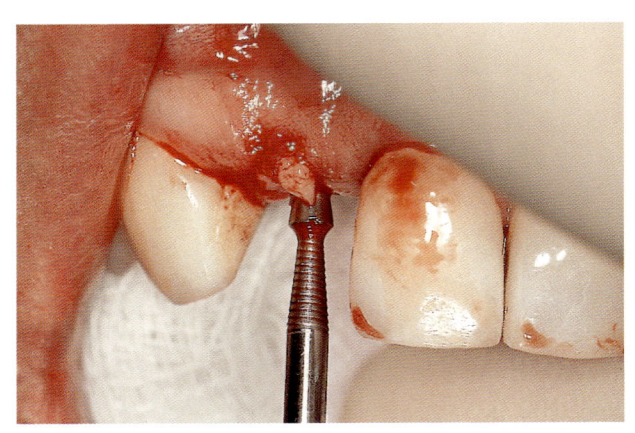

**Fig 9-8**  Labial view showing the cover screw being removed. The reverse thread on the special instrument designed for cover screw removal engages the screw thread within the cover screw. This minimises the risk of the accidental loss of the cover screw.

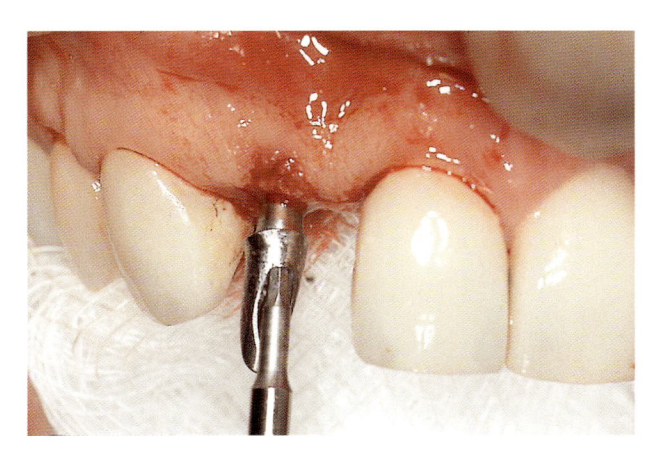

**Fig 9-9**  The abutment, modified in the laboratory (by master dental technician Mr Peter Sochor) from an impression taken at first-stage surgery, can be seen prior to attachment to the implant. The internal taper connection greatly facilitates attachment of the abutment to the implant through a minimal incision. Finger pressure is used to confirm that the conical connection is engaged prior to tightening. This ensures that there is no obstruction to the seating and engagement of the taper. Ensuring that the taper is engaged at this stage minimises the risk of abutment loosening at a later stage.

# 9 Delayed Loading: Implant Exposure

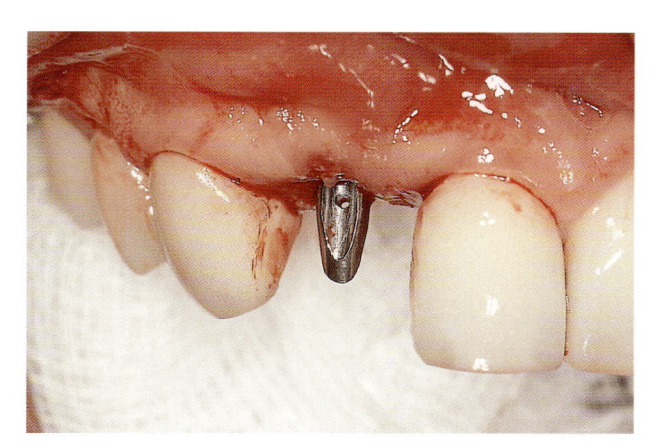

**Fig 9-10** Labial view of the abutment seated and tightened to 15 Ncm. The level of the soft tissues is visible. The labial depression that was visible earlier has been re-contoured by the labial manipulation of the soft tissues. Gauze is used to protect the airway during any stages involving small component parts.

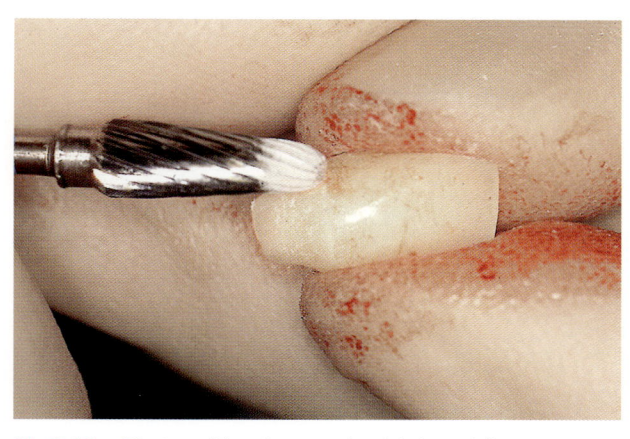

**Fig 9-11** The transitional restoration fabricated (by master dental technician Mr Peter Sochor) directly on the abutment, which has been seated from impressions taken at first-stage surgery, can be seen being modified. This will create the emergence profile for the transitional restoration and subsequently for the definitive restoration.

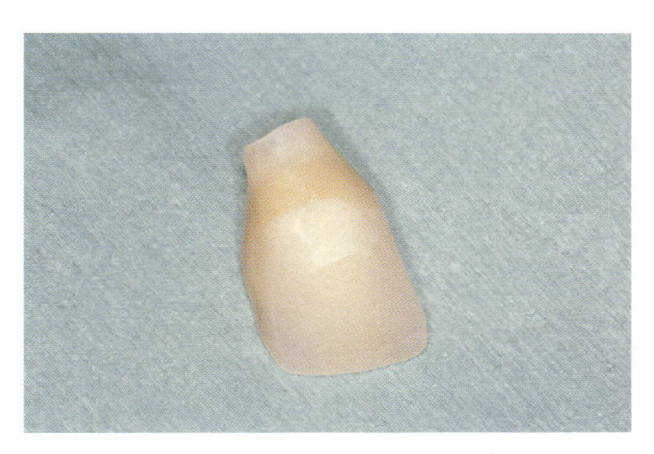

**Fig 9-12** The transitional restoration after modification showing the narrower subgingival portion. This form has been achieved by trying the transitional restoration in and observing its effect on the soft tissues.

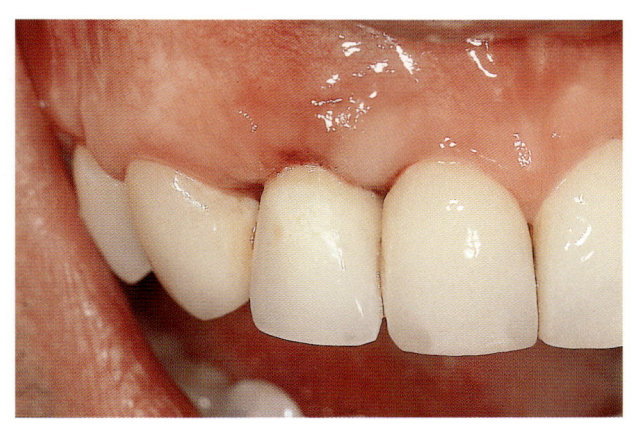

**Fig 9-13** Labial view of the transitional restoration in situ. Note that there is some blanching on the mesial aspect but none on the labial. Pressure, as identified by blanching, on the interstitial soft tissues may result in the development of a papilla. Blanching of the labial soft tissues, however, will indicate pressure that could result in recession of the soft tissues.

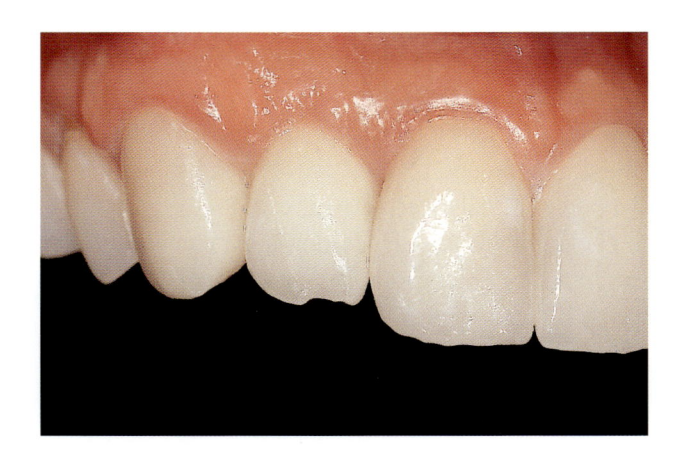

**Fig 9-14** The definitive restoration from the labial aspect showing excellent tooth form and colour. The crown can be seen emerging from healthy naturally contoured soft tissues. (Restorative work carried out by Dr Chris Parte, technical work carried out by Mr Richard Greenlees.)

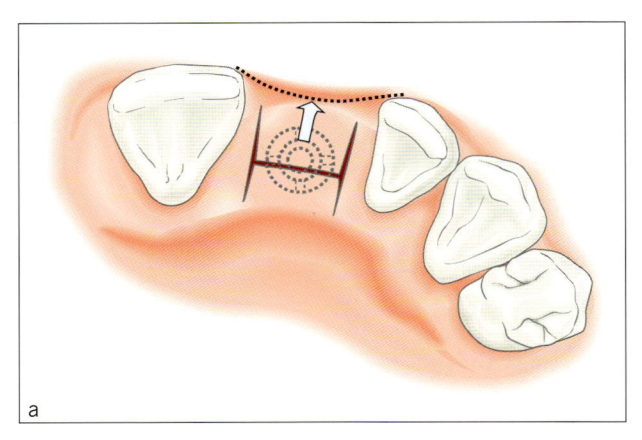

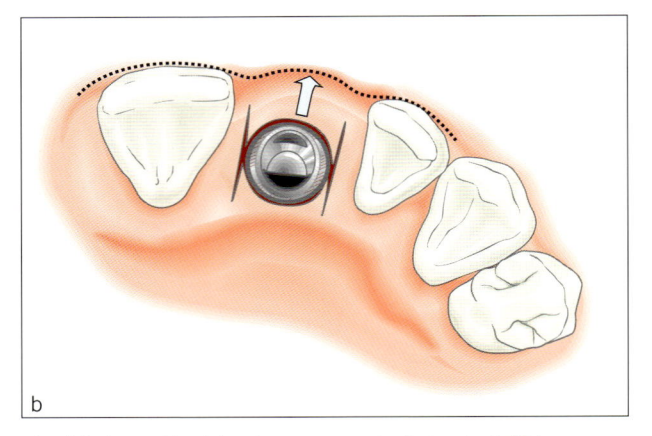

**II** Implant Placement: Surgery and Prosthodontics

**Fig 9-15** Series of two diagrams from the occlusal aspect showing the 'H'-shaped incision to expose a single implant. This incision can also be used when an implant placed into a healed site is planned to be loaded immediately. (a) The position of the incision and relationship to the implant to be exposed. Note that the papillae are not involved and that the position of the crossbar will enable tissue to be manipulated towards the labial area. (b) The abutment attached to the implant; the soft tissue overlying the implant has been displaced labially to recreate the labial contours.

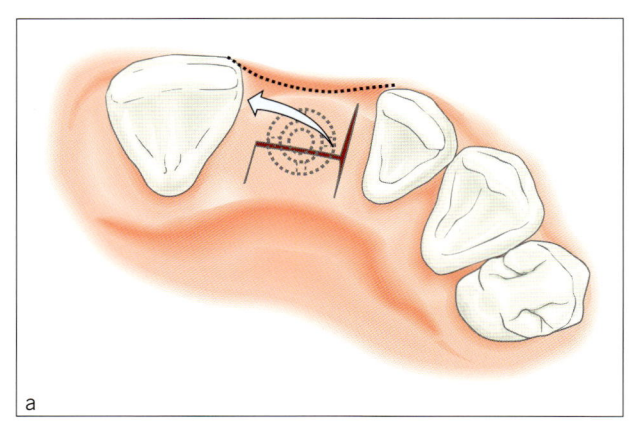

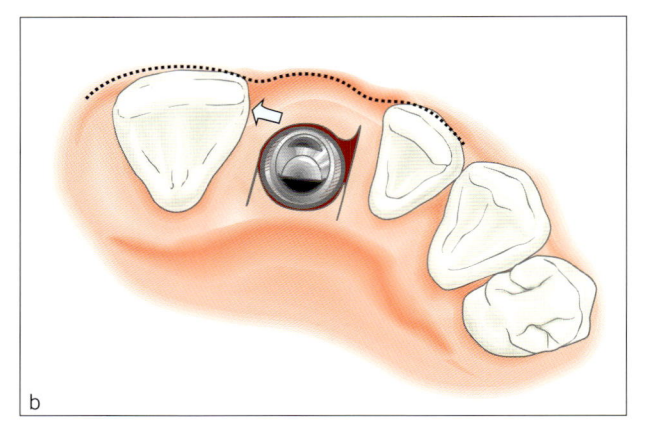

**Fig 9-16** (a and b) A variation of the 'H'-shaped incision to allow gingival tissue overlying the implant to be manipulated towards one side. This may be used to bulk out the papilla on one side.

and the parallel releasing portions next to the implant approximately 2 mm from the adjacent teeth (Figs 9-3 and 9-15). The size of the incision and its precise design will depend on the clinical circumstances (Figs 9-15 and 9-16). Undermining the soft tissue around the implant enables the access incision to be centred over the implant. The amount of tissue elevation is based on the design and size of the cover screw and abutment. There has to be sufficient access for the removal of hard and soft tissue from the top of the cover screw to enable the abutment to be seated properly. The amount of tissue that needs to be removed is also dependent on the type of connection between implant and abutment. Fitting the conical connection design requires least exposure of the surgical site, as this is mainly to gain access to the internal area of the conical connection (Fig 9-17). The abutment does not need to be seated on top of the implant but fits within it (Fig 9-18). The butt joint connection with the external anti-rotation hexagon requires the greatest attention not to damage the implant shoulder or external hex and it needs the greatest amount of exposure.

**9** Delayed Loading: Implant Exposure

**Fig 9-17** (left) The cover screw being removed via a small incision. The cover screw fits within the diameter of the implant, which facilitates its removal through a small incision.

**Fig 9-18** (right) The preselected abutment can be attached at second-stage surgery via a small incision, which is greatly enhanced by the nature of the connection between the abutment and the implant. Access to the entire top of the implant is not necessary, nor may there be any need to remove bone that has grown over the edge of the implant. It is necessary, however, to ensure that the conical connection has engaged. This is done simply by applying pressure to the abutment to engage it. Verification may be carried out by applying a minimal rotational force to confirm engagement.

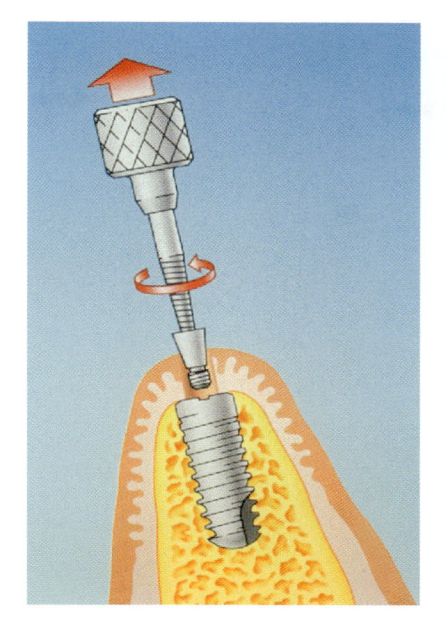

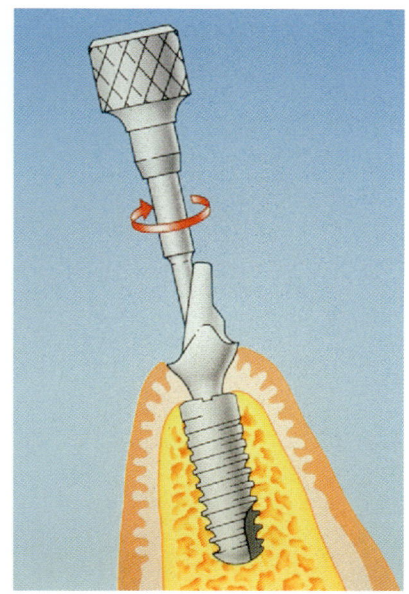

## Continuous Full-thickness Incision

Continuous full-thickness incisions are indicated for a variety of situations outlined below. This type of incision may be used in the maxilla or the mandible; there are, however, certain distinctions that relate to the type of tissue present.

### Maxilla

The maxilla has ample keratinised tissue that covers the entire palate. This tissue is well attached and more difficult to mobilise. Nevertheless, it is possible to reposition the attached tissue from the palatal to the labial aspect of the implant and to create papillae. This is fortunate, as it is the maxilla that is often more visible.

### Mandible

In the mandible, attached keratinised tissue normally atrophies with the underlying bone. As a result, there is generally a relatively narrow band of attached tissue available. Typically, in the mandible, a crestal incision is made that bisects the attached tissue, thus positioning the keratinised tissue on the lingual and labial aspects of the implant.

There is no attached tissue available for manipulation on the lingual aspect of the mandibular ridge. On occasion, however, when minimal ridge resorption has taken place, there may be a thick band of keratinised tissue on the crest and the labial aspect of the ridge. It is, therefore, sometimes possible to use this tissue for papillary reconstruction, if required. Mandibular tissue is easily mobilised and so is readily adapted around the implant. The full-thickness incision is indicated for:

- exposure of multiple implants adjacent to each other
- implants where the position cannot be accurately identified
- single or multiple implants requiring papillary reconstruction
- repositioning of keratinised tissue.

A full-thickness incision is made on the palatal aspect of the implant. The flap is reflected to expose the implant, thus mobilising the attached tissue towards the labial aspect of the implant. With the abutment inserted into the implant, this would result in a deficiency of tissue on the mesial and distal aspects of the implant. The closure of this deficiency will depend on the need to create a papilla.

A supplementary incision, either 'S' or 'C' shaped, is normally undertaken after the abutment is attached in order to assess the precise design of the incision. The size, diameter and position of the abutment will clearly influence the soft tissue contours. Narrow abutments provide the maximum space for manoeuvre, as the amount of tissue that needs to be manipulated is minimised.

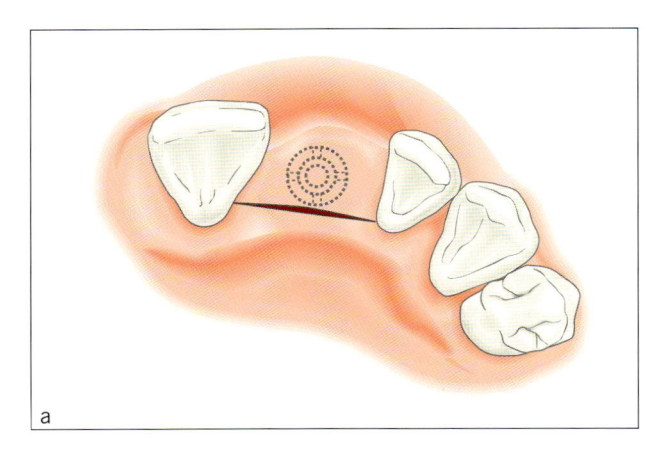

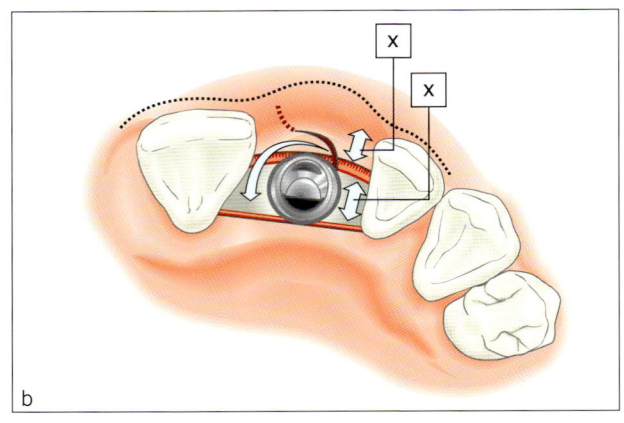

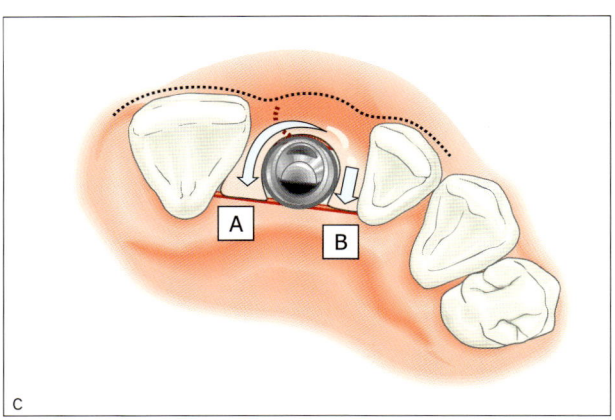

## II Implant Placement: Surgery and Prosthodontics

**Fig 9-19** Diagrams from the occlusal aspect showing the execution of an 'S'-shaped incision to expose a single implant. (a) The position of the full-thickness incision extending from one tooth to the other, positioned on the palatal aspect of the implant to be exposed. (b) Tissues are displaced to the labial side, with the abutment attached to the implant. The exposed ridge can be seen at either side of the implant. X denotes the distance that the tissues have been displaced labially. The 'S'-shaped incision is inscribed with the full-thickness component in red and the subepithelial component as a dotted line. The 'S'-shaped incision creates a small pedicled flap, which will be used to close over the exposed ridge. (c) The manner in which the pedicle flap is used to cover the exposed ridge on one side (A). This enables the elevated flap to be repositioned (B) to its original position.

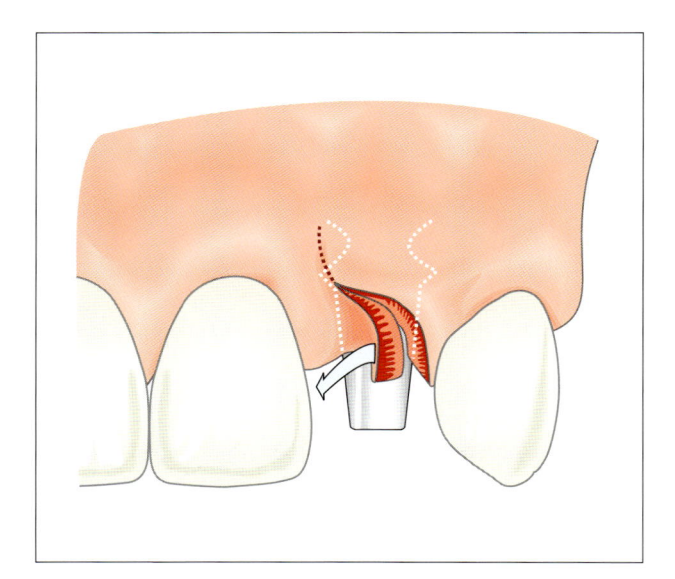

**Fig 9-20** Labial view of the 'S'-shaped incision, demonstrating both the full-thickness and the subepithelial components. The labial displacement of the flap simultaneously results in an apparent increase in the level of the mucosa.

### 'S'-shaped Incision for a Small Pedicle Flap

The 'S'-shaped incision is indicated where a papilla needs to be developed; it was first described by Palacci.[149] This type of incision is essentially designed to create a small pedicle flap, which is repositioned into the interdental area (Figs 9-19–9-31). For multiple implants placed unilaterally, the pedicle flaps are designed to position the pedicle on the mesial aspect of the implant (Figs 9-23 and 9-24). The height of the ridge, the interdental space and the thickness of the tissue influence the width of the pedicle. After attachment of the abutment, the 'S'-shaped incision is started on its distal aspect. The clinician should be able to visualise the final position of the pedicle flap on the mesial aspect of the abutment. The first part of the incision is full thickness and the second part is a split-thickness incision of the periosteum, carried out subepithelially. This provides mobility for the pedi-

**9** Delayed Loading: Implant Exposure

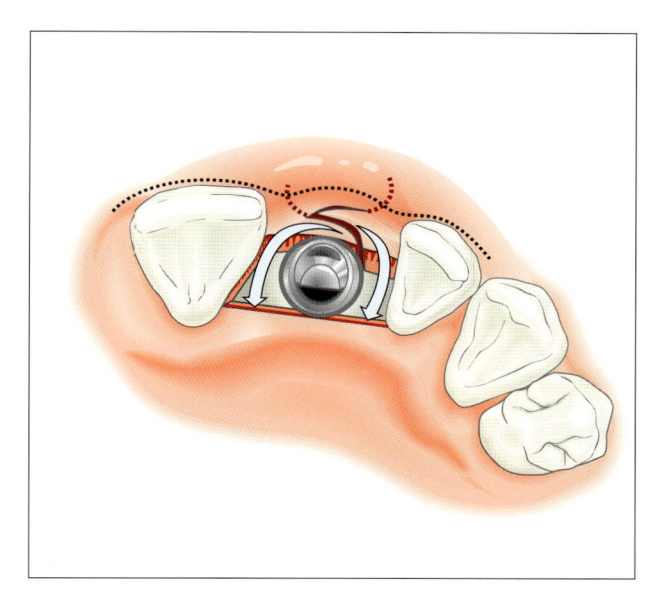

**Fig 9-21** The use of a double 'S'-shaped incision from the occlusal view. This is only possible when ample tissue is present and when augmentation of the papilla on both sides of the implant is required.

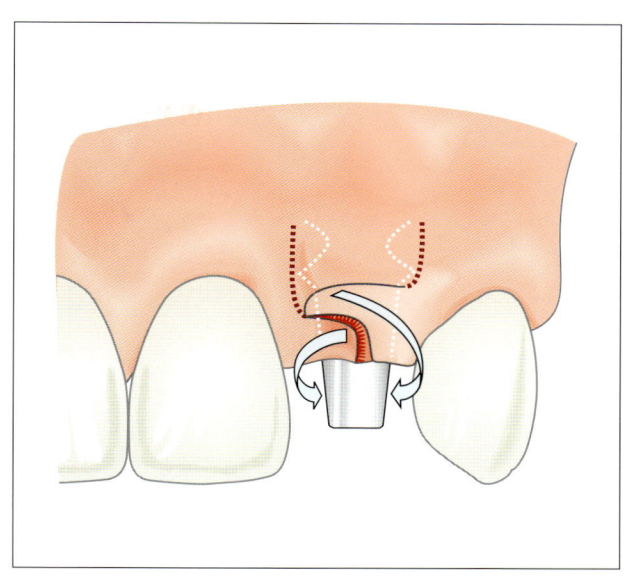

**Fig 9-22** Labial view of the double 'S'-shaped incision, demonstrating both the full-thickness and the subepithelial components, as well as the direction in which the two separate pedicle flaps will be moved.

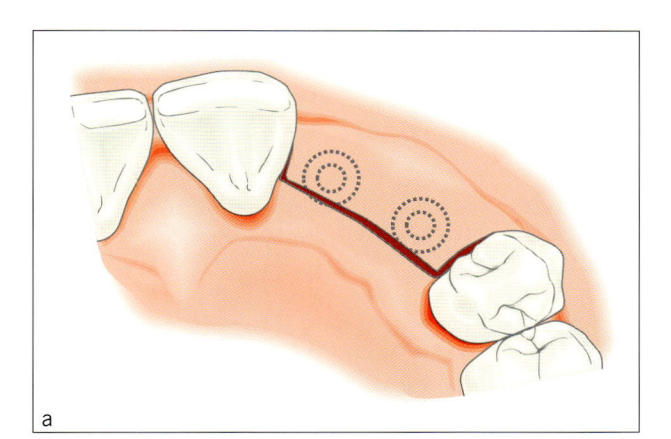

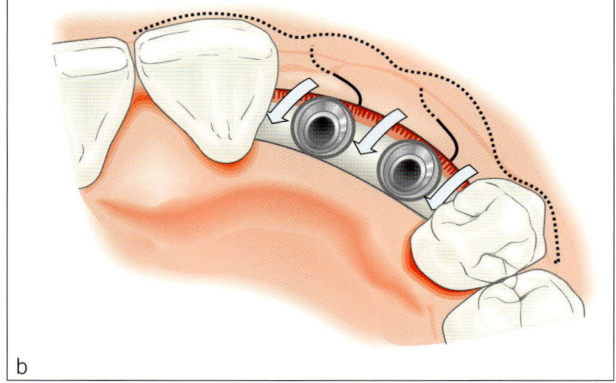

**Fig 9-23** The use of 'S'-shaped incisions for the exposure of multiple implants. The exposure of the left maxillary lateral incisor and the canine is seen from the occlusal aspect. (a) The position of the full-thickness incision on the palatal aspect of the implants. (b) The implants with the abutments attached. The incision (full thickness and subepithelial) is shown designed to move the pedicle flap towards the mesial aspect of each abutment, effecting closure as illustrated by the arrows. (c) The pedicle flaps repositioned to cover the exposed ridge and the papillae reconstructed. Note that the pedicle flaps forming the papillae have been moved towards the mesial aspect of each implant.

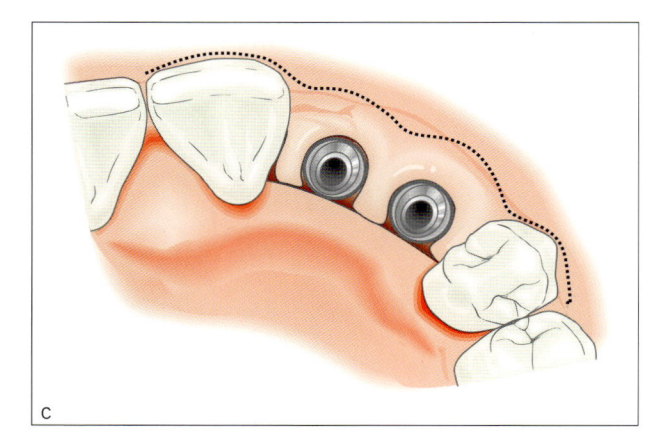

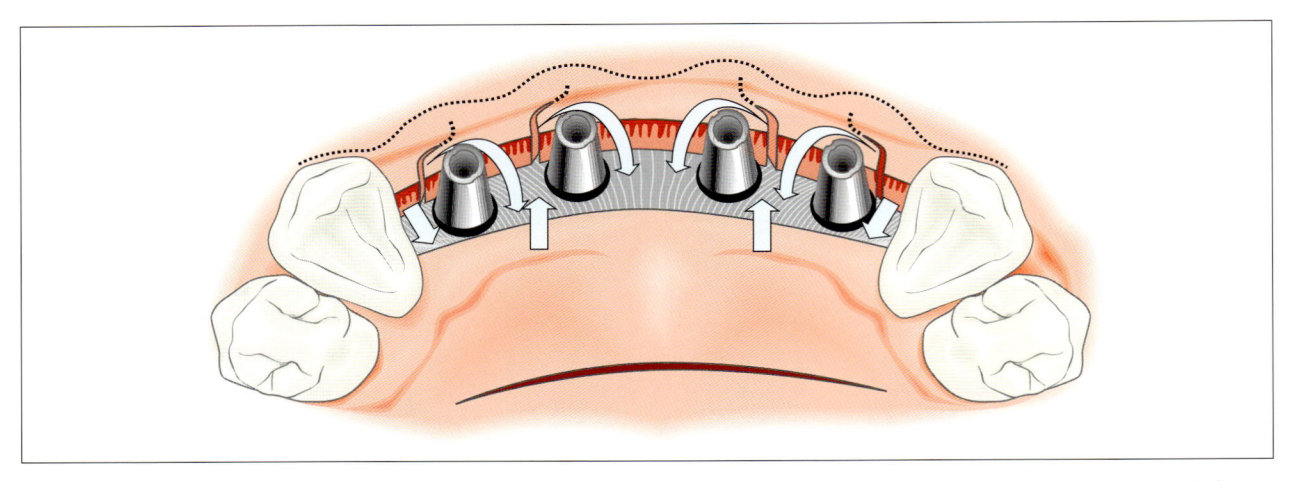

**II** | **Implant Placement: Surgery and Prosthodontics**

**Fig 9-24** The use of the full-thickness exposure with supplementary 'S'-shaped incisions for the exposure of four implants replacing the four incisors across the midline. The 'S'-shaped incisions for the pedicle flaps are arranged in the normal way so that the pedicle can be moved towards the mesial tissue. Two pedicle flaps are moved into the wider space between the central incisors in the midline. In cases where bone grafts have been used, there is a reduced amount of keratinised attached tissue. The incision is, therefore, made further towards the palate than normal. A split-thickness sliding flap (SSF) may also be advanced to cover any exposed bone. Thus, adequate keratinised tissue is available for the construction of the papillae and at the same time no exposed bone remains uncovered.

cle flap without creating a cleft within the marginal epithelium. The first pedicle should be positioned within the interdental space to accurately assess the starting point for the incision around the second abutment. On completion of the second incision and positioning of the pedicles, the flap will close spontaneously distal to the second implant. The 'S'-shaped incision can also be carried out bilaterally around a single abutment, as long as there is sufficient soft tissue present (Figs 9-21 and 9-22).

### Full-thickness Flap with a 'C'-shaped Excisional Incision

Where there is adequate soft tissue, both in terms of papillary height and labial bulk, the excision of the epithelium around the attached abutment can be carried out accurately so that the flap fits back to provide full coverage. The amount of tissue excised will influence the gingival margin of the transitional restoration, which can later be altered to further influence the marginal contours of both the labial and interstitial aspects.

### Abutment Attachment

Since the abutment shape will influence the soft tissue contours, it is important to have the shape of the abutment modified by the dental technician in preparation for the exposure. This requires that the impression is taken during first-stage surgery.

Where it is not appropriate to take an impression during implant placement, a preselected abutment may be used. The manner in which it will influence the contours can be assessed by trying in the abutment. Modifications of the abutment can be made outside the mouth by attaching it to an implant analogue. A reduction in height is most commonly required; alternatively, a reduction of the labial surface may be needed to avoid gingival recession. With implants placed at an angle,

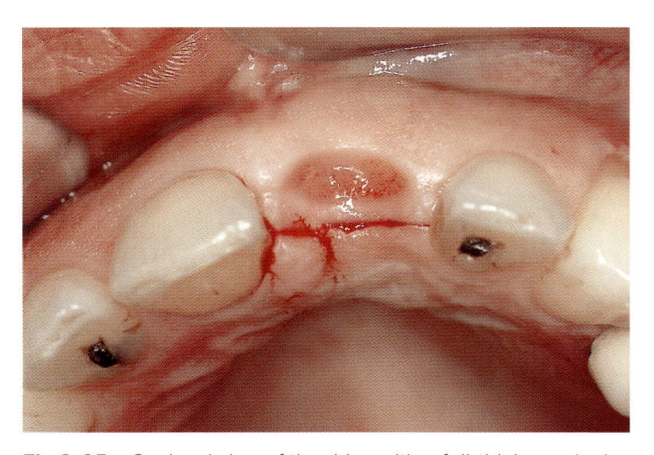

**Fig 9-25** Occlusal view of the ridge with a full-thickness incision made on the palatal aspect of the crest for the exposure of an implant placed six months previously.

**9   Delayed Loading: Implant Exposure**

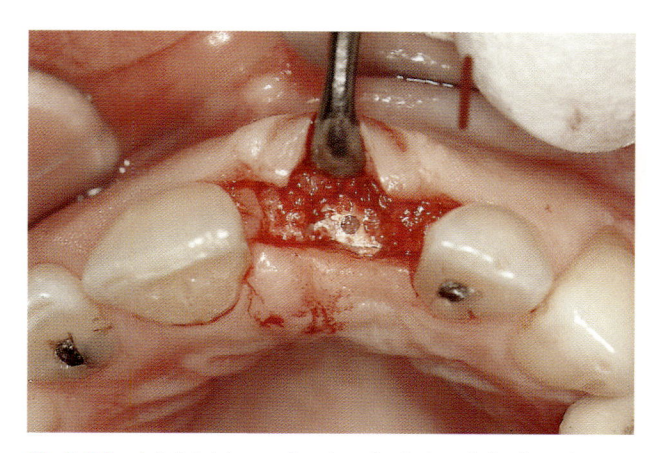

**Fig 9-26**   A full-thickness flap is reflected and displaced towards the labial. The implant is visible, as is the ridge and either side.

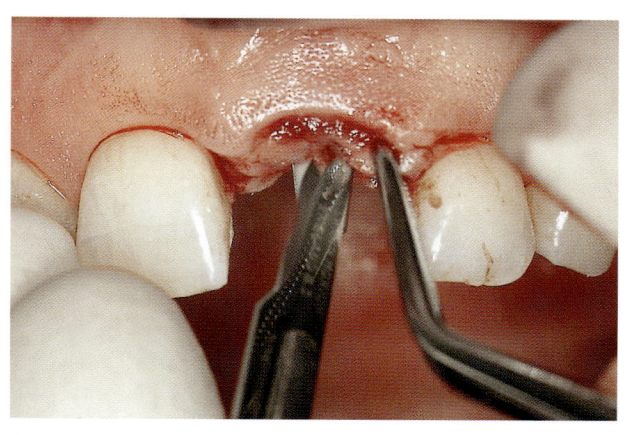

**Fig 9-27**   Labial view of the definitive abutment attached to the implant with the 'S'-shaped incision being carried out (see Figs 9-19 and 9-20).

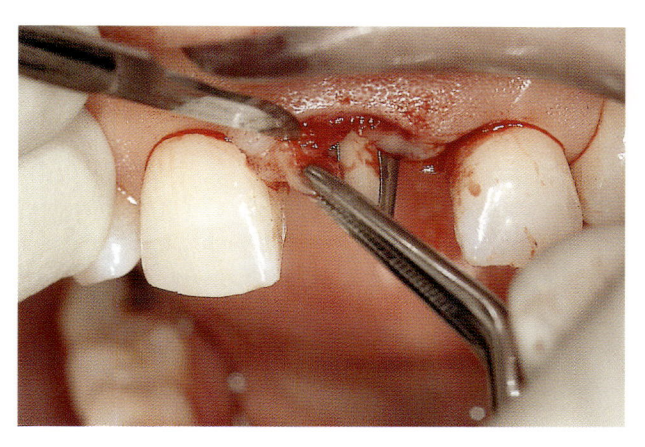

**Fig 9-28**   The subepithelial portion of the 'S'-shaped incision being completed with the pedicle flap being positioned mesial to the abutment.

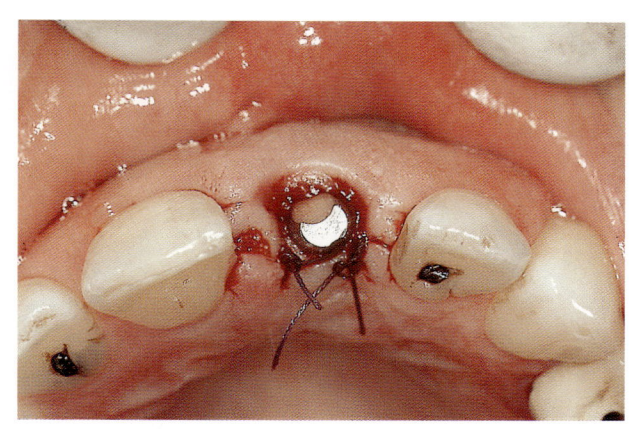

**Fig 9-29**   Occlusal view of the abutment with the pedicle flap positioned mesially and the distal part of the ridge, which had become exposed, covered by replacing the flap over the exposed ridge.

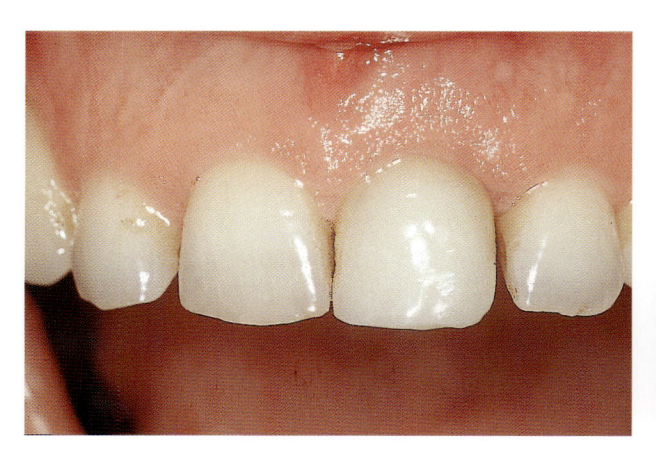

**Fig 9-30**   Labial view of the transitional restoration developing the soft tissue contours.

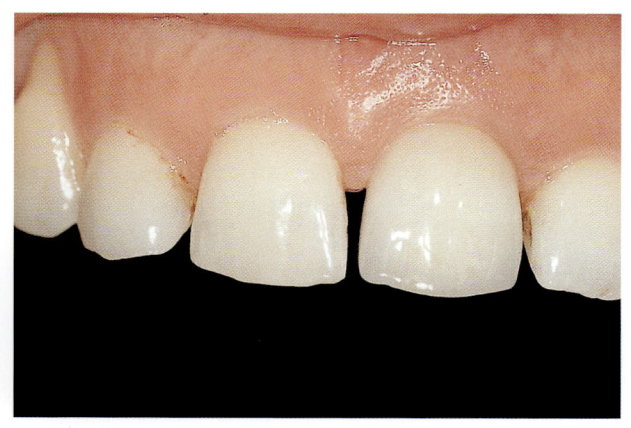

**Fig 9-31**   Definitive restoration showing the emergence profile and the soft tissue contours.

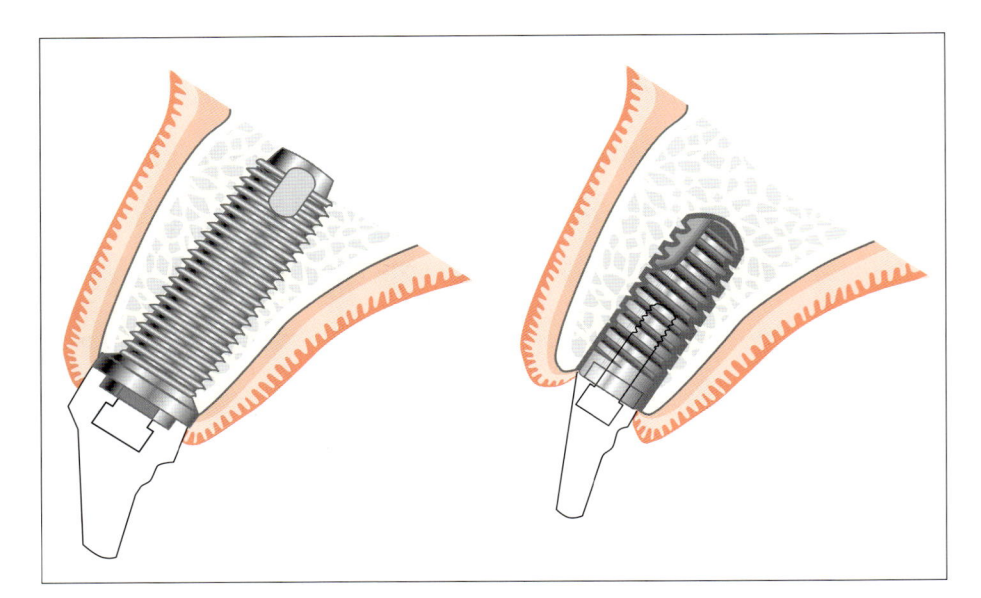

**Fig 9-32** The additional bulk of abutment required with an externally hexed implant. This becomes necessary, as the abutment has to be extended coronally to clear the hex before angular correction can take place. In contrast, an implant with an internal connection offers the facility to correct angles from the level of the implant and is, therefore, less bulky.

special care should be taken when attaching an abutment with an anti-rotational mechanism other than a conical connection. Either the rotational position of the implant should have been adjusted during placement or abutments with rotational offsets should be used. This is critical when angled abutments are being used. Reduction of the labial aspect of the abutment may also be limited by an external hex and the fixing screw (Fig 9-32).

The position of the abutment should be verified by use of the diagnostic template and should not interfere with occlusion. The abutment should fit within the prosthetic envelope. Multiple abutments should be aligned parallel to each other and adjacent teeth in order to facilitate the construction of restorations.

### Seating the Abutment

The clinician will need to ensure that the abutment is completely seated. For an external hex connection, a radiograph may be required to confirm complete seating. Abutments using a tapered connection can be tested by simply applying finger pressure to engage the taper (Ankylos). If the taper does not engage, some obstruction – such as soft or hard tissues – may be present and will need to be removed prior to tightening. The fixation screw for the abutment can be tightened to the desired torque, which may vary from 15 to more than 32 Ncm, depending on the type of connection.

The access hole for the fixation screw should then be blocked. The ideal method is to use soft wax to cover the screw, followed by glass-ionomer cement to seal the access hole of the abutment. This will eliminate the undercut to facilitate the relining or construction of a provisional restoration.

## Wound Closure

Generally the incisions designed for minimal exposure, such as the 'H'-shaped incision, do not require suturing as the abutment and the transitional restoration occlude the opening. On rare occasions, when attached tissue has been repositioned, fine labial sutures (6-0) may be used in order to close any incision lines.

Full-thickness flaps should be closed using appropriate sutures (usually 3-0). The pedicle flaps created by the 'S'-shaped incisions require finer sutures (4-0 to 6-0) to create the papillary form, which will be supported by the transitional restoration. Sliding flaps from the palate require stronger sutures (usually 3-0) and may be secured by tying them to the abutments. Supplementary dressings (such as Coepak; GC America, Alsip, IL, USA) may be used when tissues are denuded. However, this should be avoided.

## Transitional Restorations

### Impressions at First-stage Surgery

The dental technician will have modified the abutment to the desired shape and will now be able to fabricate the transitional restoration from acrylic resin directly on the abutment. Such a restoration will fit precisely and will not need relining. The contours of the restoration as it emerges from the gingival tissues may need to be modified in order to create the desired profile.

Manipulating the soft tissues with the transitional restoration is facilitated by the use of acrylic resin as the material of choice, which can be easily reduced or built up as required. Excessive pressure on the labial aspect will result in gingival recession, whereas judicious interstitial contouring will generate the interdental papillae, providing there is sufficient bone support. This technique enables the porcelain margin of the prostheses to be positioned subgingivally, thus avoiding discolouration of the soft tissues caused by uncovered metal.

### Hollow Restorations for Relining

A hollow restoration may be fabricated based on the original form determined by the diagnostic preview. This restoration can be relined on completion of the surgical phase of implant exposure. Excellent aesthetics can be achieved, with aesthetic and functional form transferred through all the phases of treatment. However, the subgingival extension of the definitive restoration is completed when the impressions are taken during the prosthetic phase.

## Chairside Fabrication

Any of the methods available for the fabrication of temporary crowns may be used in order to cover the abutment with the material of choice.

## Chapter 10

# Restorative Phase: Prosthetic Protocols

## Introduction

There are many mechanisms of varying accuracy for transferring information from the mouth to the dental laboratory.[147,150–158] There are also numerous materials that can be used for the fabrication of a prosthetic restoration. Furthermore, the means by which the restoration is attached to the abutment and retained will influence the clinical protocol and the components used (Figs 10-1–10-3).

The natural tooth form can most easily be created if there are no large screws (required for direct retention) passing through the occlusal, labial or lingual surface of the prostheses. Consequently, mainly fixed cement-retained prostheses will be described. Supplementary retention with lateral fixation screws will be addressed where indicated (Figs 10-4 and 10-5). The approach to prosthetic reconstruction will take into account the effort required to construct a restoration by the clinician and the dental technician versus the benefit that is derived by the patient.

The restorative phase starts when the soft tissues surrounding the exposed implant have matured, except where impressions were taken during implant insertion and the construction of the prostheses had started prior to implant exposure. The information that must be supplied to the laboratory can be categorised into the following broad groups:

- position of implant, abutment and metalwork and its relationship to the soft tissue contour
- jaw relations
- tooth form, position and colour.

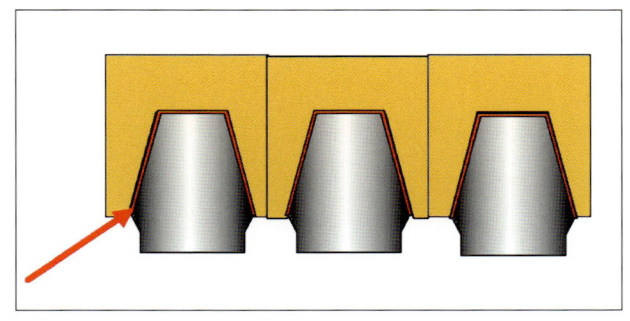

**Fig 10-1** Three abutments in alignment with a cement-retained superstructure. Alignment of the abutments without undercut is essential to provide a common path of insertion. A luting cement is used to retain the prosthesis, and the type of cement will influence the retrievability as well as the security of the prosthesis. Retention and resistance form, as well as the precision of the fit, are fundamental to the stability of the prosthesis. A space for the luting cement between 25 and 100 μm is desirable. The space for the luting cement will influence the type of cement used, in conjunction with the factors addressed above. This makes the fabrication of the prosthesis less exacting. Furthermore, no access holes are required, which are typically needed for screw-retained prostheses.

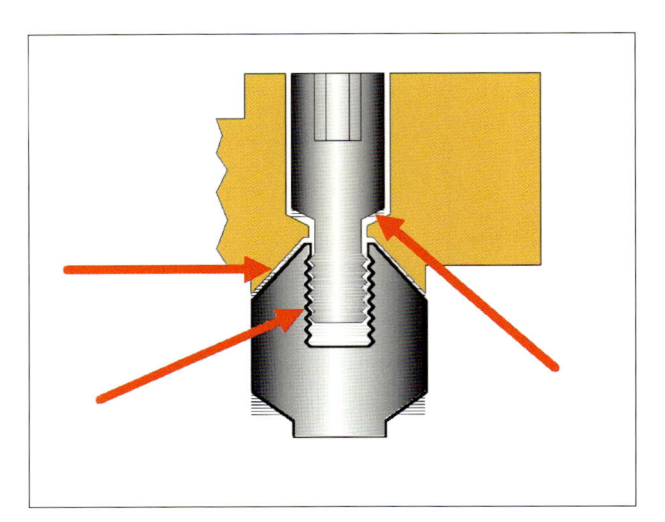

II  Implant Placement: Surgery and Prosthodontics

**Fig 10-2** The point of contact between the various component parts of a screw-retained prosthesis. Contact between the various components is depicted by red arrows. These are contacts between the fixation screw and the abutment, between the prosthesis and the abutment and, finally, between the retaining screw and the prosthesis. Transfer of information from the clinical situation to the laboratory needs to be carried out with tremendous accuracy. Inaccuracies of 10 μm can be detected by patients, which makes the construction of the prosthesis to the necessary tolerances very exacting.[18]

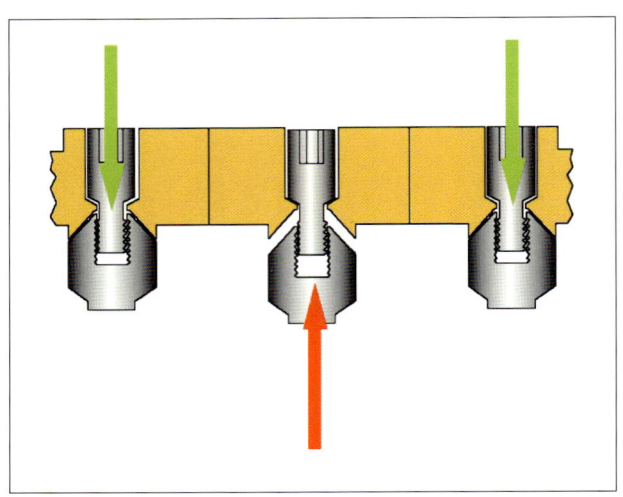

**Fig 10-3** The effect of discrepancies in the fit of a screw-retained prosthesis. Inaccuracies cause considerable forces to be transmitted to the abutments as the screws holding the prosthesis are tightened. Risks to all component parts, including the implants, are increased by parafunctional forces.

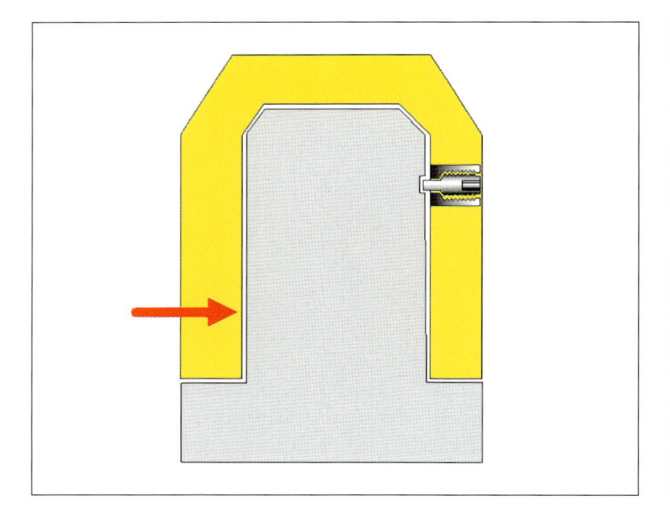

**Fig 10-4** The principle and mechanism of a lateral fixation screw. The lateral fixation screw can be seen incorporated into the prosthetic superstructure. The screw housing may be soldered or cast into the superstructure. The lateral fixation screw can be seen within the housing and is used to engage a recess within the abutment. This is suitable for the retention of smaller restorations because of its ease of fabrication. For multiple-unit restorations gold copings that are permanently cemented onto the abutment may be fabricated with a recess to receive the unthreaded part of the lateral fixation screw. The use of the gold coping enables the recess to be positioned interstitially.

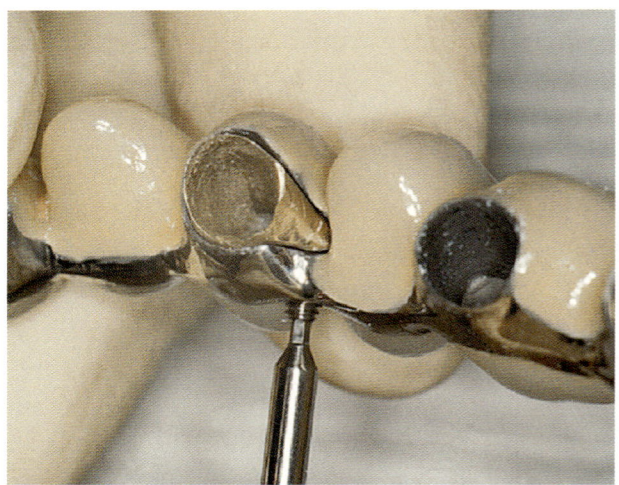

**Fig 10-5** A temporary luting cement is used as a biological seal and for the even distribution of forces; it, therefore, requires a space. Definitive and positive retention is obtained from the lateral fixation screw. Factors influencing conventional cement retention, such as alignment of abutments, resistance and retention form as well as the accuracy of fit, are also critical when using lateral fixation screws.

**10** Restorative Phase: Prosthetic Protocols

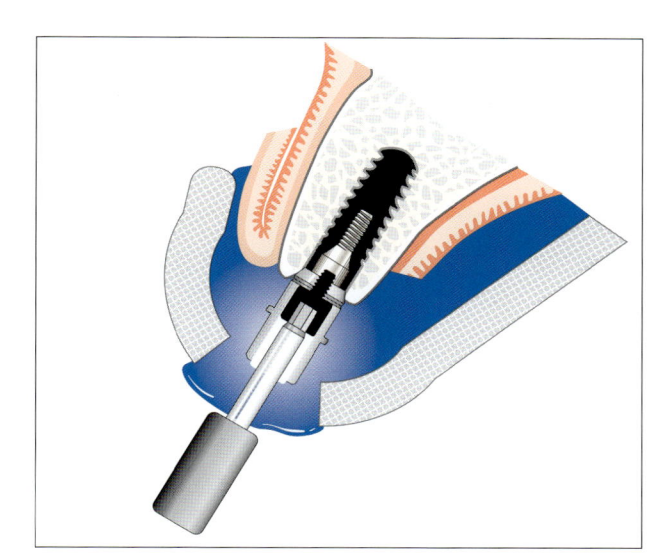

**Fig 10-6** Impressions at first-stage surgery using implant carrier with an open tray. This is particularly suitable for implant systems that are presented with the carrier of suitable shape attached to the implant (e.g. Ankylos system). The stages for this procedure are as follows.
1. Take impression with screwdriver inserted into implant carrier emerging through an open tray.
2. Unscrew and disengage implant carrier with driver once the impression material has set.
3. Remove impression with implant carrier.
4. Insert cover screw into implant analogue, if cover screw comes pre-inserted within implant.
5. Attach analogue to implant carrier and cast impression.

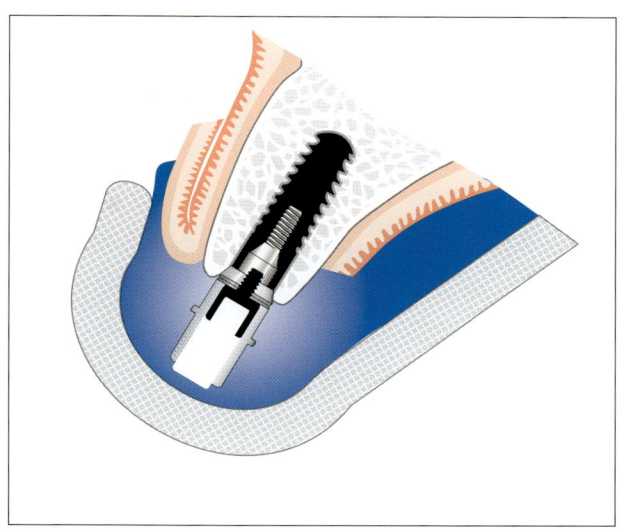

**Fig 10-7** Closed tray technique using implant carrier for first-stage surgery impression.
1. Take impression (soft material, for example Provil Monophase) of implant carrier and remove impression when set.
2. Remove implant carrier from the implant.
3. Insert cover screw into implant analogue, if cover screw comes pre-inserted within implant.
4. Attach analogue to implant carrier.
5. Reinsert implant carrier into impression and cast impression.

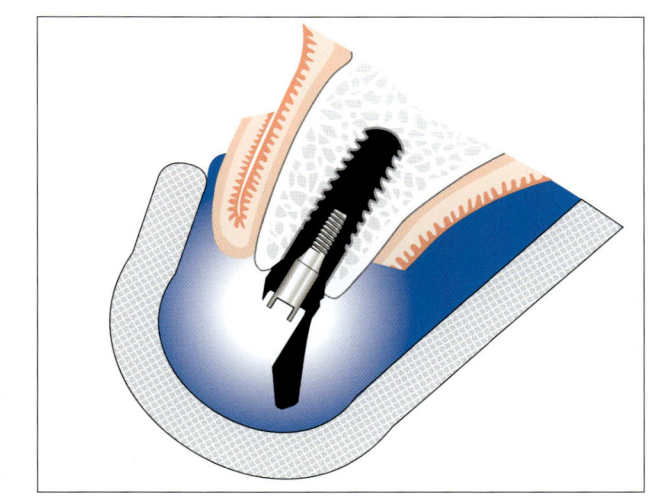

**Fig 10-8** Impressions at first-stage surgery using abutment and closed tray.
1. Select abutment using direction indicator following the insertion of implant and removal of carrier, if appropriate.
2. Remove cover screw if cover screw comes pre-inserted within implant and insert selected abutment.
3. Take impression and remove on setting.
4. Attach abutment to implant analogue or use abutment analogue, insert into impression and make cast (if immediate loading is carried out, a second abutment or an abutment analogue is used).
5. Insert cover screw into implant.

## Impressions at First-stage Surgery

This protocol starts during the surgical placement phase and can be carried out using a number of available techniques as described above. However, the preferred techniques are outlined in Figs 10-6 to 10-8. The restorative steps are summarised in Flowchart 10-1. The abutment will have been prepared to the desired shape by the dental technician based on clinical information sent by the clinician in advance of implant exposure. The acrylic resin transitional crown should also be ready to be fitted.

The framework of the definitive restoration can also be prepared by this stage (Figs 10-9–10-12).

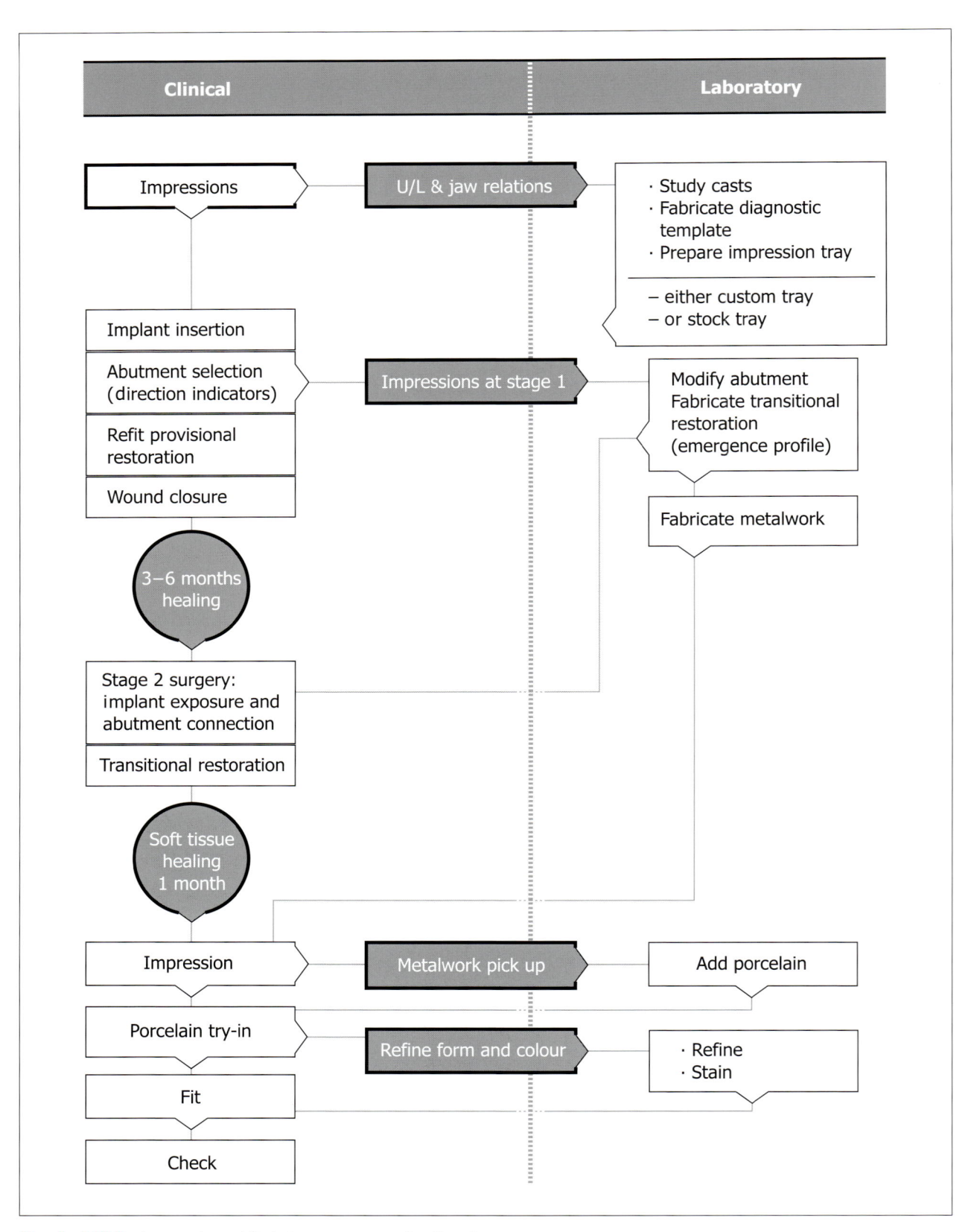

## II  Implant Placement: Surgery and Prosthodontics

| Clinical | Laboratory |
|---|---|

**Clinical flow:**
- Impressions
- Implant insertion
- Abutment selection (direction indicators)
- Refit provisional restoration
- Wound closure
- 3–6 months healing
- Stage 2 surgery: implant exposure and abutment connection
- Transitional restoration
- Soft tissue healing 1 month
- Impression
- Porcelain try-in
- Fit
- Check

**Clinical/Laboratory interface steps:**
- U/L & jaw relations
- Impressions at stage 1
- Metalwork pick up
- Refine form and colour

**Laboratory:**
- Study casts
- Fabricate diagnostic template
- Prepare impression tray
  - either custom tray
  - or stock tray
- Modify abutment Fabricate transitional restoration (emergence profile)
- Fabricate metalwork
- Add porcelain
- Refine
- Stain

**Flowchart 10-1**  Impressions at first-stage surgery: restorative phase.

# 10 Restorative Phase: Prosthetic Protocols

**Fig 10-9** Occlusal view of a cast constructed from an impression taken at first-stage surgery. Two abutments can be seen attached to the implant analogues.

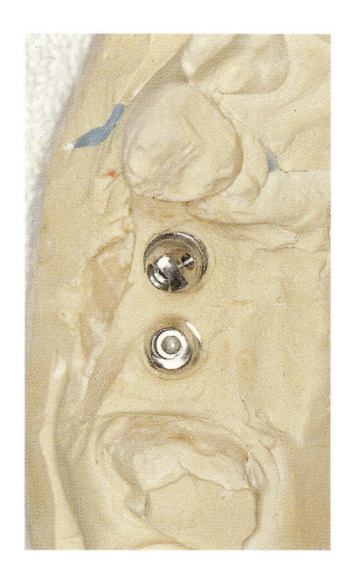

**Fig 10-10** Splinted metalwork has been fabricated directly on the two abutments. In addition two splinted acrylic resin transitional restorations have also been fabricated, which will be fitted at the time of implant exposure.

**Fig 10-11** Occlusal view of the implants exposed with the two abutments attached using an acrylic resin orientation jig. A full-thickness flap has been used to expose the implants.

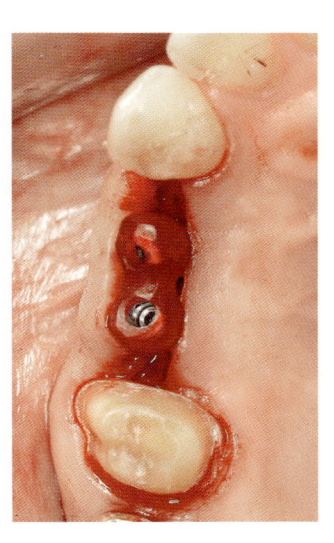

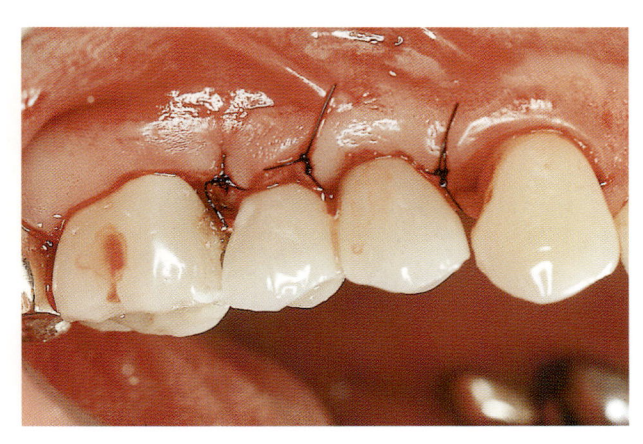

**Fig 10-12** Labial view of the abutments with the transitional restorations fitted. Soft tissue closure has been carried out using 'S'-shaped incisions.

This enables the framework to be fabricated directly onto the abutment, eliminating any potential discrepancies in the adaptation of the framework to the abutment. It will be assumed, however, that the implant will integrate and that no modifications to the abutment will be needed.

This technique is particularly useful for single or multiple unsplinted crowns in the areas of aesthetic importance and is, therefore, considered to be the technique of choice. Where there are more than two splinted crowns, the framework may need to be sectioned in order to achieve a satisfactory fit.

## Impression Taking

The transitional restoration is removed from the abutment and any excess cement removed (Figs 10-13 and 10-14). The framework is tried into place and its fit confirmed (Fig 10-15). The occlusal relationship is checked and recorded. While preparations for the impressions are made, the transitional restoration is cleaned and reseated in order to maintain the gingival contour.

The transitional restoration is removed and the framework seated on the abutment immediately before light-bodied impression material is injected into the

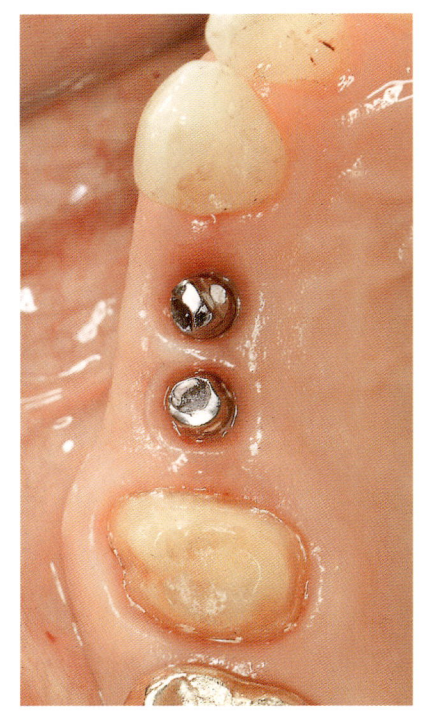

II  Implant Placement: Surgery and Prosthodontics

**Fig 10-13** Occlusal view of the healed soft tissues around the abutments. Note the contours around the abutments.

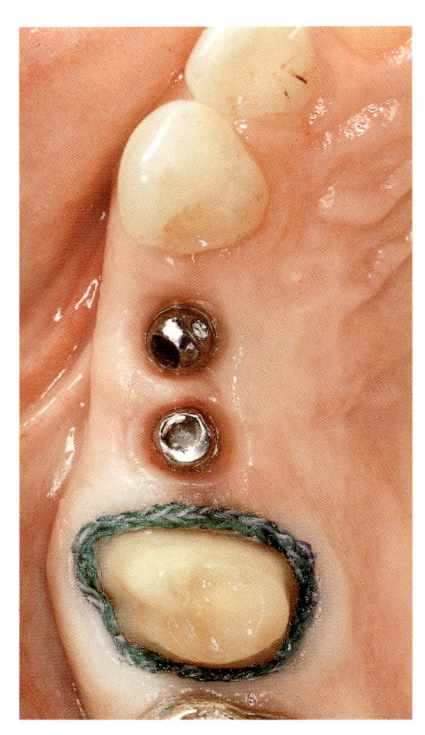

**Fig 10-14** Occlusal view of the quadrant prior to impression taking. The molar tooth has been prepared and retraction cord is in situ.

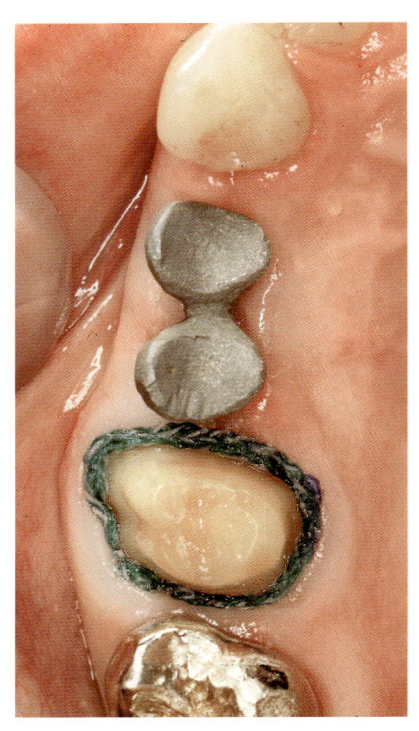

**Fig 10-15** Occlusal view showing the metalwork in situ on top of the abutments ready for pick-up using addition-cured silicone impression material.

gap between the soft tissue and framework in order to record this relationship. The medium-bodied impression material, loaded into the tray, is then inserted into the mouth to provide an overall impression relating the position of the framework to the teeth and the soft tissues (Fig 10-16). Additional information that may prove to be useful to the technician in the form of an impression of the apical area of the transitional crown can be recorded with a putty material and passed on to the laboratory. The shade of the tooth should be recorded in detail and supplemented with photographs. Alternatively, the shade can be taken directly by the dental technician.

### Try-in of the Unglazed Restoration

To confirm colour, form and occlusion, the definitive restoration in its unglazed state is tried in. Any modifications to the restoration are prescribed at this stage. Major changes in the shade may require the crown to be remade; minor changes can be achieved at the glazing stage. Changes to the form are transferred by adding composite to the restoration. The technician can then incorporate these.

### Fit of restoration

The final restoration (Fig 10-17) is fitted using temporary cement (e.g. Temp Bond; Kerr, Orange, CA, USA) (Figs 10-18 and 10-19). It is essential that the minimum amount of cement is used in order to reduce the chances of excess cement being extruded into the soft tissues. Application of Vaseline (petroleum jelly) to the outer surface of the definitive restoration facilitates removal of excess cement. Venting by holding aside the palatal soft tissue and using dental floss ensures that all of the cement has been removed. A periapical radiograph taken at this stage provides information regarding the level of the bone and the complete removal of the cement.

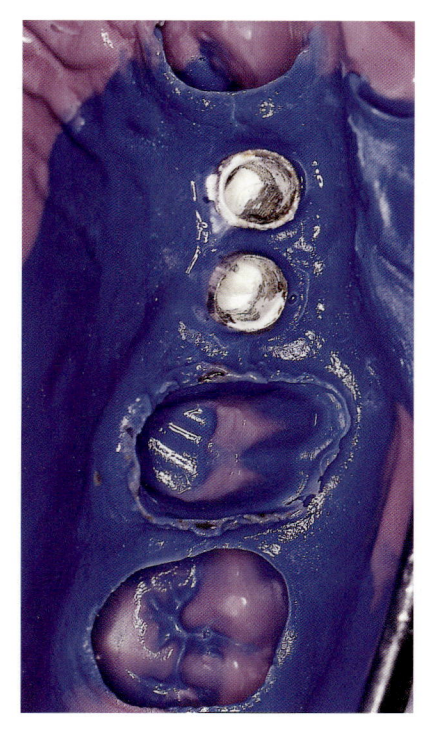

10   Restorative Phase: Prosthetic Protocols

**Fig 10-16**   The metalwork has been picked up with the impression material and the soft tissue contours around the implants recorded. At the same time, an impression of the prepared molar tooth with accurate recording of the margins has been taken.

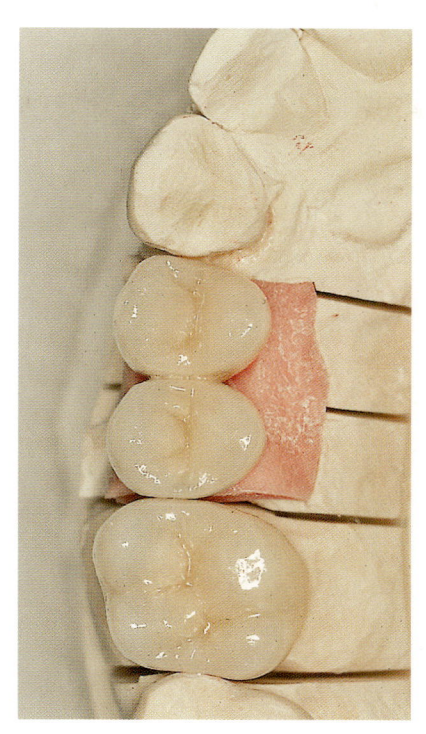

**Fig 10-17**   Occlusal view of the laboratory cast showing the two implant-supported splinted restorations replacing the premolar teeth. The soft tissue reproduction has been carried out using silicone material. The metal-ceramic restoration for the molar tooth is also visible.

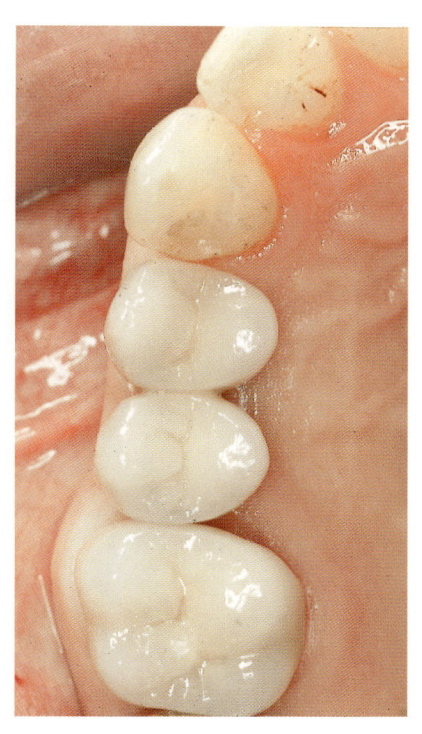

**Fig 10-18**   Intraoral occlusal view of the three restorations fitted and showing excellent occlusal form (same patient as in Fig 8-45).

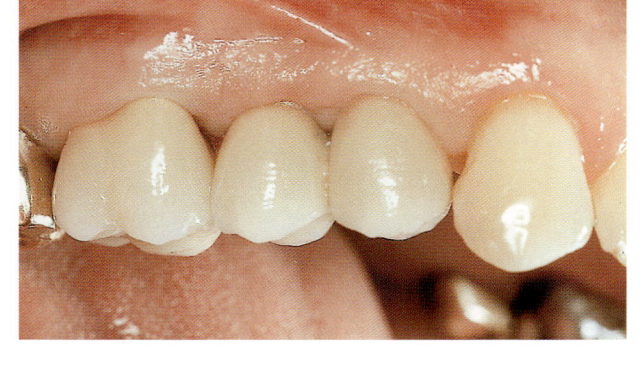

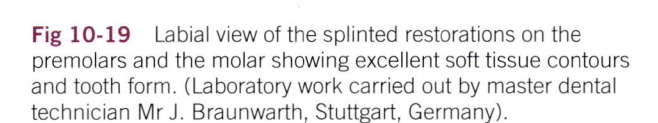

**Fig 10-19**   Labial view of the splinted restorations on the premolars and the molar showing excellent soft tissue contours and tooth form. (Laboratory work carried out by master dental technician Mr J. Braunwarth, Stuttgart, Germany).

## Conventional Direct Impressions of the Abutment

This technique is the one the general dental practitioner is most familiar with in the construction of conventional crown and bridge work. This technique allows minor modifications of the abutment, if required, the development of the soft tissue contours and the transfer of this information to the laboratory.

This technique is not suitable for patients with very thin labial gingiva around the abutment, where recession is likely to occur. It is, however, most suited to the construction of multiple splinted units and full mouth reconstruction. The clinical and laboratory stages for

173

## II  Implant Placement: Surgery and Prosthodontics

Table 10-1  Procedures and sequences for restorative phase

| Procedures and steps | Single tooth | Multiple units | Full arch reconstruction |
|---|---|---|---|
| Impression (shape and position of abutments) | Appointment 1 | Appointment 1 | Appointment 1: preliminary intermaxillary registration |
| Intermaxillary registration | Appointment 1: intercuspal position | Appointment 1: intercuspal position | Appointment 2: wax rims on acrylic framework |
| Diagnostic preview (confirm form, colour, occlusion) | Transfer from original preview | Transfer from original preview | Appointment 3: set-up of teeth on acrylic framework to confirm original preview |
| Metalwork or framework try-in (accuracy and passivity of fit, relate soft tissue to framework) | Not usually necessary | Appointment 2 | Appointment 4: cast in sections for locating or presoldered/laser-welded |
| Further try-in of metalwork (confirm accuracy and passivity of fit) | Not necessary | If required | If required; if sections located intraorally at Appointment 4 |
| Try-in of unglazed porcelain (confirm form, colour, occlusion) | Appointment 2 | Appointment 3 | Appointment 5 |
| Fit (soft cement) | Appointment 3 | Appointment 4 | Appointment 6 |
| Check and baseline records | Appointment 4 | Appointment 5 | Appointment 7 |

restorations with single crowns and short-span bridges, as well as larger restorations involving alterations of the occlusal vertical dimension, are outlined in Flowchart 10-2.

It has already been stated that the information that needs to be transferred can be categorised into certain groups. This categorisation, which is outlined more specifically below, enables the clinician to focus on precisely which information should be transferred, based on the complexity of the proposed treatment. Table 10-1 summarises the procedures and sequences for the restorative phase.

### Impression Taking

The transitional restoration, which is often undercontoured at the gingival margin, is removed. Gingival retraction using a proprietary retractor (e.g. LM-Gingival Retractor, LM-Instruments Oy, Parainen, Finland) provides access to the abutment up to approximately 2 mm below the gingival margin. A 12-fluted tungsten carbide bur in a high-speed handpiece with copious irrigation is used to modify the abutment. This produces a chamfer, which is approximately 0.5 mm deep. The aim is to create a margin that can be used by the dental technician to define the future crown margin. The subgingival depth to which the preparation is carried out will depend on a variety of local factors, such as:

- margin of the adjacent teeth
- thickness of gingival tissues
- diameter of the abutment
- position of the access hole for the fixation screw.

This procedure is carried out under local anaesthesia. Retraction cord of the appropriate thickness is used with a haemostyptic agent.

Impressions are taken using a light-bodied addition-cured material that is soft enough to allow a die stone model to be cast. Multiple abutments will require an epoxy resin cast. The light-bodied impression material is injected into the sulcus on removal of the retraction cord. Medium-bodied impression material is used in a metal-rimmed tray to perform a single-phased impression. The impression is checked to ensure marginal integrity and the absence of drags or voids.

Care should be taken not to leave any impression material behind in the subgingival tissues. The impression provides the laboratory with the precise details of the shape of the abutment in relation to the soft tissues that have been prepared and the gingival margins of the adjacent teeth (see Figs 7-74–7-77, p. 71). This will

## 10 Restorative Phase: Prosthetic Protocols

### Clinical | Laboratory

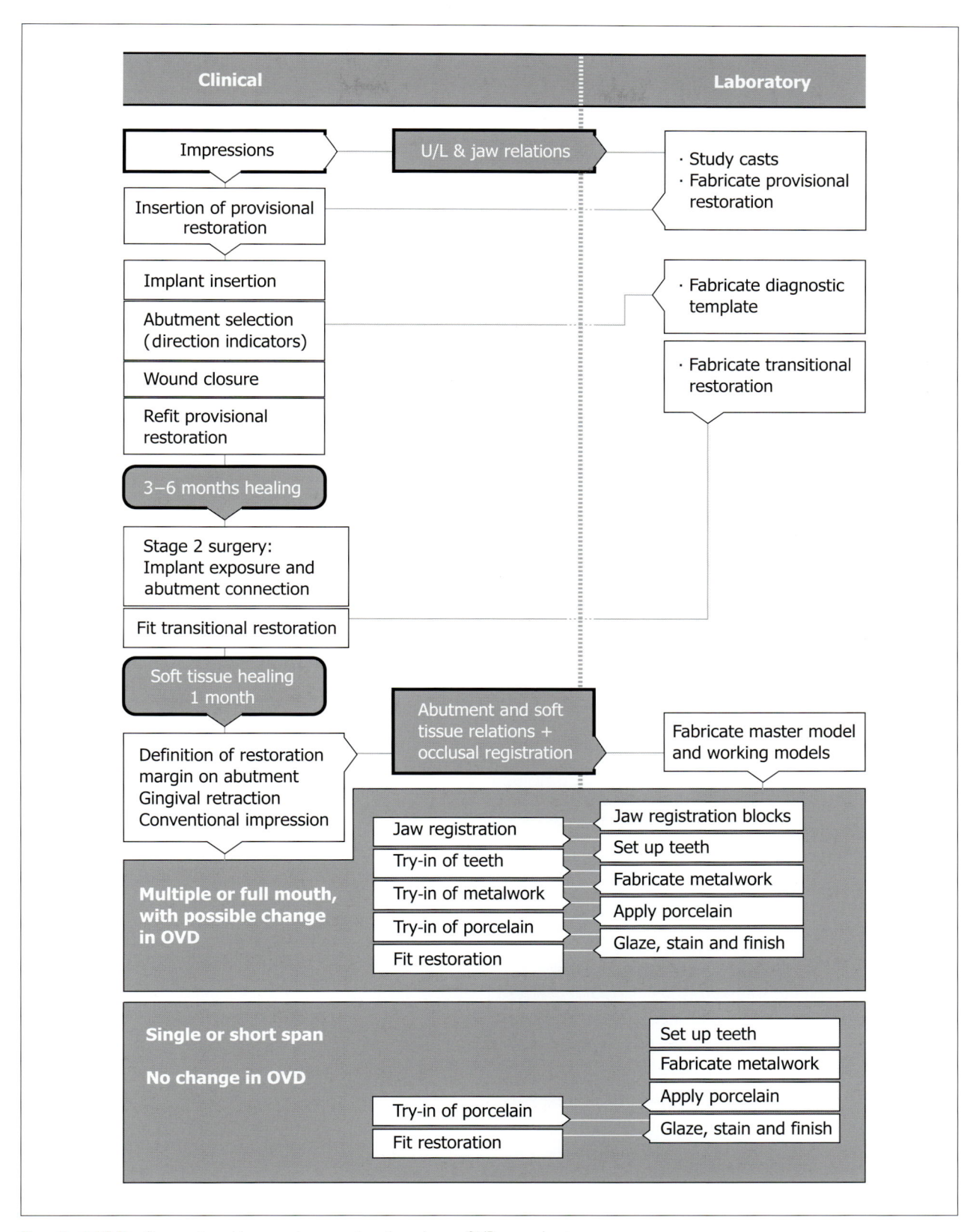

**Clinical pathway:**
- Impressions → U/L & jaw relations → Study casts; Fabricate provisional restoration
- Insertion of provisional restoration
- Implant insertion
- Abutment selection (direction indicators) → Fabricate diagnostic template
- Wound closure
- Refit provisional restoration → Fabricate transitional restoration
- 3–6 months healing
- Stage 2 surgery: Implant exposure and abutment connection
- Fit transitional restoration
- Soft tissue healing 1 month
- Definition of restoration margin on abutment; Gingival retraction; Conventional impression → Abutment and soft tissue relations + occlusal registration → Fabricate master model and working models

**Multiple or full mouth, with possible change in OVD:**
- Jaw registration → Jaw registration blocks
- Try-in of teeth → Set up teeth
- Try-in of metalwork → Fabricate metalwork
- Try-in of porcelain → Apply porcelain
- Fit restoration → Glaze, stain and finish

**Single or short span — No change in OVD:**
- Set up teeth
- Fabricate metalwork
- Try-in of porcelain → Apply porcelain
- Fit restoration → Glaze, stain and finish

**Flowchart 10-2** Conventional impressions: restorative phase. OVD, overdenture.

guide the dental technician with regard to the contours of the crown. The protocol used for multiple units is covered in greater detail in the appropriate section.

### Development of Soft Tissue Contours

The transitional restoration is cleaned with a round bur, removing the acrylic resin from the fit surface and the margin, which may have been contaminated with the temporary cement. The restoration is filled with autopolymerising acrylic resin and carefully seated on the abutment in the correct position. It must be removed from the mouth when it enters the elastic phase. Any residual acrylic resin is removed from the sulcus. The polymerisation reaction is accelerated by using hot water. The acrylic resin that extends beyond the prepared margin of the abutment is removed to prevent undercuts and overextension of the crown. The margins are polished and the restoration checked in situ to confirm that the correct gingival contours have been established. Any modifications can be made before cementing the transitional restoration with temporary cement.

### Try-in of Framework

The framework is always fabricated in accordance with a matrix produced from the original diagnostic try-in. Ideally, this would have been reconfirmed through the stages of the provisional and transitional restoration. Aesthetic and functional factors would also have been taken into account.

### Single Units

Single units do not usually require a try-in of the framework, as the fit can be achieved predictably and adjustment of the soft tissue in relation to the framework can be carried out directly from the impressions of the abutment. However, should the need arise, there is no reason why the framework cannot be tried in, particularly when the development of the soft tissue contours requires several modifications of the transitional restoration.

### Multiple Units

Multiple units require the metalwork to be tried in to confirm the accurate and passive fit of the restoration.

In the event of the framework not fitting down to the margin or if there is a rock, the metalwork will need to be sectioned and located together using acrylic resin and plaster. On completion of the soldering the metalwork is tried in again to confirm the fit and is picked up in an acrylic resin stock impression tray, thus producing a cast of the relationship of the metalwork to the soft tissues for the addition of the porcelain to create the desired contours.

### Try-in of the Unglazed Restoration

The colour, form and occlusion of the restoration must be thoroughly checked at this stage. Particular attention should be paid to the relationship of the restoration to the soft tissues, particularly if there have been changes in the contours generated by the provisional restoration.

### Fit of Restoration

The restoration is fitted with soft cement following any minor adjustments. Excess cement must always be vented by gently retracting the gingival margin by means of a fine flat plastic instrument or a periodontal probe and must not be extruded subgingivally. Additional retention and security can be achieved by the use of a lateral fixation screw. This may be engaged directly into the abutment or into a gold coping permanently cemented onto the abutment.

### Special Considerations for Multiple Units and Full Mouth Reconstruction

Large restorations, where changes in the tooth position and in the intermaxillary relationship are proposed, require special consideration. Data established during the diagnostic phase will need to be reconfirmed during the surgical phase and finally at the restorative phase. This is accentuated by the fact that implant-supported restorations have to be made with greater accuracy than conventional tooth-supported restorations. However, the bulk of the material being replaced is far greater than merely the tooth tissues that require replacement in conventional crown and bridgework. Therefore, protocols derived from restorative and prosthodontic disciplines need to be merged to satisfy the required parameters.

## Recording the Intermaxillary Relationship

The information is brought forward from the diagnostic phase in a number of well-defined and predictable steps.

- **Diagnostic preview**. During the diagnostic preview, the teeth will be arranged in their ideal position and with the correct intermaxillary relationship. The accuracy of the positioning can be confirmed using accepted guidelines such as speech, facial profile and visual appearance. This will be carried out at the try-in stage as for removable prostheses.
- **Provisional restoration**. The transfer of the information into a provisional restoration will achieve aesthetic and functional verification of the above data. Fixed provisional restorations are particularly effective at refining both aesthetic and functional design as they allow input from the patient as well as the patient's social and professional environment.
- **Diagnostic template**. The data, as verified above, are converted into the hollow prosthetic envelope (diagnostic template), which is used to identify implant position and select the abutments that fit within the envelope.
- **Transitional restoration**. The transitional restoration is fabricated as a hollow restoration according to the data established in the stages described above. It is designed to fit over the abutments selected during first-stage surgery and fitted during second-stage surgery. These abutments are fitted within the prosthetic envelope and are aligned with each other. The transitional restoration is then relined within the patient's mouth to the correct intermaxillary relationship.
- **Jaw registration blocks**. Transfer of the data from the transitional restoration to the jaw registration blocks is carried out when impressions are taken. The transitional restoration is cut in half so that the relationship between the abutments on one side of the mouth can be recorded, using a rigid registration material. This is repeated on the other side of the mouth to provide details of the relationship of the jaws to one another; this information can then be passed on to the laboratory. The position of a tooth can be transposed to the working die cast by means of a matrix produced from an impression of the transitional restoration. An acrylic resin framework is constructed to fit over the abutments on the cast, and wax is added to the framework in the matrix. This can then be used in the mouth to refine the intermaxillary distance and tooth position, size and form.

## Confirming Tooth Form and Position as Established in the Original Preview

Inherent discrepancies may become incorporated during the adaptation of the transitional restoration to the abutments at exposure. These may be in the transfer of the vertical dimension or the labio-palatal positioning of the teeth. It is essential, therefore, that the position of the tooth can be related accurately to the abutments. Use of jaw registration blocks helps to achieve this. The teeth are arranged to the established intermaxillary relationship.

The arrangement of the teeth on the acrylic resin framework can now be related accurately to the abutments. This arrangement of teeth is then transferred to the patients' mouth to confirm:

- tooth position
- tooth colour
- tooth form
- lip support
- function via speech.

This information is transferred to the laboratory; an accurate matrix can relate the tooth position at the correct dimension to the abutments, which enables the metalwork to be waxed up into the matrix.

## Try-in of Metalwork

The metalwork is cast in sections of three units and is transferred to the mouth for locating to each other using low-shrinkage resin (e.g. GC pattern [GC Corp, Tokyo, Japan] or Duralay [Reliance Dental, Worth, IL, USA]) and plaster. The soldered metalwork is tried in the mouth once again and its relationship with the soft tissue is recorded by means of an overall impression using addition-cured silicone impression material in a rigid acrylic resin stock tray. Alternatively, the metalwork can be located directly onto a solid model and soldered or laser-welded prior to try-in.

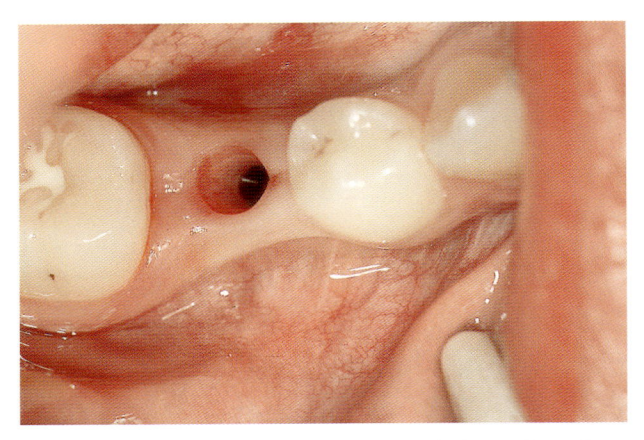

II  Implant Placement: Surgery and Prosthodontics

**Fig 10-20** This case demonstrates the technique of transferring the abutment position to the laboratory for the construction of a restoration. The occlusal view of the implant shows the healthy gingival cuff developed by the sulcus former, which was inserted at the time the implant was placed. In the posterior quadrants such as this, where aesthetics are not critical and where an angled abutment of 15 degrees or less is required, a sulcus former avoids the need for second-stage surgery.

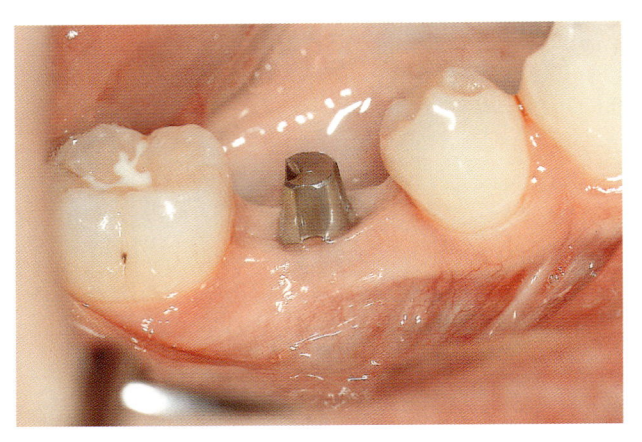

**Fig 10-21** Clinical view of the definitive (15-degree standard; Ankylos system) abutment attached, emerging through the soft tissues.

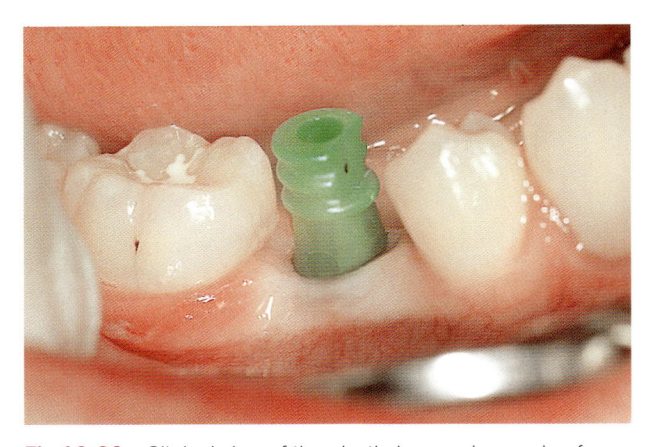

**Fig 10-22** Clinical view of the plastic impression coping for the transfer of abutment position in place on the abutment.

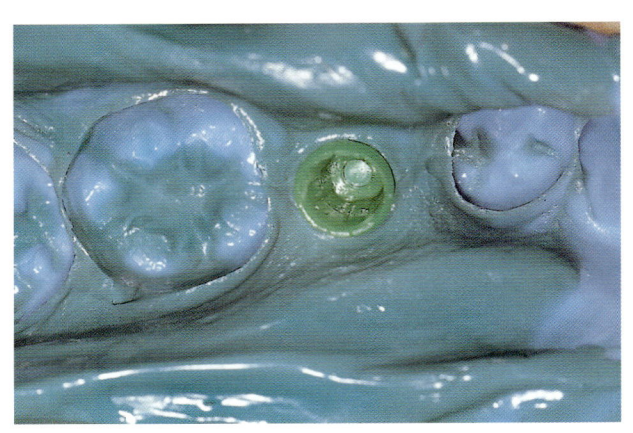

**Fig 10-23** View of the fit surface of the pick-up impression. An abutment analogue (or an abutment) may be attached to the plastic impression coping. Therefore, no changes should be made to either the abutment in the mouth or the abutment analogue in the laboratory.

### Try-in of Unglazed Restoration and Fit

The major points are outlined above, but it must be emphasised that each stage must be undertaken with the highest accuracy and greatest care, otherwise alterations in the final stages may result in severe compromises. It is recommended, therefore, that specific checklists be used at each stage to ensure that the maximum benefit is obtained. This will increase predictability and minimise complications.

## Transfer of Abutment Position

As an alternative to the conventional impression technique the transfer of the position of the abutment can be carried out (Figs 10-20–10-31). The clinical and laboratory stages using the abutment impression technique for restorations with single crowns and short-span bridges. In addition to larger restorations involving alterations to the occlusal vertical dimension, are outlined in Flowchart 10-3.

## 10  Restorative Phase: Prosthetic Protocols

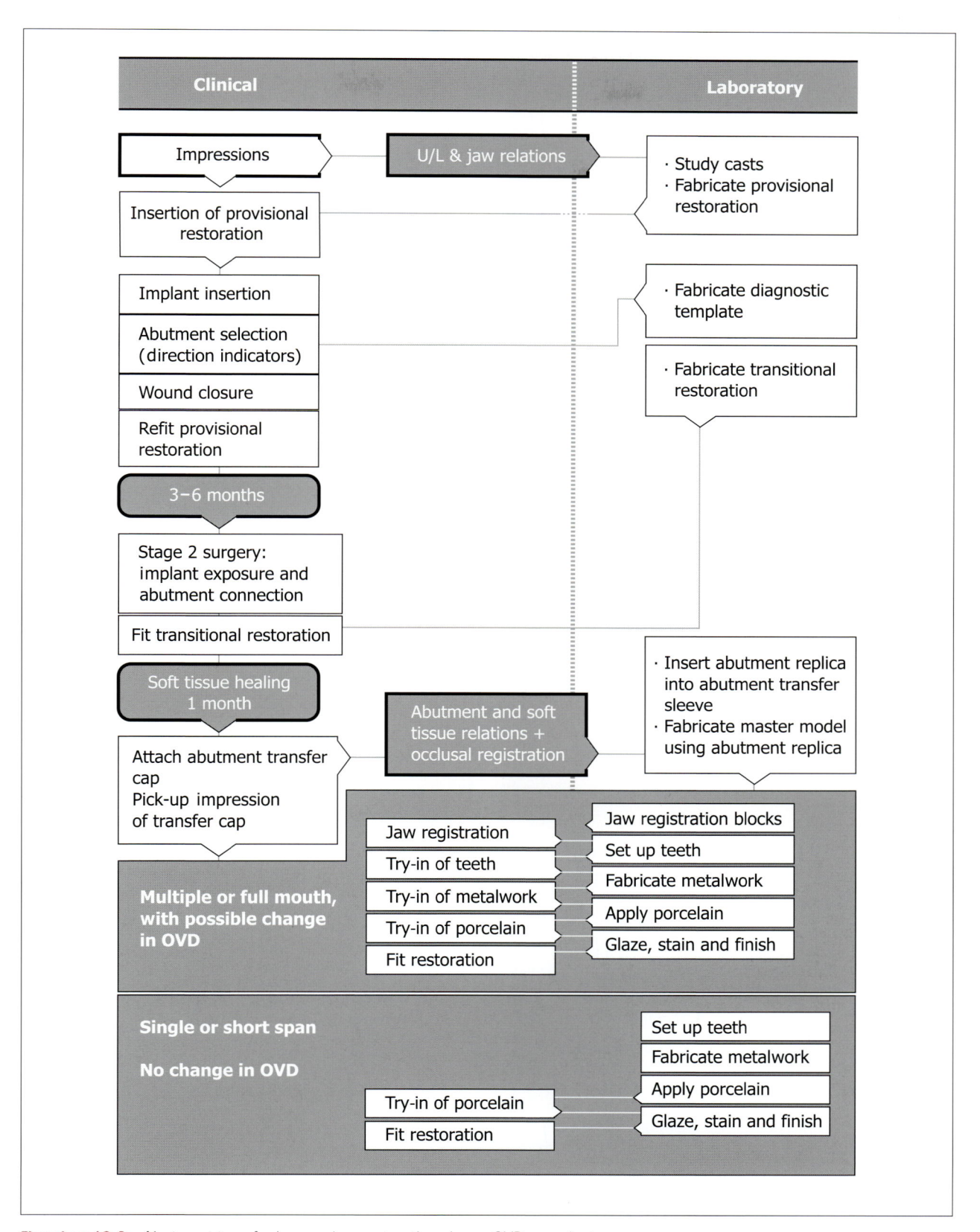

| Clinical | | Laboratory |
|---|---|---|
| Impressions → U/L & jaw relations | | · Study casts<br>· Fabricate provisional restoration |
| Insertion of provisional restoration | | |
| Implant insertion | | · Fabricate diagnostic template |
| Abutment selection (direction indicators) | | · Fabricate transitional restoration |
| Wound closure | | |
| Refit provisional restoration | | |
| **3–6 months** | | |
| Stage 2 surgery: implant exposure and abutment connection | | |
| Fit transitional restoration | | |
| **Soft tissue healing 1 month** | Abutment and soft tissue relations + occlusal registration | · Insert abutment replica into abutment transfer sleeve<br>· Fabricate master model using abutment replica |
| Attach abutment transfer cap<br>Pick-up impression of transfer cap | | |

**Multiple or full mouth, with possible change in OVD**

| Clinical | Laboratory |
|---|---|
| Jaw registration | Jaw registration blocks |
| Try-in of teeth | Set up teeth |
| Try-in of metalwork | Fabricate metalwork |
| Try-in of porcelain | Apply porcelain |
| Fit restoration | Glaze, stain and finish |

**Single or short span**

**No change in OVD**

| Clinical | Laboratory |
|---|---|
| | Set up teeth |
| | Fabricate metalwork |
| | Apply porcelain |
| Try-in of porcelain | Glaze, stain and finish |
| Fit restoration | |

**Flowchart 10-3**  Abutment transfer impression: restorative phase. OVD, overdenture.

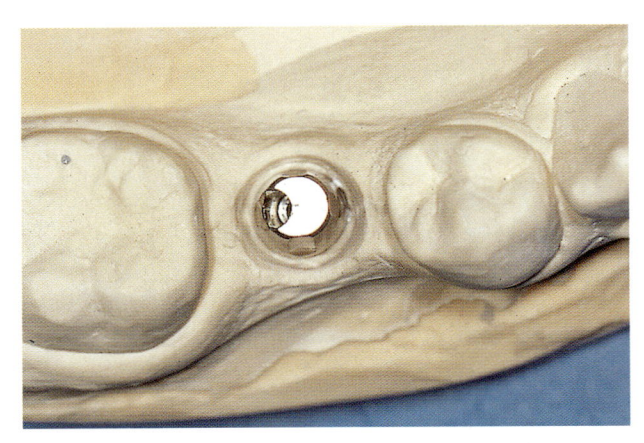

II   Implant Placement: Surgery and Prosthodontics

Fig 10-24   A laboratory cast with the abutment analogue in situ. In this case, an abutment mounted on an implant analogue has been used. The crown can be fabricated on this abutment analogue and transferred directly to the mouth for the definitive fitting. For this patient, however, an additional impression was taken with the metalwork as a pick-up to enable the soft tissue contours to be transferred to the laboratory.

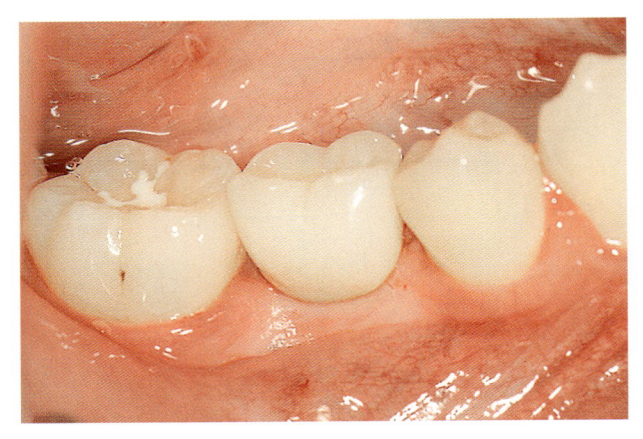

Fig 10-25   Transitional restoration in place in the form of a primary premolar which is being replaced. The transitional restoration is being used to develop the soft tissues to provide a better emergence profile.

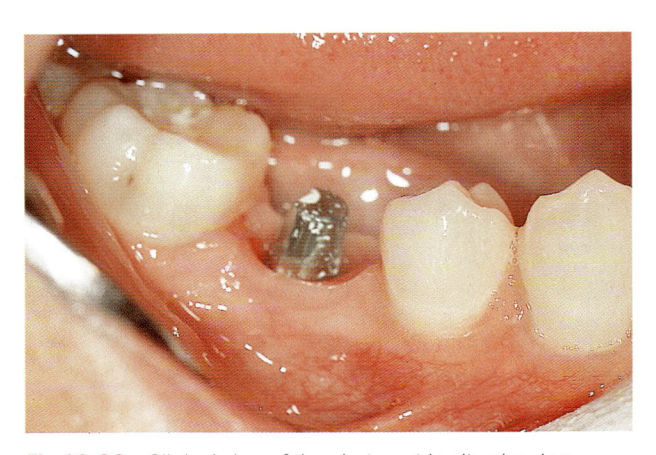

Fig 10-26   Clinical view of the abutment in situ showing improved gingival contours compared with the previous image (Fig 10-21).

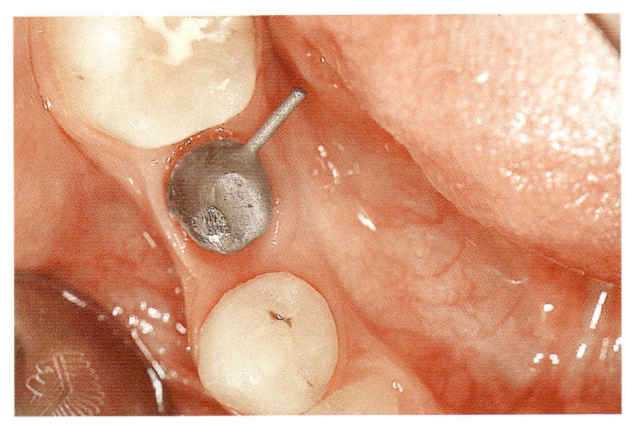

Fig 10-27   Occlusal view of the metalwork in situ, prior to pick-up.

There are specific factors that need to be borne in mind when using this technique. These originate from the fact that the abutment cannot be altered because the technician will be fabricating the prostheses on a replica of the abutment (Figs 10-32 and 10-33). The following factors need to be considered:

- the size or shape of the abutment cannot be modified
- the abutment must fit within the prosthetic envelope
- the margin of the abutment cannot be varied according to the soft tissues
- a broad range of abutments is needed (for instance, height, width and sulcus depth)
- for multiple splinted units the abutments must be perfectly aligned.

The definitive abutment is selected during implant placement and is fitted on exposure, using a template

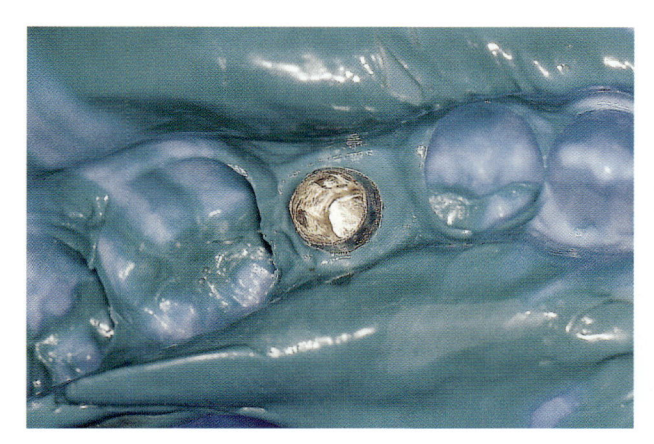

## 10 Restorative Phase: Prosthetic Protocols

**Fig 10-28** Metalwork in the silicone impression material with the newly established gingival contours being transferred to the laboratory.

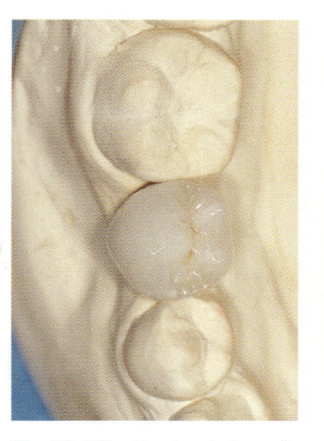

**Fig 10-29** Occlusal view of the definitive metal-ceramic restoration on the laboratory cast. Note that the form of a premolar has now been developed in order to produce a better aesthetic and functional outcome.

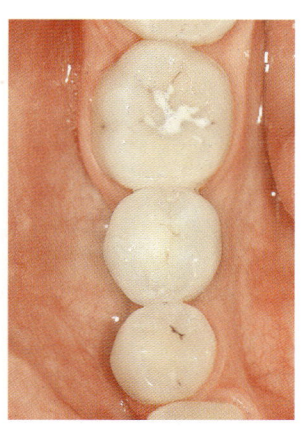

**Fig 10-30** Occlusal view of the definitive restoration in the mouth.

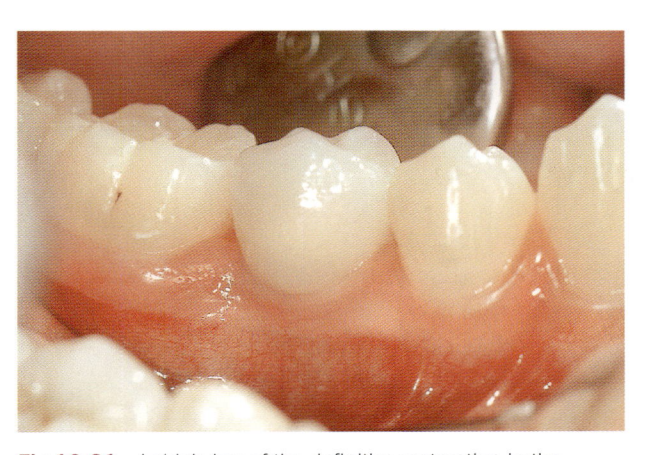

**Fig 10-31** Labial view of the definitive restoration in the mouth, showing the emergence profile developed by the transitional restoration.

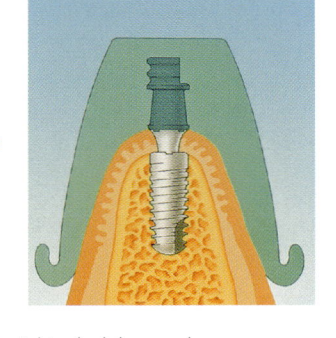

**Fig 10-32** The use of a sleeve to transfer the position of the definitive abutment to the laboratory. The plastic cap (dark green) can be seen within the bulk of the impression material (light green). The impression cap is removed with the impression, and an analogue of the abutment is positioned into the impression cap before the impression is cast. The definitive abutment remains in the mouth, attached to the implant. The dental technician works on a replica of the abutment. Neither the abutment in the mouth nor the analogue (replica) in the laboratory can be modified.

to ensure that adequate clearance is available. In addition to the height and width of the abutment being selected, the depth of the soft tissue must also be measured so that an abutment with the correct sulcus depth is chosen.

In the event that the required clearance from the template is not available, an alternative abutment needs to be selected. A transitional restoration is then inserted, as with the conventional impression method.

### Impression Taking

The impression is taken using a transfer coping that fits over the abutment (Figs 10-22 and 10-32). The transfer coping is picked up with the impression so that the replica of the abutment may be inserted into the coping (Fig 10-23). This provides a replica of the abutment in the mouth, enabling the technician to fabricate the restoration on the replica (Figs 10-24 and 10-33). The remaining stages are the same as

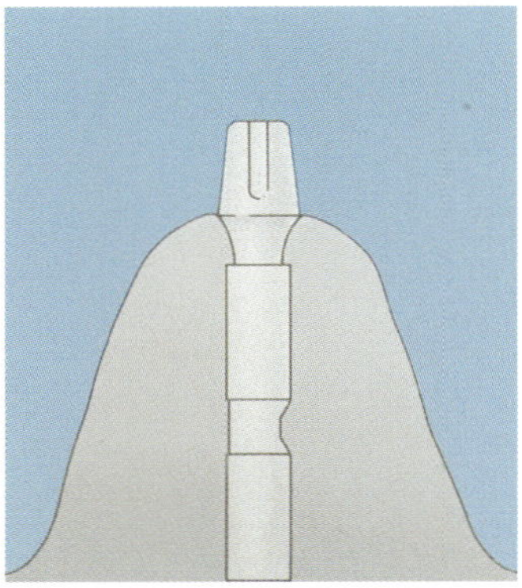

**Fig 10-33** A laboratory cast fabricated from an abutment transfer impression. The abutment analogue, which is a replica of what is fitted in the mouth, can be seen. The prosthetic work is carried out directly on this component, which is a replica of what is in the mouth in terms of both form and position.

with the conventional impression method. There are discrepancies between the dimensions of the analogue and abutment that result from engineering tolerances as well as those resulting from differences in the transfer procedure. This technique is, therefore, not recommended for use in multiple units or full mouth restorations because of the high risk of misfit. Furthermore, the aesthetic outcome might be less predictable because the abutment cannot be individualised to establish the emergence profile. However, when indicated, this technique is a very simple and effective means of transferring information. It enables the abutment position to be transferred without having to manipulate the gingival tissues with a retraction cord and so it avoids the need for local anaesthetic.

### Multiple-purpose Transfer Caps

Multiple-purpose transfer caps (Fig 10-34) have been manufactured to permit the use of one component part for:
- coping for attachment to transitional restoration for immediate loading or after exposure if a staged approach is used (Figs 10-35–10-38)
- impression taking to transfer abutment position (Fig 10-39)
- a base for waxing-up framework for the purpose of casting using the burn-out technique.

## Transfer of the Implant Position

The transfer of the implant position to the laboratory is achieved by means of an implant position transfer device (transfer post) and an implant replica. The clinical and laboratory stages for the technique are outlined in Flowchart 10-4.

Typically, at implant exposure, the cover screw will have been removed and a sulcus former (healing abutment) attached. The same provisional restoration is used with minor modifications to adapt to the presence of the sulcus former.

The technician can now work on the actual abutment that will be used and can modify it into the ideal shape to support the definitive restoration. However, this means that the abutment will need to be transferred to the mouth for the try-in of each stage. Consequently, there will be several transfers of the abutment between the cast and the mouth. It is critical, therefore, that the abutment position is reproduced accurately every time, both on the cast and in the mouth.

### Impression Taking

The impression may be taken by using the open or closed tray technique. An implant transfer device, which fits directly to the implant, will be required. The design of the transfer device will depend on the technique used.

### Open Tray Technique

The impression is taken with an implant position transfer device (transfer post), which is attached directly to the implant. The transfer post is attached to the implant by means of a screw (Fig 10-40), which is removed with the impression. It, therefore, requires the use of an impression tray, either custom made or with a metal or acrylic resin stock tray, which is adapted so that there is access to the screw attaching the transfer post to the implant. The impression is taken using an addition-cured silicone. The impression material is injected around the transfer post prior to the loaded tray being seated. Once the impression material has set, the fixation screw is detached from the implant, enabling the impression to be removed with the transfer post embedded within it. The implant replica can then be attached prior to casting the impression (Figs 10-41–10-48).

### Closed Tray Technique

The closed tray technique requires the use of either a custom-made or a stock impression tray. The impres-

**10** Restorative Phase: Prosthetic Protocols

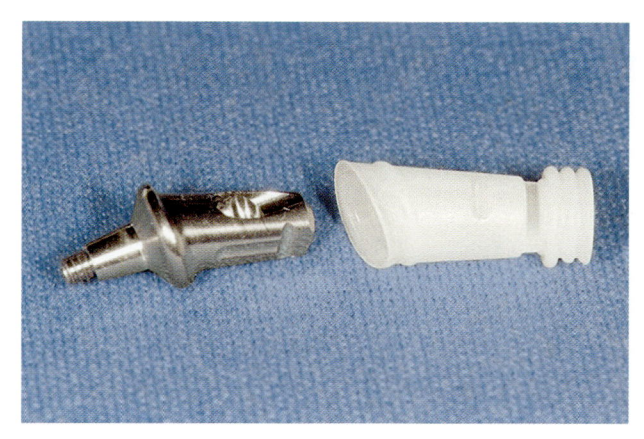

**Fig 10-34** Regular abutment and 3-in-1 cap (22.5 degree). The snap-on cap has additional retention for impression taking, which can be removed for the purpose of incorporationg it into a transitional restoration or as a base for waxing-up.

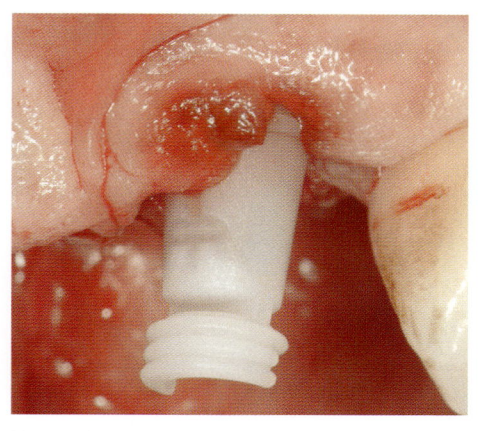

**Fig 10-35** The 3-in-1 cap seated on an abutment for the purpose of immediate loading before removing undercut extension.

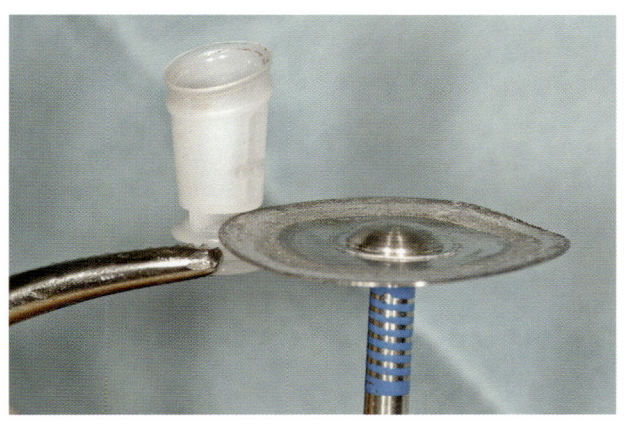

**Fig 10-36** Removal of the undercut extension is easily carried out using a diamond disc.

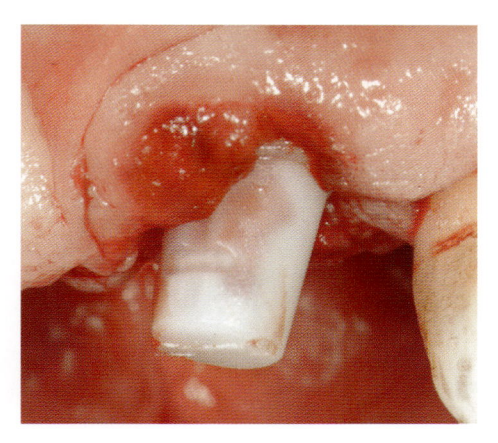

**Fig 10-37** Modified cap in situ prior to connecting to transitional restoration.

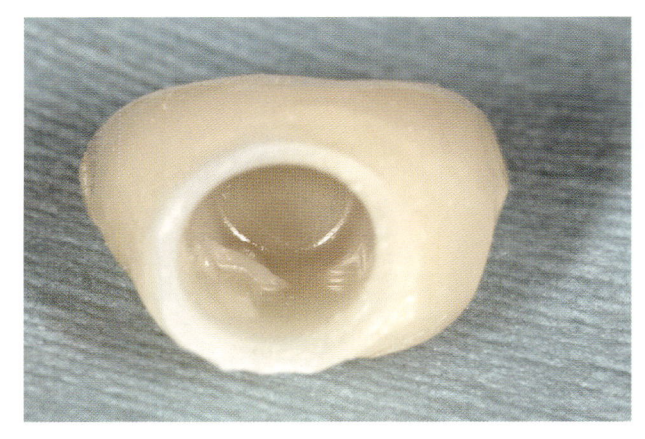

**Fig 10-38** Transitional restoration with incorporated 3-in-1 cap.

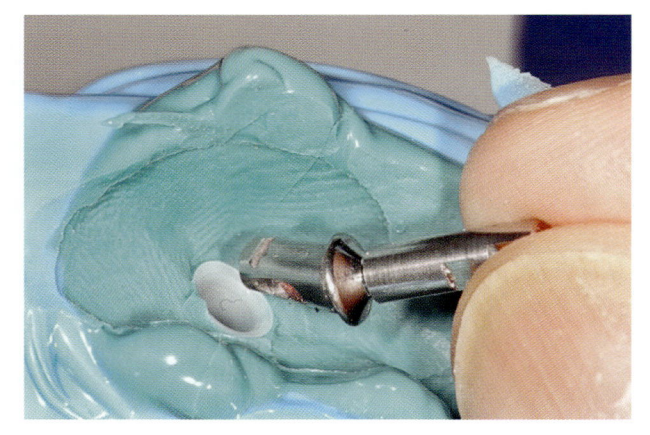

**Fig 10-39** Pick-up impression containing 3-in-1 cap with abutment mounted on an implant analogue (or abutment analogue) being inserted by the dental technician into the impression on which the restoration can be made.

183

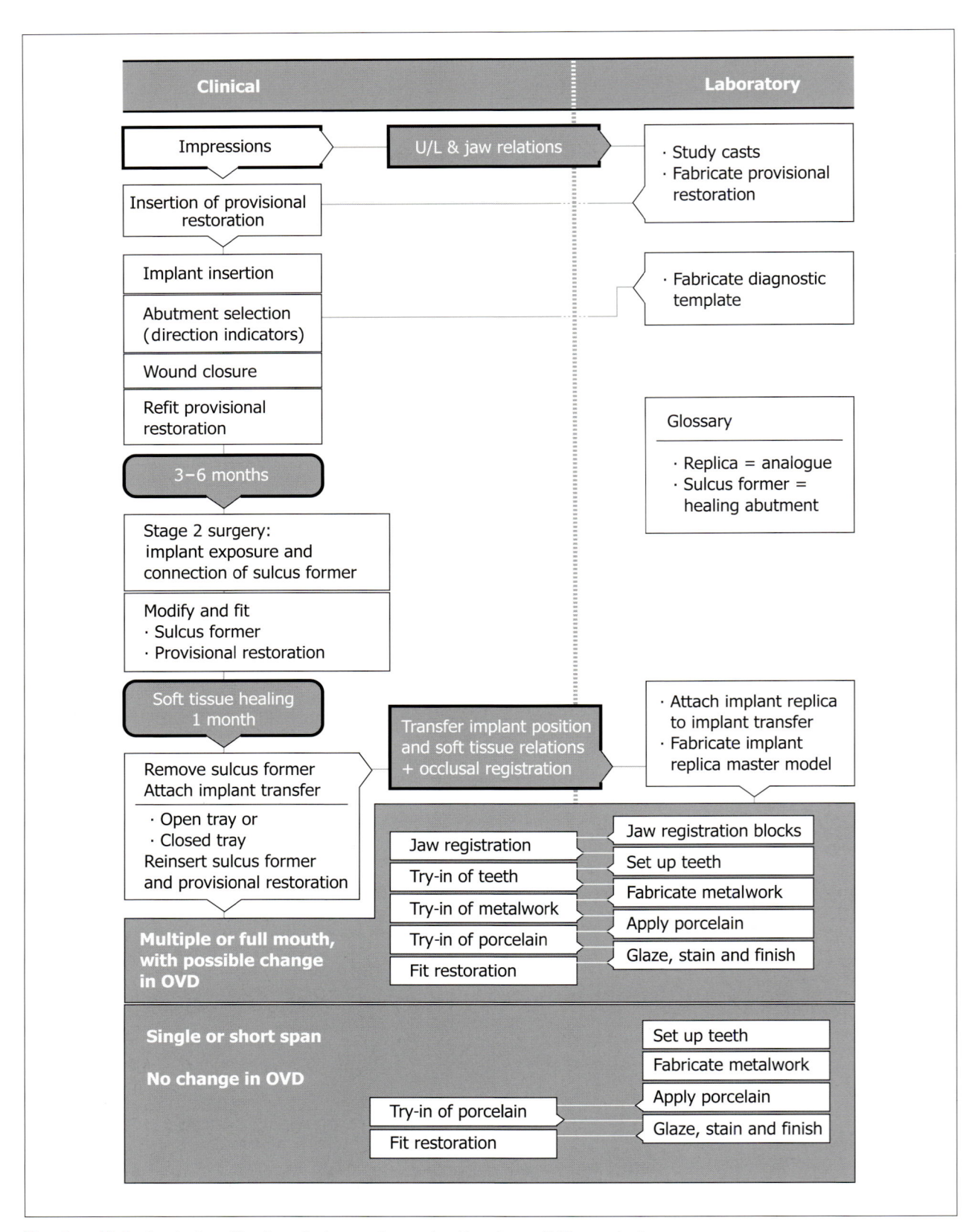

## II  Implant Placement: Surgery and Prosthodontics

### Clinical

- Impressions
- U/L & jaw relations
- Insertion of provisional restoration
- Implant insertion
- Abutment selection (direction indicators)
- Wound closure
- Refit provisional restoration
- **3–6 months**
- Stage 2 surgery: implant exposure and connection of sulcus former
- Modify and fit
  - Sulcus former
  - Provisional restoration
- **Soft tissue healing 1 month**
- Remove sulcus former / Attach implant transfer
  - Open tray or
  - Closed tray
  - Reinsert sulcus former and provisional restoration
- Transfer implant position and soft tissue relations + occlusal registration

**Multiple or full mouth, with possible change in OVD**
- Jaw registration
- Try-in of teeth
- Try-in of metalwork
- Try-in of porcelain
- Fit restoration

**Single or short span — No change in OVD**
- Try-in of porcelain
- Fit restoration

### Laboratory

- Study casts
- Fabricate provisional restoration
- Fabricate diagnostic template

**Glossary**
- Replica = analogue
- Sulcus former = healing abutment

- Attach implant replica to implant transfer
- Fabricate implant replica master model

- Jaw registration blocks
- Set up teeth
- Fabricate metalwork
- Apply porcelain
- Glaze, stain and finish

- Set up teeth
- Fabricate metalwork
- Apply porcelain
- Glaze, stain and finish

**Flowchart 10-4**  Implant position transfer impression: restorative phase. OVD, overdenture.

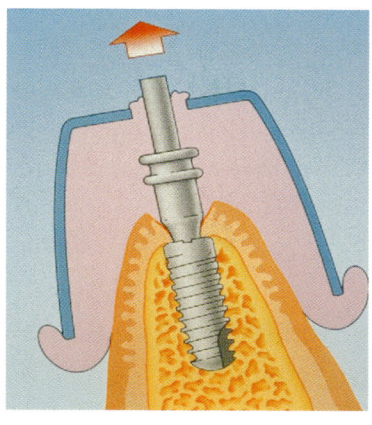

10  Restorative Phase: Prosthetic Protocols

**Fig 10-40** The open tray technique to transfer the implant position. The transfer mechanism consists of two components, the transfer post (component that is attached to the implant) and a retaining screw. Access to the screw is obtained via a hole in the impression tray, which enables the device to be unscrewed with the impression in situ. The impression is removed with the implant transfer within the impression. The implant analogue is attached to the transfer post prior to casting. This provides a replica of the implant in the laboratory cast in the correct position.

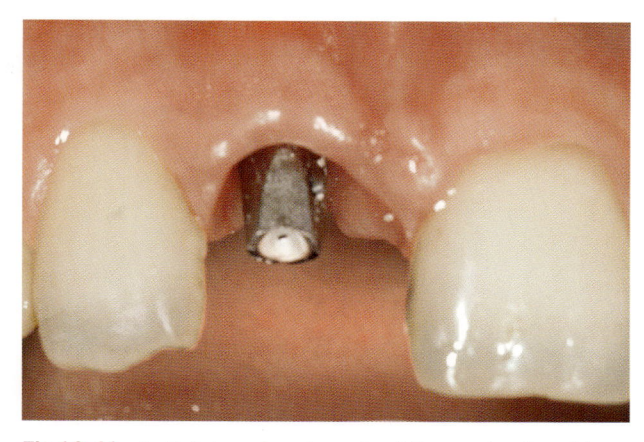

**Fig 10-41** Labial view of contoured soft tissues developed by an abutment and an acrylic resin transitional restoration. These were fashioned from impressions taken at first-stage surgery and fitted at implant exposure for the development of the soft tissues.

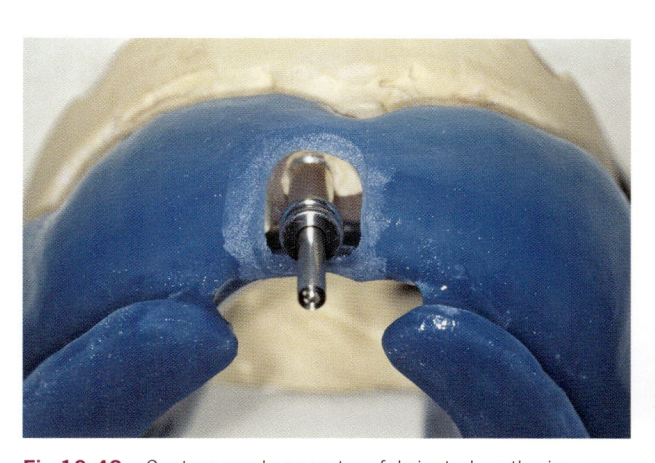

**Fig 10-42** Custom made open tray fabricated on the impressions taken at first-stage surgery.

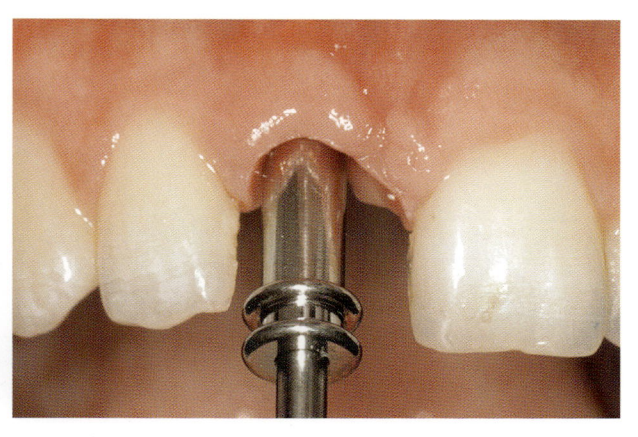

**Fig 10-43** Open tray transfer post engaging the conical connection of the implant. This is secured to the implant by means of a screw, tightened to < 10 Ncm.

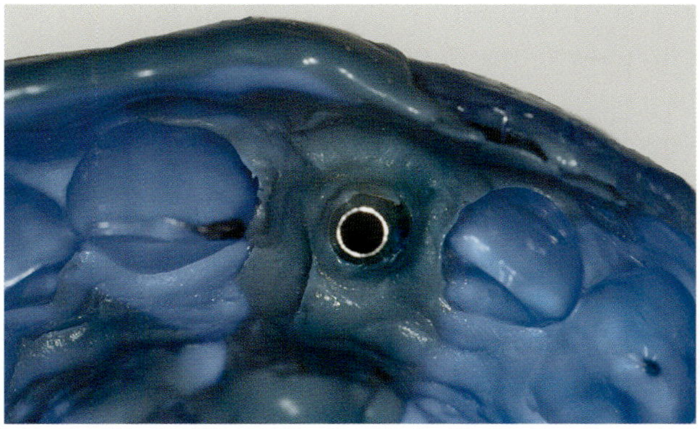

**Fig 10-44** Impression containing the transfer post is removed from the mouth by unscrewing the fixation screw, thus disengaging the transfer post.

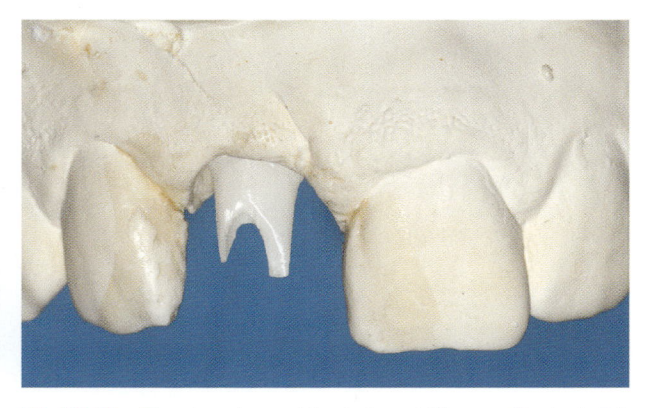

**Fig 10-45** The zirconium oxide abutment (Cercon; Dentsply Friadent) is modified by the technician to the developed soft tissue contours transferred to the laboratory using the impression. The crown margin is positioned approximately 1.5 mm below gingival margin wherever possible. Interstitially, this is often not possible especially when highly scalloped gingival contours are present.

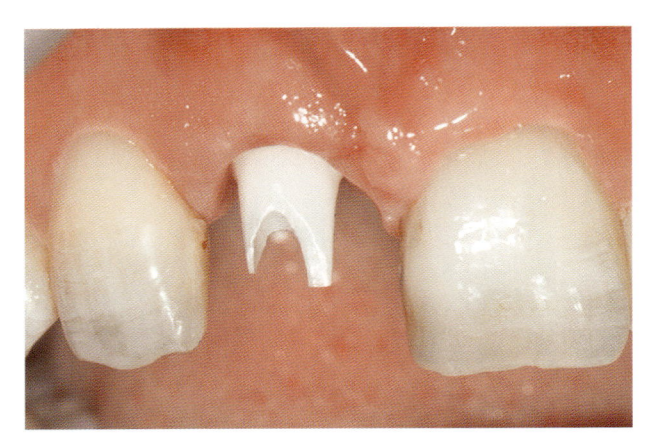

II Implant Placement: Surgery and Prosthodontics

**Fig 10-46** The zirconium abutment is transferred to the patient using a transfer jig in the absence of an internal index.

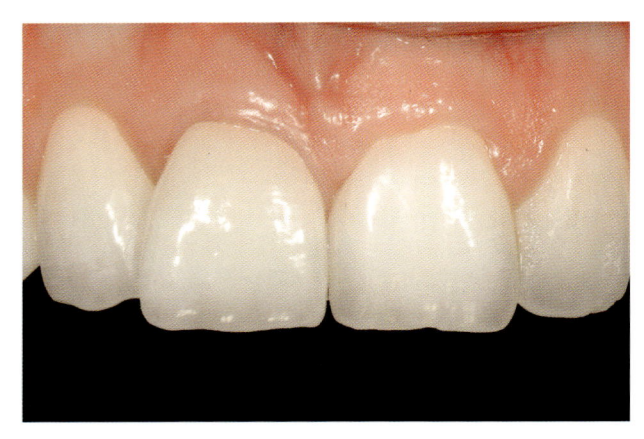

**Fig 10-47** Full ceramic crown fitted onto the ceramic abutment, emerging out of soft tissues. The cement margin is positioned close to the gingival margin. The ceramic abutment prevents the greying of gingival tissues.

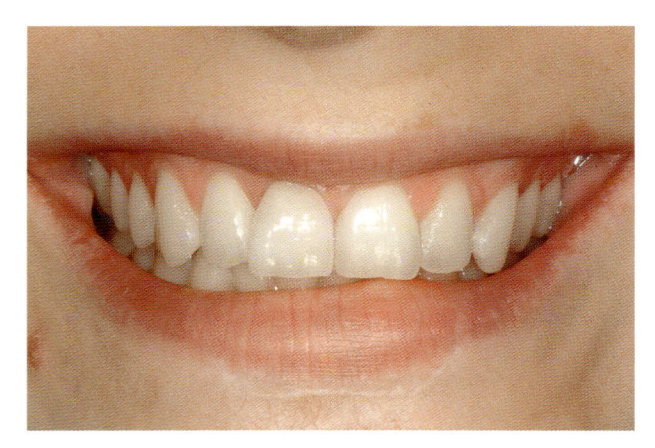

**Fig 10-48** The patient smiling showing harmonious soft tissue contours.

sion is taken over the impression device (repositioning post), which is attached to the implant (Fig 10-49). The impression is removed from the mouth leaving the repositioning post in situ. The repositioning post is then removed from the implant and reinserted into the recess created in the impression material after connecting it to an implant replica.

## Abutment Selection, Modification or Fabrication

A number of different possibilities are now available:
- an abutment, preselected in the surgery, may be attached and any modifications carried out to refine the abutment shape in accordance with the definitive restoration
- an abutment may be selected by the dental technician at this stage and modified
- an abutment may be fabricated from gold (e.g. the UCLA abutment) or milled from titanium or ceramic material (e.g. Procera [Nobel Biocare, Uxbridge, UK] or Atlantis [Astra Tech, Mölndal, Sweden]).[159–162]

The definitive restoration or framework can now be fabricated directly on the abutment (Fig 10-50). For multiple units, an index is necessary to record the orientation of the abutment on the cast and to enable this to be transferred accurately to the mouth.

### Try-in of Framework

The try-in of the framework will require the removal of the sulcus former, followed by attachment of the definitive abutment prior to the framework being tried in. The use of the index at this stage will ensure that the abutment is positioned in the correct orientation. Any discrepancy in orientation of the abutment will drastically impact the fit of the framework. Decisions on the fit of the framework, which may require the sectioning of the framework, can only be made on the assumption that the abutments are accurately positioned. It should be borne in mind that there is a possibility of a misfit of the framework every time the abutment is removed and reinserted between the cast and the mouth. This is because of the discrepancy in

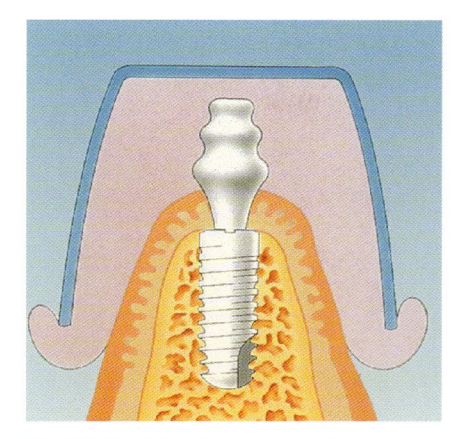

**Fig 10-49** The closed tray technique for the transfer of the implant position. The transfer post consists of one or two pieces, which is screwed into the implant. The impression is taken over the post and removed. The post is then unscrewed. The transfer post is then attached to an implant replica (analogue) and reinserted into the impression prior to casting. This provides a replica of the implant in the laboratory cast in the correct position.

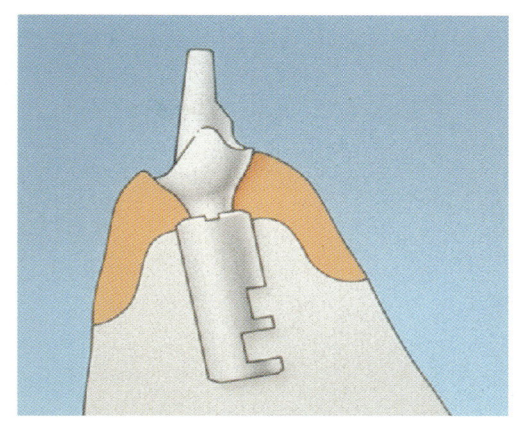

**Fig 10-50** A laboratory cast poured from any of the techniques that transfer implant position. The implant analogue is visible with the selected abutment attached. All restorative work is carried out on this abutment, which may be modified. The abutment and the prosthesis will need to be transferred to the mouth for each interim stage and the final delivery of the restoration.

the orientation of the abutment caused by engineering tolerances of the connection. It is reasonable, therefore, to leave the abutment seated once the framework has been assessed to fit accurately. In this case a transitional restoration prepared in the laboratory may now be inserted until the definitive restoration can be finished.

## Finishing the Restoration

A pick-up impression of the metalwork may now be used to relate the framework to the soft tissues (created by the sulcus formers) for the addition of porcelain, as described in the section on conventional impressions.

## Prosthetic Protocols: Clinical Cases

### Case 1: Impressions at First-stage Surgery

A 66-year-old woman required replacement of the maxillary first and second premolar teeth on the right-hand side of the mouth. A hybrid bridge with a Rochette retainer and a full preparation retainer was used as a provisional restoration during the treatment phase (Figs 8-45–8-50, p. 117).

Impressions at first-stage surgery were taken to facilitate the creation of a natural emergence profile by means of a transitional restoration (Figs 10-9–10-19; see also Fig 8-70, p. 129).

### Case 2: Conventional Impressions for Multiple Splinted Units, Cement Retention

A 65-year-old woman presented with the loss of several teeth in the maxilla and mandible. Because of excessive atrophy of the maxillary region, onlay autogenous bone grafts from the iliac crest for the reconstruction of the ridge were required. Implants were inserted 10 weeks after the augmentation and exposed six months later on completion of integration. Abutments were attached at the time of exposure and loaded by means of an acrylic resin transitional restoration (Figs 10-51–10-72).

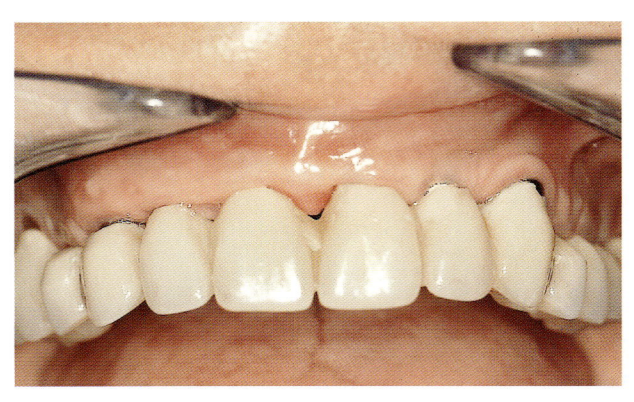

## II  Implant Placement: Surgery and Prosthodontics

**Fig 10-51**  Demonstration of the use of conventional impressions for the restoration of multiple implants and teeth in the maxilla. Labial view of the transitional restoration one month following the exposure of the implants. Note the soft tissue contours that have been developed by the transitional restoration.

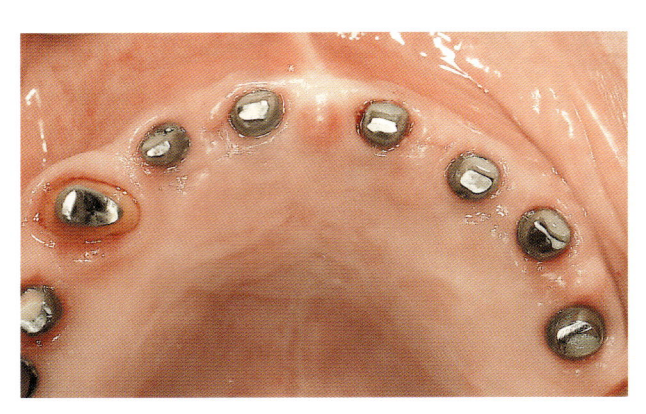

**Fig 10-52**  Occlusal view of the implants and the maxillary left canine. Once again the soft tissue contours should be observed as well as the position of the implants and the alignment of the abutments that fit within the prosthetic envelope.

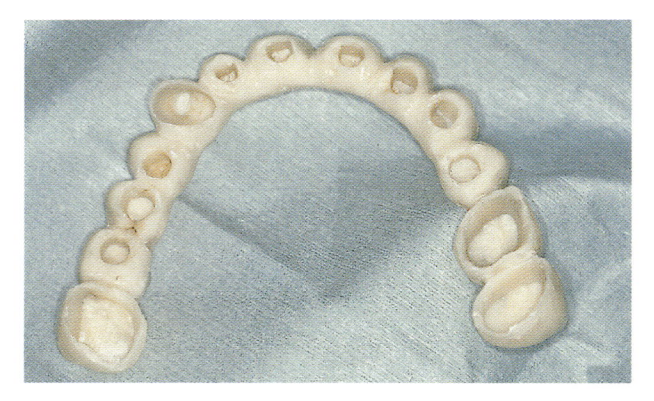

**Fig 10-53**  View of the fit surface of the transitional restoration, which has been used during the period of maturation of the soft tissues. The restoration will need to be relined following the preparation of the abutments and impression taking. The transitional restoration will, therefore, have to be adapted to the new shape of the abutments as well as the re-contoured soft tissues.

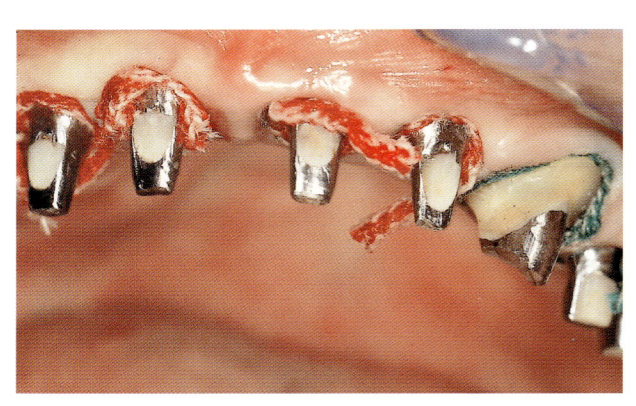

**Fig 10-54**  Clinical view of the retraction cord being used to retract the soft tissues. This is carried out after any modification of the abutments. The only modification that was deemed necessary was to prepare a margin to which the technician could work.

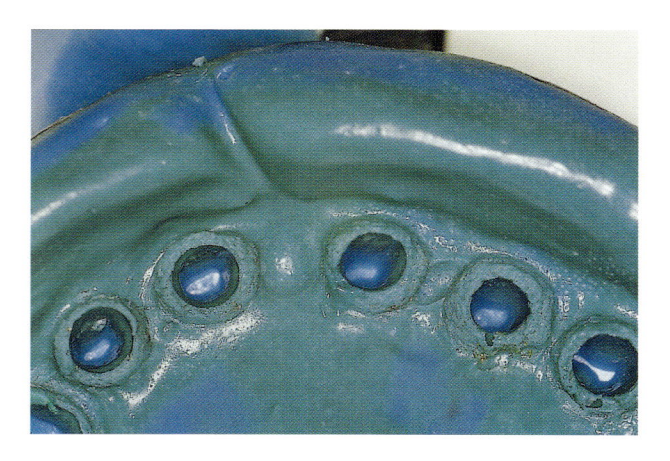

**Fig 10-55**  A view of the conventional impression taken of the abutments and the tooth, using addition-cured silicone impression material (Provil, light and heavy bodied material). The margins of the abutments are clearly visible. The impression will be cast a number of times to provide the dental technician with a solid cast as a control, a working split-die cast for waxing up the framework, two additional casts for fabricating the acrylic resin and wax registration blocks and a spare.

## 10   Restorative Phase: Prosthetic Protocols

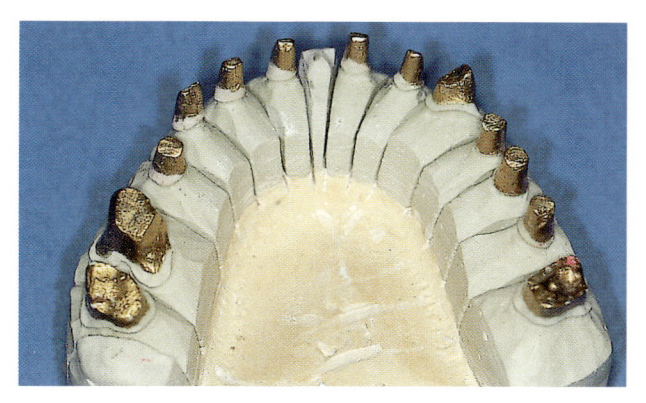

**Fig 10-56**   Die cast for waxing up the metal framework; a single layer of die spacer is used to ensure a close fit.

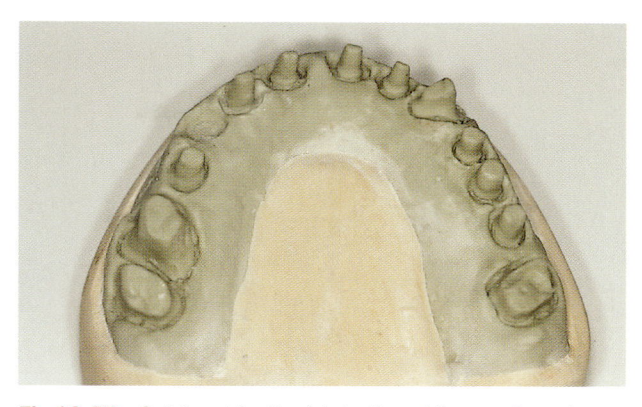

**Fig 10-57**   Solid cast for the fabrication of the acrylic resin framework, which will support the wax for intermaxillary registration.

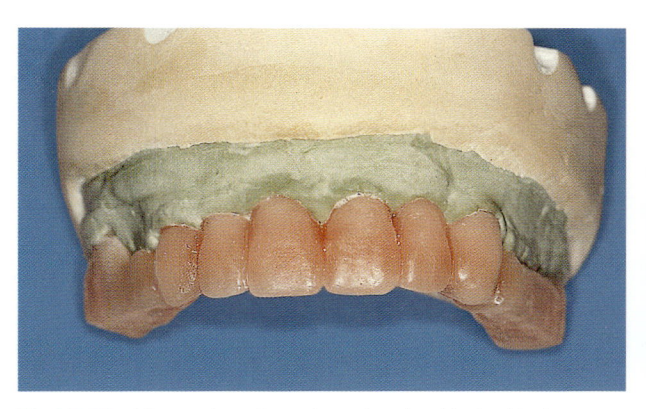

**Fig 10-58**   Wax and acrylic resin registration block with the anterior tooth form derived from a matrix of the transitional restoration, which has already been functionally and aesthetically approved. The registration block will enable all the information relating to the tooth form and position and the opposing arch to be accurately related between the cast and the abutments in the mouth.

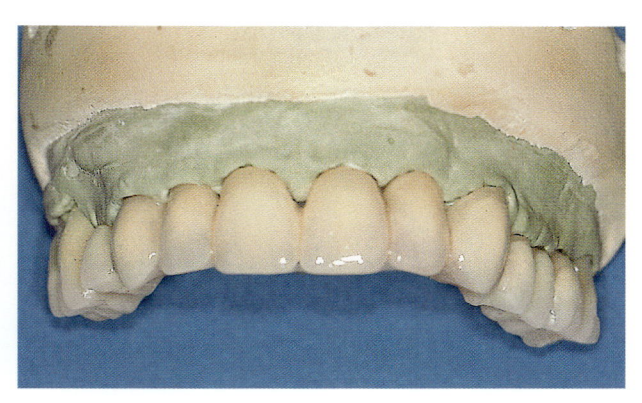

**Fig 10-59**   On completion of the recording of the intermaxillary relations, denture teeth (or wax, if preferred) are adapted to the acrylic resin framework to the established parameters forming a diagnostic preview.

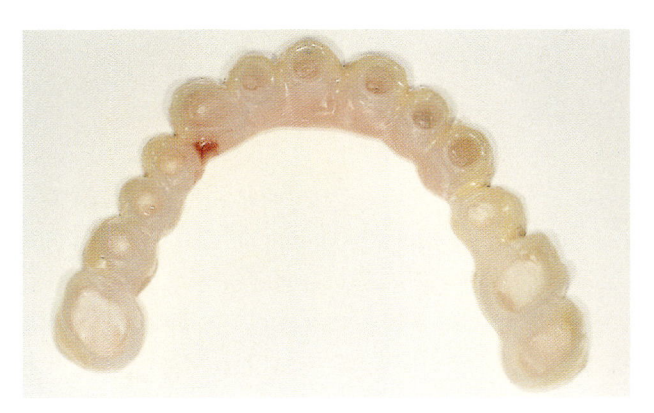

**Fig 10-60**   A view of the fit surface of the diagnostic preview showing the position of the teeth in relation to the abutments.

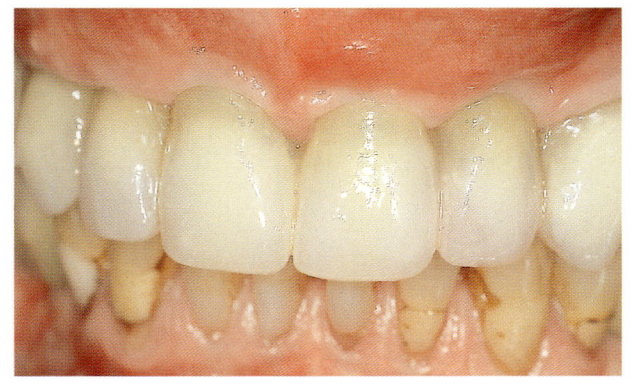

**Fig 10-61**   Labial view of the diagnostic preview being tried in the mouth to confirm the aesthetic and functional parameters. Any modifications are made at this stage prior to the commencement of the construction of the metalwork. The information gathered is recorded using a matrix for guidance during subsequent stages.

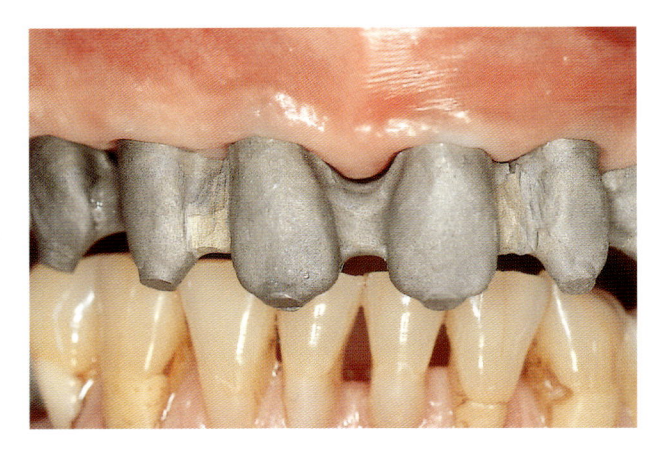

## II  Implant Placement: Surgery and Prosthodontics

**Fig 10-62** The metalwork is waxed and cast in sections, the fit of each section is checked on the master cast prior to soldering or laser welding. The sections are joined and the fit of the laser welded or soldered casting is checked in the laboratory. The three molars are constructed as individual units. The canine is incorporated within the connected units supported by the implants. A gold coping is constructed to prevent caries, and this is eventually cemented permanently with glass-ionomer cement. The metalwork is then transferred to the mouth for confirmation of the fit.

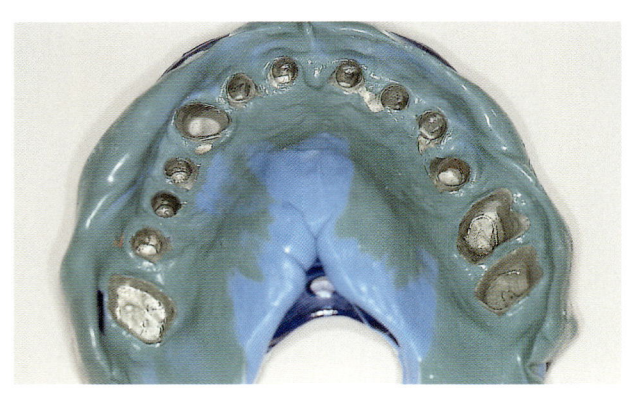

**Fig 10-63** The metalwork is then picked up using an addition-cured silicone impression material (Provil-light and heavy bodied material) in a rigid plastic stock tray relating the position of the metalwork to the soft tissue contours developed so far.

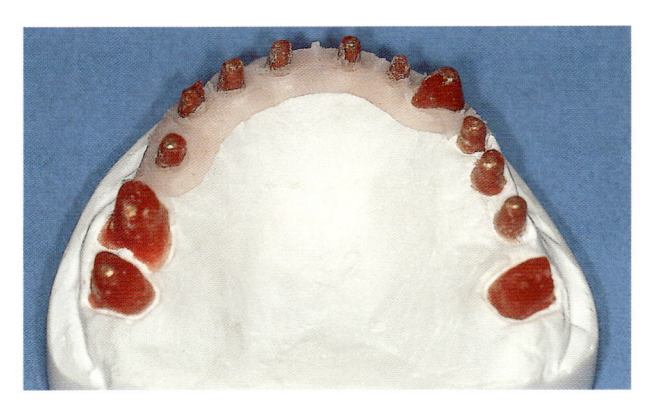

**Fig 10-64** The impression is cast using acrylic resin (GC Pattern Resin; Alsip, IL, USA) in the metal copings. This will serve as a control model to check for distortion during subsequent stages of porcelain application.

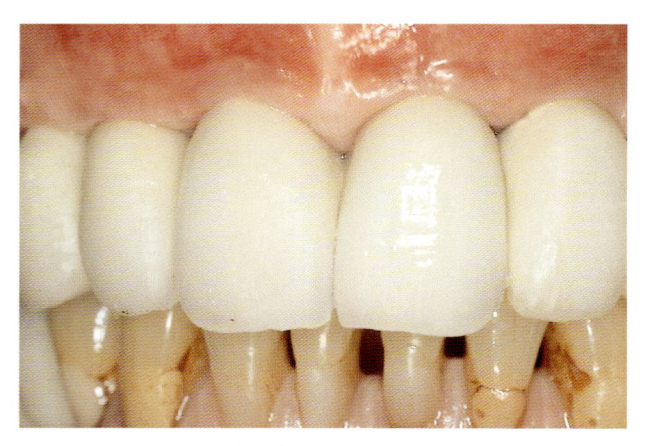

**Fig 10-65** The porcelain is applied and the teeth built into the matrix made from the diagnostic preview. The teeth are then tried in to confirm aesthetics with view to tooth form, midline, embrasures for interdental hygiene and shade.

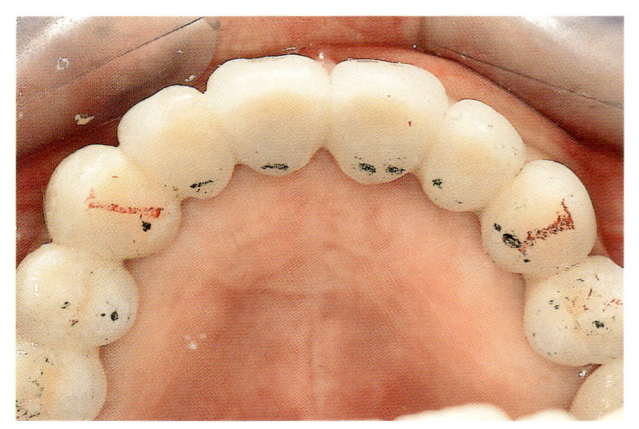

**Fig 10-66** The occlusal contacts and the lateral and protrusive excursions are checked before the porcelain is glazed. Canine guidance was the preferred occlusal scheme for this patient.

## 10　Restorative Phase: Prosthetic Protocols

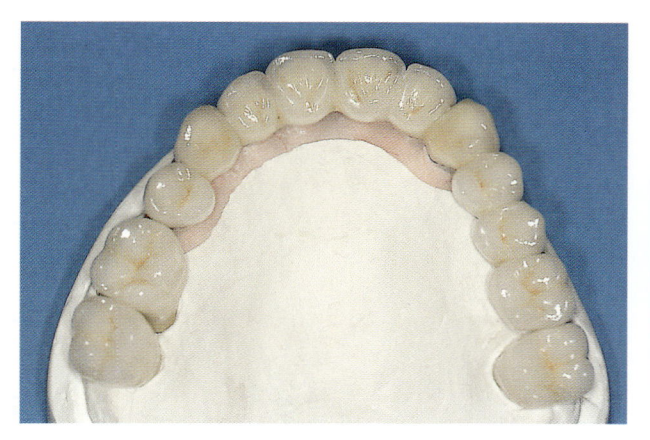

**Fig 10-67**　Occlusal view of the glazed restoration on the laboratory cast. Cement-retained restorations enable the occlusal form to be developed to ideal contours without the interference from access holes if occlusally approaching screws are used for retention.

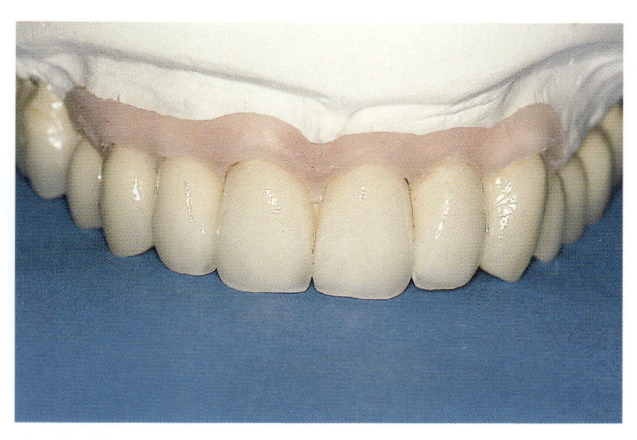

**Fig 10-68**　Labial view of the glazed restoration on the cast. The soft tissues have been reproduced using a proprietary silicone material.

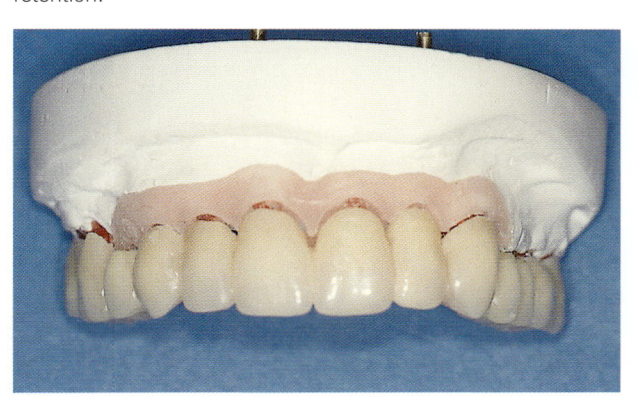

**Fig 10-69**　A comparison of the final outcome may be made with the diagnostic preview, which has been transferred to the same cast.

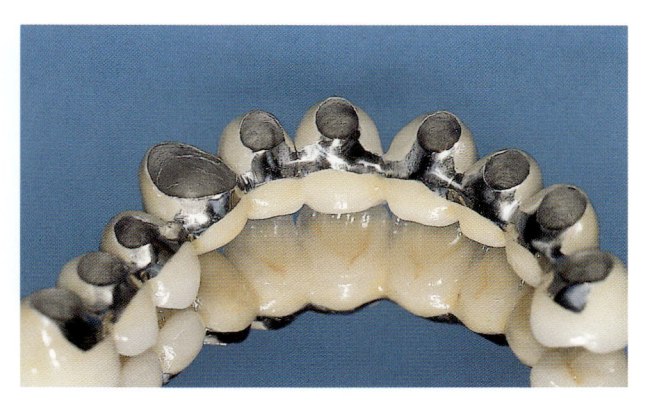

**Fig 10-70**　View of the fit surface of the metal-ceramic restoration showing the precision of the implant and abutment positioning in relation to the metal and porcelain of the restoration.

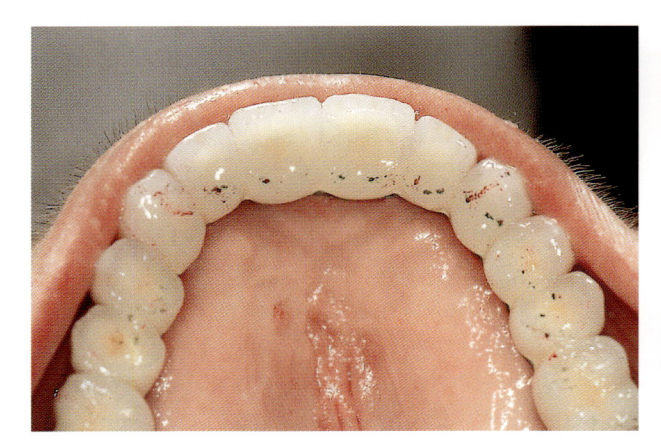

**Fig 10-71**　Occlusal view of the fitted restoration after a functional check. The connected units of the restoration were cemented with temporary cement (Temp Bond) over the permanently cemented gold coping. The individual crowns for the molars were cemented with permanent cement.

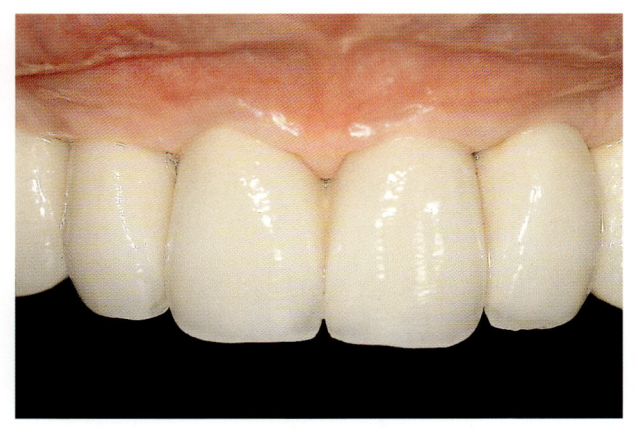

**Fig 10-72**　Labial view of the definitive restoration showing the tooth form and emergence profile contributing to the excellent aesthetics achieved by following a methodical protocol.

191

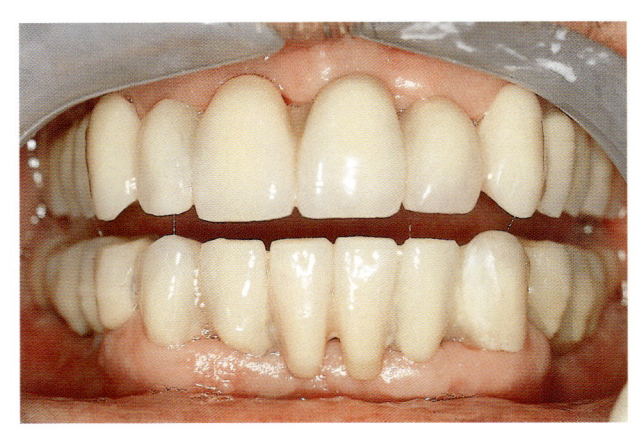

## II   Implant Placement: Surgery and Prosthodontics

**Fig 10-73**   Labial view of the diagnostic preview being tried in, supported by teeth and implants that were previously exposed and prepared for conventional impressions. The intermaxillary relationship was verified using wax blocks on acrylic resin frameworks. A facebow was used to transfer information to a semi-adjustable articulator.

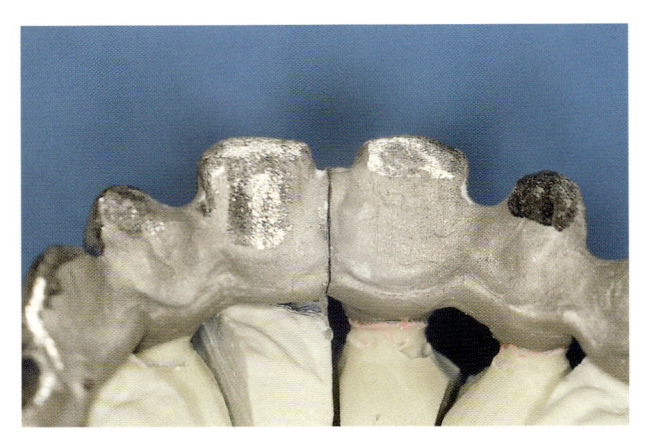

**Fig 10-74**   Metalwork waxed and cast in sections on the laboratory cast.

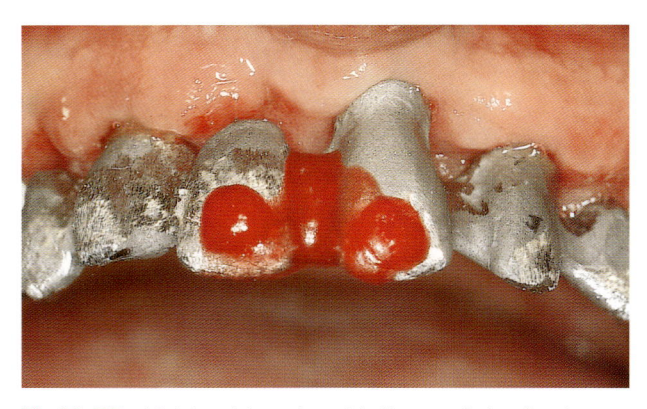

**Fig 10-75**   Metalwork transferred to the mouth for direct intraoral location of the sections. Pattern resin (GC Pattern Resin) is used to locate the segments. Stability of the metalwork on the abutments is essential and may be assured by the use of softened temporary cement.

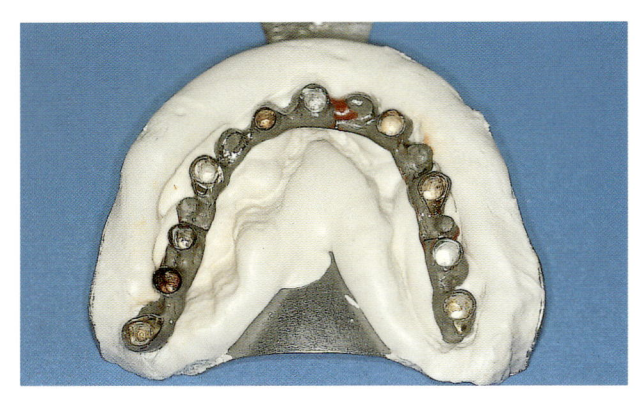

**Fig 10-76**   The metalwork is then stabilised and picked up using plaster (SnoWhite; Kerr) in a non-perforated metal stock tray.

### Case 3: Conventional Impressions for Full Mouth Rehabilitation with Multiple Splinted and Single Units, Lateral Fixation Screw in Combination with Cementation

A 60-year-old man with failing dentition as result of caries and periodontal disease presented for treatment requesting a smooth transition from the failing restorations to implant-supported fixed restorations. Provisional metal acrylic resin restorations were constructed to assess the aesthetic requirements, establish the correct intermaxillary relations and to verify the occlusal scheme. The provisional restorations were supported on teeth following the removal of all pathological lesions. Subsequently, the maxillary teeth were to be extracted and the remaining mandibular teeth to be retained following a final assessment. Augmentation of the maxillary sinuses was carried out, followed by implant placement in both jaws.

The implants were exposed six months after placement and the abutments attached at the same time. The implants were loaded via acrylic resin tran-

10 Restorative Phase: Prosthetic Protocols

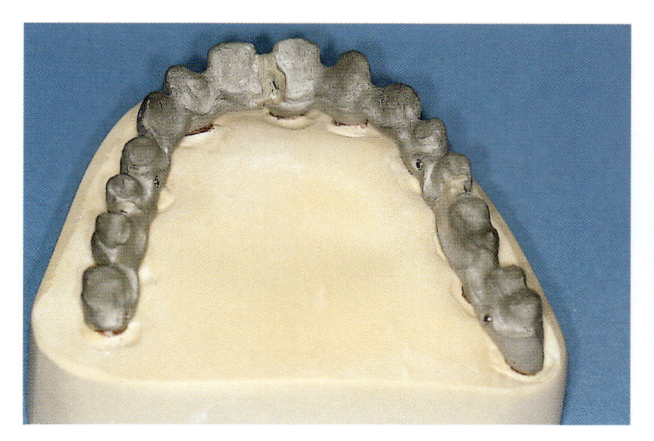

**Fig 10-77** The control model is made using pattern resin and dowel pins in the metal copings and will be used to ensure that no discrepancy has taken place during soldering. The soldered casting can be seen on the control model.

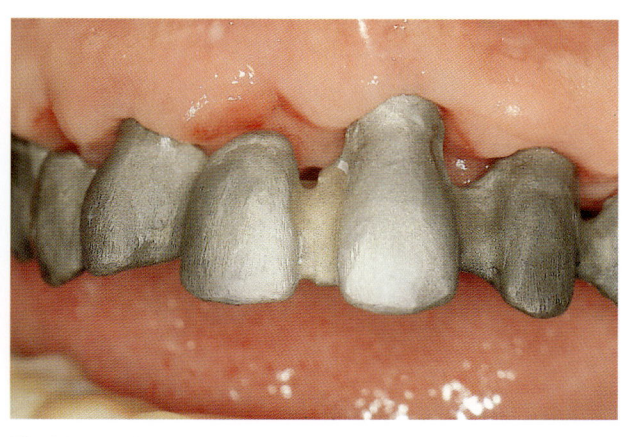

**Fig 10-78** Labial view of the soldered metalwork being tried in the mouth. The solder joint between the two central incisors is visible. The relationship between the metalwork and the soft tissues can be observed and will need to be recorded.

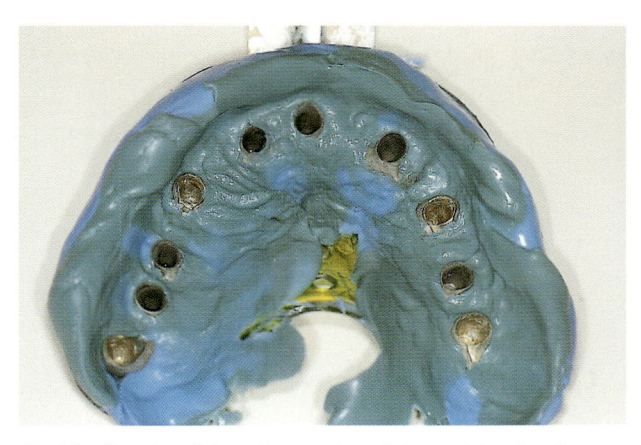

**Fig 10-79** The pick-up impression of the metalwork using a heavy and a light body silicone impression material (Provil) in a rigid acrylic resin stock tray is used to record the relationship of the metalwork to the soft tissues for transfer to the laboratory.

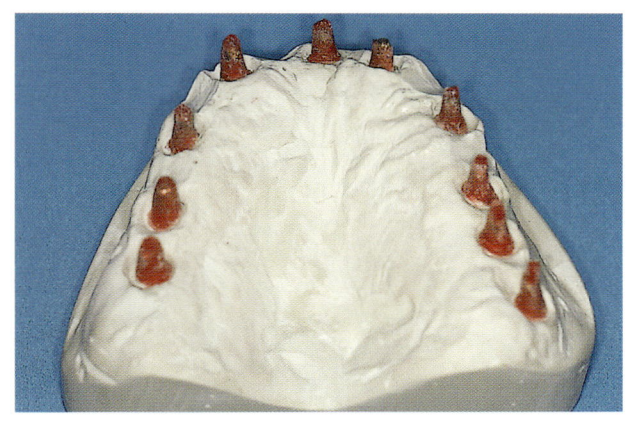

**Fig 10-80** The impression is cast using acrylic resin and dowel pins in the metal copings and plaster to reproduce the remaining soft tissues. Once again, this control model is used to ensure that distortion during the addition of porcelain to the metal can be monitored.

sitional restorations constructed from the information transferred from the provisional metal-acrylic bridges. Impressions were taken two months after implant exposure and the intermaxillary relationship confirmed. The final restoration was constructed using the protocols outlined. Gold copings were used to receive the lateral fixation screws for cementation permanently onto the abutments. The restorations were fitted and reviewed annually (Figs 10-73–10-88). After 14 years, the tissues are still stable with minor remodelling (Figs 10-89–10-91).

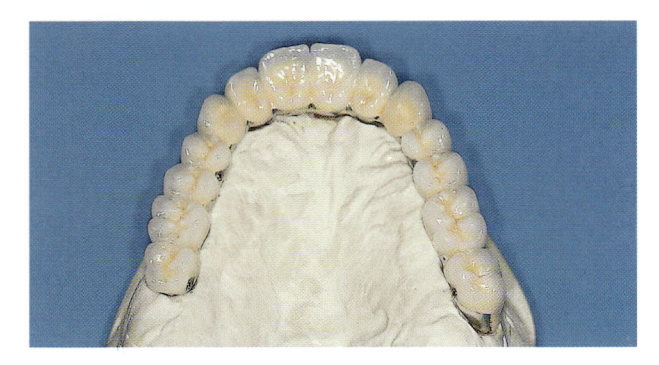

**Fig 10-81** Occlusal view of the laboratory cast with the completed full arch restoration.

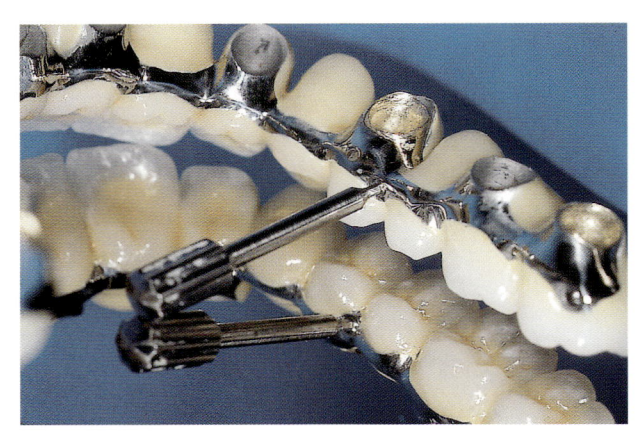

## II  Implant Placement: Surgery and Prosthodontics

**Fig 10-82**  View of the right quadrant of the restoration showing the lateral fixation screw being inserted through the palatal aspect of the bridge. The lateral fixation screw assembly consists of the screw and the housing; the housing is cast into the metalwork and the screw inserted through the housing to engage a recess in the gold coping. The gold coping constructed to fit on one of the abutments is also visible. Note that the gold coping has been constructed with a distal extension to receive the lateral fixation screw. This enables the thickness of the metalwork to be kept to a minimum (see also Fig 10-4).

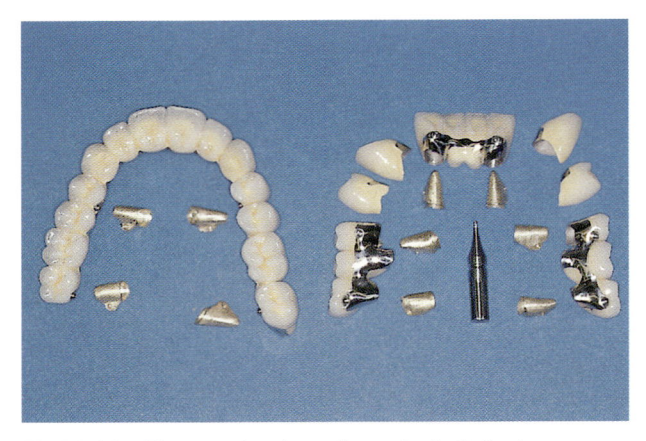

**Fig 10-83**  The completed prostheses for both the jaws are visible. In the maxilla, a full arch, single-piece construction will be supported by lateral fixation screws engaging four gold copings, which will be cemented permanently onto the abutments. The gold copings are positioned on the most distal abutments and close to the canine region. The restoration for the mandible has been planned in sections. The two implants in the anterior region support four units and will be retained by two lateral fixation screws. The four remaining teeth will be restored by four separate crowns. Both the posterior quadrants will be restored with three units supported by three implants. Two lateral fixation screws engaging copings on the mesial and distal abutments will retain each bridge.

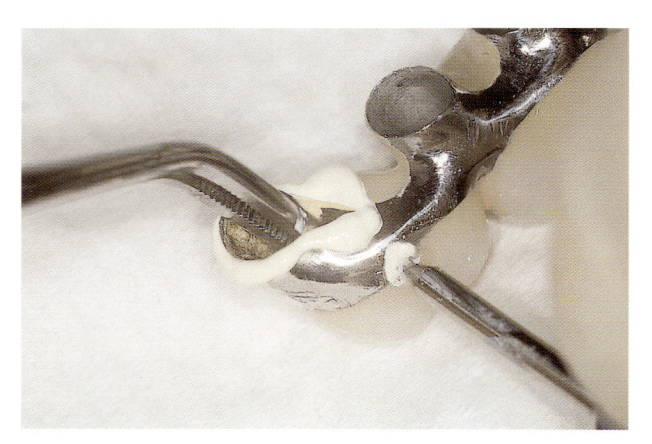

**Fig 10-84**  The gold copings and the bridgework may be assembled outside the mouth using temporary cement (Temp Bond). The lateral fixation screw, coated in Vaseline (petroleum jelly) to facilitate disengagement if required, is inserted so that it positively engages the recess that has been constructed in the gold coping to receive it. The mesial extension of the gold coping into which the recess is prepared is clearly visible and reduces bulk. The bridge will be cemented in the mouth using glass-ionomer cement to permanently cement the gold copings onto the abutments. Temporary cement will be used to secure all the rest of the bridge to the remaining abutments. This will provide retrievability.

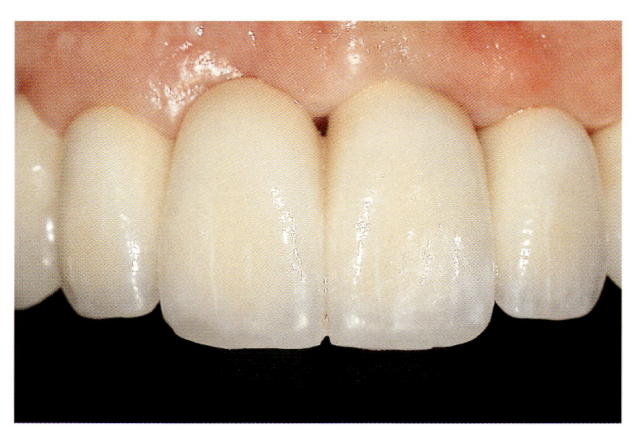

**Fig 10-85**  Labial view of the cemented bridge showing the relationship of the soft tissues to the bridge. The interdental spaces have been designed to provide access for interstitial hygiene.

10   Restorative Phase: Prosthetic Protocols

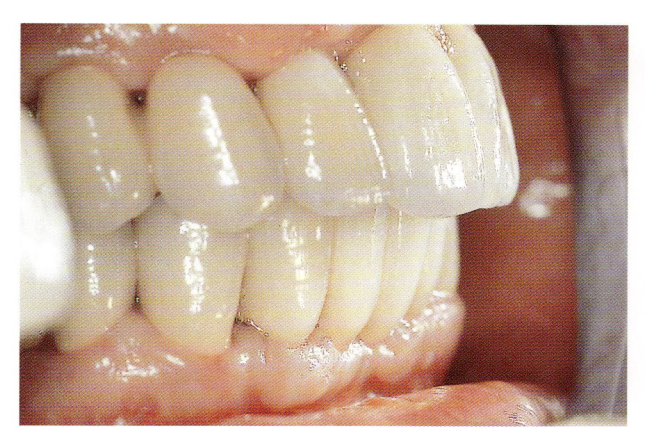

**Fig 10-86**   Right lateral view (mirror view) of the completed restoration in centric relation and maximum intercuspal position.

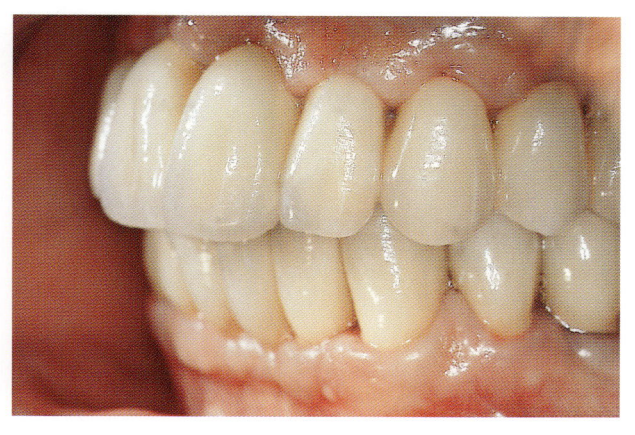

**Fig 10-87**   Left lateral view (mirror view) of the completed restoration in occlusion.

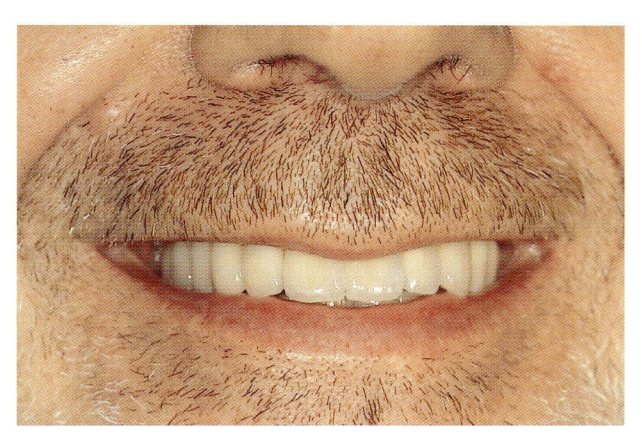

**Fig 10-88**   Anterior view of the patient smiling showing the smile line and the support obtained for these soft tissues from the restoration. An aesthetic and functional outcome has been achieved using a protocol allowing information to be transferred from one stage to the next, and checks at each stage ensure the satisfactory completion of that stage prior to proceeding to the next.

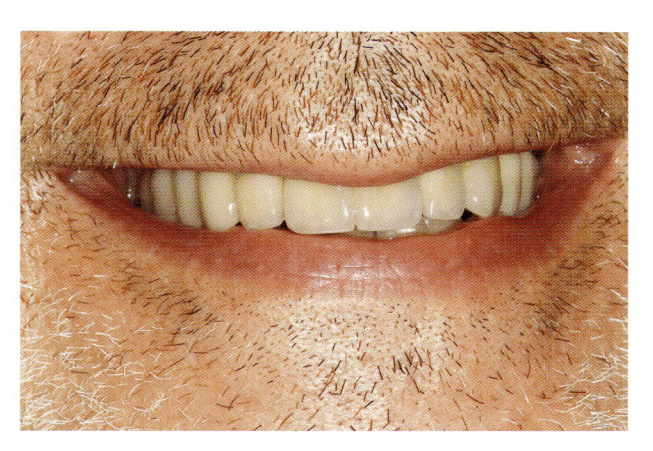

**Fig 10-89**   Patient smiling demonstrating good aesthetic appearance 14 years later.

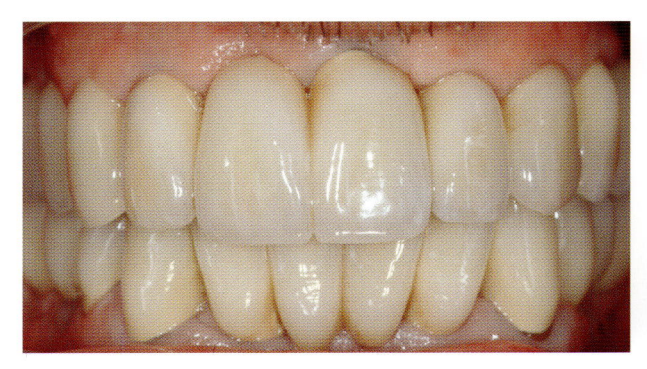

**Fig 10-90**   Labial view showing stable occlusion with no signs of adverse wear or fracture after 14 years.

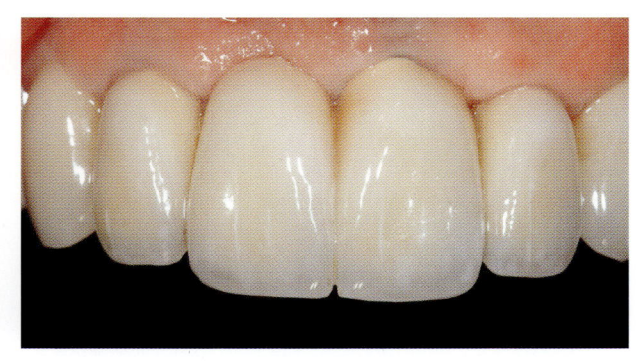

**Fig 10-91**   Close-up of the maxillary anterior teeth showing excellent soft tissue condition, with minor recession around the left central incisor after 14 years.

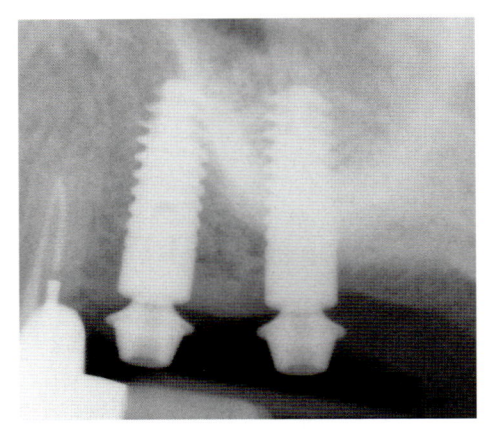

**Fig 10-92** Radiograph of the exposed implants with transmucosal abutments attached for screw-retained prostheses (balance base abutments).

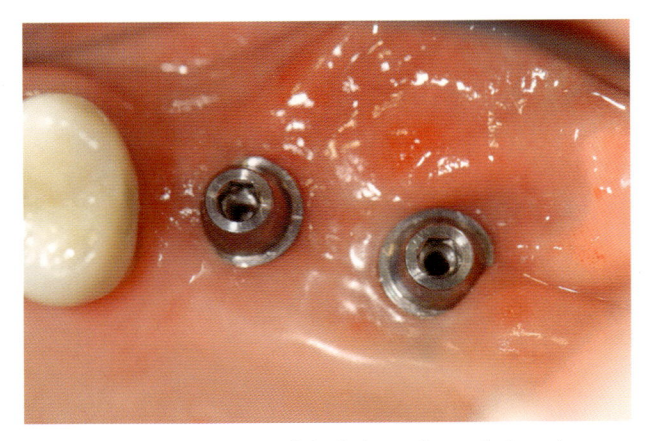

**Fig 10-93** Intraoral view of the balance base abutments.

## Case 4: Abutment Transfer for a Single Cemented Restoration

An 18-year-old man requiring the replacement of a primary premolar in the mandible had an implant placed with a sulcus former attached at the time of implant placement for transmucosal healing. A 15-degree standard abutment (Ankylos) was attached six months after implant placement. The abutment position was transferred to the laboratory for the fabrication of an abutment analogue model. The metalwork was constructed directly onto the abutment analogue. The metalwork was transferred to the mouth in order to relate the soft tissue contours created by a transitional restoration back to the laboratory so that a properly contoured crown could be constructed. This deviates from the standard protocol where definitive restoration is normally constructed directly on the abutment analogue. As mentioned above, neither the abutment nor the analogue can be modified (see Figs 10-20–10-31; p. 178, 180–181).

## Case 5: Transfer of Implant Position for a Single Cemented Restoration

A 22-year-old patient with a high smile-line and high expectations required the replacement of a maxillary central incisor and was treated using the staged approach. The implant was placed and permitted to integrate prior to exposure. Impressions were taken at first-stage surgery to prepare the abutment and a transitional restoration for the development of the soft tissue contours. The restorative phase was designed for the use of a ceramic abutment. Information of the implant position and soft tissue contours was transferred to the laboratory for the adaptation of the ceramic abutment and the fabrication of the all-ceramic crown. The aim was twofold: to prevent greying of the soft tissues and to approximate the cement and gingival margins (see Figs 10-41–10-81).

## Case 6: Transfer of Abutment Position for a Splinted Screw-retained CAD/CAM Designed Restoration

The development of modern CAD/CAM (computer-aided design and computer-aided manufacturing) technology will possibly in the future replace traditional methods of transferring information to the laboratory as well as the processes of fabricating restorations. This patient required impressions using the open tray technique to transfer data to the laboratory. Thereafter, milling, using CAD/CAM technology, was used to fabricate the framework. The accuracies required for screw-retained prostheses (10 μm) are difficult to achieve using conventional casting techniques, particularly for larger restorations. CAD/CAM technology has the potential for achieving high accuracy.

The CAD/CAM technology was used to fabricate a two-unit splinted screw-retained restoration (Figs 10-92–10-109).

## 10 Restorative Phase: Prosthetic Protocols

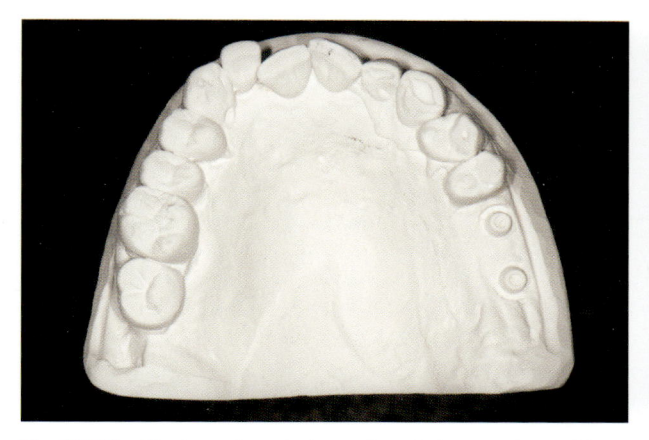

**Fig 10-94** Study cast made from alginate impressions of the abutments in situ.

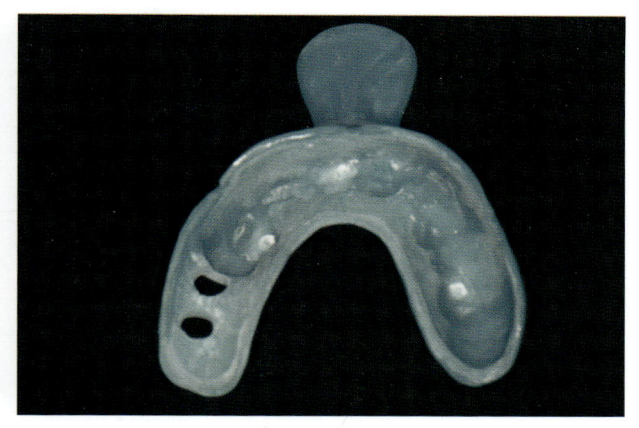

**Fig 10-95** Special tray constructed for an open tray technique to permit transfer of abutment positions to the laboratory.

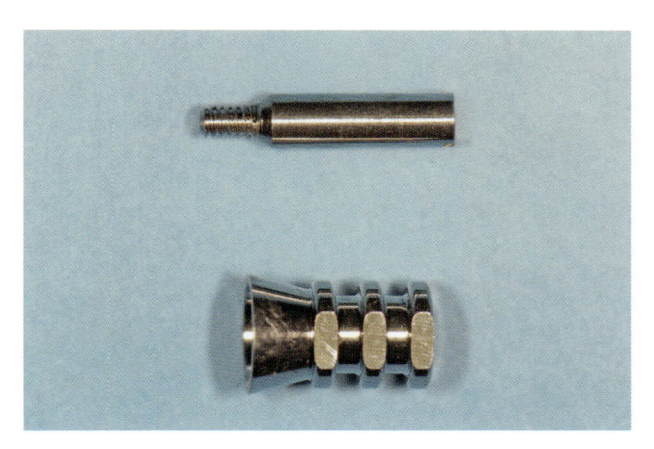

**Fig 10-96** Open tray impression coping.

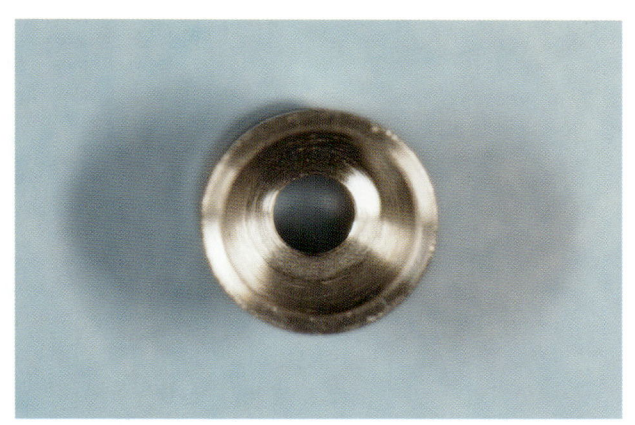

**Fig 10-97** Fit surface of impression coping, which will attach to the balance base abutment.

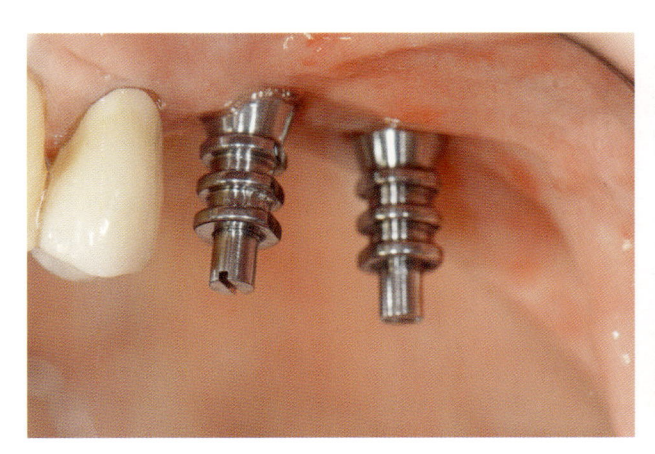

**Fig 10-98** Open tray impression copings attached to the abutments.

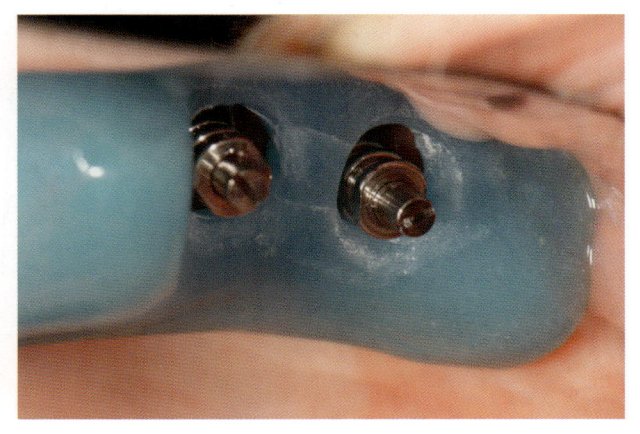

**Fig 10-99** Impression tray being tried in.

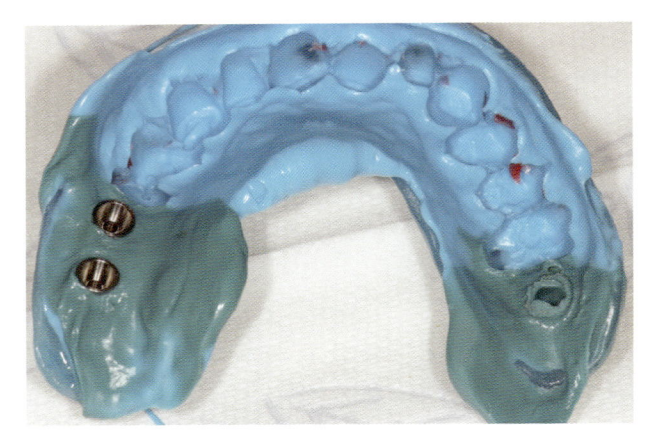

II   Implant Placement: Surgery and Prosthodontics

Fig 10-100   Impression with the copings.

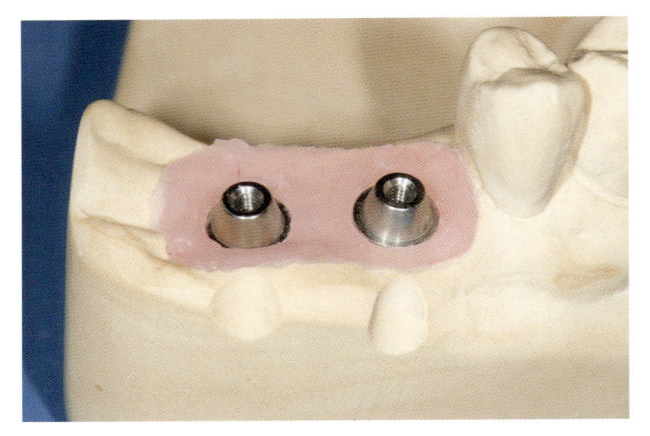

Fig 10-101   Working cast with abutment analogues and soft tissue model.

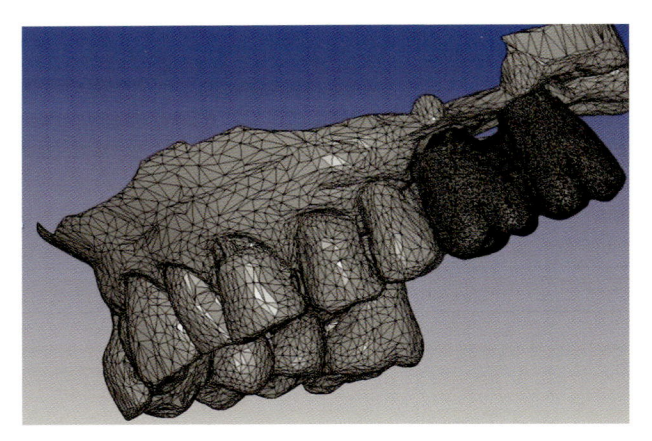

Fig 10-102   Scan of the waxup made on the study cast.

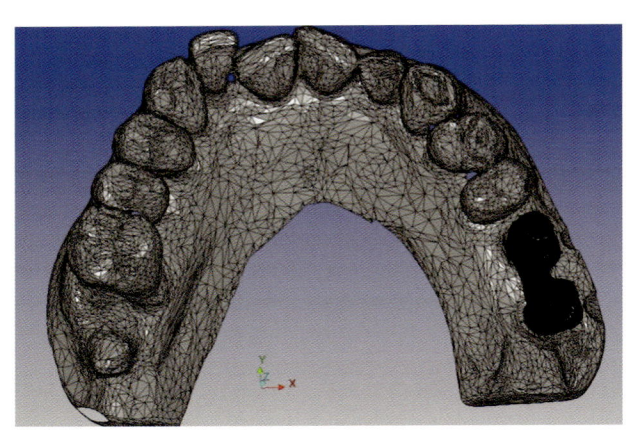

Fig 10-103   Occlusal view of the scan of the waxup, which has been cutback to allow for veneering with porcelain.

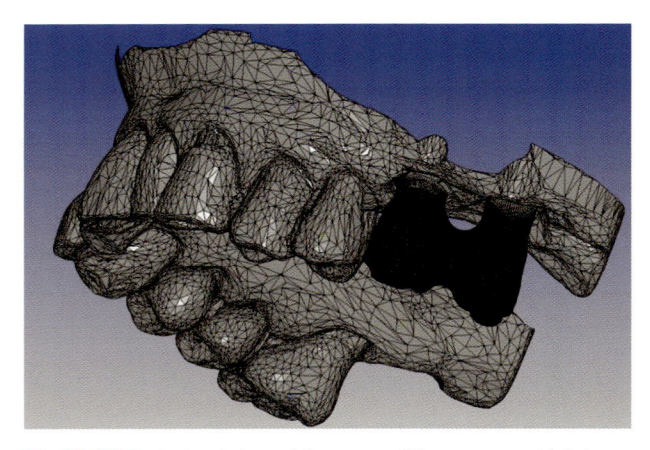

Fig 10-104   Lateral view of the scan of the waxup, which has been cutback to allow for veneering with porcelain.

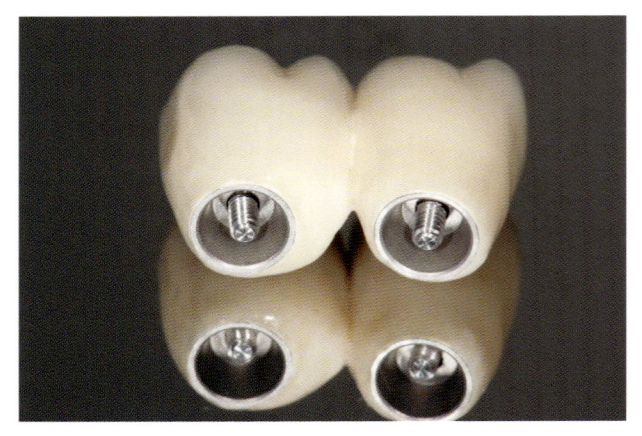

Fig 10-105   Metalwork milled using CAD/CAM technology with porcelain fused to the metal.

10 Restorative Phase: Prosthetic Protocols

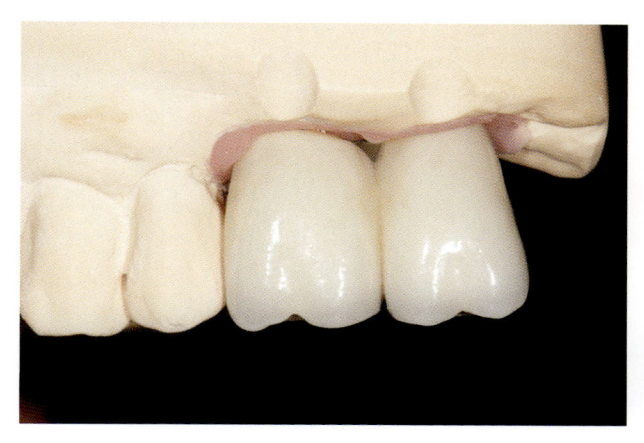

**Fig 10-106** The restoration on the working casts.

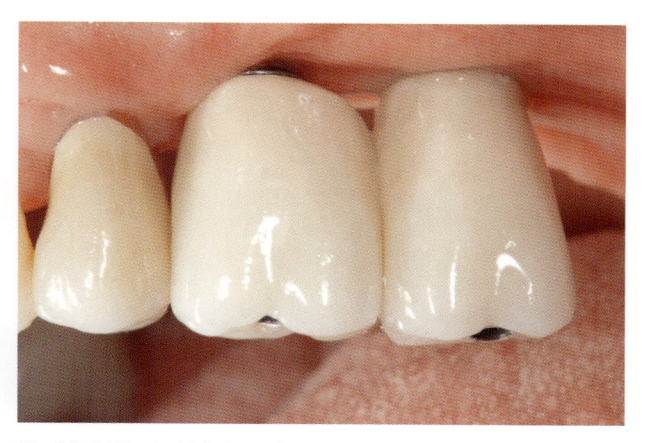

**Fig 10-107** Labial view of restoration in the mouth.

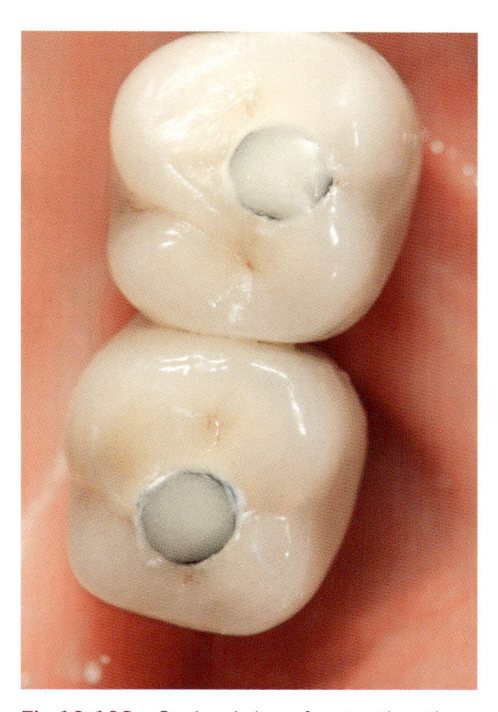

**Fig 10-108** Occlusal view of restoration, the access holes for the screws have been closed using a glass-ionomer cement.

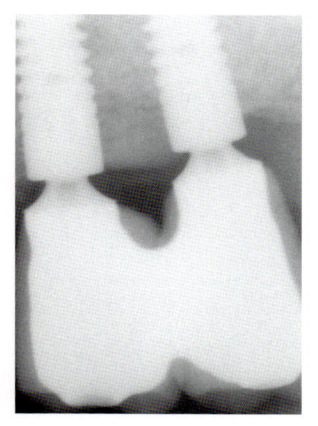

**Fig 10-109** Radiograph of screw-retained restoration generated by CAD/CAM technology. Note the accurate fit of the restoration.

# SECTION III

# Augmentation

*'Medicine is not only a science; it is also an art. It does not consist of compounding pills and plasters; it deals with the very processes of life, which must be understood before they may be guided'*

(Paracelsus, 1493–1541)

# Chapter 11

# Overview

## Introduction

A number of factors must be taken into account when treatment involving the use of implant-supported restorations is considered. Not only must the high success rate that is integral to implant dentistry be met but also the treatment should be carried out in a predictable manner. As far as patients are concerned, it is essential that their aesthetic and functional needs are met.

Therefore, the relationship of the residual ridge to the future tooth position must not be overlooked as the clinician assesses volume and quality of bone. The supporting bone will need to resist functional and parafunctional loads, and these must be assessed and related to the region being treated.

Several grafting techniques that attempt to correct bone deficiencies have been described. These include the use of resorbable and non-resorbable membranes in conjunction with the technique of guided bone regeneration (GBR).[163–172] Particulate material from a variety of sources has been used as a space maintainer with varying results. However, the best particulate material is reported to be autogenous bone.[173]

Membranes have also been used in conjunction with autogenous block bone grafts with good results.[174]

The use of titanium mesh has been reported in the literature but largely as a means of containing autogenous bone or a mixture containing other materials together with autogenous bone.[175–180] These have been used simultaneously at the time of implant placement or in a staged approach. A single-stage approach is reported to lead to poorer bone-to-implant contact than a staged approach.[181,182]

Although a variety of techniques are available, the use of an autogenous block of bone that has been shaped to correct the deficiency is considered to provide the best method of reconstructing a deficient ridge.[183–186] Here again, a two-stage approach is reported to result in a better clinical outcome than a single-stage approach.[187,188]

More recently, manipulation techniques such as bone expansion and distraction osteogenesis have been described and reported to have high success rates, but not without the incidence of complications.[189–195]

Combining manipulation and grafting may become necessary, for example where a skeletal correction needs to be made as a part of preprosthetic surgery, when a graft can be used in combination with a maxillary (Le Fort I) osteotomy.

# III  Augmentation

## Causes of Deficiencies

Extensive loss of bone, either labial or palatal, can have a number of causes. Deficiencies are traditionally classified based on aetiology:
- congenital deficiencies
- neoplasm
- trauma
- infection
- disuse atrophy
- atrophy accelerated by parafunctional load.

These are discussed below and their relevance to clinical implant dentistry addressed.

### Congenital Deficiencies

Congenital deficiencies that result in discontinuity of hard and soft tissues, such as a cleft palate, are best treated by clinicians who have experience of such repairs. Subsequent treatment with implants can provide these patients with excellent function.

Congenitally missing teeth can result in inadequately developed alveolar processes and, as a result, may require bone-grafting procedures. These respond well to treatment when implants are used to provide functional stimulus to the reconstructed ridges.

### Neoplasm

Implant dentistry has contributed significantly to the rehabilitation of patients who have undergone ablative surgery.[13] The use of implants in conjunction with bone grafts, in particular free vascularised grafts, significantly improves the quality of life for these patients and the overall outcome of the treatment at the same time. Complex treatment, often involving radiation, hyperbaric oxygen therapy and other treatments with a much higher risk of complications, should be carried out only at appropriately equipped hospitals (Fig 11-1).

### Trauma

Deficiencies resulting from trauma can vary in size and complexity. Trauma can result merely in tooth loss or the loss of alveolar bone, resulting in hard and soft tissue deficiencies. The corrective treatment will depend upon the type and size of defect.

### Infection

Infection is the most common cause of tooth loss and may present itself as caries, leading to periapical infection, or periodontal disease. Vertically fractured roots following endodontic treatment and/or post-crowns may result in substantial loss of bone. Failure of implants as a result of peri-implantitis or failure of grafts causes extensive loss of bone. This bone loss necessitates repair as, depending on the type of deficiency, spontaneous repair may not occur.

### Periapical Bone Loss

Periapical bone loss may result from untreated endodontic infections or failed endodontic treatment. The extent of bone loss will influence the degree of repair that will spontaneously take place. Accurate diagnosis prior to endodontic treatment or re-treatment should aim to prevent further bone loss.

### Periodontal Bone Loss

Periodontal disease is characterised by bone loss and may present itself as an infrabone deficiency around a specific tooth, which may repair itself on elimination of the cause or extraction of the tooth. Extensive periodontal disease may result in loss of height of the alveolar process (horizontal bone loss) around the infected teeth.

Regaining the ridge form following the loss of teeth requires autogenous onlay grafts or other supplementary procedures, which make the treatment more exacting as the alveolar ridge height is more difficult to reconstruct.

Persistent treatment – contrary to current data on the success of that treatment modality – should not be carried out if it leads to greater tissue loss. Evidence-based guidelines should be established in order to enable clinicians to make decisions that prioritise the preservation of those tissues that are most difficult to replace.

The decision-making process must take into account the consequence of any treatment that may result in further bone loss. Typically, re-treatment of endodontically treated teeth with periapical lesions and post-crowns should be reconsidered. Consideration should also be given to the persistent treatment of periodontally involved teeth with progressive bone loss.

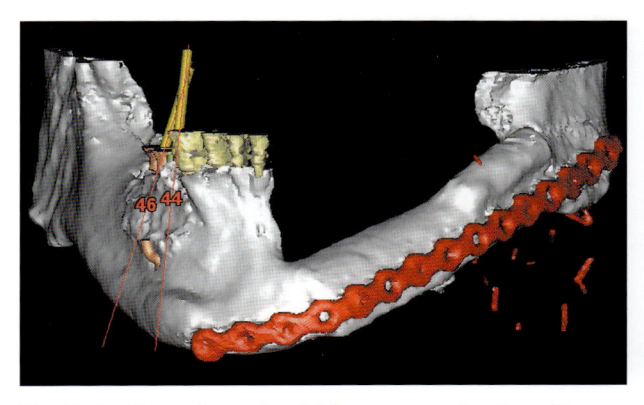

**Fig 11-1** Three-dimensional CT scan reconstruction of free vascularised fibula graft following ablative surgery for the removal of a carcinoma.

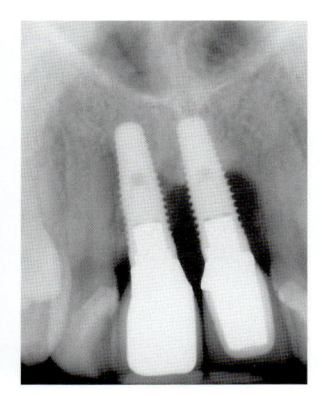

**Fig 11-2** Periapical radiograph of failing implants with progressive bone loss.

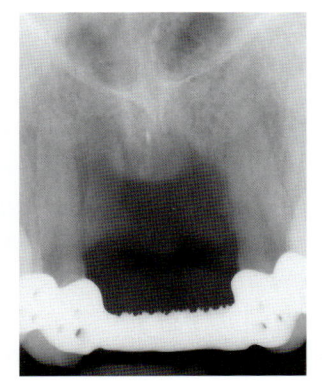

**Fig 11-3** Buccal and palatal bone loss is evident. A large block graft will be required to repair the deficiency.

### Peri-implant Bone Loss/Failure of Grafts

Substantial progressive bone loss has been recorded associated with implant designs employing porous surfaces such as beads, hydroxyapatite and titanium plasma flame-sprayed coatings. Other causes may relate to known periodontal risks such as environmental (e.g. smoking), host (genetic disposition) or bacterial factors. The use of biomaterials in conjunction with implants placed into existing bony defects may also increase the risk of infection. Inappropriately placed biomaterials into extraction sockets (e.g. infected sockets or dense packing of material) may also result in infection, causing bone loss extending into the base of the defect (Figs 11-2–11-4).

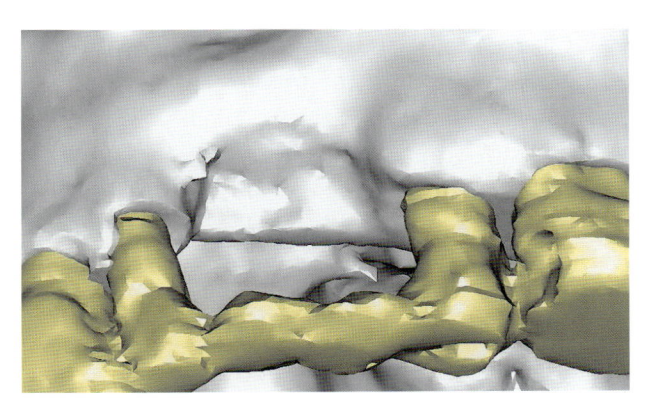

**Fig 11-4** A 3D CT scan reconstruction of a maxillary deficiency caused by failure of implants.

## Indications for Augmentation

### Aesthetics

The indication for either manipulation or augmentation may entirely be aesthetics. In such cases, relating the position of the tooth to the ridge form is fundamental to the assessment process. This is often the case in the anterior maxillary region, which is very visible. Grafting may be necessary even though there may be sufficient bone to meet biomechanical demands. There are, of course, many situations where there are multiple indications.

### Biomechanics

Biomechanics is often a matter of counter-balancing load with support and there are many complex factors that influence both of these. There is now information that will provide guidance in clinical decision making, the details of which are beyond the scope of this text. Each clinician must make these judgements based on experience and evidence.

### Load

A distinction must be made between functional and parafunctional load. Functional load is determined by activity such as mastication and is dependent upon the diet; although this type of load can be of considerable magnitude, it is generally less than the forces generated during parafunctional activities. Parafunctional activity is also influenced by factors such as personality type, stress and life events, and this should be taken into account.

# III Augmentation

Load is also influenced by the region of the mouth that is to be restored. Forces that are up to eight times greater in magnitudes may be generated in the molar region than in the anterior region.

Various studies have shown that the load is influenced by the shape of the jaws and the size of the muscles. These should, therefore, be considered within the decision-making framework.

## Support

The volume and nature of the bone that will receive the implant will have to resist the forces exerted. Bone is a living tissue that constantly remodels throughout life and, therefore, influences the long-term stability of the osseointegrated implant. The remodelling process itself depends on local and systemic factors.

Mechanical load is one of the local factors influencing the remodelling process. The amount of load that is distributed to the bone is influenced by the surface area of the implant in contact with the bone, which, in turn, is influenced by the bone density. The nature of the load, be it compressive, tensile or shear, will have an impact on bone response. It is recognised that several thresholds exist that govern the response of bone to load. The first threshold defines the point when stimulation of the bone sustains density; the second increases density and the third results in micro-fractures, which may lead to loss of bone integrity.

The remodelling of bone is also governed by metabolic factors. A number of hormones, such as adrenocorticosteroids, calcitonin, parathormone, growth hormone and insulin, influence bone metabolism. Several diseases and malfunctions of certain organs, such as renal and hepatic disorders, also affect bone metabolism, as do dietary factors. Drugs such as bisphosphonates influence bone metabolism, with potentially serious risks. Assessment of the general medical condition of the patient is, therefore, fundamental.

Finally, the gross morphology and mechanical and chemical nature of the implant surface will have an effect on the quality of the bone–implant interface that can be generated.

## Categories of Augmentation

Once the presence of a deficiency has been identified, a decision will need to be made regarding the need to alter the shape of the ridge. The nature of the procedure that is carried out must depend upon the goal that needs to be achieved. This may, in principle, be considered in two separate categories: manipulation of hard and soft tissues and grafting of hard and soft tissues. In addition, synthetic/alloplastic materials are used for augmentation.

### Manipulation of Hard and Soft Tissues

Manipulation procedures alter the position or dimension of the tissues that are already present at a particular site. Examples include:
- bone expansion or bone condensing
- manipulation of the sinus floor or of the nasal floor
- distraction osteogenesis
- repositioning of nerves
- pedicle flap
- maxillary or mandibular osteotomies to correct spatial relationship of the jaws.

### General Principles of Manipulation Techniques

The key principle with tissue manipulation is to maintain sufficient blood supply to the tissues being manipulated, so that vitality and function are sustained. This differs from other augmentation procedures, where a blood supply needs to be re-established.

This general principle applies to all the manipulation procedures listed above.

For bone expansion, it is fundamental to maintain a blood supply to the labial cortical plate and to avoid displacement fractures, which would make the bone more susceptible to resorption and possibly sequestration. It is for this reason that the periosteum is not elevated from the labial plate.

The technique for distraction osteogenesis depends upon soft tissue incisions designed to maintain the blood supply to the segment being transported. This is commonly the palatal or lingual soft tissues. Violation of this basic principle can result in the loss of the entire segment.

The repositioning of nerves aims to minimally interrupt neural function. Key to this is to maintain the continued blood supply across the epineurium and perineurium during the surgical procedure and in the final relocated position of the neurovascular bundle. This will cause the least disruption to the electrolytic balance around each axon and, therefore, reduce any interruption to nerve impulse transmission. It is for this reason that stretching and compression of the neurovascular bundle has to be avoided.

A pedicle flap depends upon its survival almost totally on an uninterrupted blood supply. The design of such a flap must consider the source of the blood supply as well as the length and base of the pedicle.

The most fundamental principle of mandibular and maxillary osteotomies is to maintain the blood supply even in this very richly vascularised region. Incisions and flap reflections are kept to the minimum that is sufficient to gain adequate access.

## Grafting of Hard and Soft Tissues

Autogenous grafting is a transpositioning of either hard or soft tissues from a donor site remote from the recipient site. It has to re-establish a blood supply at the recipient site. The aim is the addition of tissue to alter the shape of the recipient site. A range of augmentation techniques using non-autogenous material from a variety of sources has also been described.

Examples of grafting techniques are:
- bone graft
- GBR or guided tissue regeneration (GTR)
- sinus lift
- free gingival graft
- connective tissue graft.

Augmentation procedures, such as bone grafts, may further be classified into categories that describe the defect that they correct, such as
- correction of height
- correction of width
- correction of height and width
- correction of spatial relationship.

They may also be categorised according to the manner in which they are positioned at the recipient site, such as:

- onlay graft: placed on the surface of the recipient site to correct height and or width
- inlay graft: placed in a space within the bone such as the sinus cavity
- interpositional graft: placed between two pieces of bone that have been separated, such as bone splitting, or in conjunction with a maxillary or mandibular osteotomy, which may be indicated by a need to correct the spatial relationships between the jaws.

Further classification based on source, form and composition of the augmentation material is also informative.

Any biomaterial used for grafting or GBR/GTR must comply with certain properties, which will vary depending upon its application.

For bone regeneration, the main properties can be summarised as:
- biocompatible
- non-infective
- resorbable.

Following resorption and replacement with vital bone, the material should be functionally responsive and, therefore, stable.

The ideal qualities for a bone grafting material are:
- osteogenic: contains cells that can generate bone
- osteoinductive: contains factors that stimulate undifferentiated precursor cells to differentiate into osteogenic cells
- osteoconductive: provides a scaffold onto and into which bone can grow.

Autogenous bone provides all of the above properties. Materials purely for bulking (e.g. soft tissues) should ideally be non-resorbable. Grafts can be classified as autogenous (from the same individual), allogeneic (from the same species) or xenogeneic (from a different species).

## Autogenous Grafts: Examples

A graft from the same individual is the most attractive material because of its potential for bone formation, rapid healing, low incidence of infection and long-standing use. It is used in a variety of forms for a broad range of applications.

- **Vascularised graft**. A bone graft can be obtained from the donor site with its blood supply (arteries and veins) attached; it is then transplanted to the recipient site and the blood vessels anastomosed to the regional vessels. A composite graft consisting of bone, skin, muscles and nerves may be harvested for reconstruction following ablative cancer surgery.
- **Non-vascularised graft**. The graft is removed from the donor site and transplanted to the recipient site; it is, therefore, dependent upon re-establishing a blood supply at the recipient site from the local blood vessels. Bone or soft tissue grafts may be transplanted this way.
- **Cortical bone block**. Cortical plate may be transplanted when a thin veneer is required. Generally intraoral sources often provide mainly cortical bone and only a limited amount of cancellous bone.
- **Cortico-cancellous block**. A cortical plate of bone with cancellous bone attached provides several advantages. The cortical bone placed on the outside provides stability and resistance to rapid remodelling, whereas the cancellous bone is easy to adapt to the recipient site for contact healing and permits rapid union with the recipient site.
- **Cancellous bone**. Cancellous bone heals and remodels rapidly. It is, therefore, used within bony cavities such as sinuses, often supplemented with materials having lower resorption rates. It does not provide stable contours on its own when used for ridge augmentation.
- **Particulate bone.** Either cortical or cancellous bone may be particulated in a bone mill. Its use is indicated for a cavity such as a sinus or it has been described as a space maintainer with guided bone regeneration.

## Allogeneic Grafts
- **Fresh frozen bone**. This is not commonly used in dentistry for reasons of disease transmission and availability of sources.
- **Freeze-dried bone**. Allogeneic freeze-dried bone is available in a range of forms including cortical and cancellous bone. Its consists of the mineral and non-mineral matrices. It may be considered to be osteoconductive. No osteogenic or osteoinductive properties have been demonstrated. It suffers the perceived disadvantage of being biologically derived, with potential concerns of disease transmission.
- **Demineralised freeze-dried bone**. Allogeneic demineralised freeze-dried bone (DMFDB) is a collagen matrix that retains its proteins and can be used for potential osteoinduction. The osteoinductive property has not been verified. It also suffers the perceived disadvantage of being biologically derived.
- **Irradiated cortical, cortico-cancellous and cancellous bone**. Allogeneic irradiated bone is obtained from screened donors and irradiated to denature the protein, DNA and RNA components of bone, leaving the mineral structure; it is, therefore, osteoconductive but lacks osteogenic and osteoinductive properties of autogenous bone. It suffers the perceived disadvantage of being biologically derived.
- **Soft tissues**. A range of allogeneic soft tissue products are available. These include lyophilised dura mater, collagen and acellular skin tissue. A variety of applications have been described, with disease transmission risks associated with the processing employed for each of the products.

## Xenogeneic Grafts
- **Bovine**. Bovine bone is commonly used as particulate or block material. It is prepared by heat processing to leave the mineral matrix behind. It suffers the perceived disadvantage of being biologically derived and is solely osteoconductive. It is described for use as a space maintainer with GBR and for sinus augmentation. Bovine membranes derived from tendons or skin are also available and offer a variety of resorption rates based on chemical processing; these are used for various procedures.
- **Porcine**. Collagen membranes of porcine origin are widely available for use as occlusive membranes in conjunction with GBR.
- **Phycogene**. Porous particulate hydroxyapatite as a phycogenic bone substitute is available and has osteoconductive properties.

### Infectivity of Allografts and Xenografts

Manufacturers of allografts and xenografts undertake numerous processes to eliminate risks of disease transmission. These range from using a number of chemical agents, including acetone, hydrogen peroxide, ethylene oxide, sodium hydroxide, to low-dose radiation or heat. The processes are product specific to inactivate bacteria, viruses and prions as well as remove antigenicity.[196–198]

### Use of Synthetic/Alloplastic Materials

Synthetic/alloplastic materials by their nature eliminate the risk of disease transmission. They are available for a range of applications for bone and soft tissue augmentation as well as for membranes in conjunction with GBR techniques. When used on their own, these materials are osteoconductive.

- **Hydroxyapatite**. Hydroxyapatite is normally available as a non-resorbable particulate material suitable for soft tissue bulking.
- **Tricalcium phosphate**. A variety of products of varying particle sizes and porosities are available, suitable for GBR and sinus augmentation. The rate of resorption varies with particle size, processing and porosity.
- **Bioglass**. A range of synthetic bioactive materials are available. Some claim to be osteostimulative due to specific particle sizes.
- **Polymers**. These are widely used. Applications range from resorbable products made from polylactic acid or polyglycolic acid and also include membranes and fixation pins and screws. Polyacrylic products are available as non-resorbable particulate materials for bulking purposes. Polymers are also used for a broad range of non-resorbable membranes such as expanded polytetrafluoroethylene, which is prone to infection if exposed. Nanoporous polytetrafluoroethylene has a reduced pore size and may be left exposed to allow soft tissues to generate underneath it.
- **Calcium sulphate**. Although an inorganic compound, calcium sulphate has also been described as a biomaterial, with a combined use as a membrane and as a filler.

### Summary

A broad range of materials is now commercially available for the purposes of augmentation. The available documentation for these materials varies in detail, and it is beyond the scope of this book to address this issue. The clinician may choose to use any of the biomaterials that have been developed after careful assessment of their properties and the clinical evidence.[199–202]

The development of materials containing proteins to induce certain tissue reactions is quite promising (e.g. to stimulate cell differentiation) and awaits documentation of clinical applications. Factors to modulate cell proliferation and vascularisation may be derived from the patient's own blood (e.g. platelet-rich plasma).

Bone morphogenetic proteins produced by recombinant and other technologies in combination with a suitable carrier show considerable promise. These will have osteoinductive properties.

Tissue-engineered autogenous osteogenic cells seeded into a 3D polymer fleece are another example of future biomaterials (e.g. Bio Seed Oral Bone; BioTissue Technologies, Freiburg, Germany). To grow osteogenic cells, a small sample (e.g. periosteum with cambium cells) is harvested from an intraoral site and sent for culturing. These are returned for implantation after culturing and embedded in a polymer fleece. This technology is also available for soft tissue cells for oral mucosa replacement (BioSeed-M; BioTissue Technologies).

## General Principles for Grafts

### Guided Bone Regeneration

Sound surgical principles dictate that soft tissue surgery must be carried out in a manner to prevent dehiscence of the membrane or breakdown of the wound. This is particularly critical when non-collagen membranes are used. Autogenous bone as a space maintainer with its inherent properties is the most predictable method of bone formation using this technique, for reasons described above. Any micromotion of the material beyond the permissible strain levels will interfere with bone formation. Therefore, use of a block graft provides the most predictable way of repairing a defect.

III   Augmentation

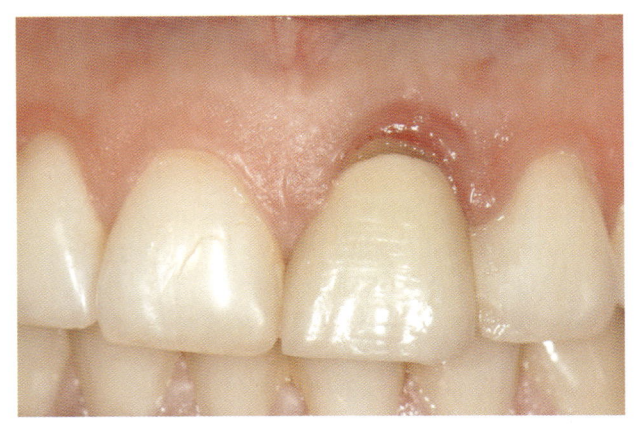

Fig 11-5   Preoperative view of a failing tooth, unsuitable for immediate replacement because of recession of the soft tissues.

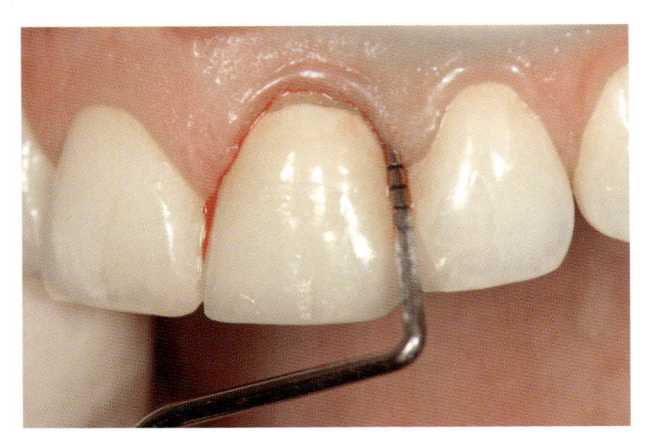

Fig 11-6   Excessive probing depths indicative of bone loss is a further contraindication for immediate implant placement.

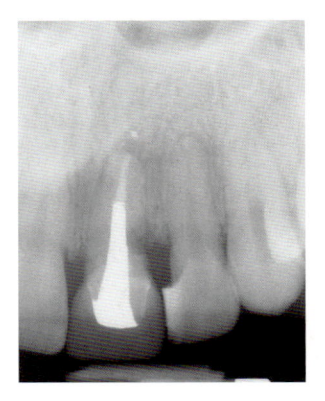

Fig 11-7   Radiograph showing external resorption and persistent pathology.

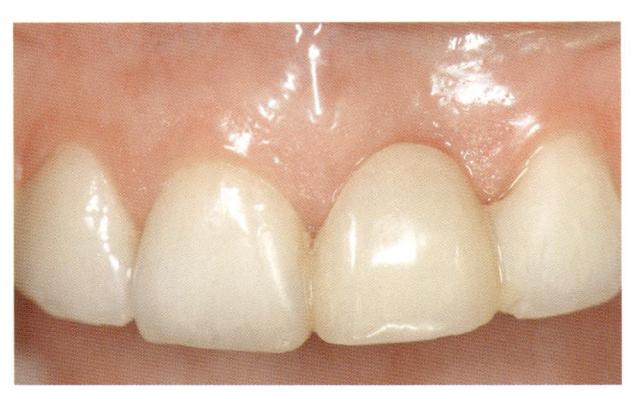

Fig 11-8   Metal-acrylic resin Rochette bridge three months after extraction, showing labial depression.

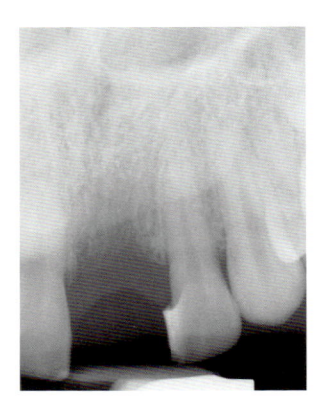

Fig 11-9   Postextraction radiograph showing healing at three months.

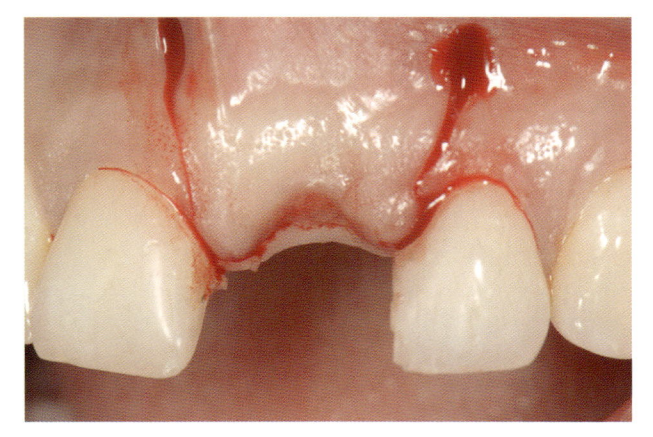

Fig 11-10   Crestal incision for implant placement three months after extraction.

However, where a minor deficiency is present, GBR provides an alternative method by which soft tissue contours can be maintained. This is particularly the case if an infrabony defect needs correction. This is depicted by the case study illustrated in Figs 11-5 to 11-31.

11  Overview

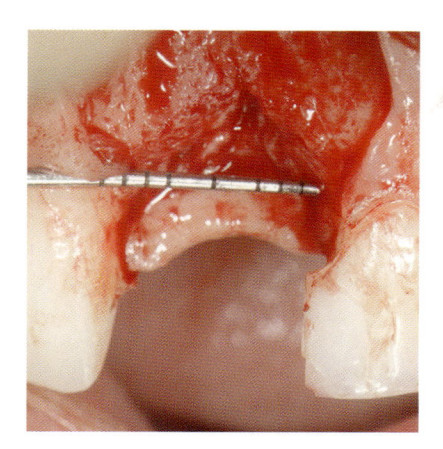

**Fig 11-11**  Bone deficiency that will require augmentation.

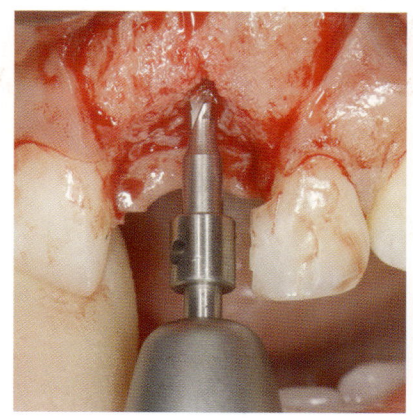

**Fig 11-12**  Osteotomy preparation using an internally irrigated Lindemann bur to establish direction.

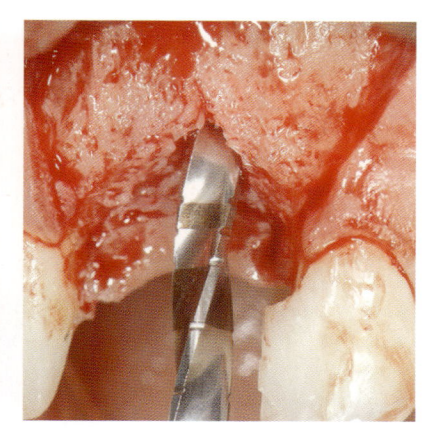

**Fig 11-13**  Internally irrigated osteotomy bur used to confirm direction and establish depth and the diameter.

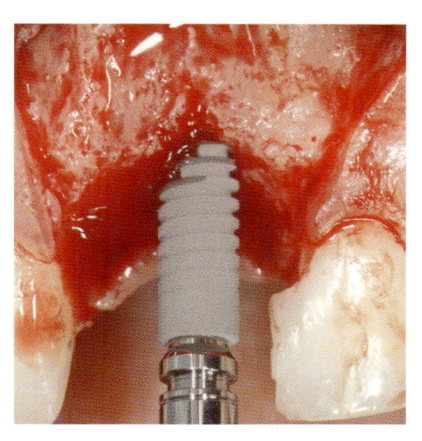

**Fig 11-14**  Implant being inserted.

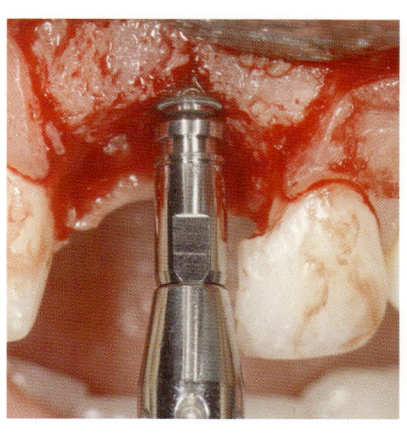

**Fig 11-15**  Implant is inserted to a depth level with the deficiency. The Ankylos CX implant is used here. Although the index does not need to be engaged, the rotational position of the implant is identified by the depression of the implant insertion instrument.

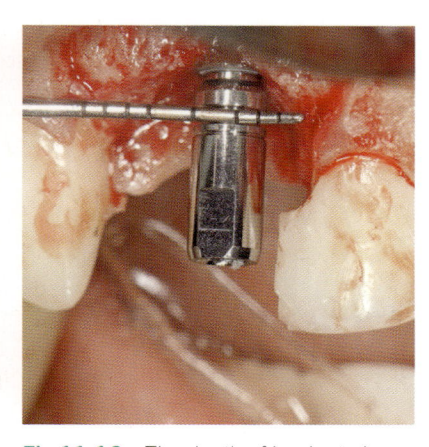

**Fig 11-16**  The depth of implant placement is measured against the bone level of the adjacent teeth.

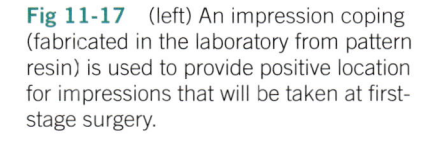

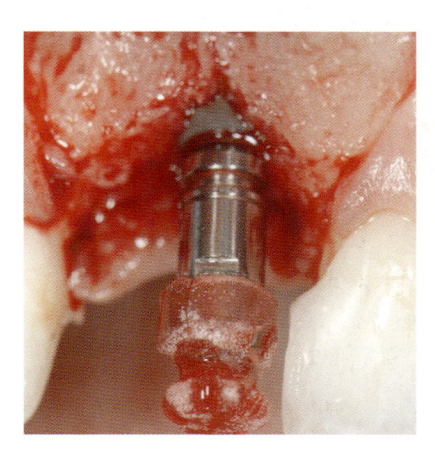

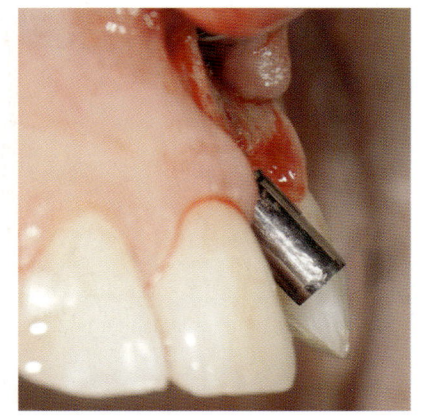

**Fig 11-17**  (left) An impression coping (fabricated in the laboratory from pattern resin) is used to provide positive location for impressions that will be taken at first-stage surgery.

**Fig 11-18**  (right) The implant carrier seen in profile, providing an indication of the angle at which it has been placed and its relationship to the adjacent teeth.

213

III Augmentation

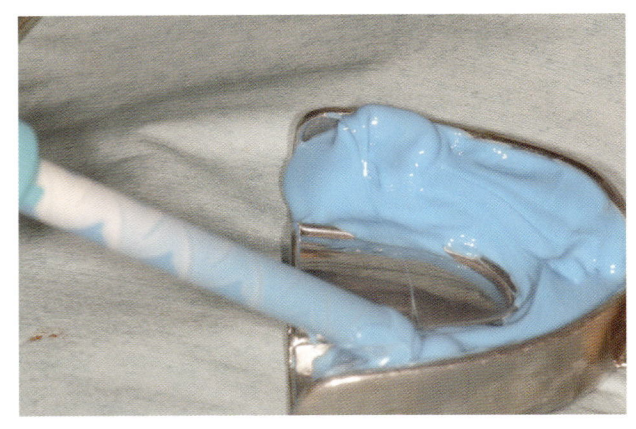

**Fig 11-19** A sterile rimmed metal tray is loaded with a medium bodied silicone impression material (Provil Monophase).

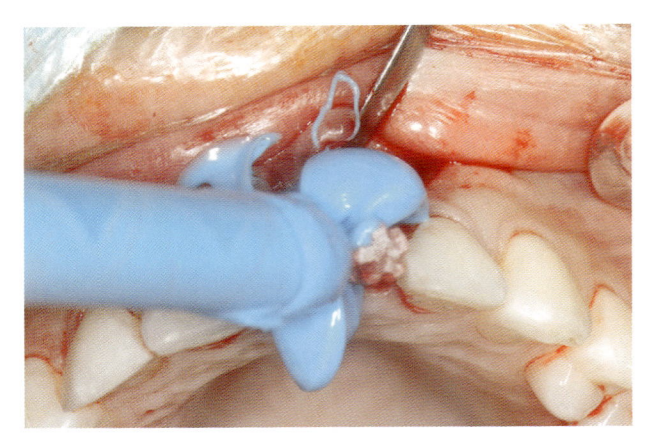

**Fig 11-20** The impression material is then injected around the resin coping and implant carrier.

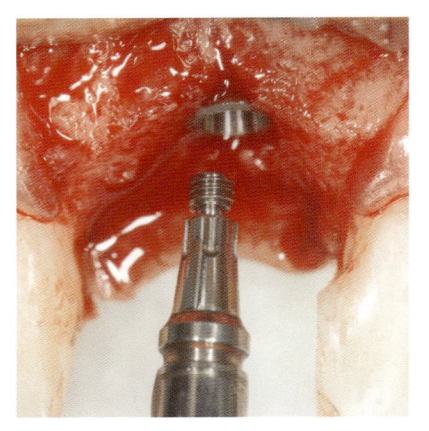

**Fig 11-21** The implant carrier is removed for insertion into the impression that has been taken. This will transfer the implant position to the laboratory.

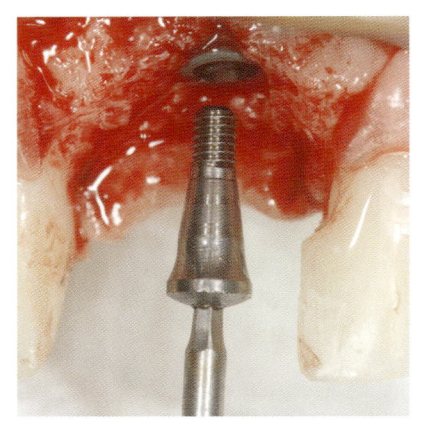

**Fig 11-22** A sulcus former is inserted into the implant to provide support for the biomaterial and the membrane that will be used to repair the defect.

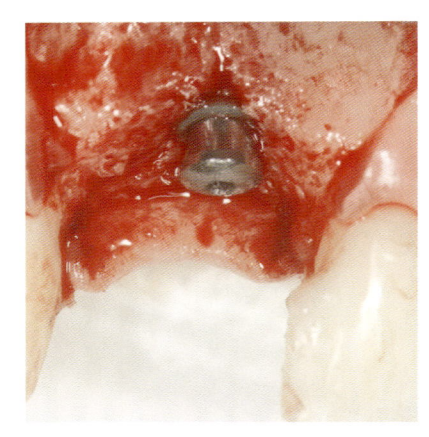

**Fig 11-23** The implant with the sulcus former in situ.

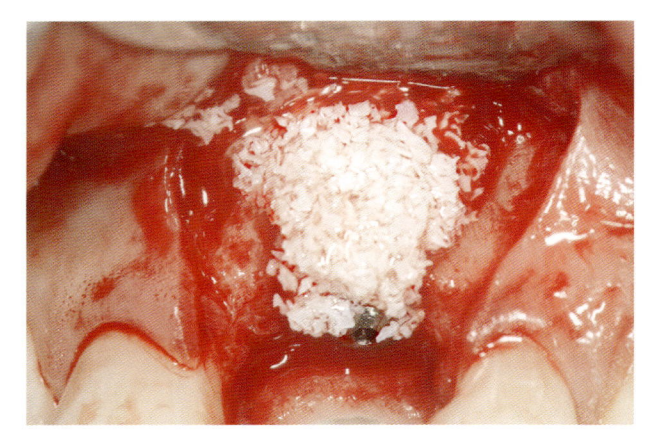

**Fig 11-24** Bovine xenograft (Bio-Oss, Geistlich Pharma, Wolhusen, Switzerland) placed around the deficiency.

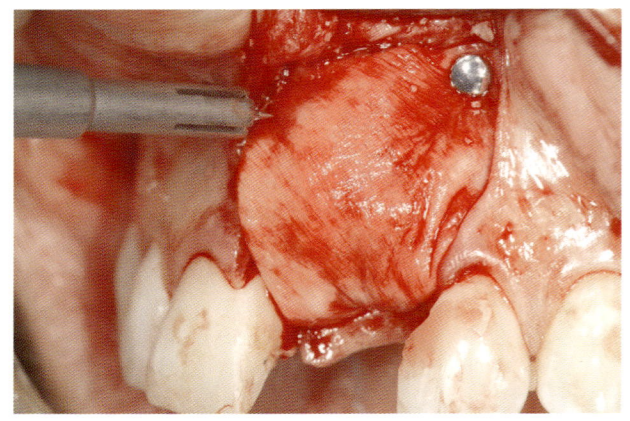

**Fig 11-25** Bovine collagen membrane (Bio-Gide, Geistlich Pharma) will be used to contain the biomaterial. FRIOS titanium tacks (Dentsply Friadent) being used to secure the membrane. The tack is carried in the pre-tensed carrier to the site, held perpendicular and inserted with the mallet using a light tap.

11 Overview

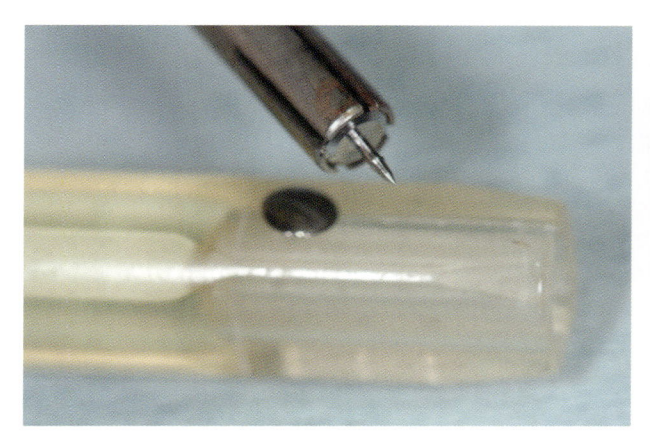

**Fig 11-26** FRIOS tacks being loaded onto the insertion instrument from the dispenser.

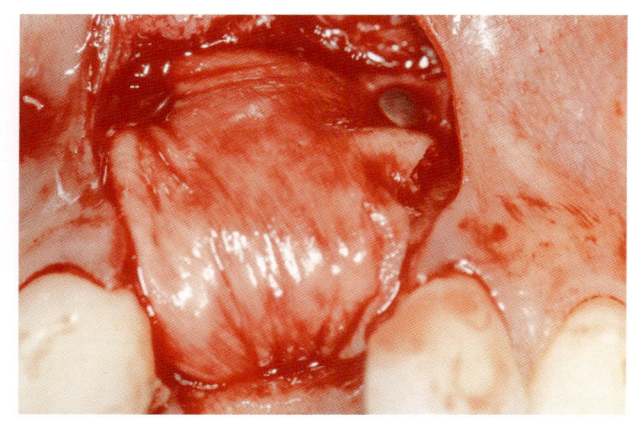

**Fig 11-27** The membrane securely positioned and tucked under the palatal flap.

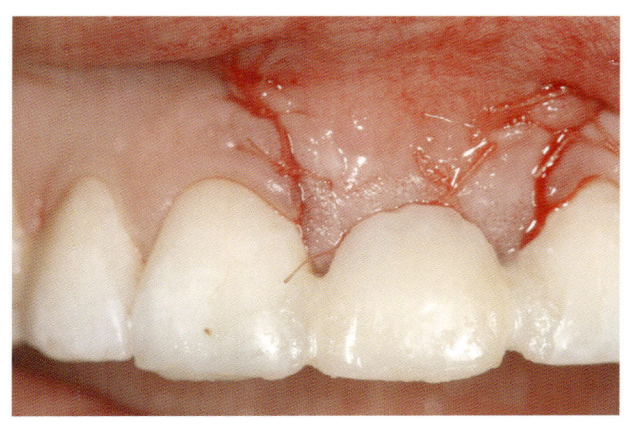

**Fig 11-28** The provisional restoration recemented after suturing the wound (6-0 Vicryl). Note the overcontoured soft tissues.

**Fig 11-29** Post-operative radiograph; the implant with the sulcus former and the titanium tacks can be seen.

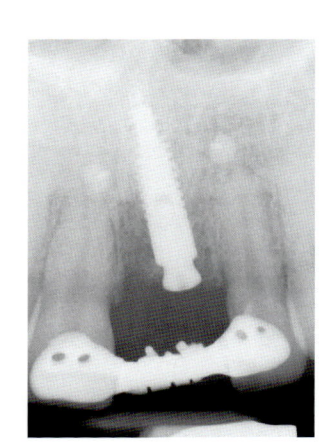

**Fig 11-30** The impression prior to insertion of the implant carrier and analogue. This can be done either in the surgery or at the laboratory.

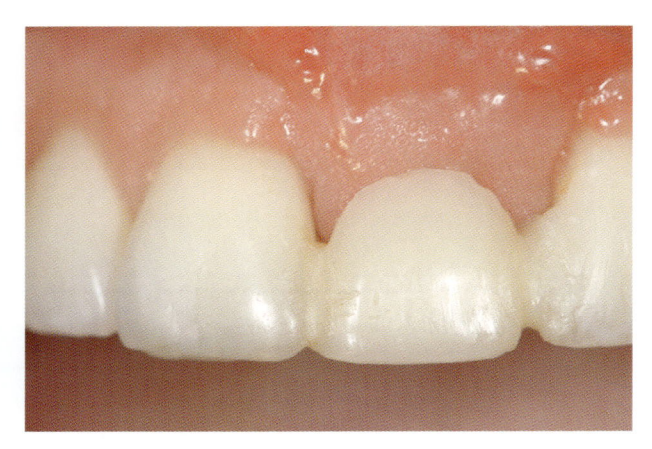

**Fig 11-31** Healing of the wound at one week. Implant exposure and attachment of the definitive abutment as well as the fitting of the transitional crown will be carried out at three months.

III   Augmentation

**Main decision criteria for the assessment of possible augmentation – hard and soft tissue manipulation:**

1. Relationship of ridge to future tooth position
2. Volume and quality of bone
3. Functional and parafunctional load
4. Jaw relationship

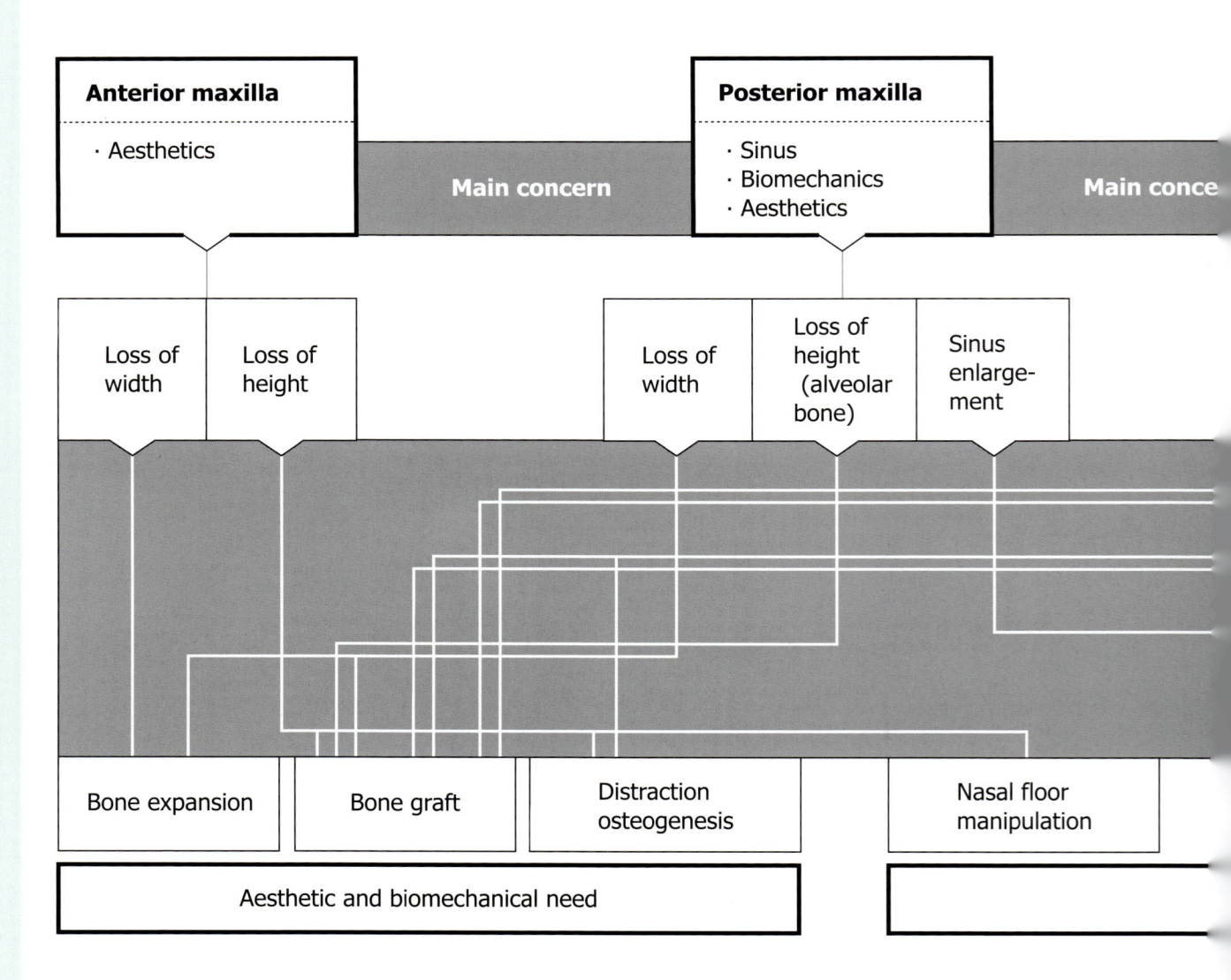

| Anterior maxilla | Main concern | Posterior maxilla | Main conce... |
|---|---|---|---|
| · Aesthetics | | · Sinus<br>· Biomechanics<br>· Aesthetics | |

Anterior maxilla: Loss of width | Loss of height

Posterior maxilla: Loss of width | Loss of height (alveolar bone) | Sinus enlargement

Treatment options: Bone expansion | Bone graft | Distraction osteogenesis | Nasal floor manipulation

Aesthetic and biomechanical need

Possible treatment options – see specific flowcharts for further details and decision criteria

**Flowchart 11-1**   Main decision criteria for the assessment of possible augmentation - hard and soft tissue manipulation or grafting.

## 11 Overview

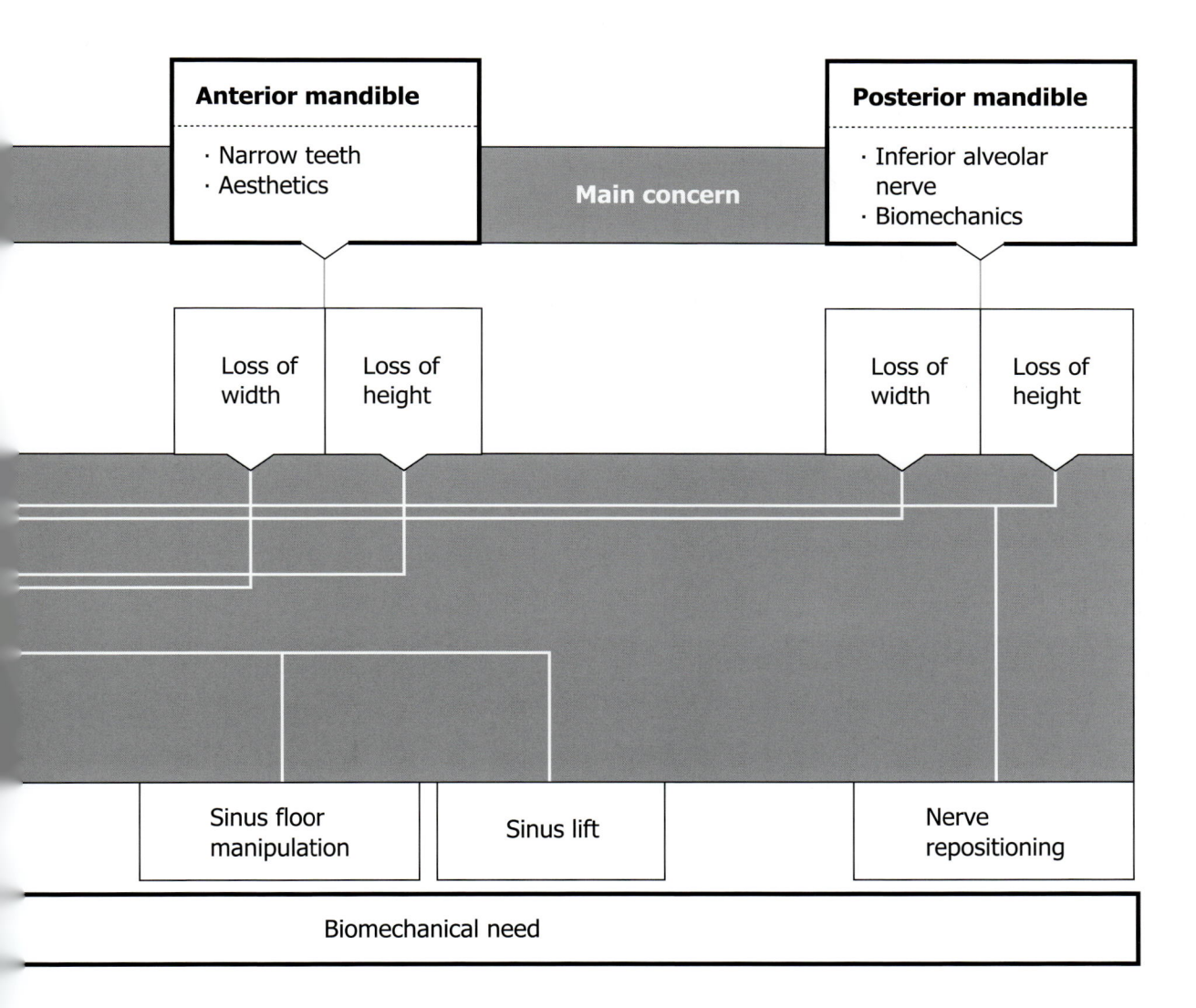

| | Anterior mandible | Main concern | Posterior mandible |
|---|---|---|---|
| | · Narrow teeth<br>· Aesthetics | | · Inferior alveolar nerve<br>· Biomechanics |

| Loss of width | Loss of height | | Loss of width | Loss of height |

| Sinus floor manipulation | Sinus lift | | Nerve repositioning |

Biomechanical need

## III Augmentation

### Block Bone Grafts

The rationale behind use of block bone grafts is to use a block of cortical or cortico-cancellous autogenous bone of a shape that re-establishes the required contour of the ridge, ensuring that it is overcontoured to compensate for remodelling during the revascularisation.

The fundamental clinical principles and technique are as follows to optimise outcome:

- **Soft tissue management**. The design and handling of the mucoperiosteal flap must allow for tension-free closure to prevent breakdown at the incision line or over the graft, thus facilitating revascularization from the overlying soft tissues. Whenever possible the incision should be remote from the graft site.
- **Graft adaptation**. The graft should be closely adapted to the recipient site to permit contact osteosynthesis, which allows for a more rapid incorporation of the bone graft and reduces the risk of soft tissue intervening between the graft and recipient site. Margins that are not closely adapted should have supplementary procedures carried out to prevent soft tissue ingress, such as the use of particulate materials and occlusive membranes.
- **Graft fixation**. Good graft adaptation by modifying graft or recipient site will increase graft stability. It should subsequently be rigidly fixed with screws using the lagged principle, which will increase the contact surface area and ensure immobility. Osteosynthesis plates or wires may be used when the use of fixation screws is not possible, but a less rigid fixation may result. We consider graft adaptation to the recipient site an important factor contributing to rapid and predictable healing without the need for decortication.[203] Decortication of the recipient site is often not possible in severely resorbed cases (e.g. Case 7 in Chapter 14). The only rationale for modifying the recipient site is to improve graft adaptation.

### Decision-making Process for Augmentation

The overview flowchart to assess possible hard tissue procedures is designed to facilitate the decision-making process for the various regions of the mouth and the range of defects that are likely to be present (Flowchart 11-1 see pages 216–217). The procedures for augmentation of hard tissues are designed so that soft tissues at the site can be developed simultaneously. The anatomical changes that take place as a result of atrophy will alter the jaw relations and, therefore, consideration must be given during planning of augmentation to the reconstruction of the ridges in the correct jaw relationships.

In the event that soft tissue deficiencies cannot be adequately corrected, additional soft tissue procedures may need to be carried out.

Procedures designed for use on soft tissues will be addressed in Chapter 17, which also contains a flowchart used to facilitate the decision-making process.

# Chapter 12

# Bone Expansion

## Introduction

Maxillary bone expansion allows a narrow maxillary ridge to be widened for the simultaneous insertion of implants. Specific criteria that need to be assessed are:
- relationship of residual ridge to planned tooth position
- bone width and ridge morphology
- height of available bone.

A summary of the assessment is shown in Flowchart 12-1. This procedure may be carried out in situations where there is insufficient width of bone for an implant to be inserted (Fig 12-1). Conventional osteotomy would lead to a dehiscent implant, which would be compromised. The loss of bone takes place at the expense of the labial plate, and consequently the procedure is designed to manipulate the labial plate in attempt to reconstruct the ridge.[204–206]

It is clear that the implant must be placed between the cortical plates. The angle at which the implant is placed is, therefore, dictated by the orientation of the residual ridge. This often differs from the longitudinal axis of the tooth that needs to be restored (Figs 12-2 and 12-3). A wide range of angled abutments should be available so that the implant can be restored without compromising the aesthetic outcome.[204] This procedure may also be used to re-contour the labial plate where sufficient bone is present but is not in a position suitable for producing ideal aesthetics because of the collapse of the labial plate (Figs 12-4 and 12-5). This would otherwise result in an implant being placed too far towards the palate, leading to poor aesthetics or to the ridge lapping of the crown.

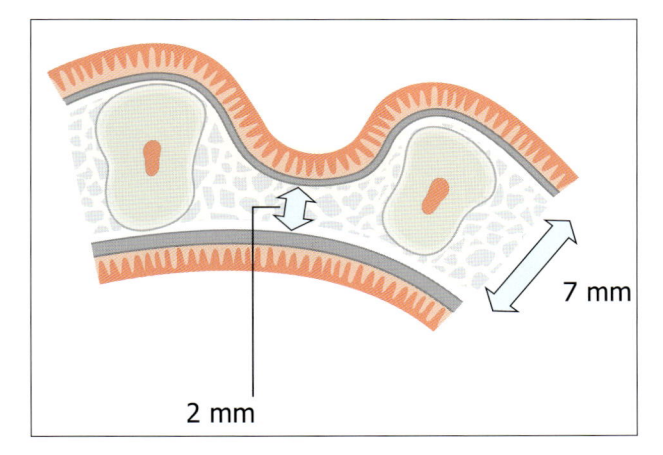

**Fig 12-1** Diagram of a severely resorbed maxillary ridge requiring expansion. Two separate cortical plates with intervening cancellous bone are considered to be a requirement for maxillary bone expansion. Note the severe loss of ridge width at the expense of the labial plate, which is typical of patients with prominent roots with large interdental depressions.

III  Augmentation

```
Missing tooth — healed hard and soft tissues
                    ↓
        Assessment of residual ridge
        Clinical assessment
        Diagnostic imaging
        Diagnostic preview
                    ↓
    Main decision criteria for the assessment of
    possible bone expansion:
    ─────────────────────────────────────────
    1. Sufficient height of bone in relation to future
       tooth position
    2. No fused cortical plates (according to CT scan)
       or >3 mm of width (according to
       ridge mapping)
    3. More than 12 mm of bone height
                    ↓
        Bone expansion possible?
        (Criteria 1–3 = Yes)
    Yes ←                    → No
```

**Yes branch:**
Bone expansion procedure
─────────────────
· Bone expanders
· Bone condensers

**No branch:**
· Further assessment necessary
· Treatment decision based on type of deficiency (loss of height or width), location, aesthetic and functional needs

Augmentation procedure
─────────────────
· Bone graft
· Sinus lift
· GTR
· Ti Mesh

Hard and soft tissue manipulation
─────────────────
· Sinus manipulation
· Distraction osteogenesis

**Flowchart 12-1**  Assessment for bone expansion.

## 12 Bone Expansion

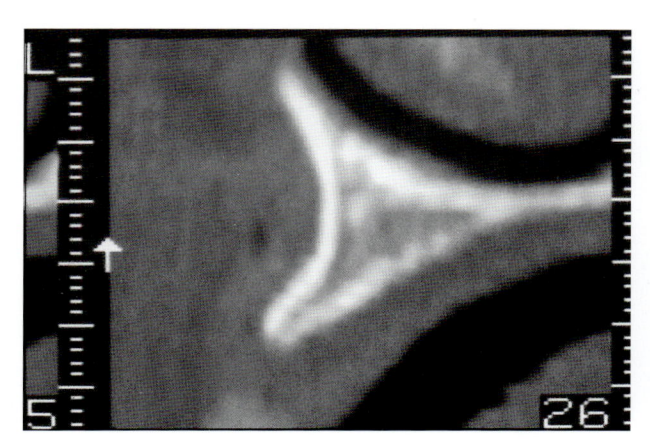

**Fig 12-2** Oblique cross-sectional CT image showing a narrow maxillary ridge, which widens rapidly. The angulation of the maxillary ridge should be noted as it will influence the position of the implant and its relationship to the restoration.

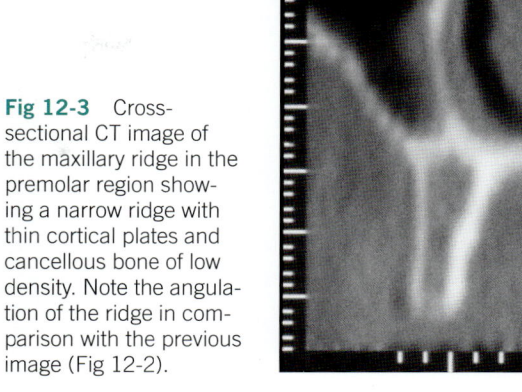

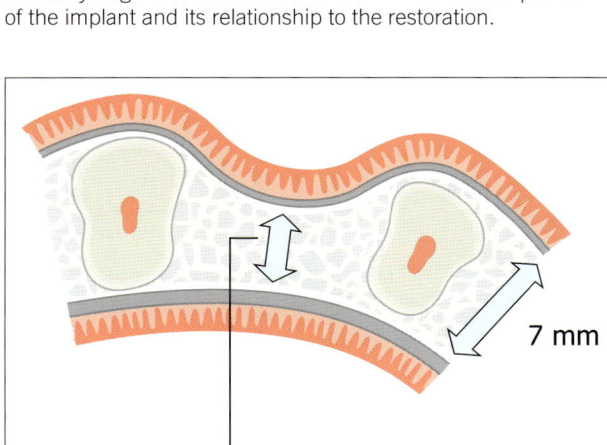

**Fig 12-3** Cross-sectional CT image of the maxillary ridge in the premolar region showing a narrow ridge with thin cortical plates and cancellous bone of low density. Note the angulation of the ridge in comparison with the previous image (Fig 12-2).

**Fig 12-4** Axial cross-section of a typical ridge following tooth loss and collapse of the labial plate. Typically such a ridge may result in the labio-coronal part of the implant being dehiscent or the implant being positioned too far palatally.

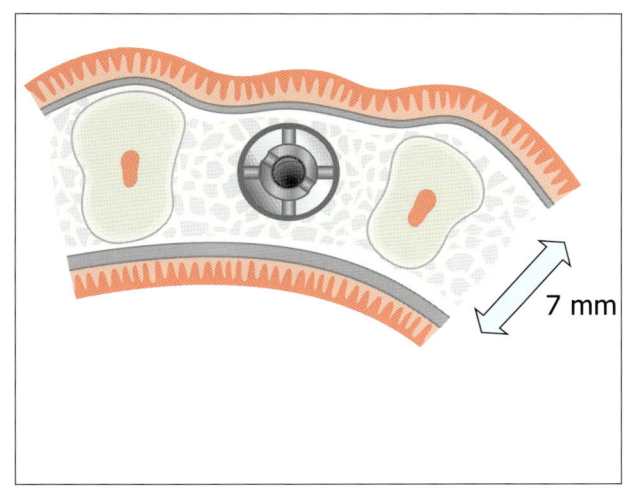

**Fig 12-5** The re-contouring of the labial plate, using bone condensers or bone spreaders to ensure that the correct emergence profile as well as the correct position of the implant can be achieved.

Tatum originally developed the technique for the insertion of 'D'-shaped finned transmucosal implants.[206] The technique has evolved and the version described here has been modified for the insertion of screw-form two-stage submergible implants that are allowed to integrate in a closed environment.[204,205] Other techniques with varying success rates have been described in the literature.[207–212]

### Height of the Crestal Ridge

The technique described here is designed to increase the width of the ridge and cannot be used to increase ridge height. The crestal ridge height needs to be assessed, taking into account the level of the bony ridge and the level of the soft tissues.

The level of the soft tissue can be assessed visually and should ideally be the same as the papillae of the adjacent teeth. This is particularly important for multiple implants, where it is difficult to create natural contours when the implants have been placed adjacent

# III Augmentation

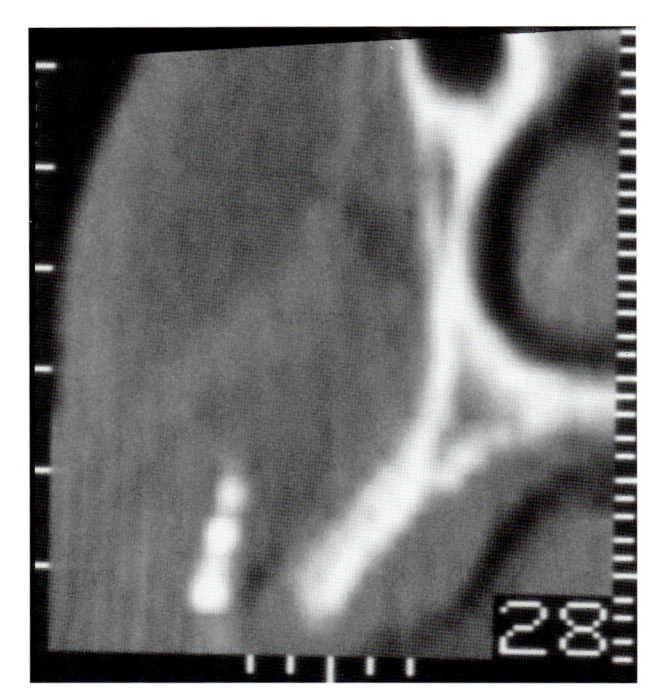

**Fig 12-6** Fused cortical places of a maxillary ridge, which would not be considered suitable for maxillary bone expansion.

to each other. This assessment can be facilitated by reference to the diagnostic preview and the provisional restoration made from it. The diagnostic preview has to be used judiciously, projecting an increase in width of approximately 2 mm. For multiple units, an assessment of the lip support should also be made.

Periapical radiographs give a good indication of ridge height for single-tooth implants or short spans. The level of bone attachment to the adjacent teeth should be noted, as well as the midcrestal level.

CT scans should have reference radiopaque markings so that tooth position can be assessed in relation to the future implant position.

## Bone Width and Ridge Morphology

In order to undertake ridge expansion, the ridge must constitute two separate cortical plates with intervening cancellous bone. This can best be assessed by means of a CT scan or conventional tomograph, which will provide information regarding the width of the ridge, the thickness of the cortical plate, the density of cancellous bone between the cortices and the angulation of the ridge (Figs 12-2, 12-3 and 12-6). Where a CT scan is not possible, ridge mapping should be carried out to provide details of the width of the bony ridge. Several points starting at 3 mm from the crest of the ridge and moving towards the base of the ridge should be measured. This will indicate whether the ridge narrows or widens towards the base. If a minimum ridge width of 3 mm can be found, separate cortical plates with intervening cancellous bone, suitable for ridge expansion, are likely to be present. Although a 2 mm ridge can also be expanded, the likelihood of fused cortical plates is higher and a CT scan is desirable prior to proceeding.

## Height of Available Bone

The ridge should be a minimum of 12 mm in height to ensure adequate primary stability and sufficient bone support. If the height of the ridge is marginally less than 11 mm, sinus or nasal floor manipulation may be carried out in combination with the expansion procedure.

## Treatment Sequence

Bone expansion should be carried out in a healed site with matured cortical plates. A healing period of three to six months after implant insertion is recommended to ensure that integration takes place. Immediate loading is not generally recommended because of the fragility of the labial plate, which has just been repositioned, and because primary stability may well have been compromised. It is for this reason that this protocol has been developed for submergible implants (two stage) in order to minimise trauma from occlusal forces during healing. An exception to this may be where minimal re-contouring of the labial plate has been undertaken and sufficient primary stability has been achieved to enable early or immediate loading, as determined by the criteria described above. The use of a two-stage implantation procedure with the implant being submerged at first-stage surgery to allow integration has additional benefits. These relate to the ability to develop the desired emergence profile by manipulating the soft tissue at the time of implant exposure.

## 12  Bone Expansion

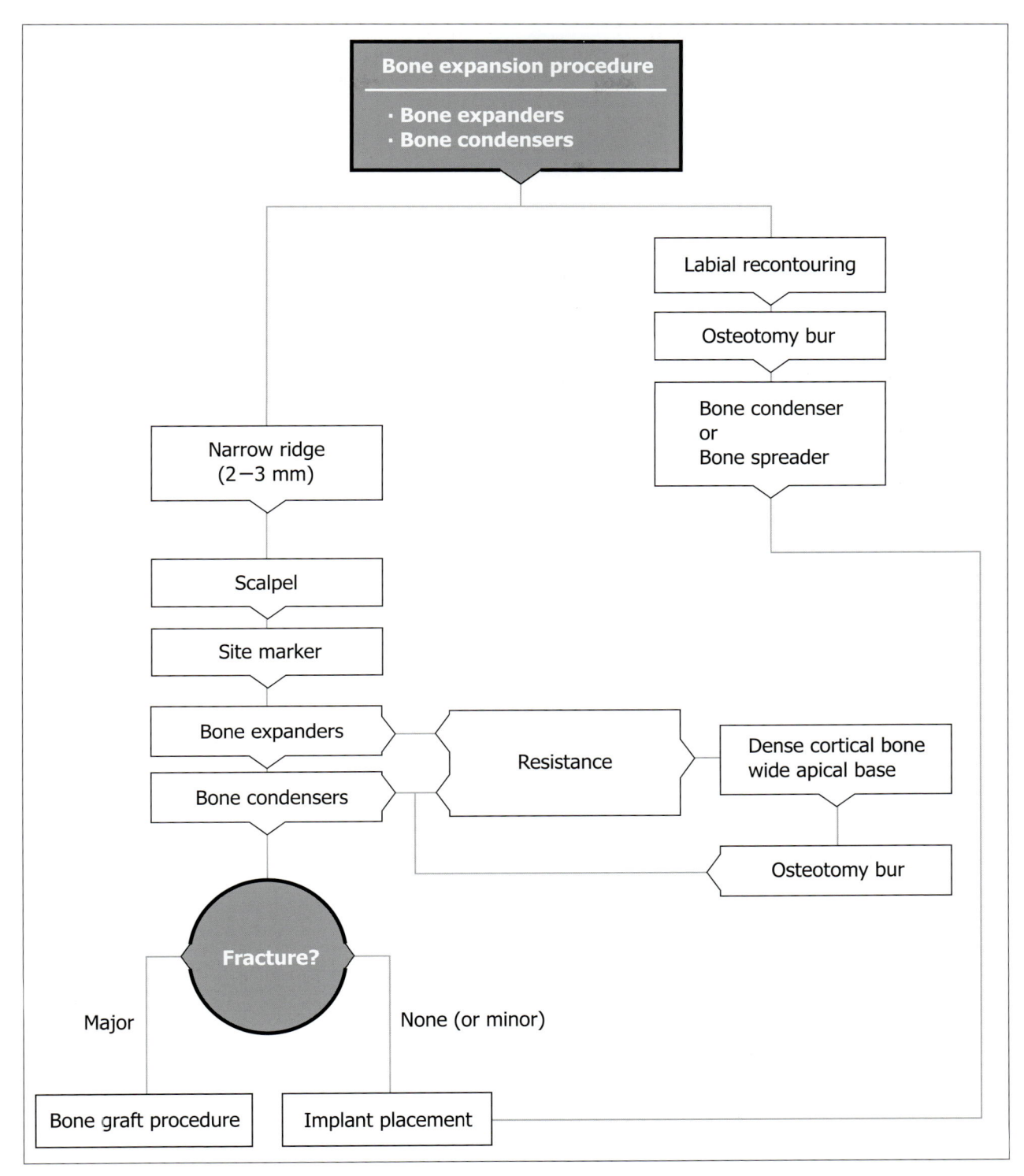

```
                    Bone expansion procedure
                    • Bone expanders
                    • Bone condensers
```

**Flowchart 12-2**  Bone expansion and labial recontouring.

## Surgical Protocol

Flowchart 12-2 summarises the sequence of instruments needed for either bone expansion or labial recontouring.

# III  Augmentation

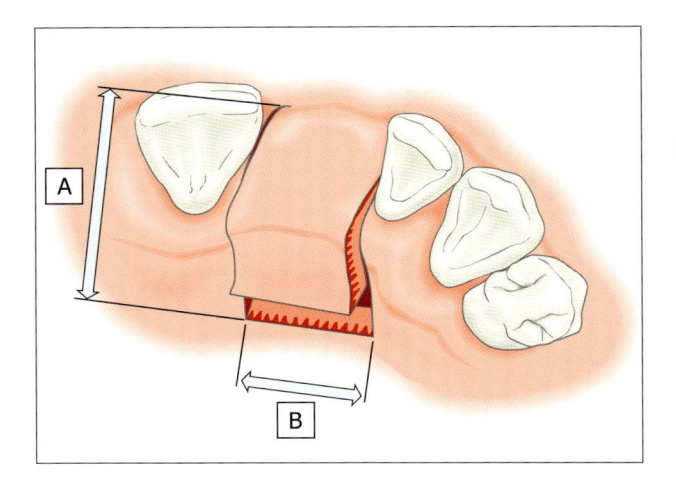

**Fig 12-7**  The outline of the remote palatal incision for the exposure of a healed maxillary ridge in the region of an incisor. The incision consists of two components. First, two incisions are extended into the palate to a distance of approximately 10 mm each (A). These incisions are designed to include the papilla and to extend within the gingival sulcus towards labial aspect. The second component (B) is a bevelled incision made parallel to the ridge joining the incisions. A Blake's knife is the most suitable instrument for this. This produces a full-thickness flap with a bevelled component, which is buccally based. The labial periosteum is not elevated to ensure that an adequate blood supply is maintained to the labial cortical plate, which will be manipulated during the procedure of maxillary bone expansion.

## Remote Palatal Incision

Access to the ridge is gained via a remote palatal incision made approximately 1 cm from the crest of the ridge. The perpendicular component of the incision is made with a number 15 blade in a conventional handle. The palatal incision is made with a Blake's knife (blade number 15) and is bevelled towards the crest to allow for closure of the wound after expansion (Fig 12-7). The buccally based flap is elevated using a curved elevator (Dentsply Friadent) to expose the crest of the ridge. To ensure that the blood supply to the labial cortical plate, which is supplied by the periosteum, is not interrupted, the labial periosteum is not reflected.[213]

The rationale behind a remote palatal incision is that it enables closure of the wound in a predictable manner after expansion. In addition, this is the appropriate incision for a bone graft should that be required in the event of a fracture of the labial plate.

## Instrument Sequence

Ridge expansion is a surgical art form in which a specific protocol should be followed in order to attain a successful and predictable expansion. A sequence of instrument use has been developed, which is outlined below. Use of this specific sequence coupled with appropriate surgical skills results in a high success rate.[204] The skills required for the use of the protocol outlined below should be obtained before attempting treatment on severely resorbed ridges. There are several animal models that may be used to become familiar with the behaviour of bone and mode of employment of the instruments. It is advisable that the clinician be familiar with the use of instruments, such as bone expanders and bone condensers, for the preparation of osteotomies in maxillary bone.

## Scalpel

The scalpel is used with good finger support to score the crest of the ridge, defining the plane of expansion (Fig 12-8). It should be possible to visualise the labial displacement of the buccal plate at this point. Accurate marking of the ridge is very important (Fig 12-9).

## Position Marker

The position marker (site marker) is used to select the implant site (Fig 12-10). It is introduced into the ridge to identify the direction of the proposed osteotomy. The position marker is aligned between the labial and palatal cortical plates parallel to adjacent teeth or adjacent implant. The position marker is inserted to a depth of about 10 mm, but this will depend on the amount of bone available. The position marker directs itself between the cortical plates along the line of least resistance, ensuring that there is no perforation.

For a single implant, the site should be selected in the middle of the ridge, taking the local anatomical structures (such as incisive canal) into account. The site can be selected visually with sufficient accuracy.

For multiple implants, a minimum distance of 7 mm from the centre of each implant site is necessary for

## 12  Bone Expansion

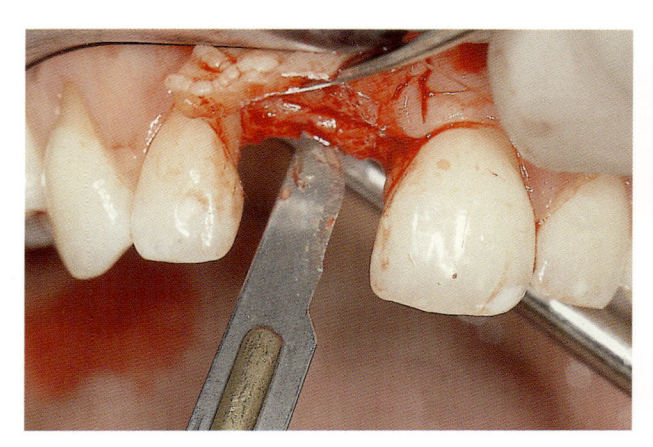

**Fig 12-8**  The ridge is exposed via a remote palatal incision and a scalpel is used to define the plane along which the bone expansion is to be carried out.

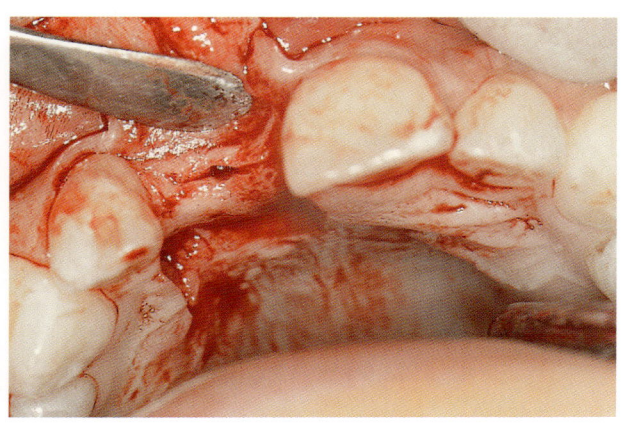

**Fig 12-9**  Occlusal view of the ridge, which has been marked using a scalpel and a position marker. Note the width of the ridge (2 mm at the crest) in comparison with the width of the adjacent teeth (7 mm).

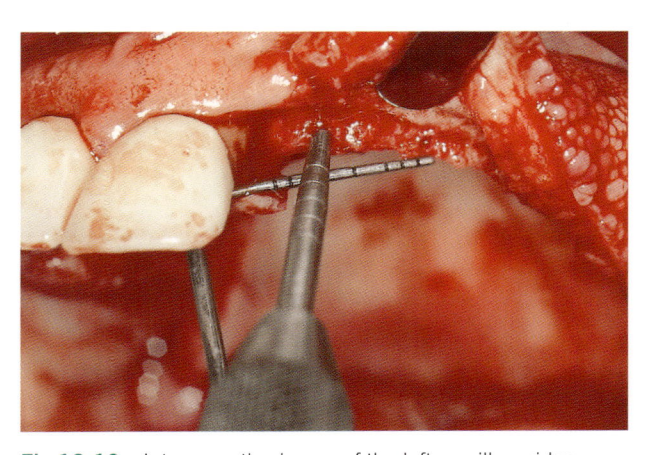

**Fig 12-10**  Intraoperative image of the left maxillary ridge showing the selection of sites. The lateral incisor is positioned 4 mm from the central incisor and the canine is positioned 7 mm from the lateral incisor to provide adequate interdental spacing. The position marker can be seen marking the implant site as well as establishing the direction of the osteotomy between the cortical plates.

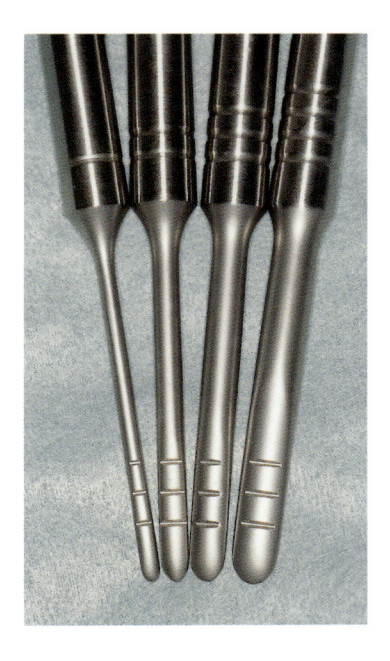

**Fig 12-11**  Series of four bone expanders with marks at 10, 15 and 20 mm to enable the depth of insertion to be gauged. The 'D'-shaped cross-section of the four instruments of increasing width is visible.

3.5-mm implants in order to sustain an adequate inter-implant bone height. A surgical template may be useful in selecting implant sites to coincide with tooth positions.

### Bone Expanders (Ridge Expanders)

Bone expanders are used to separate the cortical plates (Figs 12-11 and 12-12). The principle behind the use of these instruments is to facilitate bone expansion over a larger area without the formation of sharp angles, thus minimising the risk of fracture (Figs 12-13 to 12-16). During the course of the expansion procedures, the

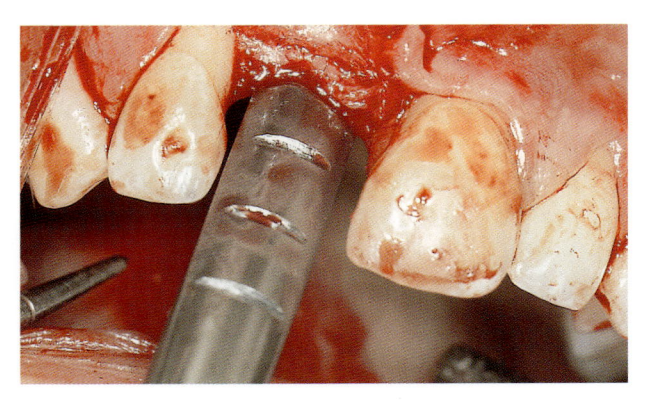

**Fig 12-12**  Labial view of a bone expander being used to separate the cortical plates.

225

# III Augmentation

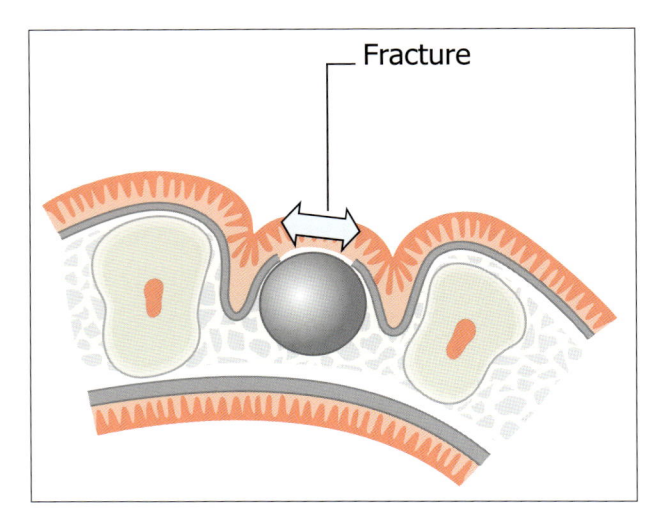

**Fig 12-13** Attempts to manipulate a narrow ridge such as that shown here are likely to increase the chances of fracture, caused by exceeding the elastic limit of the labial plate.

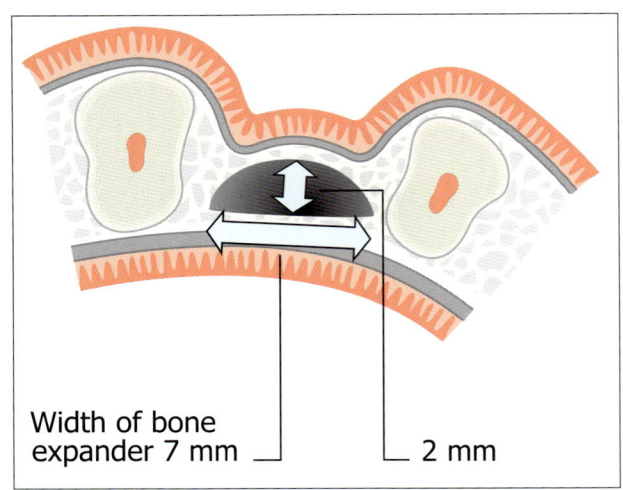

**Fig 12-14** The use of 'D'-shaped bone expanders enables the two cortical plates to be a separated with a reduced risk of fracture. The bone expander, which is used with the convex side towards the labial aspect, repositions the labial cortical plate.

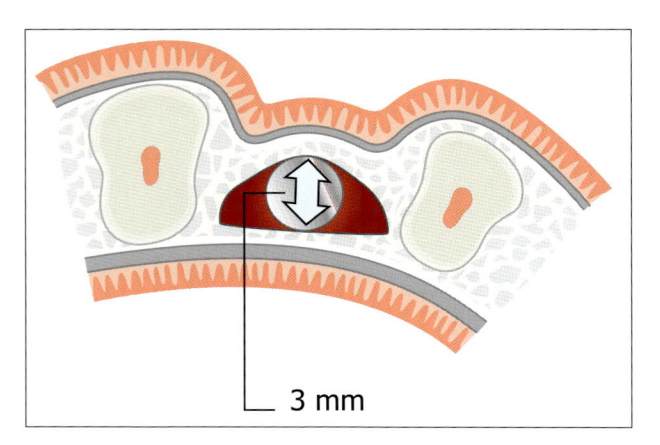

**Fig 12-15** The separation of the cortical plates by a bone expander allows the introduction of a series of bone condensers, which are round in cross-section, to create an osteotomy progressively that is matched to the diameter and length of the selected implant.

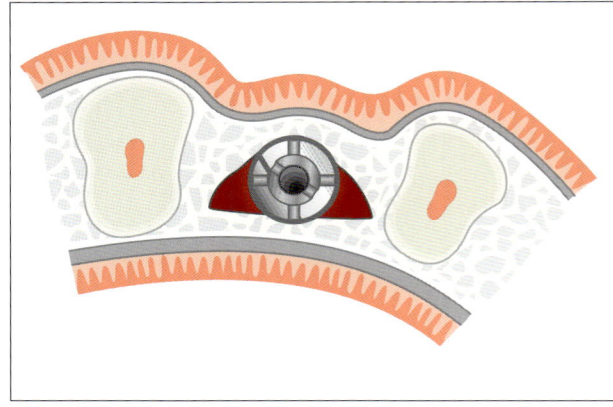

**Fig 12-16** The implant may then be placed into an osteotomy lying between the two cortical plates that have been separated, with the labial plate being repositioned towards the buccal.

labial and palatal cortical plates are supported firmly to prevent fracture. Particular attention should be paid to supporting the palatal bone. Loss of the palatal bone in the event of a fracture results in a loss of height, which is more difficult to rectify.

Bone expanders are 'D' shaped in cross-section and have sharp paraboloid tips. They are used with the convex surface towards the labial aspect so that the labial plate can be re-contoured. A series of four expanders with widths ranging from 3 to 7.5 mm is available. They are used in sequence to a depth of 5–10 mm and are inserted with the aid of a surgical mallet, using a controlled (pulled) tap. Benign paroxysmal vertigo has been reported as a rare result of the use of percussive instruments in the maxilla. Judicious controlled use of the mallet is, therefore, recommended.[214,215]

Acoustic and manual feedback is used to determine the depth to which the expanders are being inserted. The instruments are alternated if necessary. The bone expanders are removed from the osteotomy

## 12  Bone Expansion

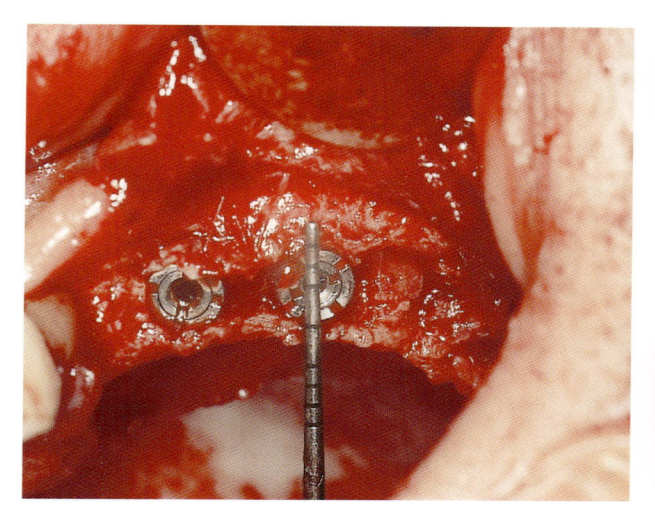

**Fig 12-17**  Occlusal view of the expanded ridge, showing the separation of the cortical plates and the presence of trabecular bone between the implants within the separated cortical plates. A 6-mm ridge width has been achieved.

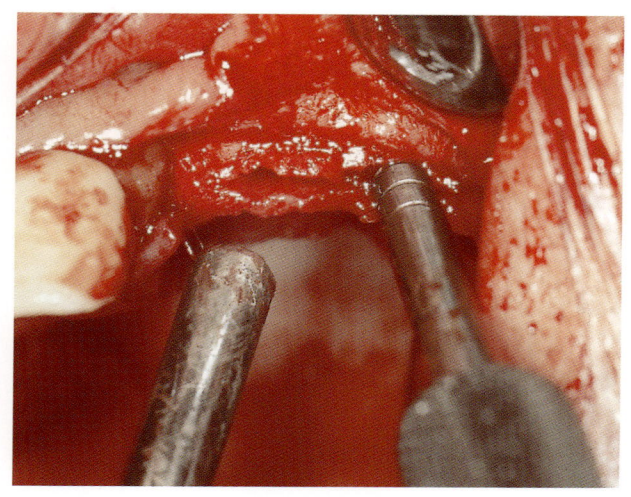

**Fig 12-18**  The bone condenser is used to establish the osteotomy for each implant to ensure that primary stability can be achieved.

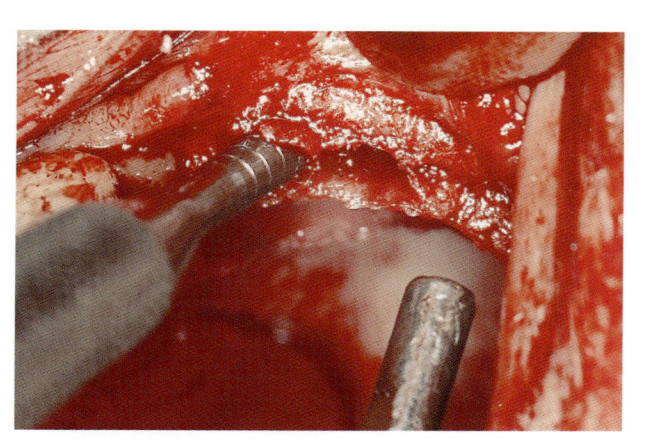

**Fig 12-19**  The development of osteotomies adjacent to each other results in a separation of the cortical plates in the coronal aspect of the ridge. The bone condensers, however, produce osteotomies within the maxillary ridge, which are specific to implant position.

by mesiodistal movement to release them. For single teeth, the interdental distance will dictate the size of the bone expander that can be used. For lateral incisors, the use of expanders greater than 6 mm in width is unusual.

For multiple implants, the osteotomies often coalesce, leading to a separation of the labial and palatal cortical plates along the length of the ridge (Fig 12-17). However, the continuity of the crestal bone does not extend to the base. Separate osteotomies are made, with the bone condensers providing the primary stability and individual positioning that is required by the implants (Figs 12-18 and 12-19). This is because cancellous bone is manipulated into the interimplant space by the bone condensers.

### Pilot Bone Condenser

The pilot bone condenser is inserted to a depth determined by the diagnostic procedures, and the direction of the insertion follows that established by the site marker. It will also direct itself between the cortical plates without perforating them.

Should resistance be met, identified by a sharper sound or resistance to insertion, the use of this instrument should be terminated. Further development of the site with bone expanders should be carried out before continuing with the pilot bone condenser.

The pilot bone condenser widens the osteotomy to enable the first of the bone condensers to be inserted without damaging the thin crestal bone. All bone condensers are removed by rotational movements.

Where the bone density is high, excessive force would have to be used to prepare the osteotomy and here a pilot osteotomy bur (Lindemann bur) may be used to determine the depth of the osteotomy. The bur follows in the direction previously determined by the site marker or pilot bone condenser. This procedure

III    Augmentation

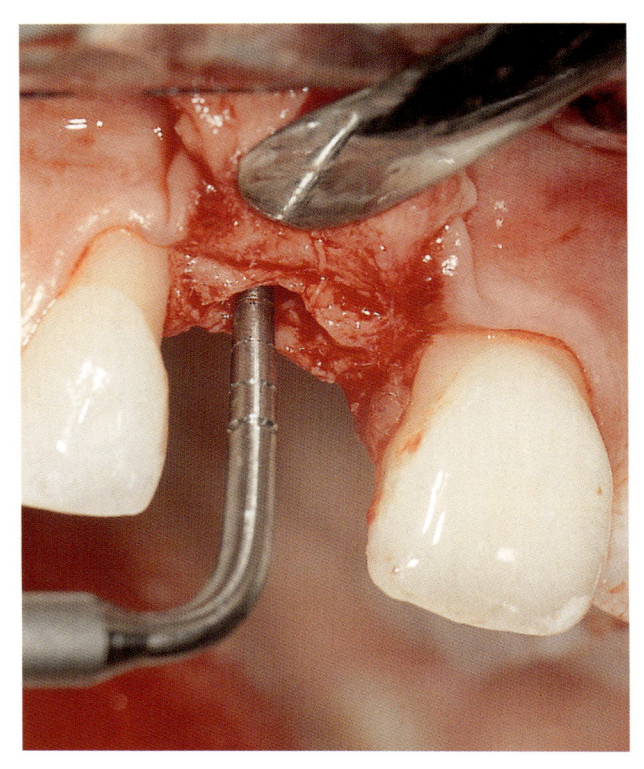

**Fig 12-20** A probe is used following each instrument to ensure that the integrity of the prepared socket has not been compromised.

should only be carried out if there is adequate width in the apical region into which the osteotomy may need to be extended. The pilot bone condenser must not be used to manipulate the sinus or nasal floors because of the risk of perforation. It is prudent to prepare the depth of the osteotomy to approximately 2 mm longer than the length of the selected implant. This will allow the implant to be seated accurately according to the prosthetic needs and will provide room for manoeuvre without the need to remove the implant and enlarge the osteotomy where insertion at a greater depth becomes necessary.

### Pilot Osteotomy Bur (if necessary)

The pilot osteotomy bur is aligned with the bone condenser, which is then removed, and the bur is introduced into the osteotomy site before drilling is started in order to prevent damage to the crestal bone. The bur is used to establish the depth of the osteotomy and is inserted to a predetermined depth established from the diagnostic procedures. The pilot osteotomy bur is internally irrigated.

### Osteotomy Probe

The osteotomy probe is inserted each time a different instrument has been used; its function is twofold: (a) to ensure that the osteotomy walls have not been fractured or perforated and (b) to confirm the depth of the osteotomy (Fig 12-20).

### Bone Condensers

Bone condensers are a series of titanium alloy instruments with a round cross-section that correspond to various implant diameters. They are used in sequence beyond the predetermined depth, as described above (Fig 12-15). Ridge expansion using the bone condensers is stopped when resistance to expansion is met, as determined by acoustic and manual feedback. Alternative instruments, as described above, are used to complete the osteotomy. The implant of selected diameter and length can then be inserted (Fig 12-16).

### Implant Insertion

The implant is mounted on to the long-handled implant driver (Ankylos) and judiciously inserted into the osteotomy to prevent damage to the fragile marginal bone of the osteotomy. It is then tapped lightly with a mallet until the cutting flutes are below the crest of the ridge (Fig 12-21). Finally, the implant is rotated until it is below the level of the crest of the ridge. The depth will need to be confirmed using direction indicators. However, judgements based on the angle of the abutment and the pivot point likely to be used will assist in positioning the implant at the correct level at this stage.

### Direction Indicators

Direction indicators are used to select the correct angled abutment and to position the implant precisely for the correct emergence profile (Figs 12-22 and 12-23). The implant may also need to be rotated to increase or decrease its depth. The direction indicator should ideally be in line with the adjacent teeth or other abutments and should fit within the prosthetic envelope defined by the diagnostic template.[6,7,204]

12 Bone Expansion

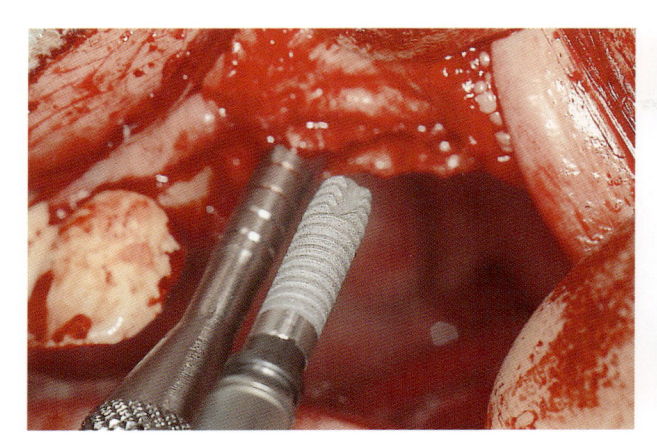

**Fig 12-21** The implant is inserted directly as the bone condenser is removed to prevent the separated ridges from collapsing.

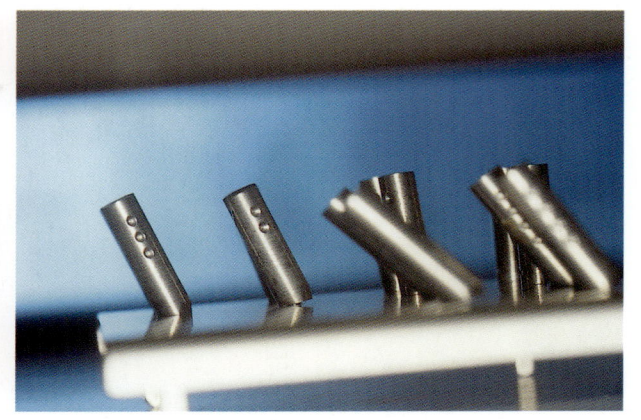

**Fig 12-22** A series of prototype direction indicators used to select abutments and measure the angle between the long axes of the implant and the long axes of the proposed restoration as indicated by the prosthetic envelope.

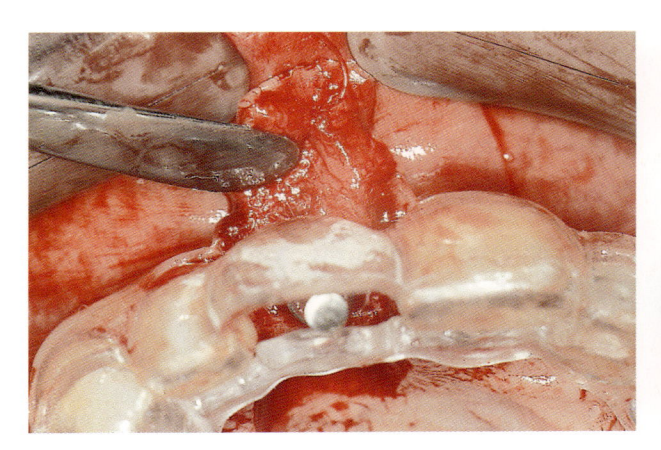

**Fig 12-23** Occlusal view of a diagnostic template being used to select the abutment at the time of implant placement.

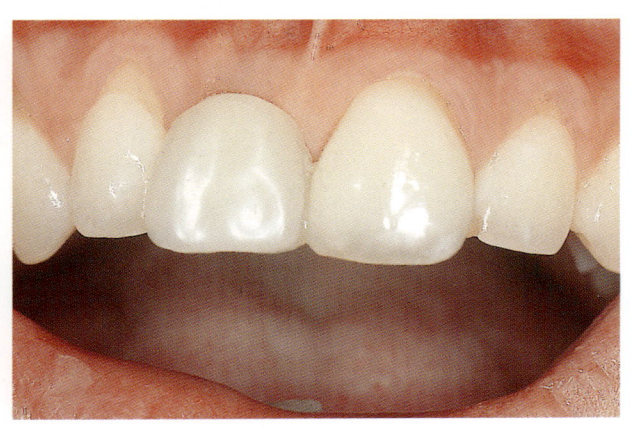

**Fig 12-24** Labial view of the metal-acrylic Rochette bridge fitted after implant placement. Note that the ridge has been contoured favourably and the pontic has had to be modified to allow for this.

### Impression at First-stage Surgery

Impressions may be taken at this stage, as described above.

### Wound Closure

Dense hydroxyapatite (OsteoGraf D-300 or D-700) may be used under the flap. Some of this material will become incorporated into the surface of the bone and the remainder into the soft tissue, thus forming a thick fibrous layer below the gingival margin. The intention is to reduce the incidence of gingival recession around the neck of the abutment. The wound is closed, using sutures, once the flap is accurately repositioned applying finger pressure to the labial aspect of the ridge.

### Provisional Restoration

The provisional restoration is modified before it is fitted to ensure that there is no blanching, indicative of pressure, of the expanded ridge when it is seated. Fitting the provisional restoration will show the amount of augmentation that has been achieved (Fig 12-24) and will also give an indication of what the final restoration will be like in terms of gingival contours.

III   Augmentation

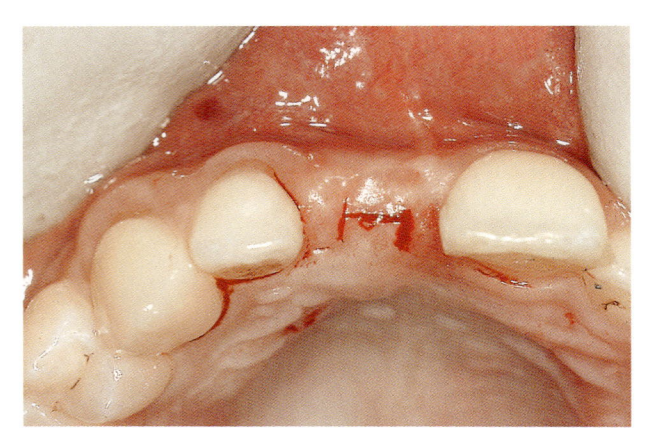

**Fig 12-25** Occlusal view of the healed site at the time of exposure. An 'H'-shaped incision is used to expose the implant. The crossbar of the H is positioned more towards the palatal aspect of the implant. This will enable further repositioning of the soft tissues to create an ideal emergence profile.

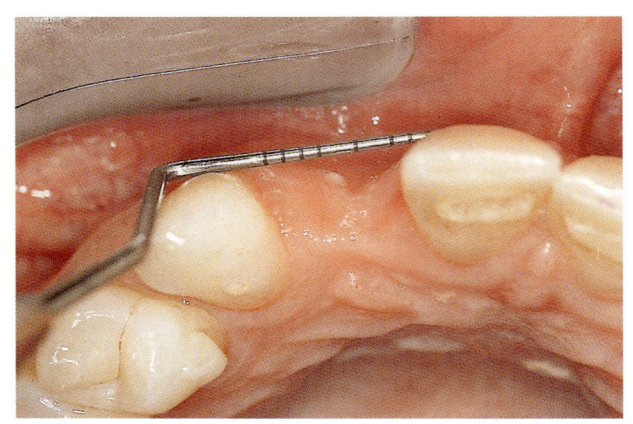

**Fig 12-26** Occlusal view of a ridge with collapsed labial plate following tooth loss. The extent of the depression is visible, and a poor aesthetic result would be obtained without re-contouring the ridge.

## Healing Phase

When expansion of narrow ridges is carried out, it is not considered appropriate to immediately load implants inserted using this technique. This is because the load-bearing capacity of the displaced labial plate may be reduced. However, where minor labial re-contouring has been carried out, immediate loading may be considered as long as the primary stability has been achieved and other criteria, such as the type of incision, permit immediate loading.

The implant is allowed to heal for a period of up to six months to allow osseointegration to take place. The provisional restoration is used as a point of reference from which the changes in soft tissue contours can be monitored. This will assist in the planning of second-stage surgery.

## Implant Exposure

The type of incision required is based on the assessment of the soft tissue carried out following the healing phase (Fig 12-25). The protocols described in Chapter 9 are used to develop the emergence profile. Incisions are utilised to manipulate tissues either to increase the bulk of the labial gingiva or to create papillae.

The definitive abutment, selected at first-stage surgery, may now be attached to the implant. Care should be taken when using angled abutments to ensure that the incision is made in the region where the abutment should emerge. This should allow for any soft tissue manipulation as well as the shape of the transitional restoration. The transitional restoration can be used to further develop the soft tissues and may be extended below the gingiva to achieve this.

## Restorative Phase

The restorative phase is completed according to the guidelines outlined in Chapter 10. Preference is given to cement-retained restorations made from impressions taken at first-stage surgery for single units and conventional impressions for multiple units.

## Bone Expansion: Clinical Cases

### Case 1:
### Bone Expansion for Re-contouring the Labial Plate

The procedure is illustrated in Figs 12-26–12-30.

12  Bone Expansion

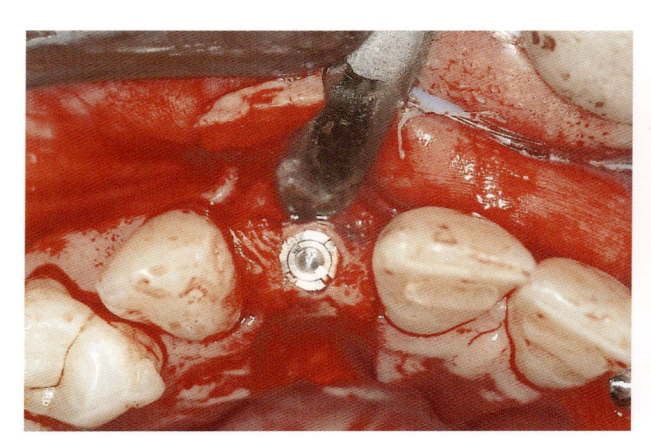

**Fig 12-27**  Occlusal view of the implant in situ following ridge expansion, which was completed using a Lindemann (pilot) bur followed by bone condensers. The re-contoured labial plate can be seen.

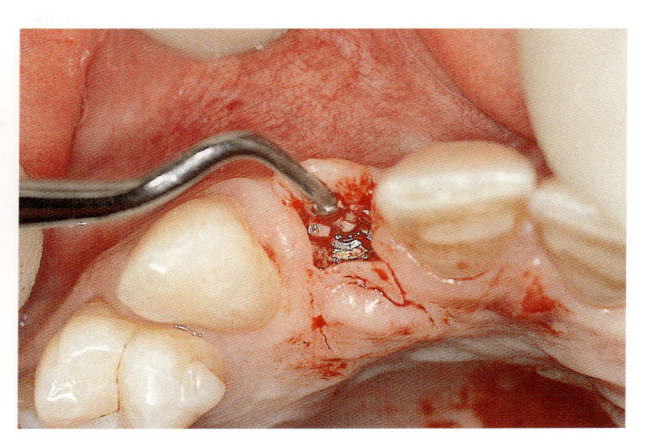

**Fig 12-28**  Occlusal view of the 'H'-shaped incision being used to expose the implant six months after it was placed. The 'H'-shaped incision is used for the manipulation of the soft tissues towards the labial to further compensate for the labial plate collapse.

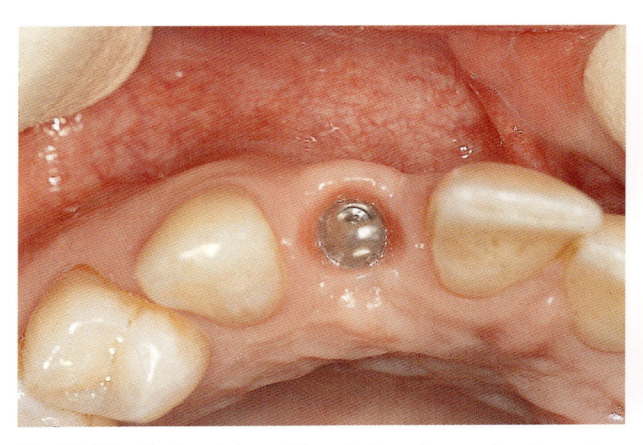

**Fig 12-29**  Occlusal view of the abutment emerging through the healed soft tissues one month after it was fitted at the time of exposure. Note the re-contoured soft tissues. Conventional impressions were taken for the construction of the definitive restoration.

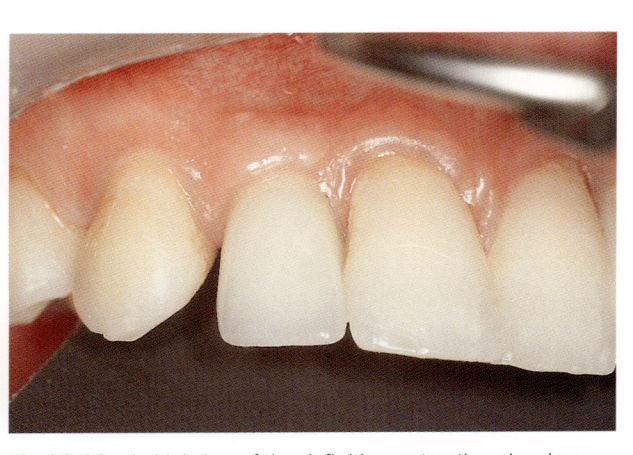

**Fig 12-30**  Labial view of the definitive restoration showing good tooth form and position as well as a satisfactory emergence profile.

## Case 2:
## Bone Expansion for a Single Implant

The procedure is illustrated in Figs 12-31–12-53.

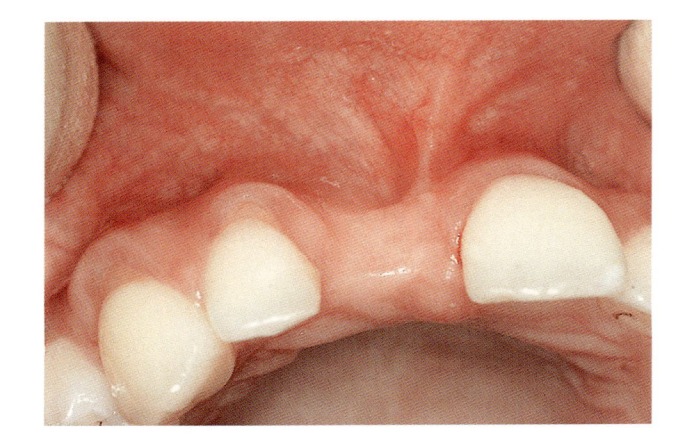

**Fig 12-31**  Occlusal view of a maxillary ridge six months following the loss of the central incisor. A severe resorption of the labial plate has taken place.

231

III Augmentation

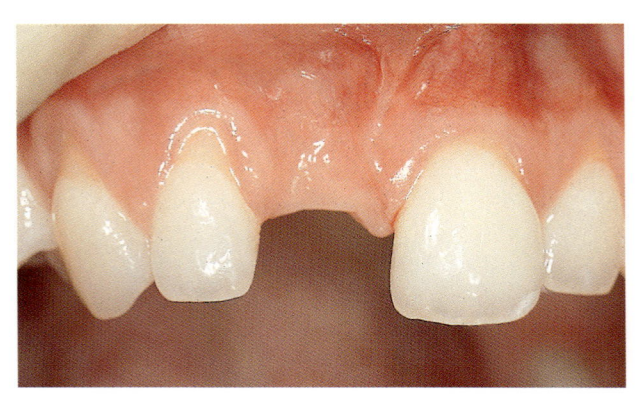

**Fig 12-32** Labial view of the healed ridge showing adequate height. The level of the soft tissues is consistent with that of the adjacent papillae. Note the gingival marginal level around the lateral incisor, which is indicative of this patient's predisposition to gingival recession.

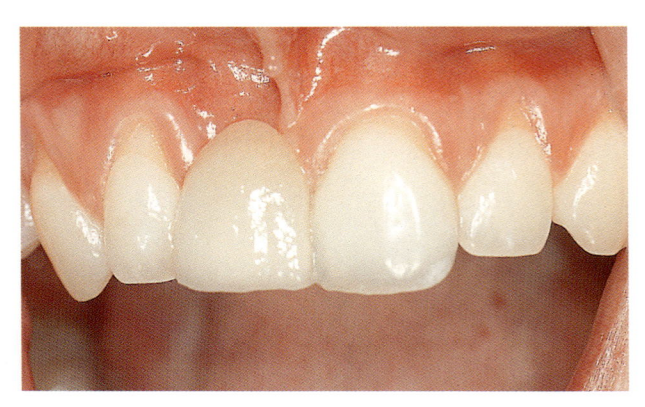

**Fig 12-33** The use of a metal-acrylic resin Rochette bridge to assess the aesthetic outcome prior to the commencement of treatment. A ridge width increase of approximately 2 mm is estimated. The Rochette is also used for functional verification of the selected tooth position.

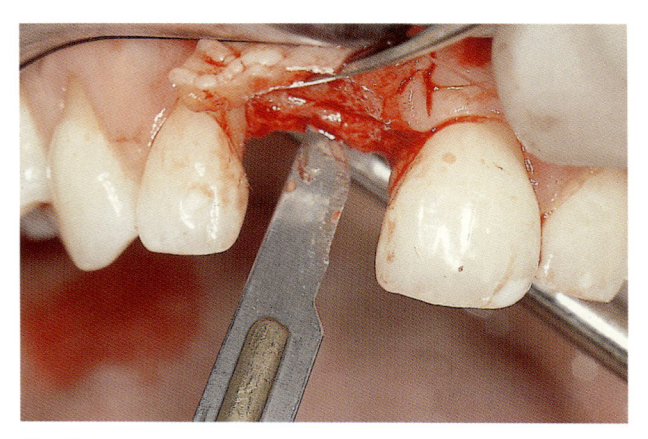

**Fig 12-34** The ridge is exposed via a remote palatal incision and a scalpel is used to define the plane along which the bone expansion is to be carried out.

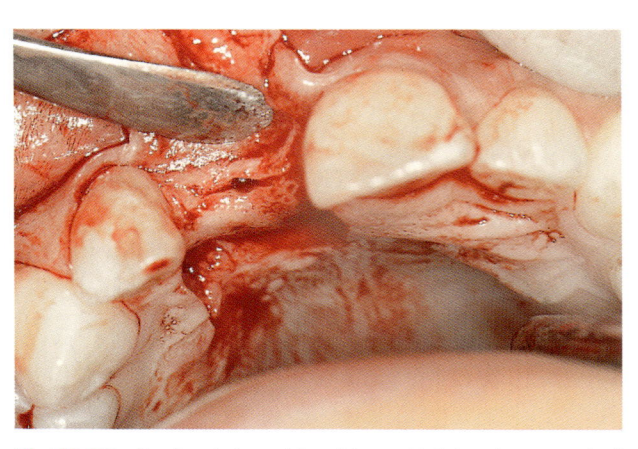

**Fig 12-35** Occlusal view of the ridge, which has been marked using a scalpel and a position marker. Note the width of the ridge (2 mm at the crest) in comparison with the width of the adjacent teeth (7 mm).

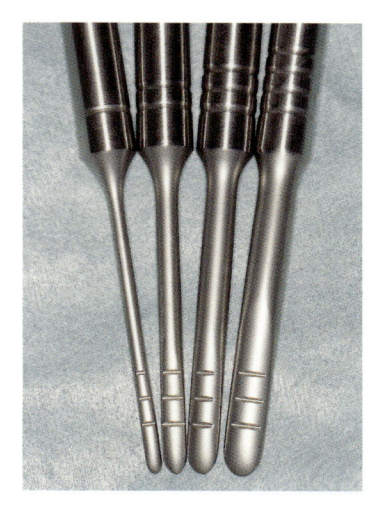

**Fig 12-36** Series of four bone expanders with marks at 10, 15 and 20 mm to enable the depth of insertion to be gauged. The 'D'-shaped cross-section of the four instruments of increasing width is visible.

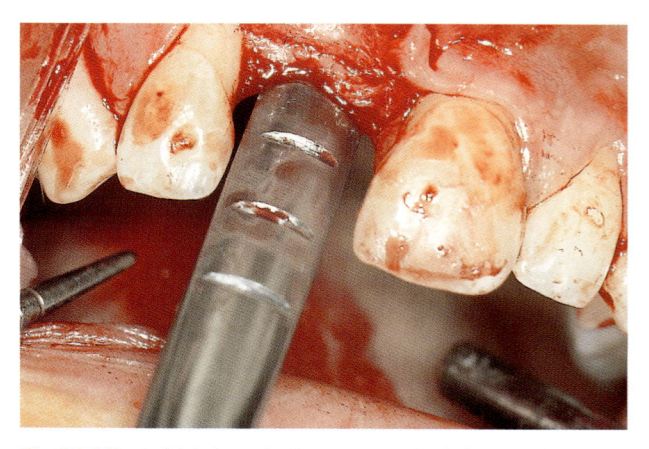

**Fig 12-37** Labial view of a bone expander being used to separate the cortical plates.

12  Bone Expansion

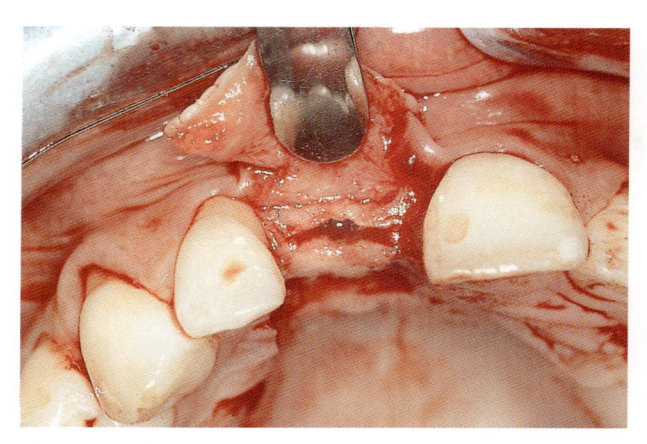

**Fig 12-38**  Occlusal view of the ridge with the separation created by the bone expander.

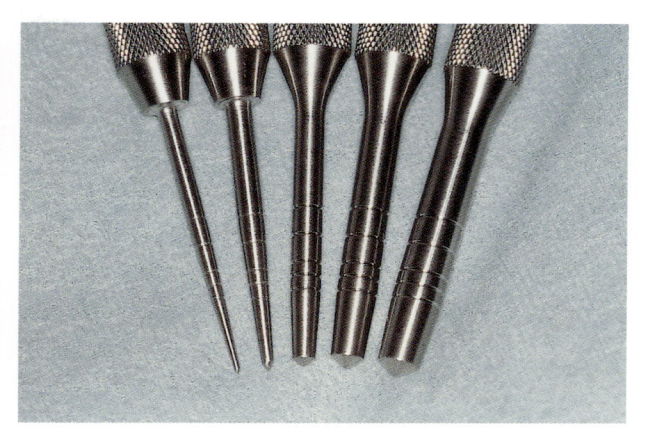

**Fig 12-39**  Series of five bone condensers (Ankylos implant system). The position marker is visible on the left-hand side and has a sharp tip to enable a site to be marked. Adjacent to this instrument is the pilot bone condenser and the remaining condensers, which are matched to implant diameter and length for the range of implants available within the Ankylos system. These correspond to diameters of 3.5, 4.5 and 5.5 mm.

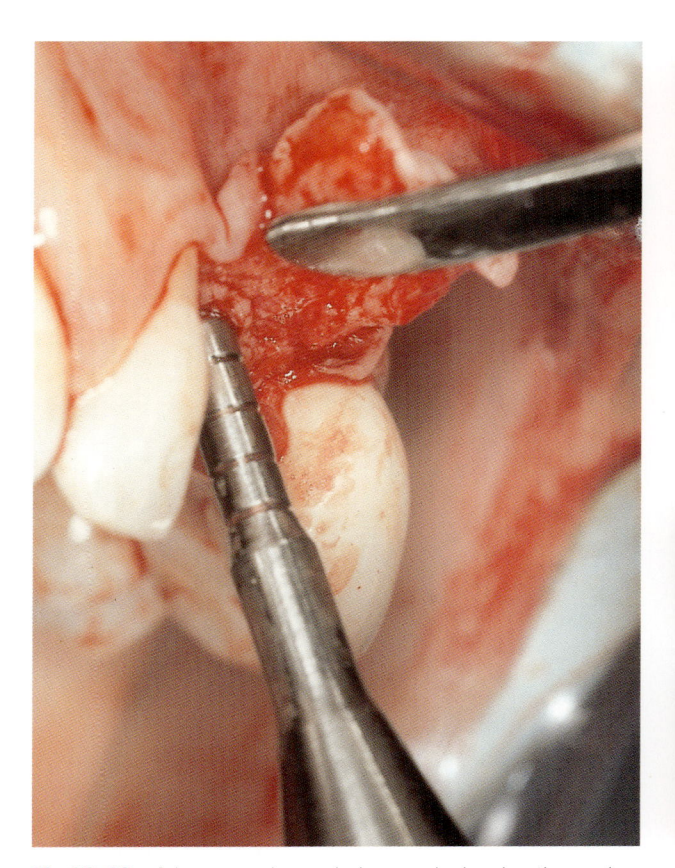

**Fig 12-40**  A bone condenser being used, showing the angle at which the osteotomy is being prepared between the separated cortical plates.

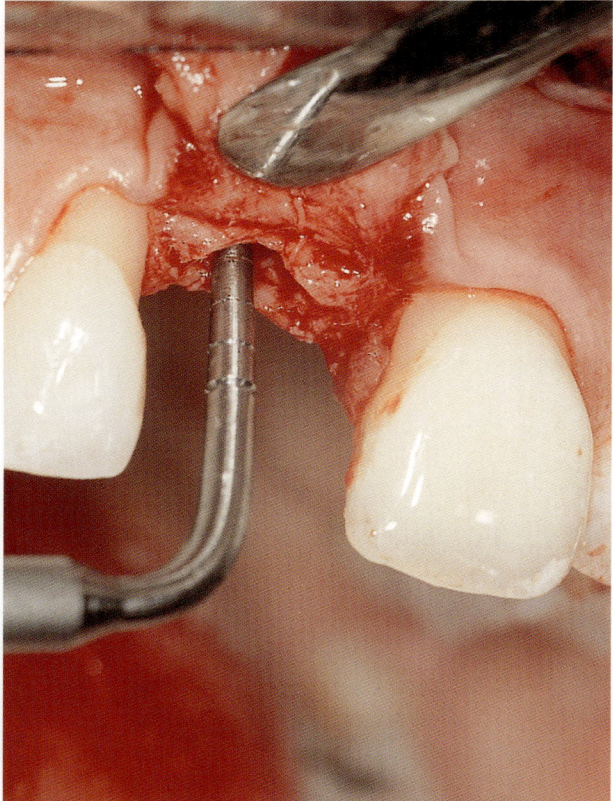

**Fig 12-41**  A probe is used following each instrument to ensure that the integrity of the prepared socket has not been compromised.

III   Augmentation

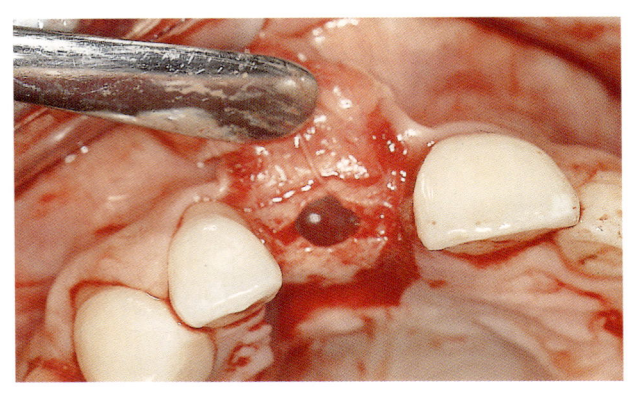

**Fig 12-42**  Occlusal view of the ridge following the completion of the osteotomy prior to implant insertion. Note the labial displacement of the collapsed cortical plate.

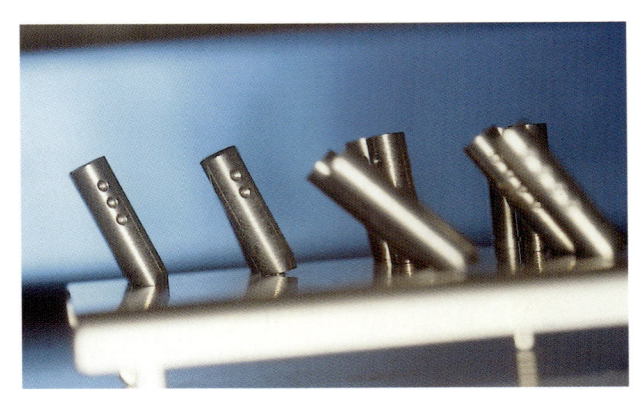

**Fig 12-43**  Series of prototype direction indicators used to select abutments and measure the angle between the long axes of the implant and the long axes of the proposed restoration as indicated by the prosthetic envelope.

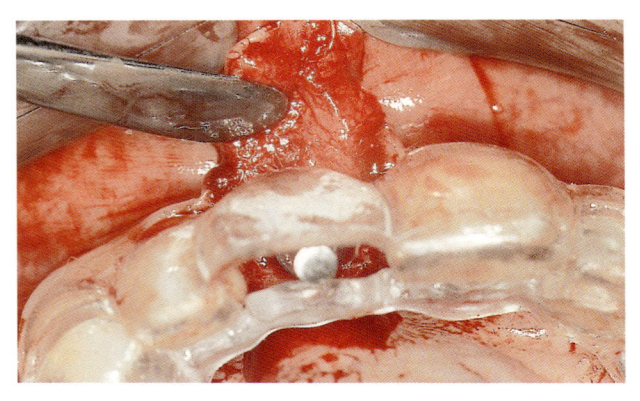

**Fig 12-44**  Occlusal view of a diagnostic template being used to select the abutment at the time of implant placement.

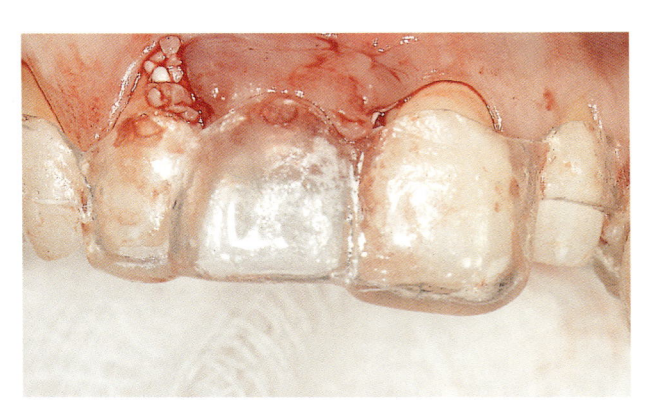

**Fig 12-45**  Labial view of the diagnostic template being used to assess the established contour. Supplementary hydroxyapatite particles (Osteograf 700 µm) are used to stabilise the soft tissues against future recession.

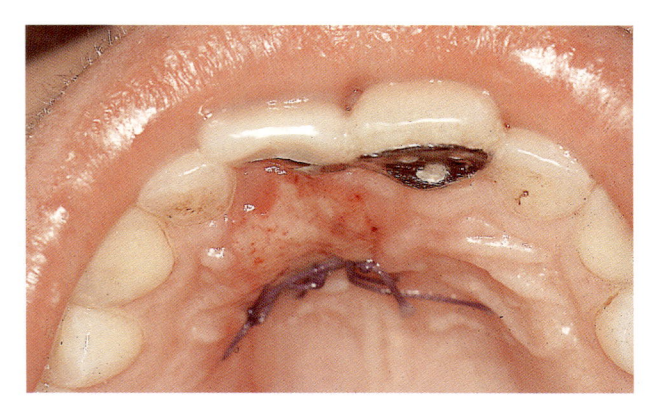

**Fig 12-46**  Occlusal view of the palate one week after surgery, showing the healing of the soft tissues. Note the area of secondary healing with a small region of loss of epithelium, which may sometimes occur with remote palatal incisions.

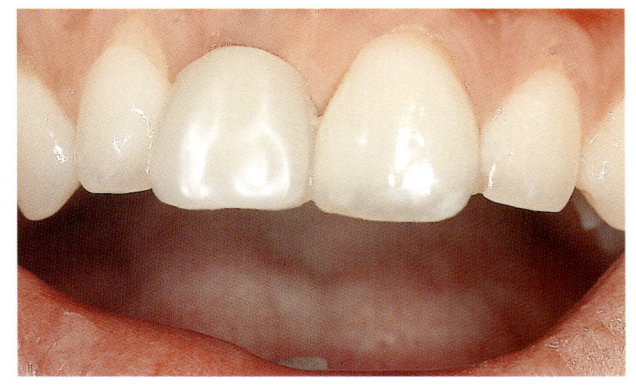

**Fig 12-47**  Labial view of the metal-acrylic Rochette bridge fitted after implant placement. Note that the ridge has been contoured favourably and the pontic has had to be modified to allow for this.

## 12  Bone Expansion

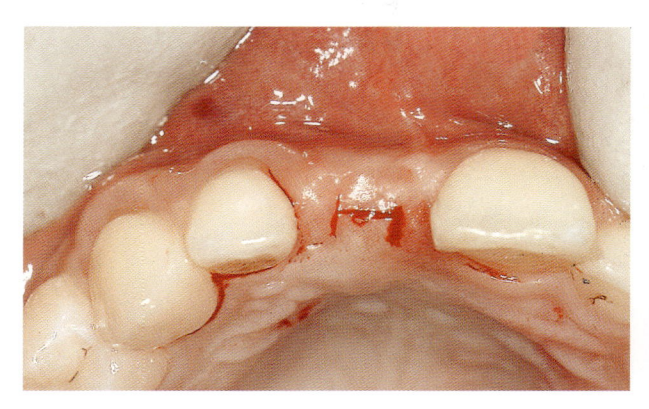

**Fig 12-48**  Occlusal view of the healed site at the time of exposure. An 'H'-shaped incision is used to expose the implant. The crossbar of the 'H' is positioned more towards the palatal aspect of the implant. This will enable further repositioning of the soft tissues to create an ideal emergence profile.

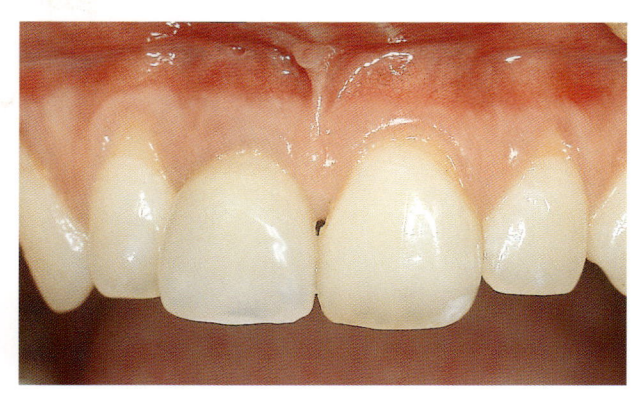

**Fig 12-49**  Labial view of the acrylic resin transitional restoration constructed from an impression and taken at first-stage surgery. The transitional restoration was fitted at the time of exposure directly onto the preselected customised abutment.

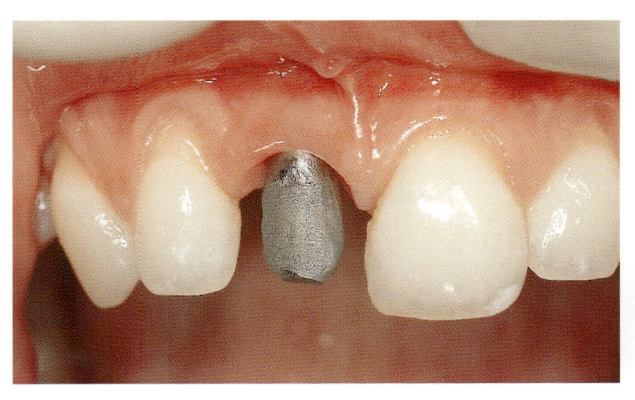

**Fig 12-50**  Labial view of the metal coping at the time of impressions. Note the soft tissue contours established by the transitional restoration. This information will be transferred to the laboratory to enable the porcelain to be added to support the established contours.

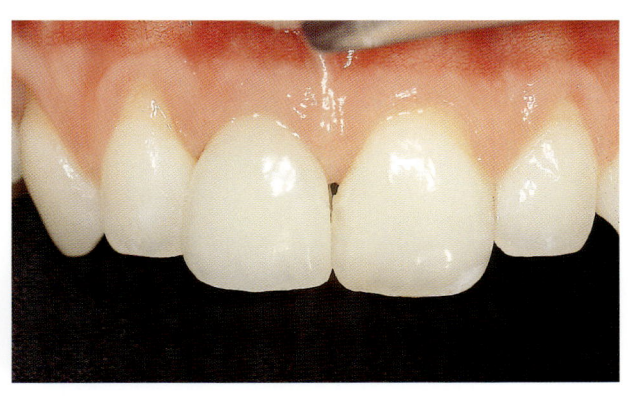

**Fig 12-51**  Labial view of the definitive metal-ceramic restoration showing the re-established labial contours, good tooth position, form and colour and a harmonious emergence profile.

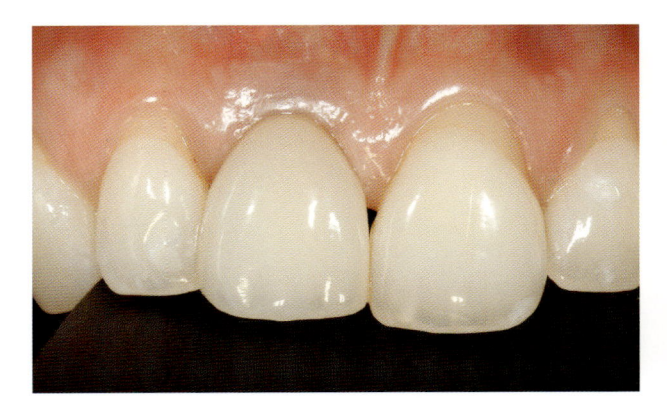

**Fig 12-52**  The labial view 10 years after the procedure, showing stable soft tissues resulting from the use of hydroxyapatite at the time of implant placement. Changes in the incisal tip level are evident and result from ongoing facial development. Note also the ongoing recession around the natural teeth in this patient, who had a thin bony and soft tissue biotype.

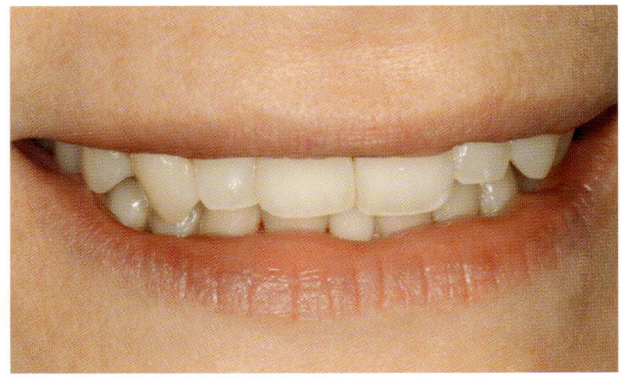

**Fig 12-53**  The patient smiling, demonstrating the exposure of the incisors.

# III  Augmentation

## Case 3:
## Bone Expansion for Multiple Implants

The procedure is illustrated in Figs 12-54–12-61.

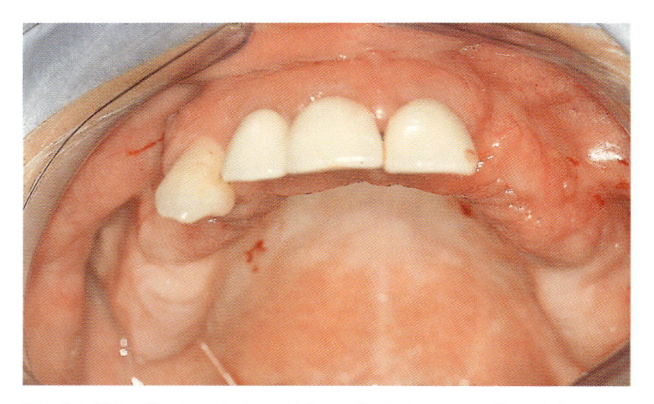

**Fig 12-54** Occlusal view of the edentulous maxillary ridges, which are apparently of sufficient width.

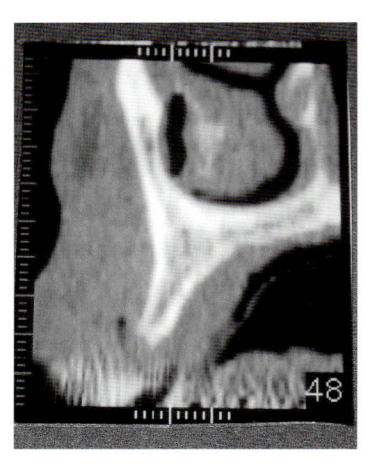

**Fig 12-55** Oblique cross-sectional view of a CT scan showing the narrow maxillary ridge present under the mucosa. A ridge width of approximately 2 mm can be measured. Note the thickness of the soft tissue on the palatal aspect of the ridge, which is visible on the right-hand side of the image.

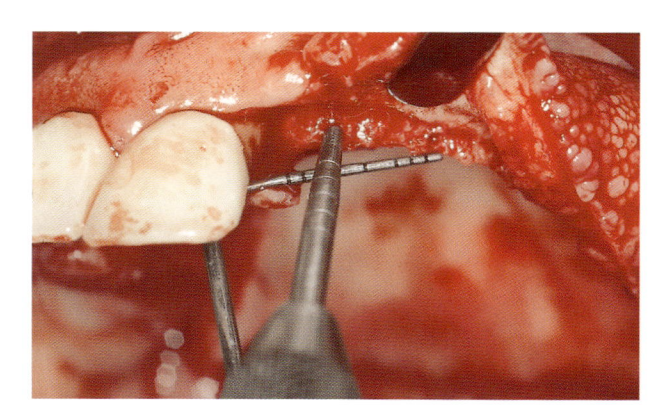

**Fig 12-56** Intraoperative image of the left maxillary ridge showing the selection of sites. The lateral incisor is positioned 4 mm from the central incisor and the canine is positioned 7 mm from the lateral incisor to provide adequate interdental spacing. The position marker can be seen marking the implant site as well as establishing the direction of the osteotomy between the cortical plates.

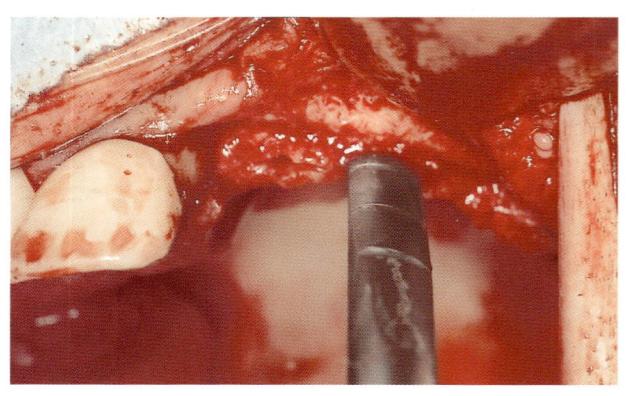

**Fig 12-57** Clinical view of a bone expander being used to separate the thin cortical plates.

12 Bone Expansion

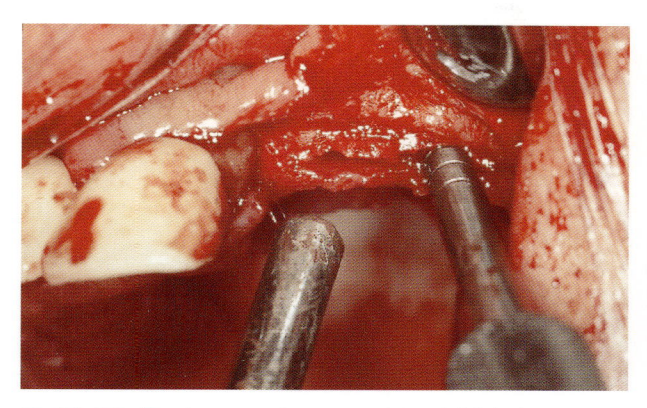

**Fig 12-58** The bone condenser used to establish the osteotomy for each implant to ensure that primary stability can be achieved.

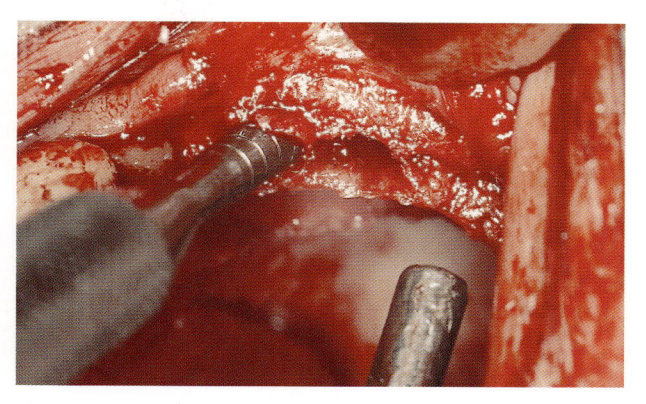

**Fig 12-59** The development of adjacent osteotomies results in a separation of the cortical plates in the coronal aspect of the ridge. The bone condensers, however, produce osteotomies within the maxillary ridge, which are specific to implant position.

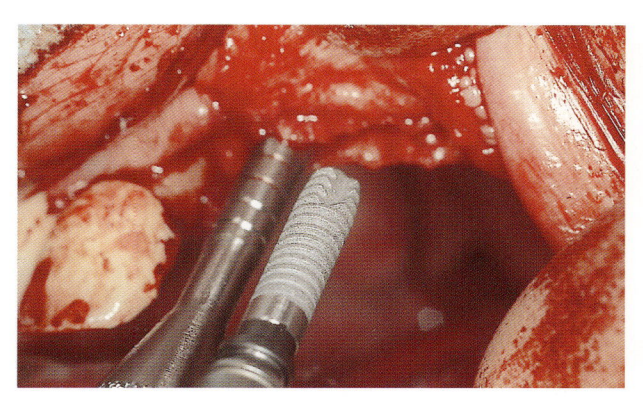

**Fig 12-60** The implant is inserted directly as the bone condenser is removed to prevent the separated ridges from collapsing.

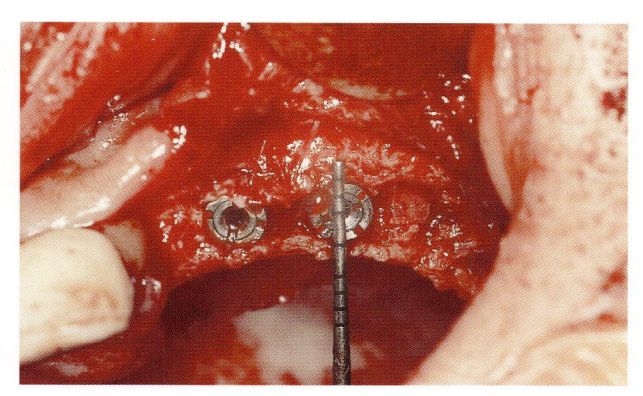

**Fig 12-61** Occlusal view of the expanded ridge showing the separation of the cortical plates and the presence of trabecular bone between the implants within the separated cortical plates. A 6-mm ridge width has been achieved.

# Chapter 13

# Localised Onlay Bone Grafts

## Introduction

Autogenous onlay block grafts are required to reconstruct a minor deficiency of the alveolar ridge for aesthetic and/or biomechanical reasons. The likely causes of minor deficiencies are:
- congenital deficiencies: caused by congenitally missing single teeth
- disuse atrophy: caused by tooth loss, which is likely to be more pronounced in specific biotypes
- minor trauma: leading to tooth loss and possibly alveolar bone loss
- infection: caused by localised periodontal issues, endodontic failures, fractured roots or failed implants and bone grafts.

## Assessment of Localised Bone Deficiency

Assessment of the residual ridge should be carried out as described above, using appropriate diagnostic measures. The quantity of bone should be measured in relation to the future position of the tooth. Local bone deficiencies may be classified very simply according to practical requirements (Fig 13-1):

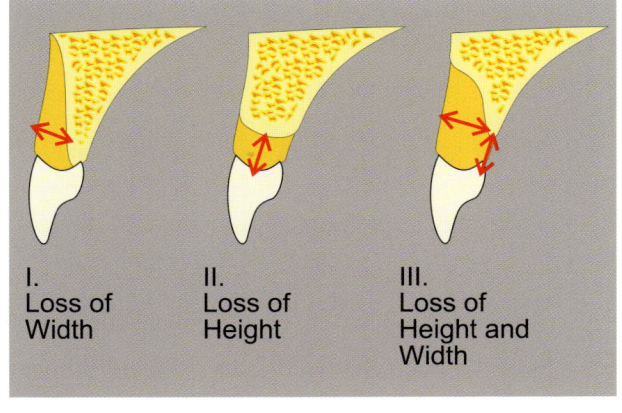

**Fig 13-1** Classification of bone deficiencies based on the type of defect, namely height, width or height and width.

- loss of width
- loss of height
- loss of height and width.

For larger deficiencies, the volume of bone that needs to be replaced must also be assessed in relation to any of the available classifications of jaw atrophy that the clinician is familiar with. This will be dealt with in a separate chapter (Chapter 14). The type of bone reconstruction and the position of the bone graft will influence the design of the flap used to ensure wound closure.

III   Augmentation

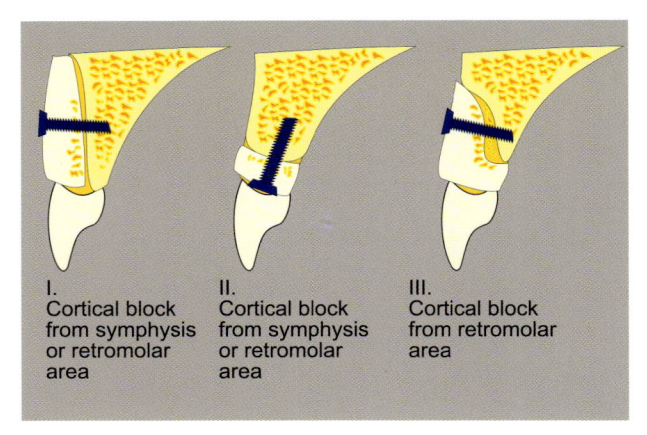

**Fig 13-2** The type of graft required for the correction of the three types of deficiency illustrated by the classification in Fig 13-1. Screws are illustrated here as the primary form of fixation, to prevent micro-movement and sequestration of the graft.

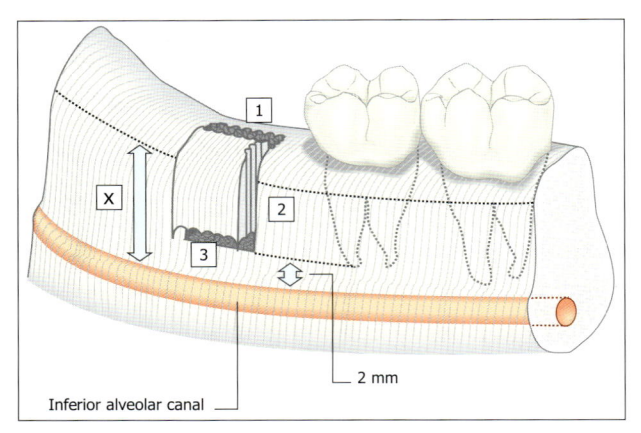

**Fig 13-3** The harvesting of a bone graft from the ramus (lateral aspect). Measurements, clinical and radiographic, must be made from the external oblique ridge. A clearance of 2 mm from the inferior alveolar canal must be allowed. In addition, compensation for any distortion of the radiograph must be made. Bone cuts must not be extended beyond the critical depth X (see also Fig 13-6).

### Loss of Width

Deficiencies in ridge width may be corrected using bone from either of the two intraoral donor sites: the ramus or the symphysis (Fig 13-2, I).

Sufficient bone can usually be obtained from each ramus for up to four implants and from the symphysis for four implants. An increase in width of 2–6 mm can be achieved with bone from the ramus and between 2 and 6 mm with bone from the symphysis. This, however, depends on the actual anatomy of the region, the assessment of which will be covered in a subsequent section (Figs 13-3–13-5).

### Loss of Height

Sufficient bone for up to four implants can be harvested from the symphysis and for up to four implants from each ramus. An increase in height of up to 4 mm can usually be achieved (Fig 13-2, II).

### Loss of Width and Height

Although it is possible on occasion to use the symphysis to increase height and width, its morphology does not always lend itself to the 3D reconstruction of a deficient ridge. The ramus with its external oblique ridge, however, is ideally shaped to provide a graft that will reconstruct a ridge deficiency (Fig 13-2, III). Typically, it is possible to achieve an increase in width of up to 6 mm and an increase in height of 4 mm. Each ramus will provide sufficient bone to construct the ridge for two implants. The local morphology of the ramus will, of course, need to be assessed carefully.

Careful assessment of the width of the entire alveolar ridge must be made in order to ensure that sufficient bone is available to extend the graft towards the basal part of the ridge should the entire alveolar ridge be insufficient in width. This will influence the selection of the donor site.

Where the tooth is present, certain indicators will determine the likelihood of having to use bone grafts prior to or at the time of extraction of the tooth. Loss of more than half of the labial plate increases the likelihood of a bone graft being necessary, particularly where aesthetics are critical. Loss of palatal bone is a significant indicator for a deficiency in height, requiring a bone graft.

Assessment of the adjacent teeth and the interdental bone level must not be overlooked as bone can only be built up to or marginally above the level of bone attachment of the adjacent teeth. This is because the graft must not be in direct contact with the tooth.

## Assessment of Donor Site

### Symphysis

Assessment of the symphysis as a donor site is carried out radiographically, using panoramic radiographs and lateral cephalographs following correction for magnification. A clearance of 5 mm below the tips of the roots is advised to minimise the risk of damage or the interruption of sensory innervation. The position of the canine root tips should be established accurately if extensive grafts are going to be required. The lower limit of the graft should not extend beyond the maximum convexity of the mental process in order to maintain the patient's facial profile (Fig 13-4).

### Ramus

A panoramic radiograph is used for the assessment of the ramus in conjunction with a physical examination of the external oblique ridge. When CT is available, interpretation of the distance between the inferior alveolar ridge and the external oblique ridge should be undertaken, but with caution as the orientation of the cross-sectional images may not be perpendicular to the external oblique ridge or the inferior alveolar canal. This would give an incorrect measurement of the distance between the two structures. The position of the inferior alveolar nerve in the bucco-lingual dimension is useful information that can be obtained from this investigation.

Other factors that should be taken into account are:

- all measurements must be made from the external oblique ridge and not the alveolar ridge (Fig 13-3); the height of the bone available for harvesting will affect the size of the surface area of the recipient site that can be covered
- the presence of wisdom teeth will limit the width and length of the bone graft that can be obtained
- the width between the external oblique ridge and the lingual wall of the mandible will also determine the width of the bone graft that can be harvested (Figs 13-5 and 13-6).

### Extraoral Sites

When insufficient bone is available at one or more intraoral donor sites an extraoral donor site should be considered (Chapter 14).

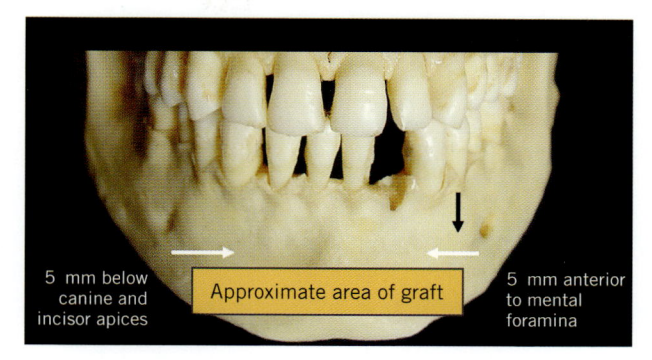

**Fig 13-4** Anterior view of the mandible outlining the area where a graft can safely be harvested, depending upon the local anatomical limitations.

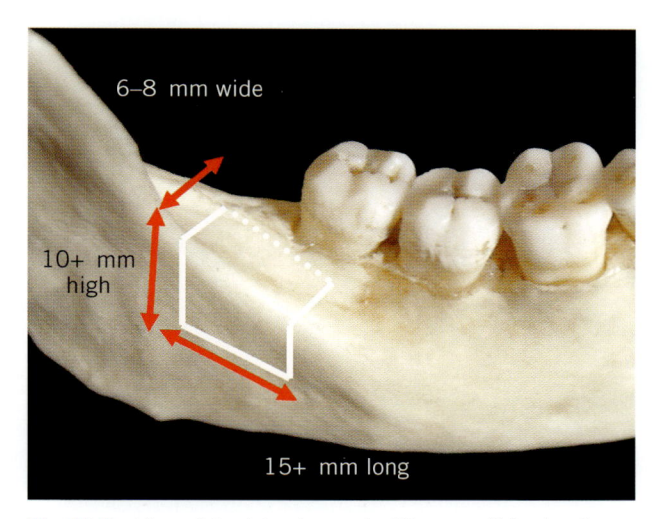

**Fig 13-5** View of the lateral aspect of the mandible showing the typical dimensions for a graft designed to correct a deficiency in height and width (Class III).

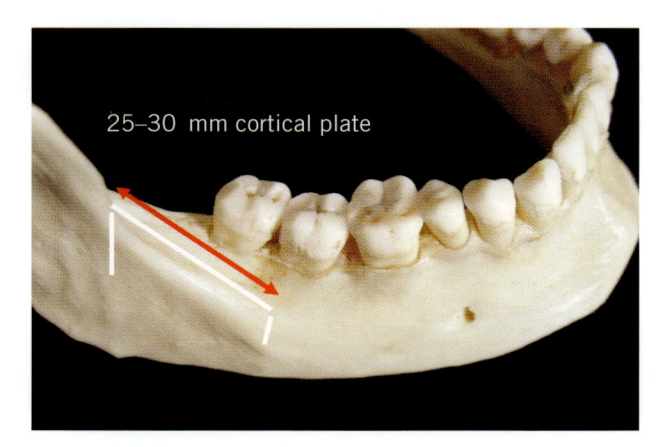

**Fig 13-6** Lateral aspect of the mandible showing the typical dimensions of a graft designed to correct a deficiency in either width or height (Class I or II). Generally deficiencies requiring repair for up to four implants can repaired.

## III  Augmentation

Table 13-1  Sequencing of treatment

| Step | Sequence |
|---|---|
| 1 | Extraction (assessment) |
| 2 | Soft tissue healing (8–12 weeks) |
| 3 | Recipient site: incision, reflection, measurement |
| 4 | Donor site: incision, reflection, marking |
| 5 | Harvest graft (oversized) |
| 6 | Fit graft (modify graft and recipient site) |
| 7 | Fix graft (screw or plate) |
| 8 | Close recipient site (advance soft tissue) |
| 9 | Close donor site |
| 10 | Assess bone healing (radiograph); remodelling: 2–4 months, up to 6 months for membrane |
| 11 | Implant insertion into grafted and recipient bone (3–6-month integration period), assess for soft tissue surgery |
| 12 | Corrective soft tissue surgery if necessary (2–4 months after implant insertion) |
| 13 | Expose |
| 14 | Corrective soft tissue surgery if necessary |
| 15 | Soft tissue healing (4 weeks) |
| 16 | Restore |

## Treatment Sequence

Treatment can be started on a healed site once the diagnostic procedures have been completed, providing that the mouth is free of disease.

Following extraction and where a bone graft is anticipated, a period of 8 to 12 weeks should be allowed for soft tissue healing and adequate blood supply to establish. Completion of healing should be monitored, and the mucosa covering the ridge should be free of depressions and fissures. This period may be used to confirm the need for a bone graft based on radiographic examination and the appearance of the provisional restoration in relation to the gingival tissues. Flowchart 13-1 summarises the main criteria that can be used to assess the need for a bone graft.

Where there is uncertainty about the need for a bone graft, a healing period of six months allows the bone to mature sufficiently that an appropriate decision can be made. Assessment can then be made as to whether conventional placement or bone expansion is possible. The likelihood of healing is much higher where the labial cortical plates are thicker and is likely to be poorer where thin vestibular cortical bone overlies prominent roots with interdental depressions. In the latter, patients often have scalloped gingival contours, whereas patients with thick labial cortical plates generally have flat gingival contours. The sequence of treatment is shown in Table 13-1.

## Surgical Protocol

The preoperative assessment should have determined the amount of bone that will be required and have identified a potential donor site. Based on the information gained, a decision regarding the type of incision has to have been made before starting surgery to ensure closure without tension over the graft. This will also be influenced by which region of the mouth is being treated.

### Access to Recipient Site

Surgery is started at the recipient site in order to identify the precise shape of the graft that will be required and to measure the dimensions of the deficiency. Once the recipient site has been prepared, donor-site surgery can be started and the bone harvested and transferred to the recipient site within a minimum period of time.

### Maxilla

The most common bone deficiency of the maxilla occurs on the labial aspect of the ridge. A remote palatal incision is used to expose the deficiency in the ridge and labial aspect of the maxilla (Fig 13-7). If the loss of bone is on the palatal aspect of the maxilla, a palatal incision must not be used. A crestal or labial incision is indicated under these circumstances (Figs 13-8–13-13).

Access to the ridge is gained via a remote palatal incision made approximately 1 cm from the crest of the ridge. The perpendicular component of the incision into the palate is made with a number 15 blade in a conventional handle. The incision is extended within the cervical margin to the distal papilla of the adjacent teeth. A vertical release incision on the labial aspect, one tooth away from the recipient site, is made to include the papilla. The vertical release incision is extended into the unattached mucosa. The palatal incision parallel to the crest is made with a Blake's knife (blade number 15)

**13** Localised Onlay Bone Grafts

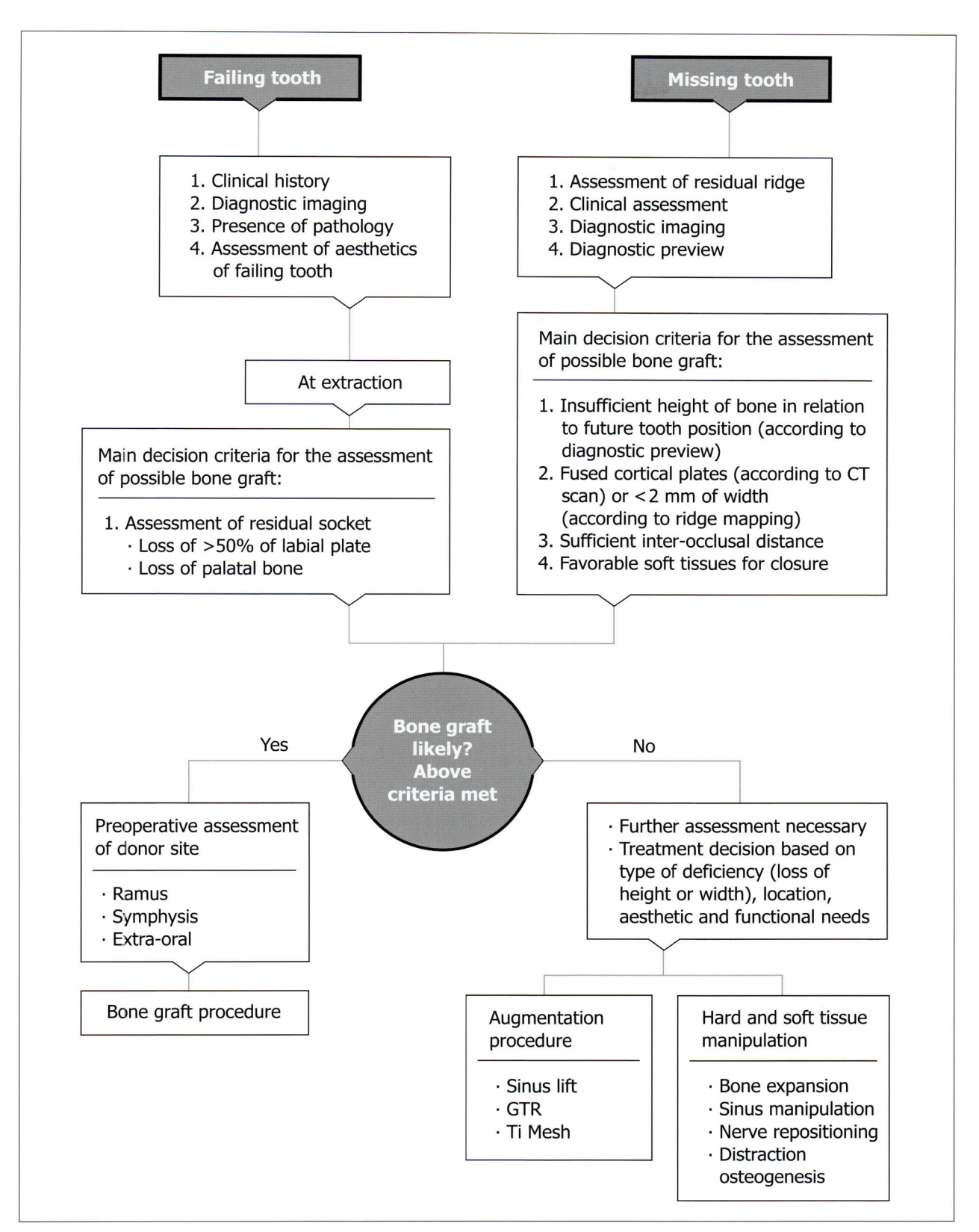

## Failing tooth

1. Clinical history
2. Diagnostic imaging
3. Presence of pathology
4. Assessment of aesthetics of failing tooth

At extraction

Main decision criteria for the assessment of possible bone graft:

1. Assessment of residual socket
   · Loss of >50% of labial plate
   · Loss of palatal bone

## Missing tooth

1. Assessment of residual ridge
2. Clinical assessment
3. Diagnostic imaging
4. Diagnostic preview

Main decision criteria for the assessment of possible bone graft:

1. Insufficient height of bone in relation to future tooth position (according to diagnostic preview)
2. Fused cortical plates (according to CT scan) or <2 mm of width (according to ridge mapping)
3. Sufficient inter-occlusal distance
4. Favorable soft tissues for closure

**Bone graft likely? Above criteria met**

Yes → Preoperative assessment of donor site
· Ramus
· Symphysis
· Extra-oral

Bone graft procedure

No →
· Further assessment necessary
· Treatment decision based on type of deficiency (loss of height or width), location, aesthetic and functional needs

Augmentation procedure
· Sinus lift
· GTR
· Ti Mesh

Hard and soft tissue manipulation
· Bone expansion
· Sinus manipulation
· Nerve repositioning
· Distraction osteogenesis

Flowchart 13-1   Assessment for bone grafts.

III  Augmentation

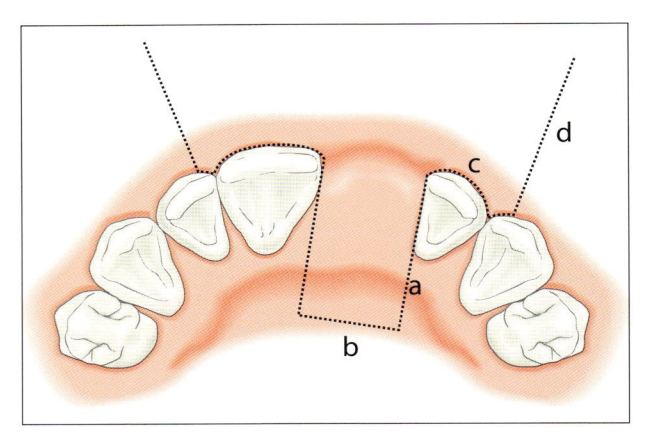

**Fig 13-7**  Remote palatal incision required for the recipient site for a deficiency in the anterior maxilla. The incision was made in the following sequence: a, the vertical component, approximately 10 mm; b, the horizontal bevelled component made with Blake's knife; c, the intrasulcular incision; and d, the vertical release incision, including papilla.

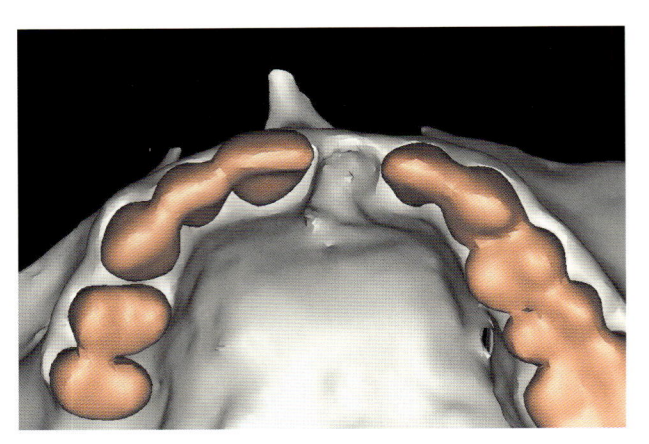

**Fig 13-8**  CT 3D view showing the palatal defect.

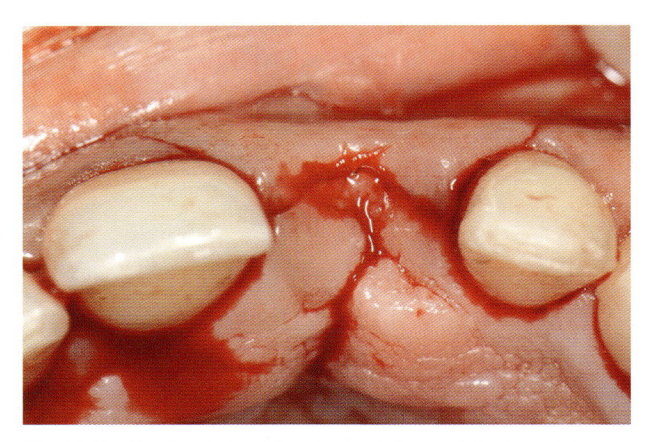

**Fig 13-9**  Occlusal view showing soft tissue defect overlying the bony defect as well as the outline of the crestal incision.

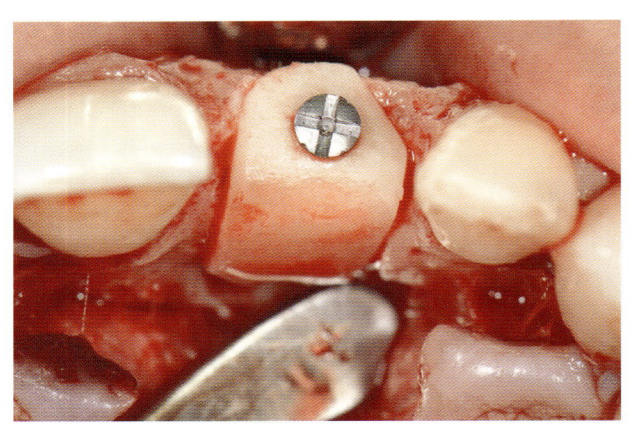

**Fig 13-10**  Block graft harvested from the ramus in situ for repair of the palatal defect.

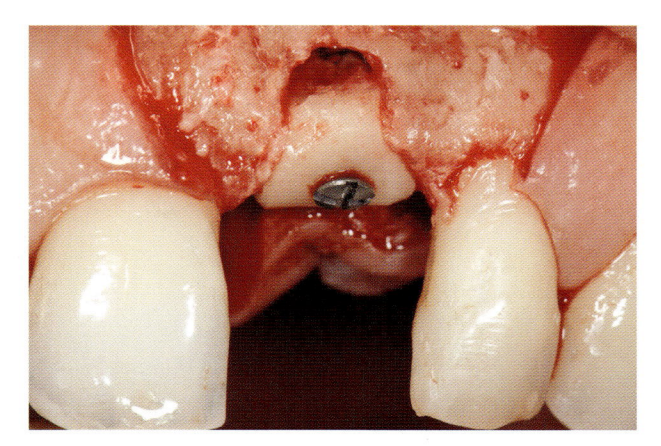

**Fig 13-11**  Labial review of the graft in situ showing a residual defect, which will be filled with particulate cortical chips.

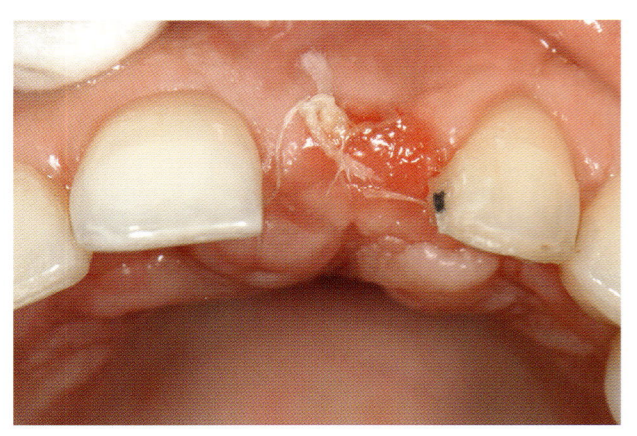

**Fig 13-12**  Healing of soft tissues at one week, showing no exposure of the graft and demonstrating the efficacy of everted tissue closure using horizontal or vertical mattress sutures.

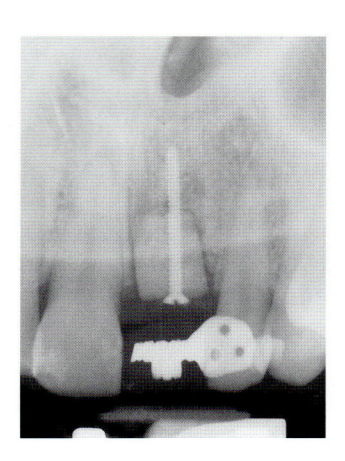

**Fig 13-13** Post-operative radiograph showing graft and the fixation screw. This baseline radiograph will be used to monitor the maturation of the graft.

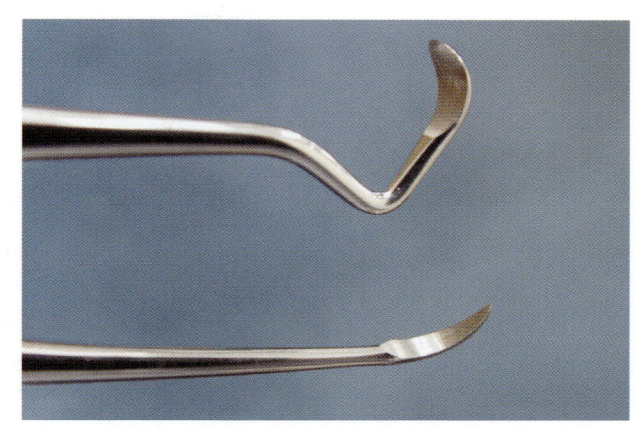

**Fig 13-14** Curved elevator (top instrument) for the elevation of a buccally based flap. Papilla elevator (bottom instrument) for the atraumatic elevation of papillae in an aesthetically critical zone. These instruments are also part of the sinus lift kit (Fig 15-22, p. 314).

and is bevelled towards the crest to allow for easy closure of the wound. The buccally based flap is elevated using a curved elevator (Dentsply Friadent) to expose the crest of the ridge.

A fine periosteal elevator is used to lift the periosteum from the area of bone loss and to elevate the gingival margin from the adjacent teeth without perforating this critical area. The papillae are carefully elevated using a papilla elevator (Fig 13-14).

The reflection of the buccally based flap is extended and reflected off the appropriate anatomical structures.

- **Anterior maxilla**. For grafts in the anterior region, the reflection of the buccally based flap is extended towards the anterior nasal spine and the piriform rim. For grafts that are more laterally placed the flap is extended towards the zygomatic arch. This will normally provide sufficient tissue for closure without the need for periosteal release incisions. Care must be taken while making vertical release incisions and reflecting the flap in the region of the infra-orbital foramen to avoid damage to the structures emanating from the foramen.
- **Posterior maxilla**. Any palatal incision in the posterior maxilla must be carried out with care in order to avoid severing the branches of the greater palatine vessels or nerves. A split-thickness incision should be used here, the periosteum being incised near the crest of the ridge. No distal vertical release incision in an unbound saddle is needed in the posterior maxilla, as the parallel component of the palatal incision can be extended distally over the ridge distal to the tuberosity. Any periosteal release carries the risk of damage to the parotid duct, which must be identified and avoided.

## Mandible

For localised bone deficiencies of the mandibular ridge, a crestal incision is usually the approach of choice. Care needs to be exercised whenever a vertical release incision needs to be made in the area of the mental foramen.

- **Anterior mandible**. In the anterior mandible, flap advancement can be carried out using a periosteal release on the labial aspect and periosteal reflection on the lingual side. Clearly care must be taken not to damage any vital structures in this area, such as the mental nerve, branches of the sublingual artery, muscle attachments and the sublingual duct.
- **Posterior mandible**. A periosteal release incision in the labial and lingual area of the posterior mandible is fraught with serious risk to several vital structures, and sharp dissection should, therefore, not be contemplated. Some of the structures of particular concern are the lingual nerve, the facial artery and the mental nerve. This makes the posterior mandible a difficult area to treat, particularly when the defi-

# III   Augmentation

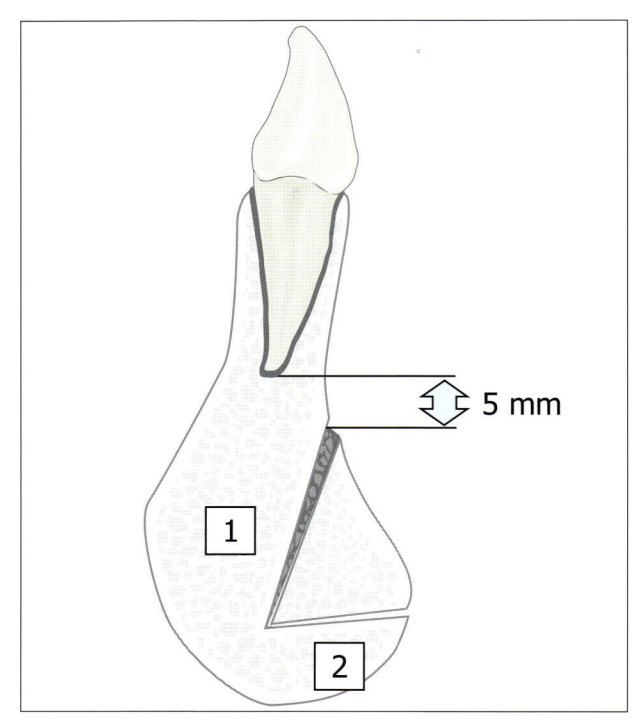

**Fig 13-15** Bone harvesting from the symphysis. Two horizontal cuts are made (as shown in the diagram), which normally extend between the roots of the canine and are parallel to the lower border of the jaw. When larger grafts are required that extend beyond the apices of the canine, the risk of damage to the longer roots of the canine teeth increases.
1. This osteotomy is made 5 mm from the apices of the incisor teeth. The osteotomy bur is inclined so that it is parallel to the teeth to avoid interrupting the neurovascular supply to the teeth.
2. This osteotomy is made with the bur perpendicular to the bony surface and should not be made beyond the maximum prominence of the pogonion. Two vertical cuts will be used to connect the horizontal components (not shown).

cient ridge has a distal tooth present. In those cases where the ridge has a free end, the deflection can be extended along the ramus and the tissue mobilised for easier closure.

## Measurement of Bone Deficiency

The deficiency should be measured in all relevant dimensions – length, width and height – to allow the measurements to be transferred to the donor site. This will enable an adequate size of block graft to be harvested to correct the deficiency. Allowance should be made for the dimensions of the harvesting instruments (bur or saw) and the area oversized by the appropriate amount. Compensation should also be made for the remodelling of the graft during the healing phase.

## Access to the Donor Site
### Symphysis

A labial or a cervical incision can be used to gain access to the symphysis.

When using a labial approach, an incision is made in the sulcus between the canine teeth. The tissues are dissected toward the coronal aspect of the ridge, resulting in a split-thickness flap. A periosteal incision is then made at the insertion point of the muscles and a full-thickness flap is reflected toward the inferior border of the mandible and toward the mental foramen. For a cervical approach, an incision is made that extends from premolar to premolar, with vertical release incisions distal to the mental foramen. The periosteal reflection is carried out, exposing the mental foramen and extending the reflection to the inferior border of the mandible.

### Ramus

The incision to expose the external oblique ridge is made approximately 1 cm distal to the second molar. It is made over the external oblique ridge and extended mesially towards the buccal of the second molar. Care has to be taken to ensure that the incision is not extended too far lingually, which would risk damage to the structures on the lingual aspect of the mandible. The external oblique ridge is exposed reflecting the periosteum and extended to expose the retromolar region and the lateral aspect of the ramus.

## Harvesting the Graft
### Symphysis

The size and the shape of the graft required may be marked with a surgical marker or a straight handpiece using fine fissure burs and abundant irrigation. Alternatively, rotary saws with a guard (e.g. Micro-Saw, Dentsply Friadent) or piezosurgery units (e.g. Piezosurgery [Mectron, Carasco, Italy] or Piezotome [Satelec Aceton, Merignac, France]) may be used. A superior horizontal osteotomy must be made at a minimum distance of 5 mm from the apices of the incisor and canine teeth if an extensive graft is required (Fig 13-15). This may restrict the size of the graft, as the canine teeth are longer.

In order to avoid damage to the neurovascular supply to the teeth, the osteotomy should be prepared almost parallel to the long axis of the teeth. The vertical incisions for the osteotomy are made through the cortical bone. Preparation of an inferior horizontal osteotomy is carried out parallel to the inferior border of the mandible and does not extend beyond its maximum convexity. This is often the thickest region of cortical bone, and an indication of thickness can be obtained from a lateral cephalograph. The graft required is then elevated from the symphysis with bone chisels or elevators.

### Ramus

The size of the graft and its precise position is selected with reference to the measurements of the size and position of the area of bone loss at the recipient site. Small fissure or round burs may be used to mark the size of the graft (Fig 13-16). The contour of the external oblique ridge is more rounded towards the mesial aspect and becomes more acute as it extends towards the coronoid process. The 3D shape of the graft can thus be matched to the shape required. A fine fissure bur is used to outline the graft dimensions on the superficial surface of the retromolar region, thus providing the required width of bone at the recipient site. Care must always be taken not to extend the osseous incision too far lingually or to extend the depth to which the bur is used beyond the measurement that allows adequate clearance above the inferior alveolar canal. Cuts on the lateral aspect of the mandible must be made using the measurements that ensure no damage takes place to the neurovascular bundle. These will provide the vertical cuts, which can be joined using a large round bur. Typically a number 8 round bur using copious irrigation requires minimum access and creates a groove along which the controlled fracture of the graft can be effected as it is elevated without overextension. The groove does not extend through the cortical plate and is positioned above the inferior alveolar canal, as measured from the distortion-compensated radiograph. If there are difficulties in elevating the graft, the osteotomies outlining the graft can be reconfirmed using the appropriate burs prior to further attempts to elevate the graft. This ensures that the graft is removed in one piece. Once again, micro-saws or piezosurgery instruments can be used following the precautions outlined above.

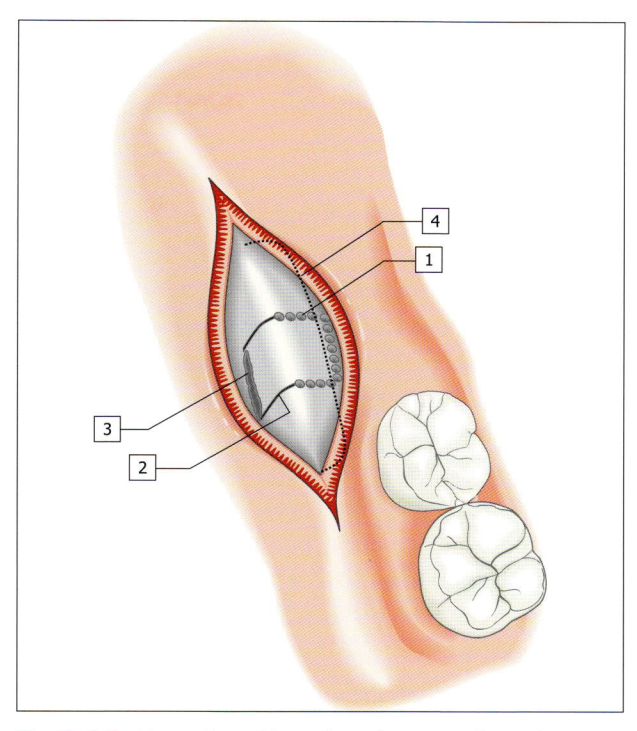

**Fig 13-16** Harvesting of bone from the ramus (superior aspect) situated buccal to the molar teeth. The soft tissue incision (red line) is kept approximately 5 mm away from the molar teeth.
1. Perforations are made with a small fissure bur and are joined with the fissure bur extended through the cortex but not beyond the critical depth.
2. Cuts are made through the cortical plate with a fine fissure bur and must remain 2 mm clear of the inferior alveolar nerve (critical depth).
3. A groove is made with a large round bur connecting the two vertical cuts and creating a line of least resistance for the fracture.
4. Mesial and distal extension (thin black line) may be used to harvest a larger piece of bone but this results in narrower thickness of graft.

### Fitting the Graft

The graft is then tried in to assess the modifications that need to be made. Modifications are made to either the recipient site or the graft. In the maxilla, hand instruments such as chisels may be used to create a socket into which the graft will fit accurately. In the mandible, rotary instruments may be necessary to create a bed in the dense cortical bone to allow the graft to be positioned without rocking. Rotary instruments may be used to alter the graft to provide the clearance from the neighbouring teeth and to produce smooth rounded contours. Certain criteria need to be met in order to ensure the proper incorporation of the graft.

- Maximum contact between the graft and the host bone is considered important to provide early primary fixation by means of contact healing.
- There should be no direct contact between the graft and the adjacent teeth. This is because of concerns regarding the possibility of infection or dehiscence in situations where a seal between the tooth and soft tissues cannot be established.
- The graft has to be overcontoured to compensate for bone remodelling (by approximately 20–25%). It is, therefore, necessary to visualise the future position of the implant. The healed site has to meet the criteria for conventional implant placement without the need to manipulate the bone.

## Graft Fixation

Once stable, the graft should be held firmly in position while the procedures to secure it are implemented. The use of a clamp facilitates this. It is strongly recommended that the lagged principle be used for securing the graft with a screw in order to facilitate accurate seating with the minimum amount of compromise. This involves preparing a slightly larger hole than the screw so that the screw passes through the hard cortical graft without binding against the sides and risking either fracturing or rotating the graft.

The twist drill is used to pass through the graft and directly into the host bone. The hole through the cortical graft is then enlarged. The length of the screw required is then measured and the screw inserted. In the event of any displacement the graft can be aligned with a probe to enable screw insertion.

One screw is normally sufficient if close adaptation of the graft to the underlying recipient site has been achieved producing inherent stability. Additional screws may be needed for larger grafts. Multiple screws should not be used as a way to compensate for poor adaptation of the graft to the recipient site. Grafts correcting a deficiency in bone height may need to be secured by means of a screw that is positioned precisely in the position of the future implant and the screw may need to be quite long. On occasion, there may be no bone available for the direct fixation of the graft and in this case osteosynthetic plates may be used.

Any small spaces at the edge of the graft are best filled with cancellous bone or cortical bone chips. In the absence of autogenous bone beta-tricalcium phosphate or other synthetic material may be used to pack the edges.

In the event that supplementary pieces of bone are required to pack larger spaces, a membrane may be used as an occlusive barrier primarily for containment purposes. The membrane, however, increases the risk of complications and prolongs the healing time as it interrupts the blood supply from the overlying soft tissues to the grafted bone. The blood supply from the area of bone contact then becomes the sole source of revascularisation and this will prolong treatment.[216]

## Wound Closure
### Recipient Site

Since the closure of the wound must be carried out without any tension, the flap is repositioned before particulate material or a membrane is put in place to ensure that passive closure is possible. This is to make sure that no displacement of the material takes place as the soft tissues are manipulated for closure.

If passive closure of the wound can be accomplished, any additional materials required are added and the wound sutured. Where wound closure cannot be achieved, periosteal release incisions may be used before placing the membrane. Maxillary palatal flaps can be secured with interrupted sutures, using a 3-0 suture with a 22 mm half-round reverse cutting needle. The interdental papillae of the adjacent teeth are secured by means of interrupted sutures using 3-0 or 4-0 sutures. Closure of the labial vertical release incisions may require finer sutures (6-0).

In the mandible (or the maxilla), the crestal incision is closed using horizontal or vertical mattress sutures

**13** Localised Onlay Bone Grafts

**Fig 13-17** (left) Periapical radiograph taken immediately after augmentation with an onlay bone graft. The outline of the bone graft is clearly visible.

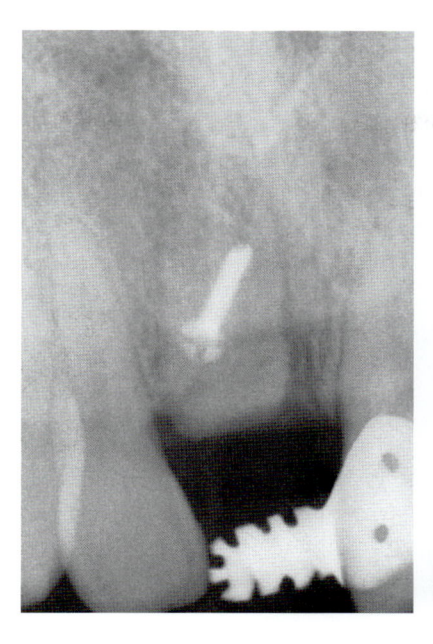

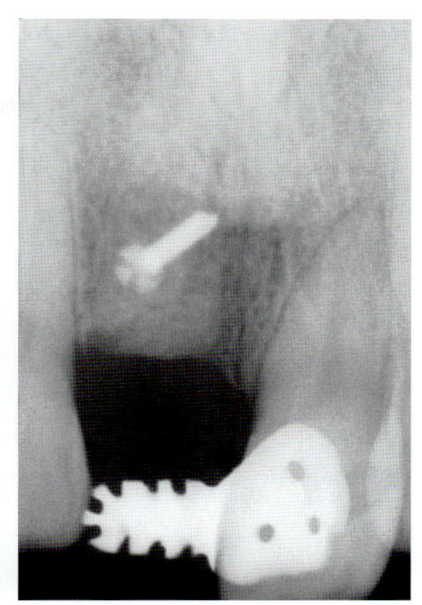

**Fig 13-18** (right) Periapical radiograph taken three months after augmentation (same patient as in Fig 13-17). Signs of remodelling and incorporation are clearly visible.

to oppose the everted edges and is supplemented with interrupted sutures. Provisional restorations will require to be modified before fitting in order to ensure that the tissues overlying the graft are not traumatised.

### Donor Site

- **Symphysis**. Two types of incision will require closure:
  - cervical incisions are closed by using either continuous or interrupted 3-0 sutures to secure each papilla accurately into its appropriate position; vertical mattress sutures may be used on occasion to position the papilla accurately
  - labial incisions are best closed by a two-layer procedure; vertical mattress sutures are used to appose the periosteal edges and supplementary interrupted sutures are used to close the wound margins.
- **Ramus.** The incision in the retro-molar region is self-apposing, and a continuous suture effectively closes the wound.

## Assessing Bone Healing

Bone healing is assessed clinically and radiographically. Techniques that measure metabolic activity or the establishment of a blood supply are currently being developed and may be used in the future to provide additional information regarding the healing process.

### Radiographic Assessment

Periapical radiographs are taken immediately after surgery using radiograph holders and a paralleling long-cone technique, which gives reproducible orientation. These are repeated two to three months after surgery. Changes in the cortical and trabecular bone patterns are indicative of integration of the graft (Figs 13-17 and 13-18).

### Clinical Assessment

Radiographs are used in conjunction with clinical evaluation of the changes in the contour of the grafted site. In the event that no changes are visible on the original radiograph, additional radiographs are taken one to two months later.

Assessment of the remodelling of the contours is facilitated when a fixed provisional restoration is present, since the contact between the pontic and the ridge allows the remodelling process to be evaluated accurately. The shape and size of the fixed provisional restoration is a good indicator of the final aesthetic outcome. At this stage, the cervical margin of the pontic is invariably shorter than the intended final restoration due to the overcontouring of the graft. This will impact on the depth to which the implant is positioned.

### High Metabolic Activity

Patients with a high metabolic turnover (e.g. younger patients) are likely to heal at a faster rate, and it is advisable to schedule implant insertion at two months, ensuring that the above-mentioned criteria have been met.

### Additional Membranes

Where occlusive membranes have been used for containment purposes, the period of healing will be longer because of the slower revascularisation of the graft. The time will, however, depend on the type of membrane used. Resorbable membranes vary in their rate of resorption, and consequently more rapid revascularisation may take place. When using resorbable membranes (e.g. Collagen, Bio-Gide; Geistlich, Wolhusen, Switzerland), adequate graft maturity has typically been achieved by four months after treatment. The use of non-resorbable membranes such as polytetrafluoroethylene sheets (e.g. Gore-Tex; Gore Medical, Flagstaff, AZ, USA) will result in slower maturation and a more stable graft during the initial healing phase; in this case the graft usually takes approximately six months to mature (Figs 13-19–13-25).

## Implant Insertion

Methods of access to the ridge for implant placement should be designed for delayed loading; therefore, remote palatal incisions in the maxilla and crestal incisions in the mandible are suitable.

The crestal portion of the graft and ridge are exposed and examined for adequate healing. The margins of the graft and the ridge should be confluent; the edges of the graft should show signs of remodelling, as observed on the radiograph. Signs of vascularity should be evident, such as bleeding from the surface of the graft. There is also a characteristic change in the colour of the graft. In the event that adequate maturation of the graft has not taken place, closure of the wound and an additional period of healing are advisable.

Adequate exposure of the site to permit removal of the screws or plates should be planned. However, if the fixation screw has been placed in the labial aspect of the graft, access to the screw may be obtained via a small incision overlying the screw. The fixation screw or plates can then be removed.

The implant site is selected with a diagnostic template, when appropriate, and the osteotomy is prepared using internally irrigated burs. However, attention needs to be paid to the proximity of the completed osteotomy to the edge of the graft. The direction of the osteotomy is selected so that it passes through the graft and engages the bone in the recipient site. Sequential enlargement of the osteotomy with incrementally wider diameter burs is essential because of the hard nature of the cortical bone. Support should be provided to the graft during osteotomy preparation to prevent accidental displacement.

The entire sequence of instruments to complete the osteotomy should be used. This includes hand reamers and bone taps. For more accurate control of these instruments, it is advisable to use them by hand as this will reduce the likelihood of fracturing the bone.

The implant should be inserted according to the standard protocol. The depth to which the implant is positioned is critical with respect to the emergence profile and abutment selection, as described above. This may result in the implant being positioned below the level of the crest. Impressions may be taken at this stage to record the position of the implant. The abutment is selected using direction indicators in conjunction with the occlusion and diagnostic template, thus confirming the implant position. The flap is repositioned and the soft tissue level assessed with a view to gauging the appearance of the final restoration.

The height of the soft tissues covering the graft at the peak of the crest should be at the level of the papillae of the adjacent teeth. Hydroxyapatite may be used at this stage for additional soft tissue support, as described above. In the event of any concerns regarding the nature or the level of the soft tissues, corrective soft tissue surgery can be planned.

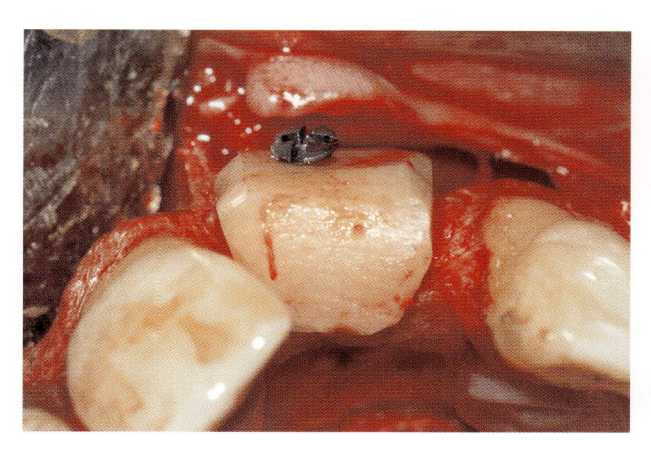

**Fig 13-19** Intraoperative view of a block graft from the ramus at the time of insertion. Note the texture of the surface of the graft.

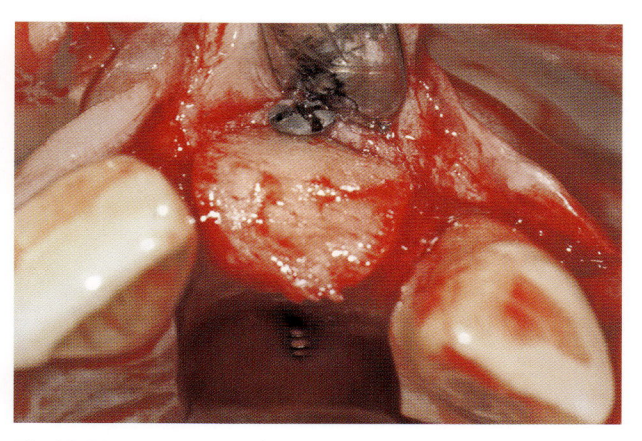

**Fig 13-20** The graft three months after insertion at the time of implant placement. Note the bleeding surface of the graft and the lack of confluence.

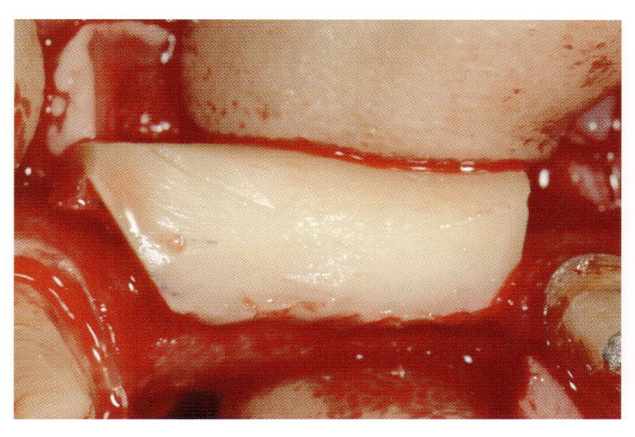

**Fig 13-21** The bone graft from the retromolar region at insertion. A resorbable collagen membrane was used to prevent soft tissue ingrowth into the spaces between the graft and the recipient site.

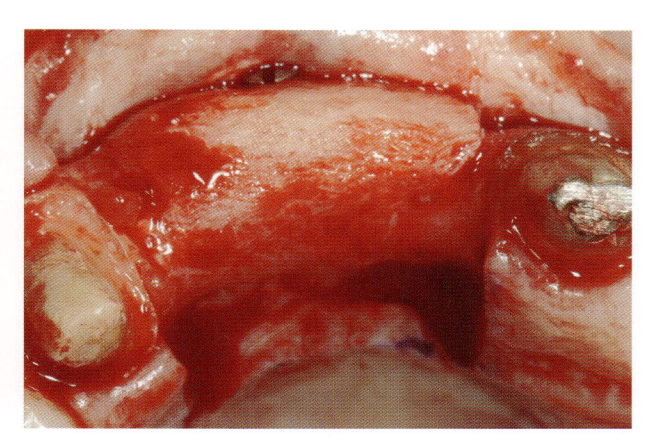

**Fig 13-22** The graft four months later. Note the bleeding surface, which appears more mature. Also note the greater degree of confluence with the recipient site.

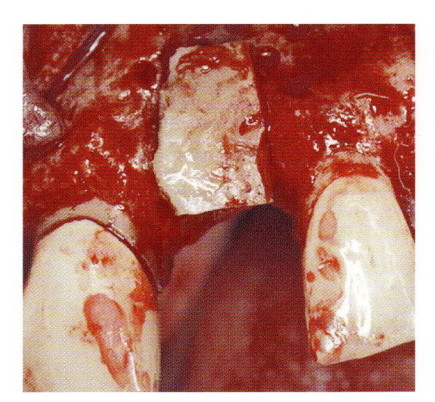

**Fig 13-23** The bone graft at insertion prior to the placement of the non-resorbable membrane.

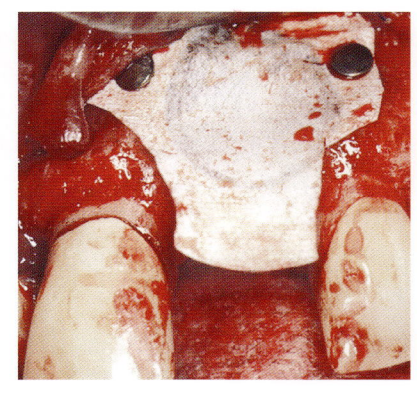

**Fig 13-24** The membrane being inserted. Note the adaptation of the membrane away from the tooth margins to prevent exposure to infection.

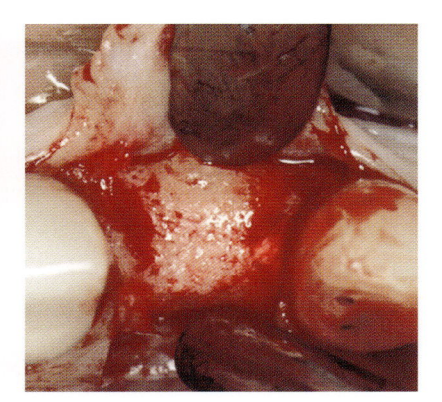

**Fig 13-25** Healing of the graft six months after surgery, at the time of implant placement. Note the maturity and the complete confluence of the graft with the adjacent bone.

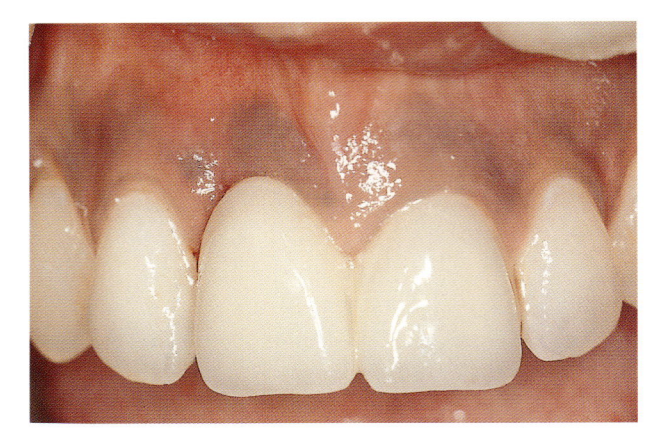

**Fig 13-26** Labial view of a metal-acrylic hybrid bridge six weeks after tooth extraction, showing the healed soft tissues prior to grafting the bone deficiency.

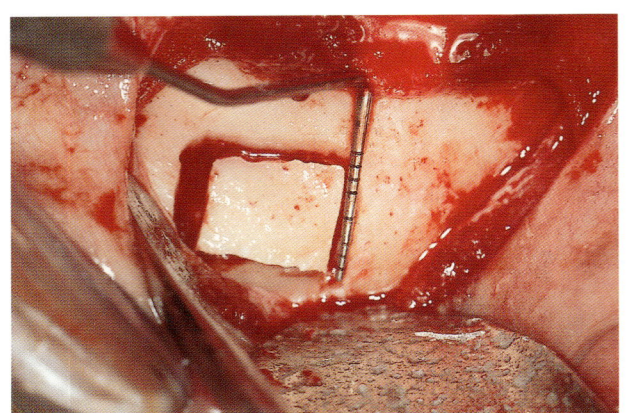

**Fig 13-27** Symphyseal donor site with the graft outlined.

## Wound Closure

The technique used for wound closure is similar to that described for conventional implant placement for delayed loading. The provisional restoration is replaced and re-contoured, if necessary. Contact with the pontic accompanied by minimal blanching of the soft tissues is acceptable at this stage to initiate the process of development of the emergence profile.

## Corrective Soft Tissue Surgery

Corrective soft tissue surgery should not be required if the appropriate protocol has been followed and healing has progressed as predicted. Nevertheless, in the event of corrective surgery being necessary the procedure will need to be assessed according to Flowchart 17-1 for corrective soft tissue surgery (p. 354–355). Depending on the type of procedure required, the correct timing for its implementation can be selected. The period in the middle of the healing phase between implant placement and exposure provides the ideal conditions with respect to the vascularisation of the graft and soft tissues.

Typically, the removal of an amalgam tattoo that has been advanced during the grafting procedure may be carried out at this stage. Its replacement with a connective tissue graft at this stage provides sufficient time for its maturation and confluence with the adjacent tissues.

## Implant Exposure

After a healing period of four to six months, exposure of the implant can be undertaken. Standard protocols should be followed for the exposure and connection of the abutment as well as for the insertion of a transitional restoration. In the maxilla, a larger amount of keratinised tissue may generally need to be repositioned labially in cases where closure during the grafting procedure resulted in the keratinised tissue being advanced toward the palate. The management of soft tissues around multiple implants at exposure is discussed in Chapters 9 and 14.

The process of developing the correct gingival profile can be carried out at this stage. The preferred method is to use the transitional restoration to either reposition the cervical gingiva apically by increasing the labial contour of the restoration with acrylic resin or to develop the interdental papilla by adding acrylic resin to the approximal subgingival area of the crown. A connective tissue graft may be used to add to the bulk of labial or interdental regions at the time of exposure.

## Restorative Phase

The soft tissues should be allowed to mature for at least four weeks; in the event of any additional re-contouring being necessary, the restorative phase should

13   Localised Onlay Bone Grafts

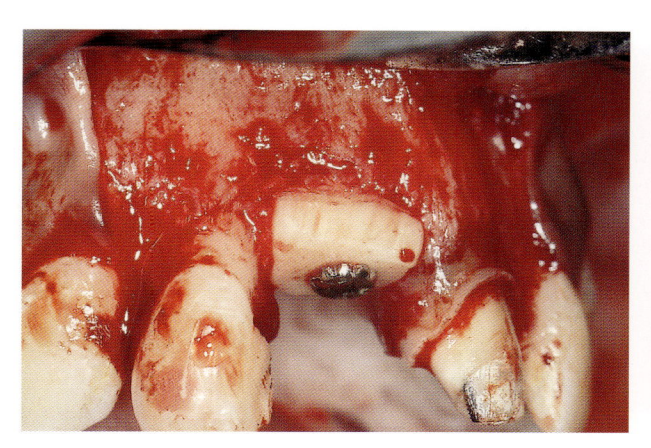

**Fig 13-28**  Recipient site with the graft in situ increasing the ridge height. Note the position of the screw has been selected so that it will coincide with the implant position on integration of the graft.

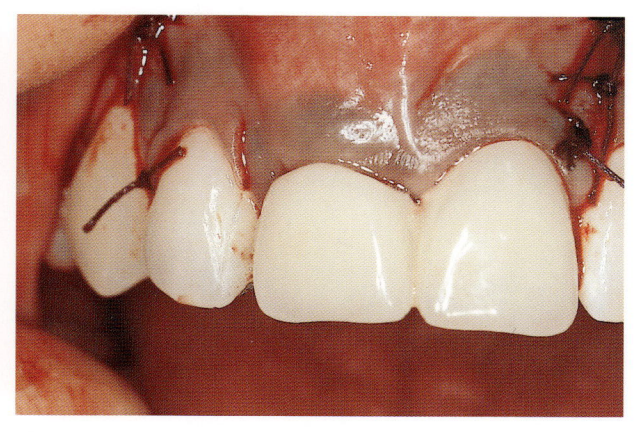

**Fig 13-29**  Replacement of the metal-acrylic bridge following surgery. Note that the pontic has had to be modified to compensate for the increased ridge height. The graft was allowed to heal for two months prior to the implant being placed. The implant was allowed to integrate for a further six months prior to exposure.

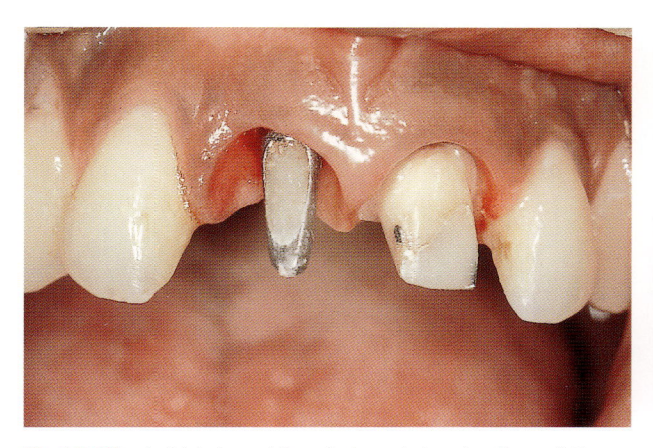

**Fig 13-30**  Labial view of the abutment showing the soft tissue contours established by the transitional restoration. The abutment was attached at the time of implant exposure and the transitional crown fitted at the same time.

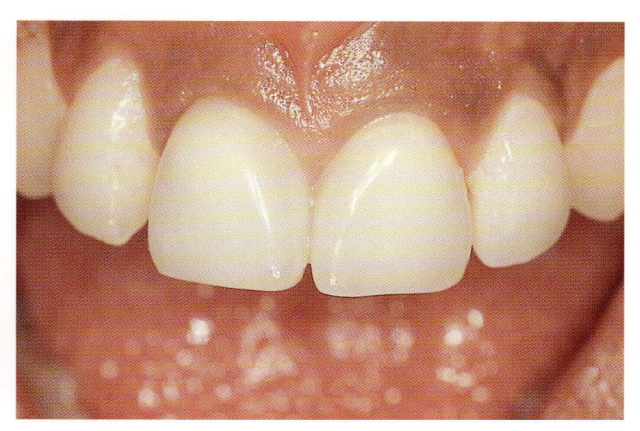

**Fig 13-31**  Labial view of the implant and the adjacent central incisor with the restorations in situ. Note the gingival margins and the level of the papilla with respect to a harmonious emergence profile.

be delayed until the gingival tissues have matured sufficiently. Further conditioning of the soft tissues can also be carried out during the restorative phase, as described above in the section on conventional impressions.

## Localised Bone Grafts: Clinical Cases

### Case 1:
### Bone Graft from the Symphysis

This case study illustrates the use of a bone graft obtained from the symphysis for the correction of a bone deficiency in height in the maxillary central incisor region (Figs 13-26–13-31).

253

III   Augmentation

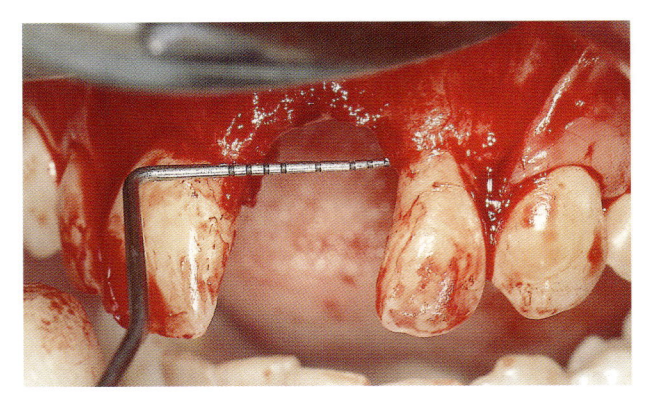

**Fig 13-32**  Labial view of the recipient site showing the loss of height and the level of the attachment of the bone to the adjacent teeth. Measurement of the deficiency enables the bone to be harvested accurately.

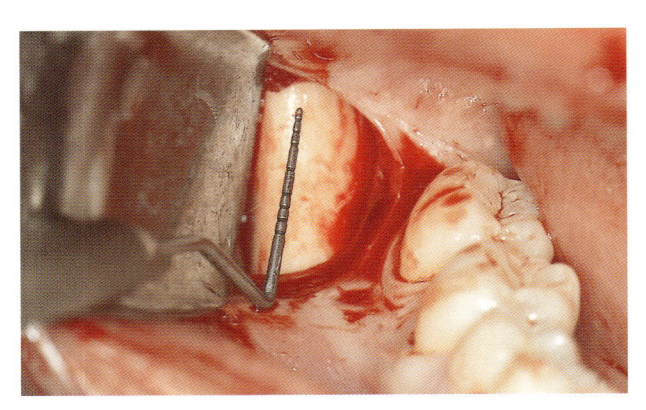

**Fig 13-33**  The right retromolar region exposed via an incision, as described in Fig 13-16. The form of the external oblique ridge is ideally suited for the reconstruction of a ridge. The periodontal probe can be used to measure the size of the graft to be obtained and to select the precise site, which will provide the desired contour.

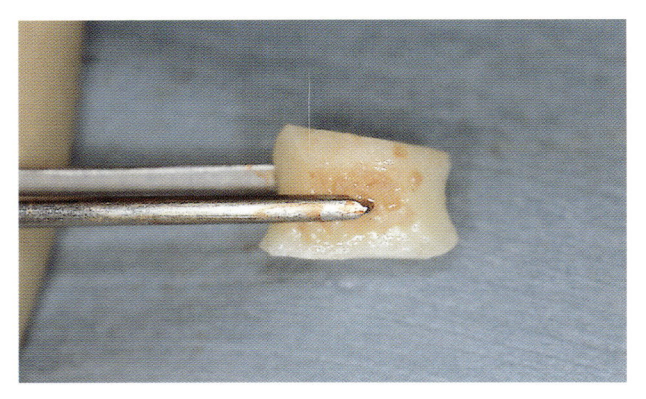

**Fig 13-34**  The undersurface of the graft showing the contour created to enable the graft to be fitted accurately onto the residual ridge.

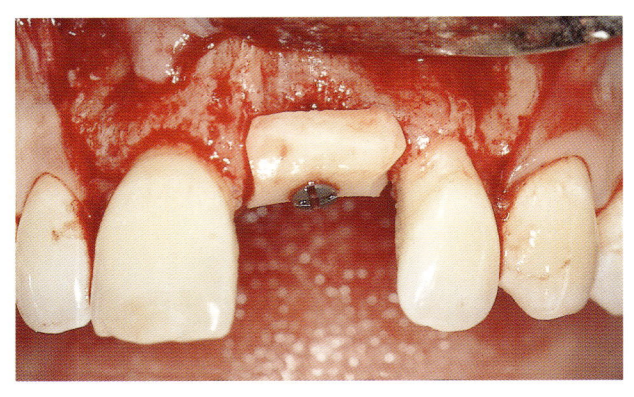

**Fig 13-35**  Labial view of the graft in situ showing the adaptation of the graft to the residual ridge. Note the adaptation of the graft to the adjacent teeth and the residual space, avoiding direct contact with tooth.

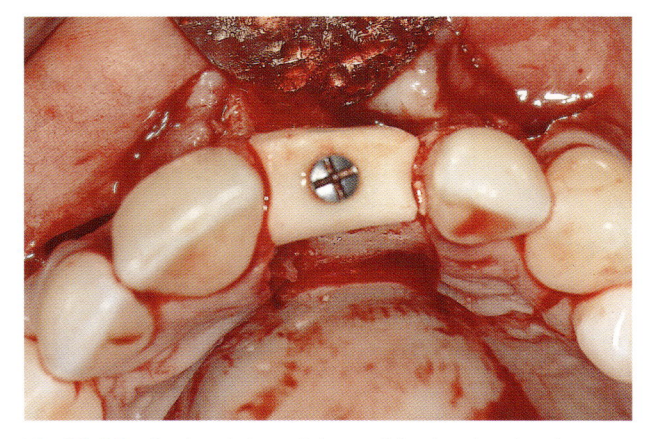

**Fig 13-36**  Occlusal view of the graft in situ showing the proximity of the graft to the adjacent teeth and the positioning of the fixation screw to be coincidental with the implant position.

## Case 2:
## Bone Graft from the Ramus

A bone graft obtained from the ramus is used to correct a deficiency in height in a maxillary central incisor area (Figs 13-32–13-36).

13   Localised Onlay Bone Grafts

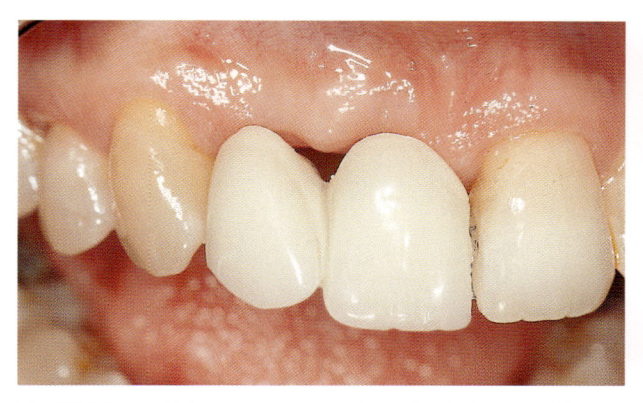

**Fig 13-37**   Labial view of the metal-acrylic Rochette bridge replacing the right central and lateral incisor, indicating the ideal tooth position and the soft tissue deficiency.

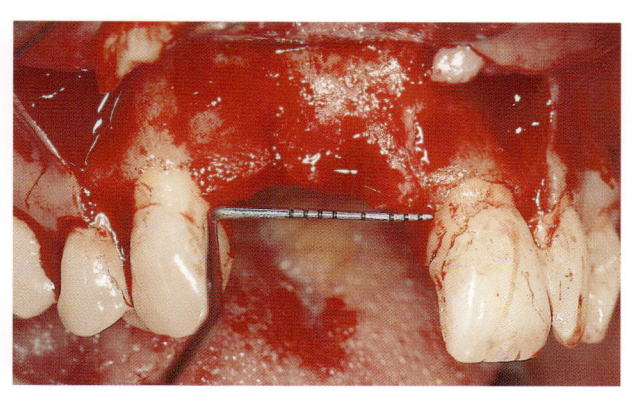

**Fig 13-38**   Labial view of the exposed ridge showing a deficiency in height and width. The deficiency is being measured between the two teeth at a level where there is contact of the bone to the adjacent teeth.

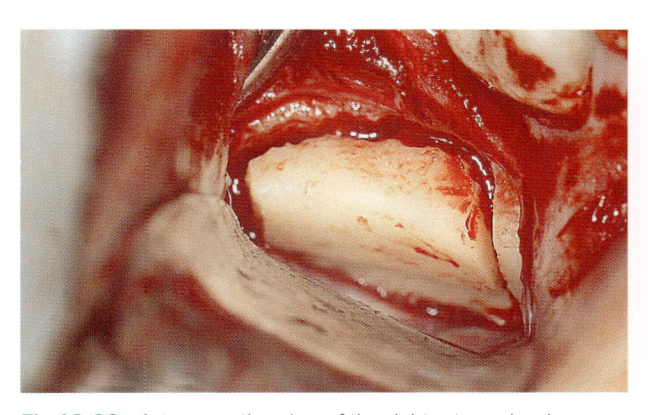

**Fig 13-39**   Intraoperative view of the right retromolar donor site. The graft has been outlined using a fine fissure bur. The groove created by the large round bur on the lateral surface of the jaw is visible.

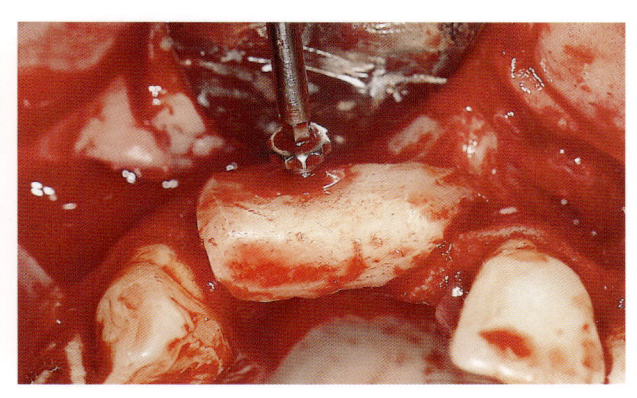

**Fig 13-40**   Clinical view of the recipient site showing the bone graft being secured by means of one screw placed between the central and lateral incisors. The contour obtained from the ramus is suitable for the reconstruction of a ridge.

## Case 3:
## Bone Graft from the Ramus

A bone graft obtained from the ramus is used to correct a deficiency in height and width where a central and lateral incisor needed to be replaced by means of implants (Figs 13-37–13-44).

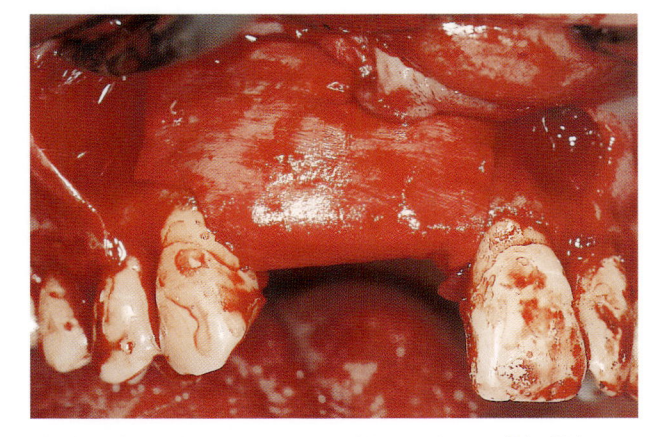

**Fig 13-41**   In this case a resorbable membrane (Bio-Gide, secured with FRIOS tacks) was used to compensate for some minor deficiencies at the edge of the graft. The graft was allowed to heal for three months prior to implant placement.

255

III  Augmentation

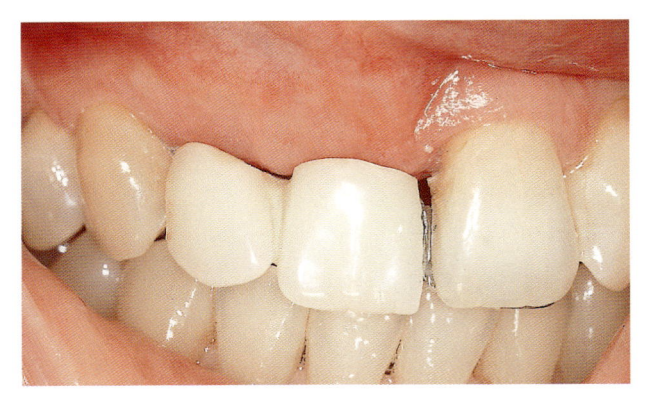

**Fig 13-42** The implants were placed and allowed to integrate for six months prior to implant exposure.

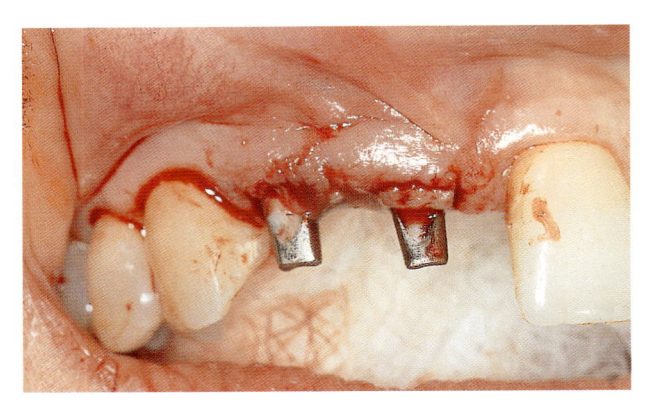

**Fig 13-43** Labial view of the implants exposed via an 'H'-shaped incision and the preselected abutments attached with a minimal exposure of the ridge.

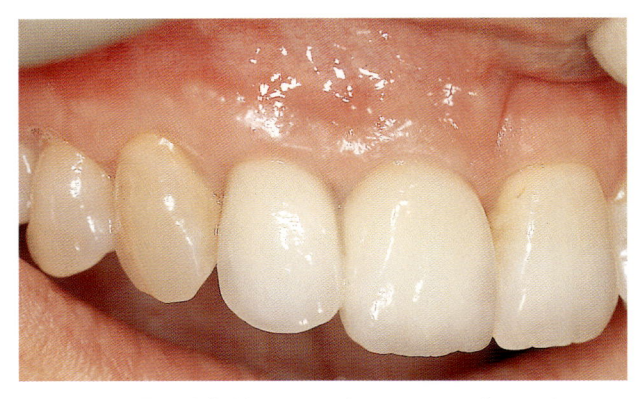

**Fig 13-44** The definitive restorations cemented on to the abutments using temporary cement. Note the soft tissue contours and the emergence profile.

## Case 4:
### Bone Graft from the Symphysis

This case study demonstrates the use of a bone graft obtained from the symphysis to correct a deficiency in both height and width. The need to use the symphysis as the donor site arose because there was insufficient bone available in the region of the ramus. This case also demonstrates the need for preoperative assessment of the restorative outcome (Figs 13-45–13-61). Follow up at 10 years is shown in Figs 13-62 and 13-63.

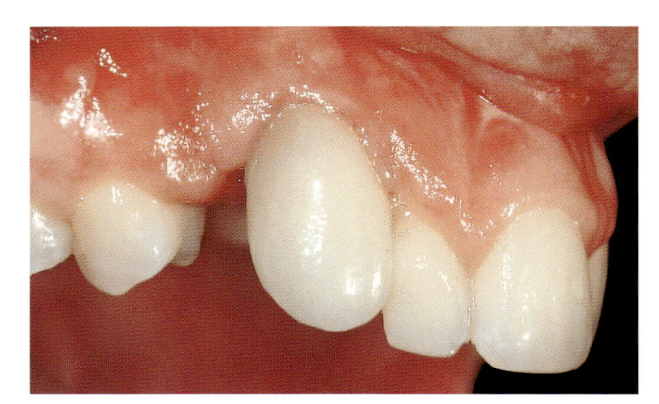

**Fig 13-45** Preoperative view of the patient showing the length and position of the failing tooth.

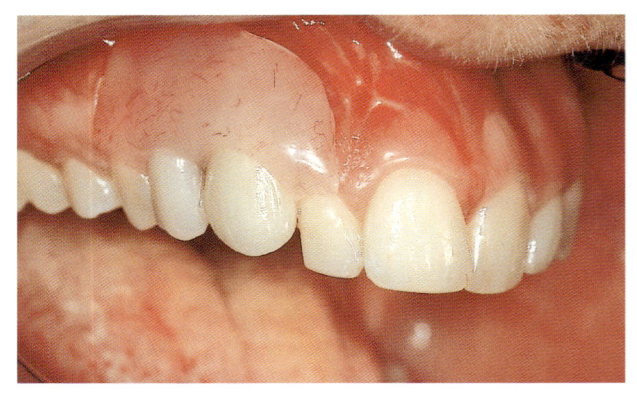

**Fig 13-46** Preoperative view with the acrylic partial denture in situ. The tooth is mesially positioned with a gap distal to that tooth that was restored previously by means of a partial denture with an acrylic resin flange to mask the increased length of the canine.

256

13   Localised Onlay Bone Grafts

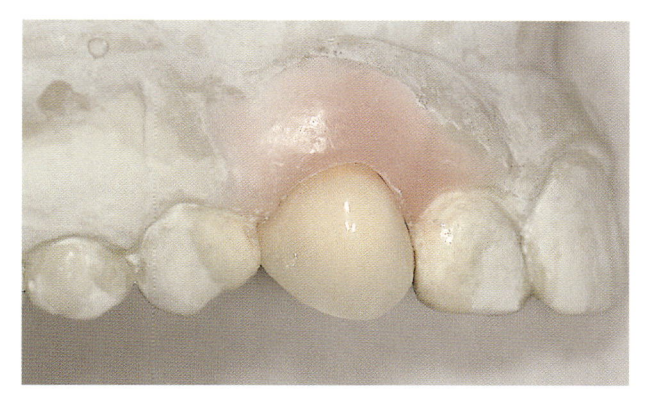

**Fig 13-47**   Diagnostic preview to establish the possibility of using a single implant and the middle of the space with an increase in width of the adjacent teeth. Note the use of pink wax to predict the eventual soft tissue contours.

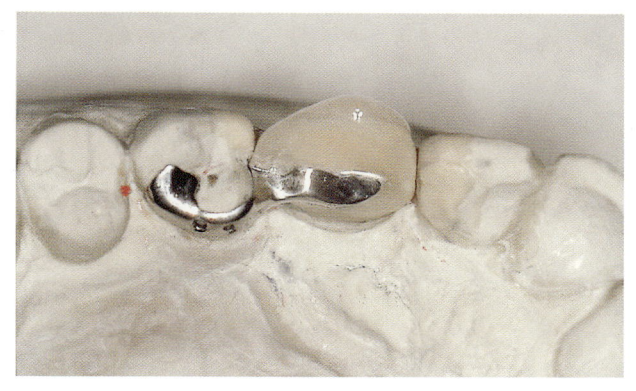

**Fig 13-48**   The construction of a metal-acrylic Rochette bridge to be used as a provisional restoration. A single wing and rest supported by the premolar was considered sufficient support and retention for the restoration. Note the position of the metal, allowing sufficient space for adjustment of the pontic as the ridge is built up.

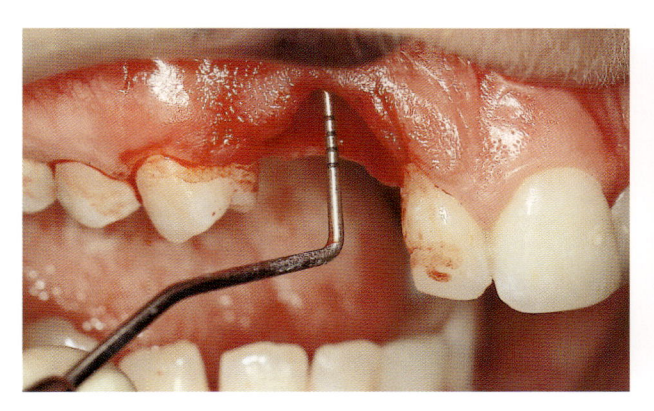

**Fig 13-49**   Labial view with a periodontal probe being used to measure the bone deficiency on the labial aspect of the socket in order to gather information about the nature of the defect.

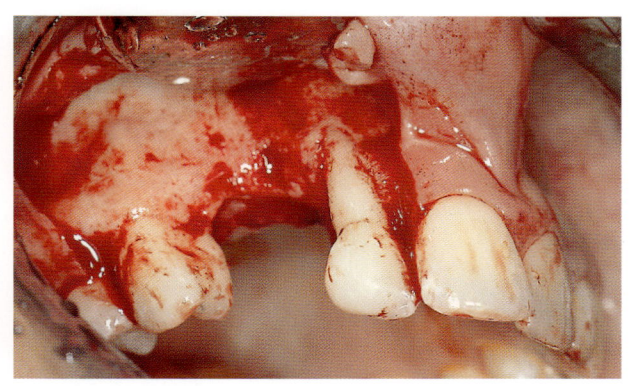

**Fig 13-50**   Clinical view of the recipient site following the reflection of a flap created by a remote palatal incision. Note the denuded root of the lateral incisor but the level of bone attachment on the distal and towards the palatal aspect of the root. A deficiency in height and width is evident, which will need correction.

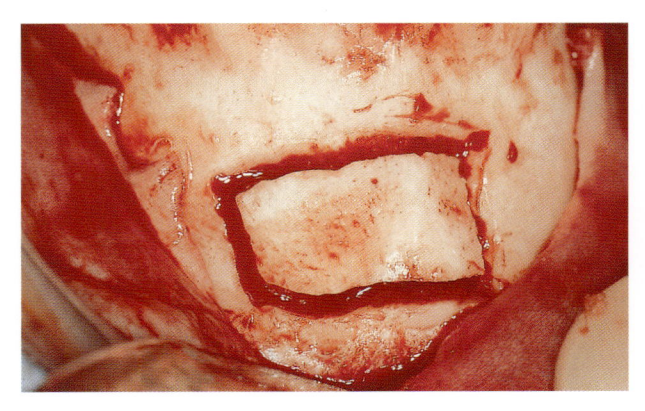

**Fig 13-51**   The symphysis has been selected as donor site because of the unavailability of bone in the ramus. The 3D form of the bone graft required is obtained by using the natural curvature of the symphysis.

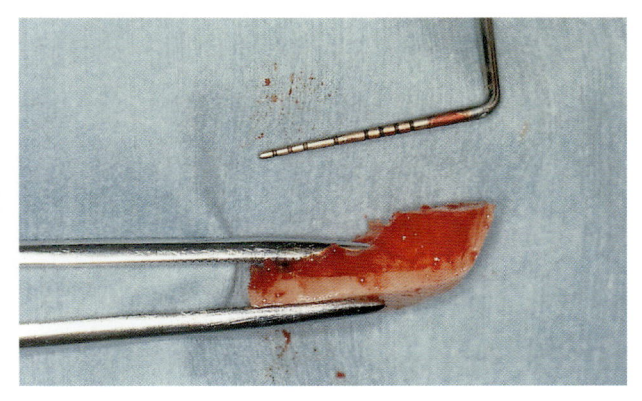

**Fig 13-52**   The cortico-cancellous bone graft harvested, showing the shape and dimensions.

III  Augmentation

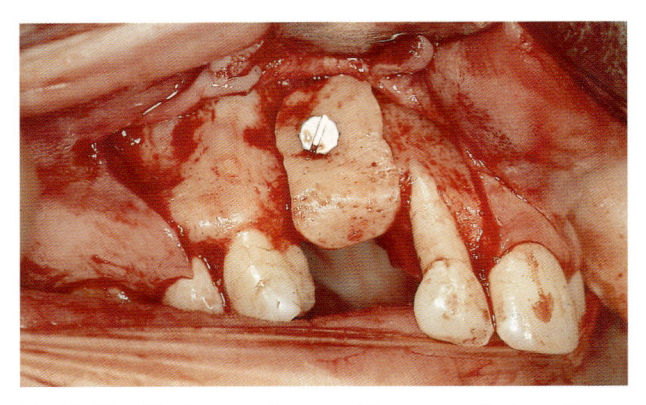

**Fig 13-53**  The bone graft secured by means of a bone fixation screw, thus restoring the width and height of the ridge.

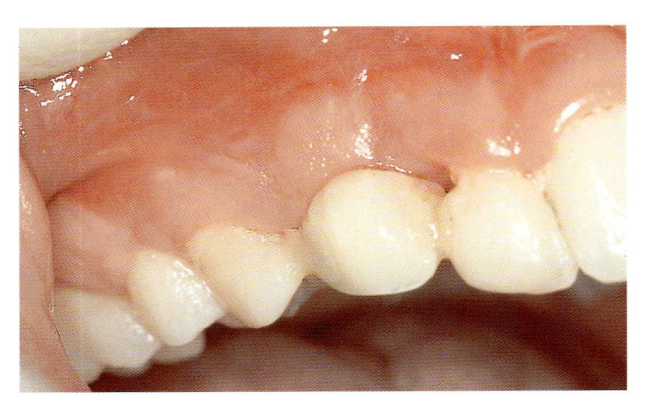

**Fig 13-54**  Post-operative view of the provisional metal-acrylic Rochette in situ following soft tissue healing after placement of the bone graft. Note that an acceptable contour has been obtained; this and subsequent restorative stages will be used to confirm the final aesthetic outcome.

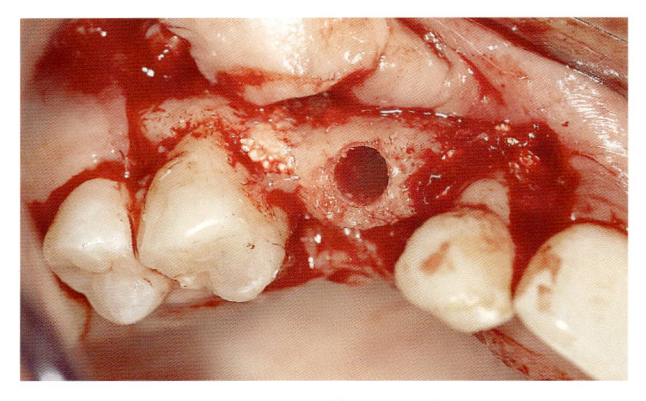

**Fig 13-55**  The ridge exposed 10 weeks after the placement of the bone graft and osteotomy prepared prior to implant placement. The bleeding surface of the bone is indicative of the fact that vascularisation has taken place. Careful preparation of the bone is essential to prevent dislodgement. Threads for the implant should also be tapped before insertion to prevent undue forces on the graft.

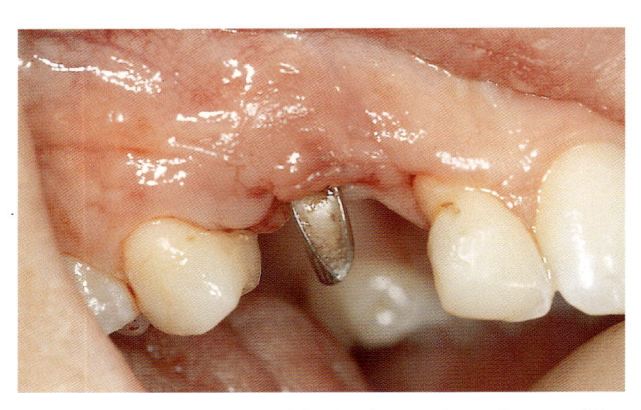

**Fig 13-56**  The exposure of the implant and attachment of the preselected angled abutment six months after implant placement.

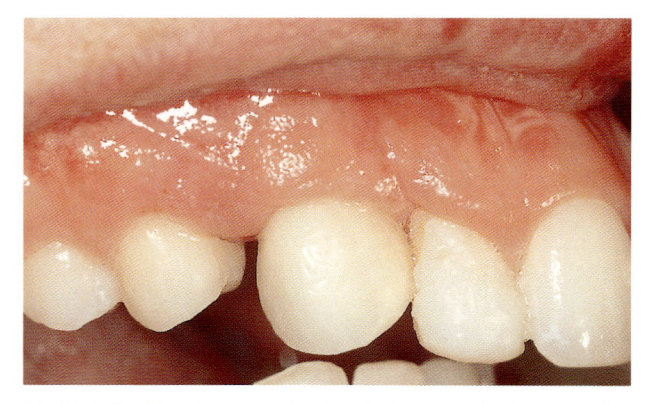

**Fig 13-57**  Transitional restoration being used to develop soft tissue contours and a papilla on the distal aspect of the lateral incisor.

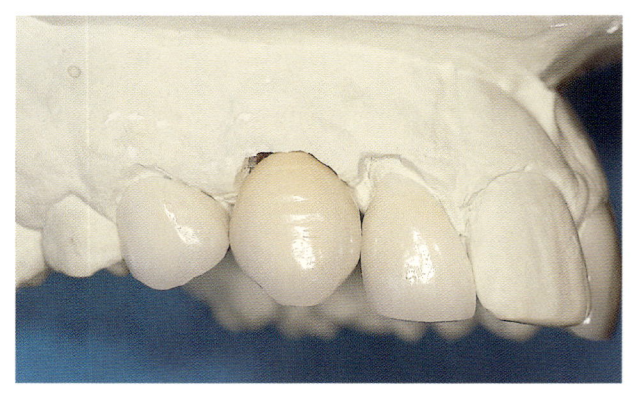

**Fig 13-58**  Laboratory cast showing the construction of the definitive restorations, a metal-ceramic crown for the implant replacing the canine, and two porcelain veneers for the adjacent teeth.

13   Localised Onlay Bone Grafts

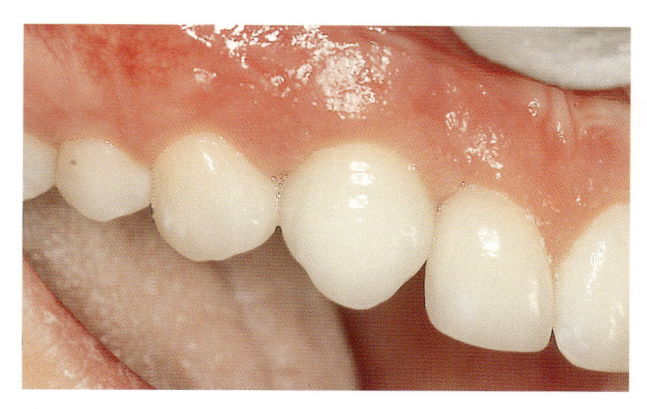

**Fig 13-59**  Definitive restorations in situ showing the contours of the soft tissues and the re-proportioned teeth, which produce a harmonious appearance.

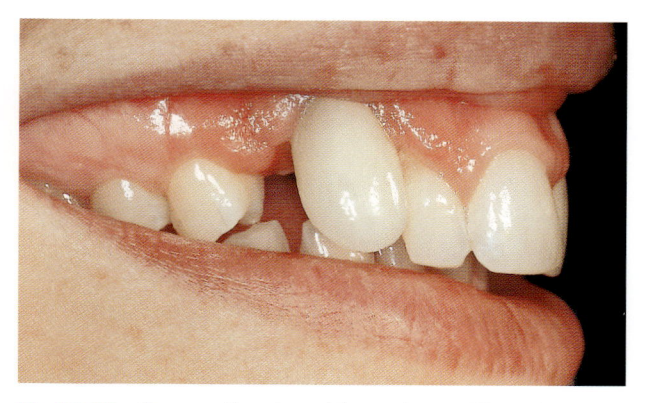

**Fig 13-60**  Preoperative view of the patient smiling, showing a high lipline and an unacceptable preoperative appearance.

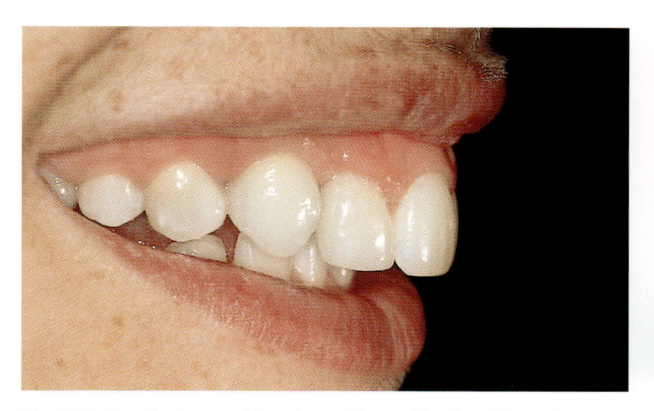

**Fig 13-61**  Post-operative view of the patient smiling, showing an acceptable aesthetic outcome with reconstructed ridge contour.

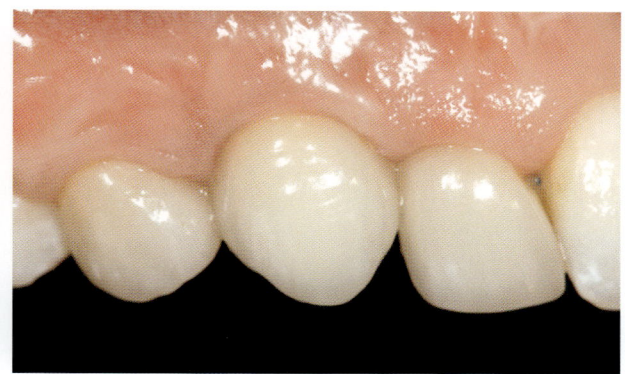

**Fig 13-62**  Follow-up at 10 years, showing stable soft tissues with minimal changes.

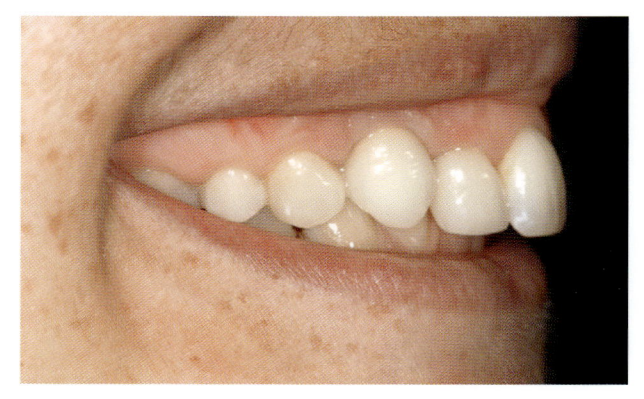

**Fig 13-63**  Follow-up at 10 years, showing the appearance of the patient smiling broadly.

# Chapter 14

# Extensive Bone Grafts

## Introduction

Extraoral bone graft donor sites include the Iliac crest, tibia, skull and rib.

## Iliac Crest

The iliac crest provides ample cortical, cortico-cancellous and cancellous bone and has contours that are easy to manipulate for use in the jaws; it is, therefore, the donor site of choice. The lateral aspect of the anterior iliac crest offers the most suitable shape and reduces the risk of peritoneal perforation. It is preferred to the posterior iliac crest to avoid turning the patient over and it permits simultaneous donor and recipient site surgery. Bicortical grafts for the reconstruction of class V and VI jaws can be harvested. The use of 'J'-shaped grafts offering two cortical surfaces is available for the management of class IV jaws. In addition, cancellous bone can also be obtained for the augmentation of the sinuses. The iliac crest is superficially placed, thus allowing easy access. The lateral femoral cutaneous nerve normally traverses anterior to the anterior iliac spine. However, in 10% of individuals, it traverses directly across the crest. Surgery must be carried out carefully to avoid damage to this nerve and subsequent paraesthesia of the skin over the lateral aspect of the thigh. Post-operative pain is associated with movement because of the disturbance of the abdominal and thigh muscles. Recovery is complete following a period ranging from one to four weeks. This does, however, depend on careful layered suturing of periosteum, muscle, adipose tissue, and skin. Otherwise, there are relatively few risks and the resulting scar can be easily concealed. Removal of bone from this site results in the least morbidity and risk.

## Tibia

There is a limited amount of bone available from the tibia, even though access is excellent. As this is a stress-bearing bone, availability is limited and there is a risk of subsequent fracture through increases in stress in the harvest area. Patients may object to the potential visible scar.

## Skull

The parietal bone offers monocortical grafts that are difficult to adapt to the recipient site and are of limited thickness. The density of the cortical bone increases the healing time for vascularisation to be completed. No cancellous bone is available and there are obvious concerns about the proximity of the brain. The presence of hair and the proximity to the oral cavity pose further operational difficulties.

## III Augmentation

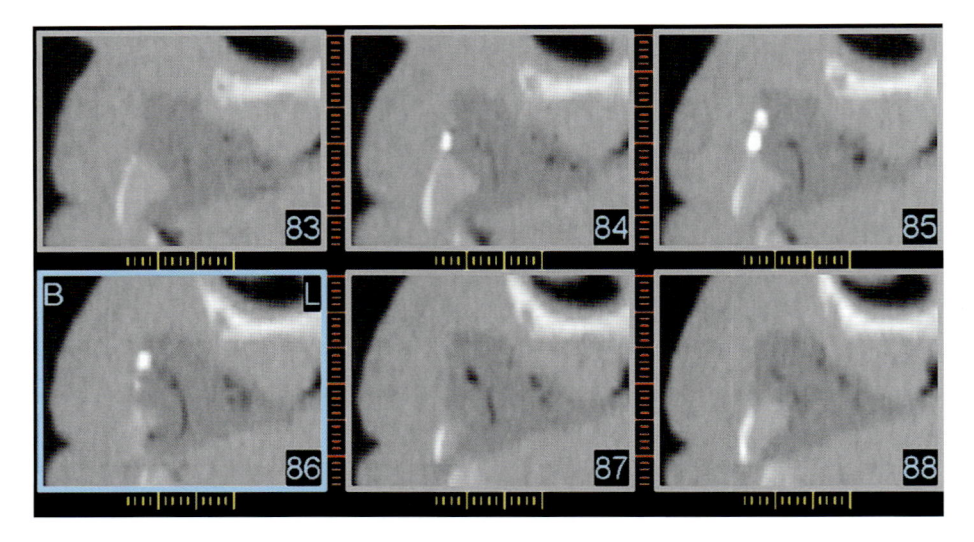

**Fig 14-1** CT scan reconstruction of the anterior maxilla in the canine and lateral incisor region (Class VI). The radiopaque markers to identify the tooth position (cross section 85/ lateral incisor with two markers, buccal side on the left-hand side) can be seen. The outline of the future tooth position can also be identified to relate it to the residual bone for purposes of planning the harvesting and positioning of the graft.

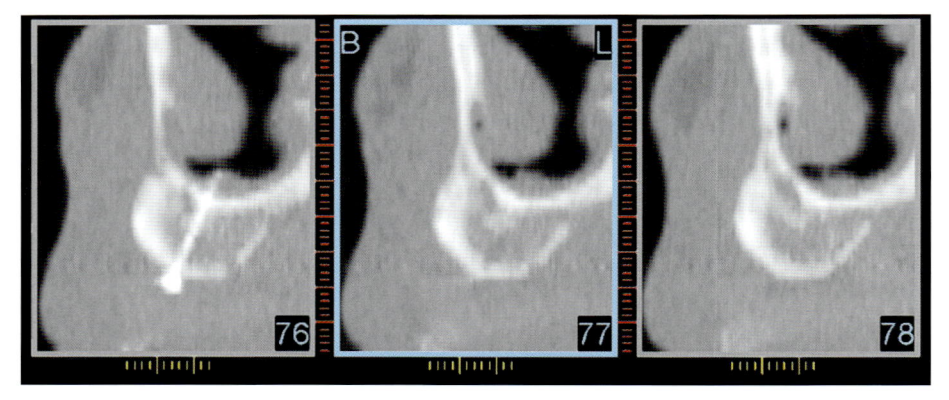

**Fig 14-2** CT scan reconstruction of the anterior maxilla in the canine region showing the reconstructed alveolar ridge prior to implant placement. The fixation screw is visible. The radiopaque marker identifying future tooth position is only just visible at the bottom of each image. The CT scan provides essential information for the planning of implant placement.

### Rib

Ribs comprise monocortical tubular bone with little or no cancellous bone, but because of its shape and composition, a graft is difficult to adapt. Risk of perforation of the pleural cavity and post-operative pain exclude the use of the rib in most cases.

### Assessment

Assessment for extensive bone grafts involves observing the patient's facial profile as an indicator of the extent of the atrophy of both the hard and soft tissues that has taken place. Examination of the intraoral soft tissues with the potential for covering the graft must also be assessed.

Assessment of the bone volume and its relationship to the ideal tooth position is fundamental to the outcome and planning. This is achieved by using radiopaque markers to identify tooth positions that can be related to the images obtained from the CT scan (Figs 14-1 and 14-2).

### Classification

Classification of the degree of atrophy is useful for deciding which corrective procedures should be implemented, and there are several accepted systems available for this purpose. We use the classification of Cawood and Howell (see Chapter 6)[50] as a guideline for the clinical management of atrophied jaws:

1. Class IV: loss of width, which includes ridges with loss of height of up to 5 mm (Figs 14-3 and 14-4)
2. Class V: loss of entire or substantial part of the alveolar process (Figs 14-5 and 14-6)
3. Class VI: loss of entire alveolar process as well as erosion of the basal bone (Figs 14-7 and 14-8).

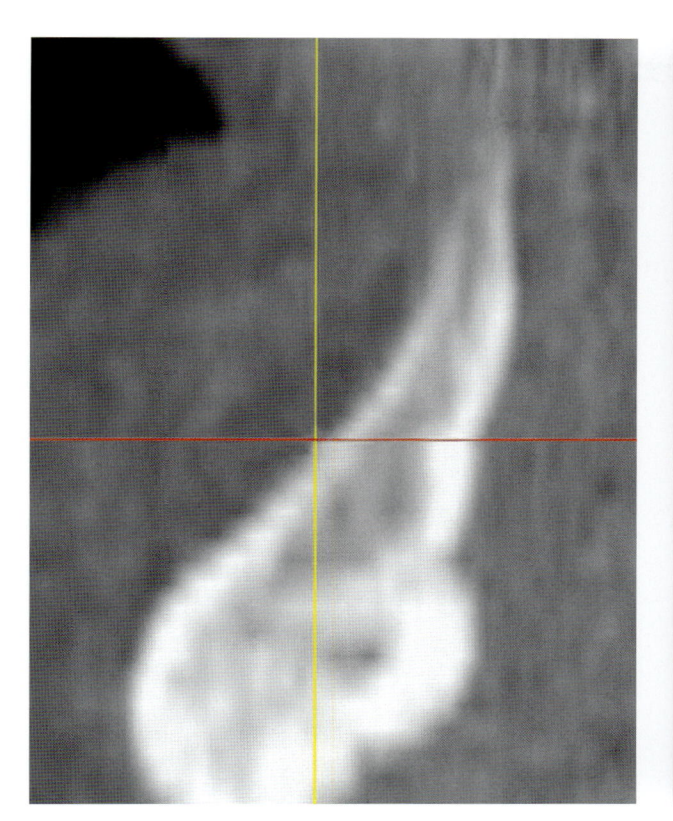

**Fig 14-3** CT cross-section of a class IV mandible.

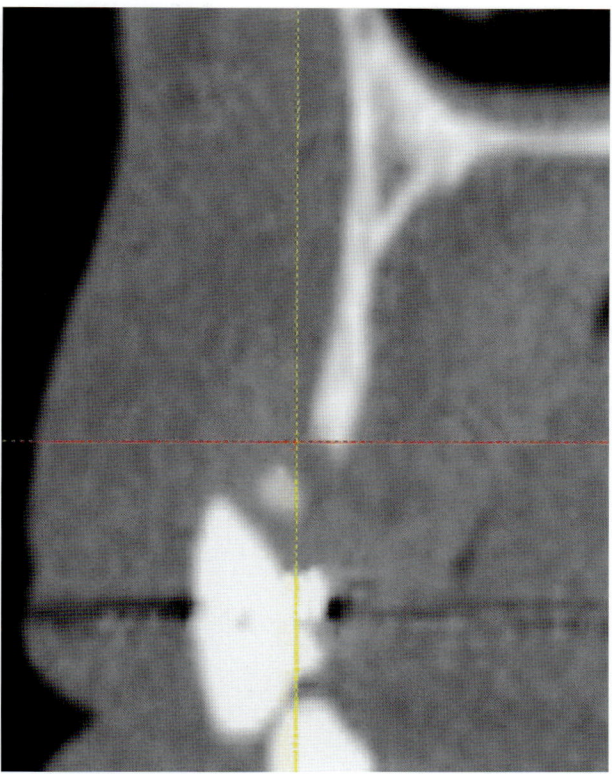

**Fig 14-4** CT cross-section of a class IV maxilla, with fused cortical plates.

## Loss of Width (Class IV)

Ridges that are not suitable for expansion (with fused cortical plates) but are of an acceptable height will require a bone graft for the purpose of increasing the width as well as offering circumoral soft tissue support.

## Loss of Width and Height (Class IV)

Narrow ridges that require an increase in width and up to 5 mm in height may be placed within this category. The decision is based on bone volume and on the relationship of the desired tooth position to the ridge. Aesthetic considerations often play a fundamental role in the decision-making process.

## Substantial Loss of Height: The Entire Alveolar Process (Class V)

A substantial loss of height is linked with a loss of facial form and function. The reconstruction of the entire

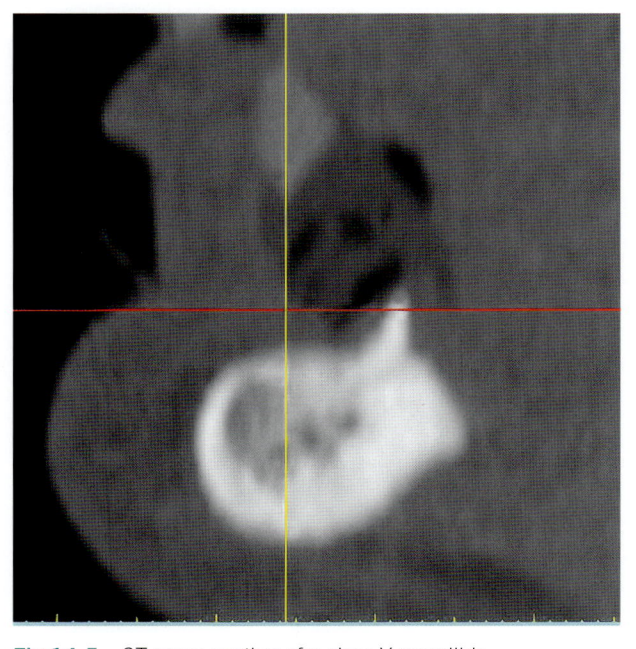

**Fig 14-5** CT cross-section of a class V mandible.

14 Extensive Bone Grafts

## III  Augmentation

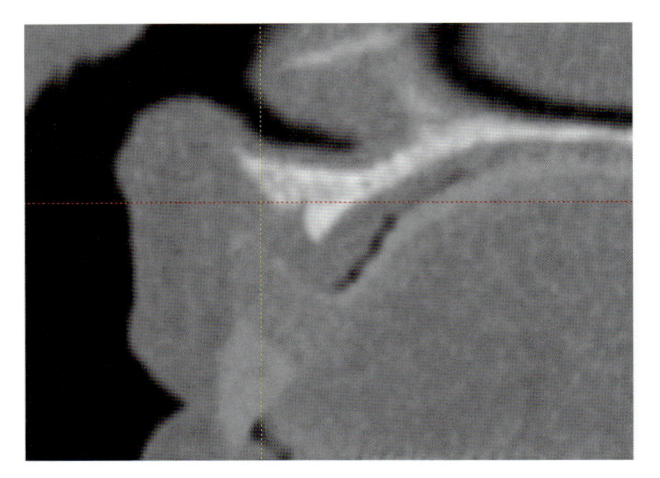

**Fig 14-6**  CT cross-section of a class V maxilla.

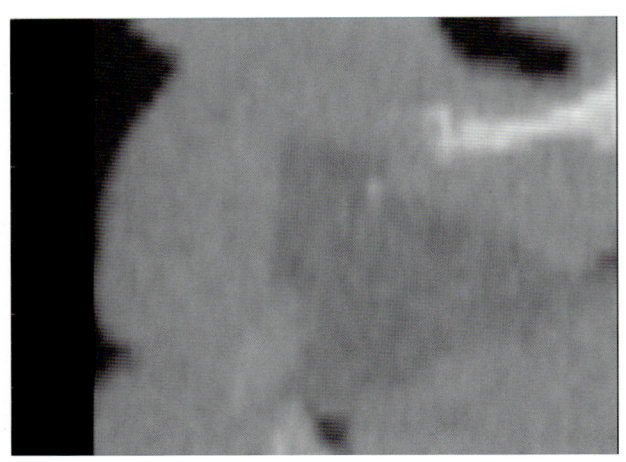

**Fig 14-7**  CT cross-section of a class VI maxilla.

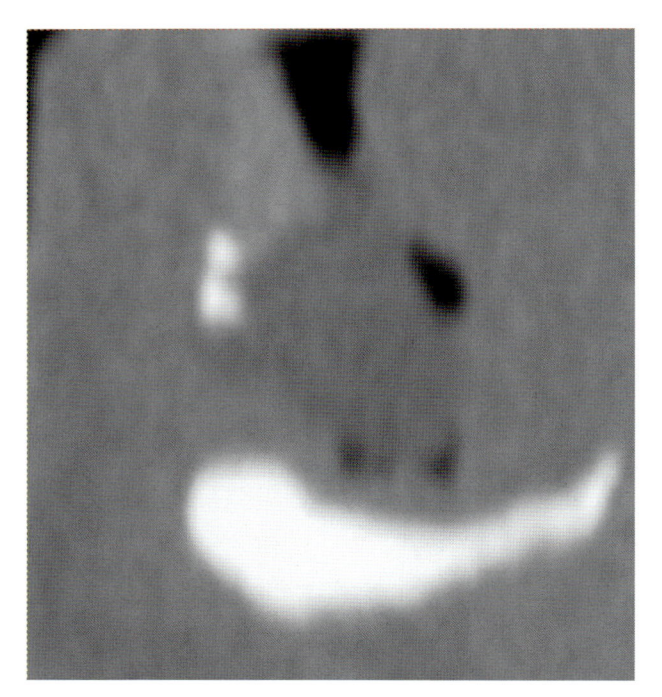

**Fig 14-8**  CT cross-section of a class VI mandible.

alveolar ridge requires treatment planning directed at the positioning of the bone graft, relating it to the tooth position, correcting the facial form and bringing the patient into function.

### Substantial Loss of Height: The Entire Alveolar Process and Basal Bone (Class VI)

In addition to the challenges of managing a Class V jaw, additional difficulties relating to availability of sufficient bone, graft fixation and soft tissue coverage of the graft make this class challenging to manage. Invariably, supplemental soft tissue surgery is required. The definitive restoration often has increased prosthetic tooth length.

## Planning of Treatment

The diagnostic phase involves positioning teeth on a wax baseplate in a position that provides the required support for the circumoral soft tissues to achieve the correct facial profile. The size, shape and position of the teeth have to meet the patient's aesthetic needs and expectations and eventually have to enable the patient to function. Some assessment of the patient's function may be carried out at this stage by using speech as an indicator of habitual muscular activity. Once the above criteria have been met, the teeth are painted with a radiopaque varnish to enable their position to be transferred to the CT images.

To obtain information about the quantity of bone that will need to be harvested, the selected tooth position is related to a stone cast of the edentulous ridge by means of a plaster matrix, and the wax of the try-in is eliminated. The space thus created between the teeth, set in the plaster matrix and the edentulous ridge, gives an indication of the amount of bone necessary to reconstruct the ridge. Silicone can be used to form a template that the orthopaedic or maxillofacial surgeon may use in determining the shape and size of the graft that is required.

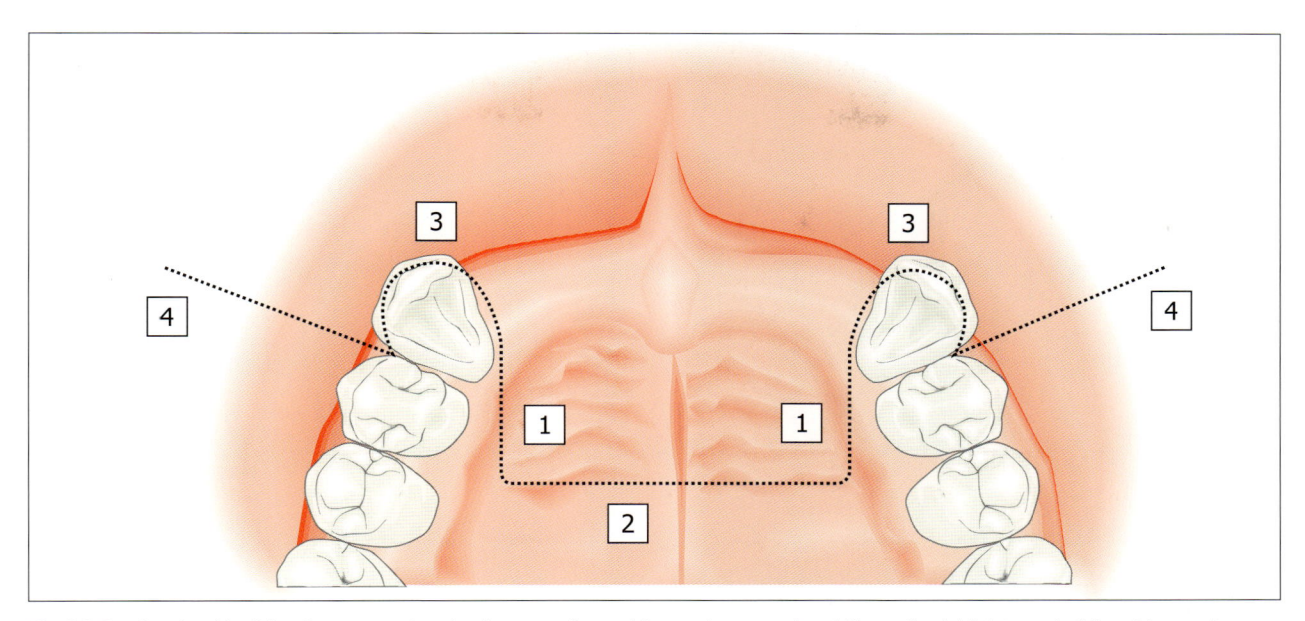

**Fig 14-9** A palatal incision for more extensive bone graft requiring an increase in width on the labial aspect of the ridge and an increase in height of <5 mm (Class IV).
1. Component extending into the palate by approximately 10 mm is made almost perpendicular to the ridge.
2. Bevelled component connecting the two incisions made with a Blake's knife.
3. Intrasulcular cervical incision.
4. Vertical release incision including the papilla.

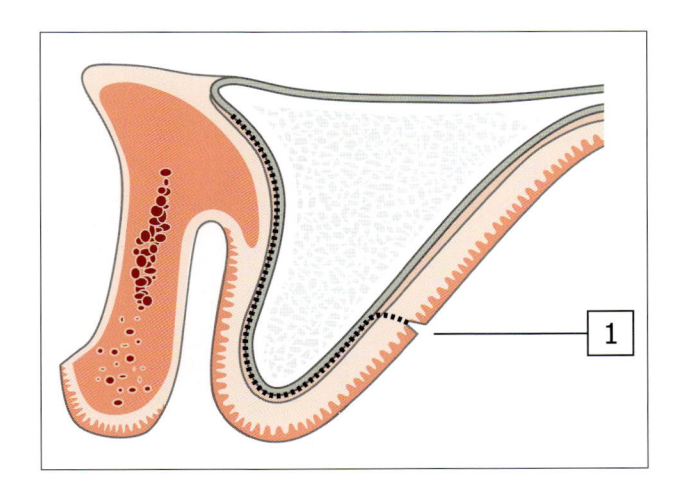

**Fig 14-10** Cross-sectional view of the anterior maxilla depicting a remote palatal incision suitable for an increase in width and an increase in height of up to 5 mm on the labial aspect of the ridge. The extent of periosteal reflection is also shown. The periosteal reflection is extended to the anterior nasal spine, the piriform rim and the zygomatic process to enable the soft tissues to be closed over the graft.

# Surgery

The surgical approach to treatment of the bone deficiencies outlined above depends on the extent and location of the atrophy.

## Loss of Width and Height

Loss of width and minimal loss of height requiring reconstruction on the labial aspect of the ridge (up to 5 mm) can be treated by using an incision made in the palate creating a buccally based flap (Figs 14-9–14-11). Bone deficiencies on the palatal aspects of the ridge require the incision to be made on the labial aspect.

## Substantial Loss of Height

A labial incision made close to the vermilion border of the lip producing a palatally based flap is used whenever a substantial increase in ridge height is required (up to 15 mm) (Figs 14-12–14-14).

III  Augmentation

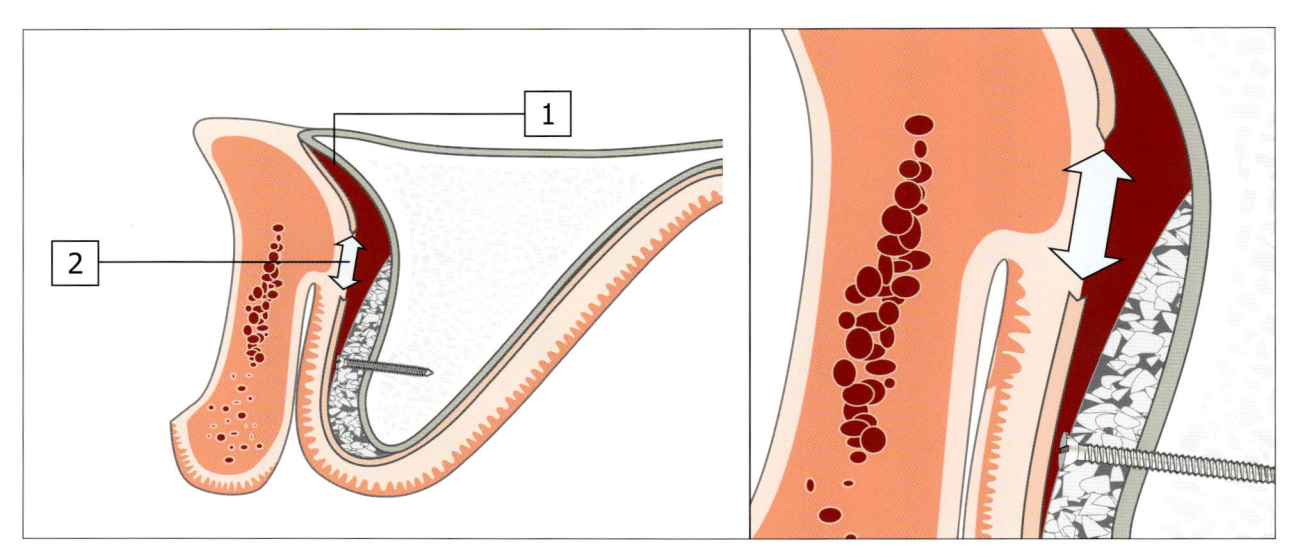

**Fig 14-11**  Creation of tissue for passive closure over a bone graft.
1. By reflection of the periosteum allowing tissue to be advanced.
2. By periosteal release incision. A reduction in the vestibular sulcus depth will result, with the labial tissue being advanced towards the palate.

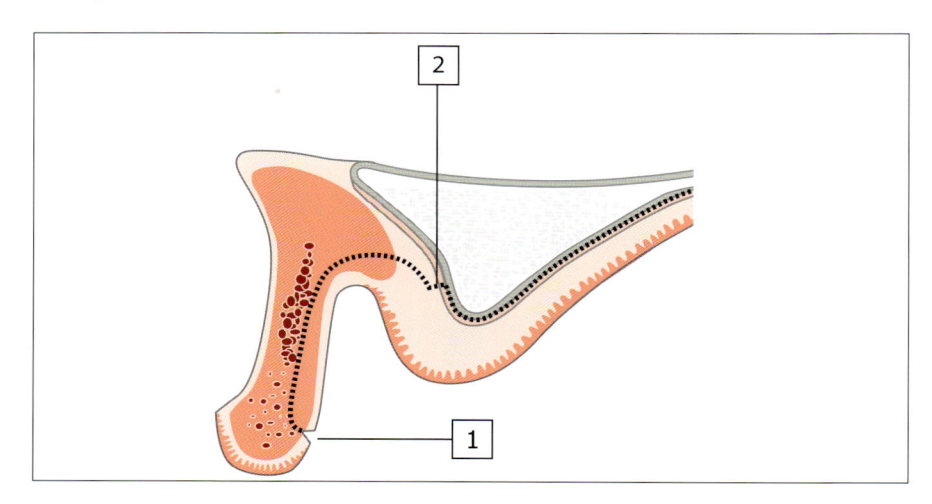

**Fig 14-12**  Cross-section of maxilla requiring augmentation in height (Class V and VI). A remote labial incision for an onlay graft requiring an increase in height of more than 5 mm on the crest and labial (most common) or palatal aspect of the ridge.
1. Split-thickness labial incision.
2. Periosteal incision and reflection of a full-thickness flap to expose crest of ridge.

Opening of parotid duct

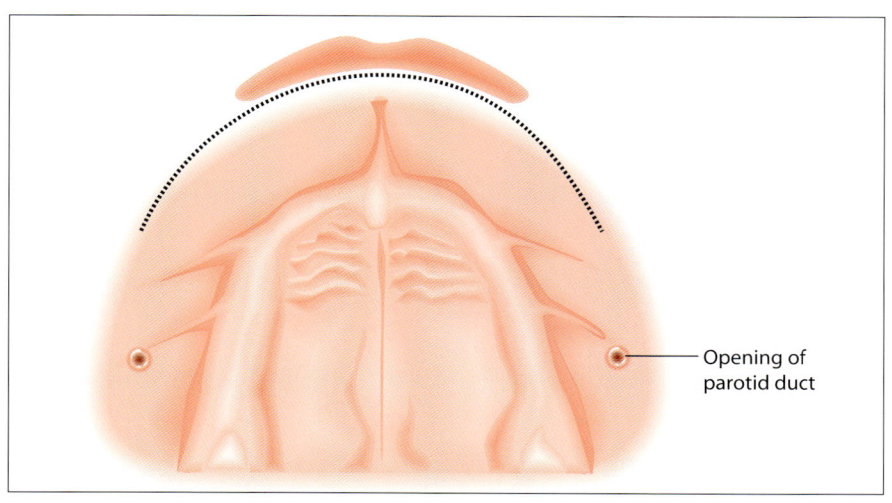

**Fig 14-13**  The remote labial incision (occlusal view) that will produce a palatally based flap. Care needs to be taken to avoid the opening of the parotid duct (parotid papilla).

14   Extensive Bone Grafts

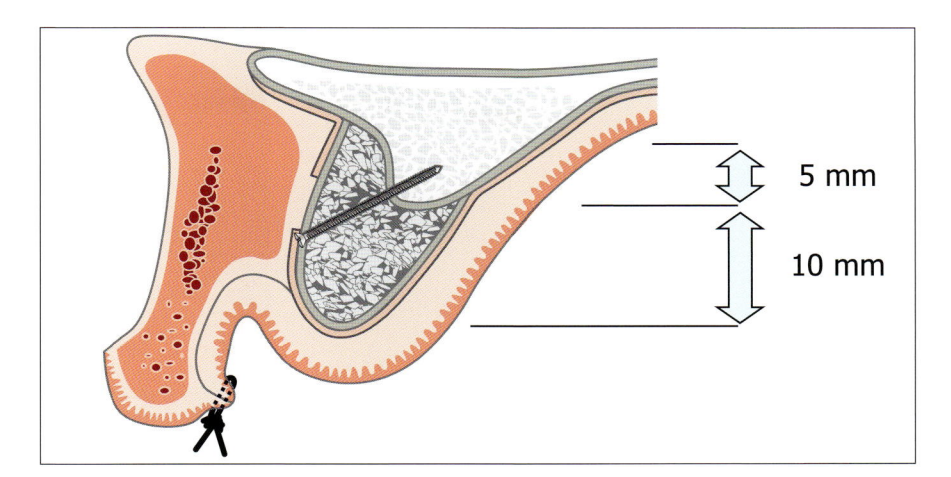

**Fig 14-14**  Closure of the soft tissues over a large onlay bone graft. The wound is closed using mattress sutures, with a substantial reduction in sulcus depth.

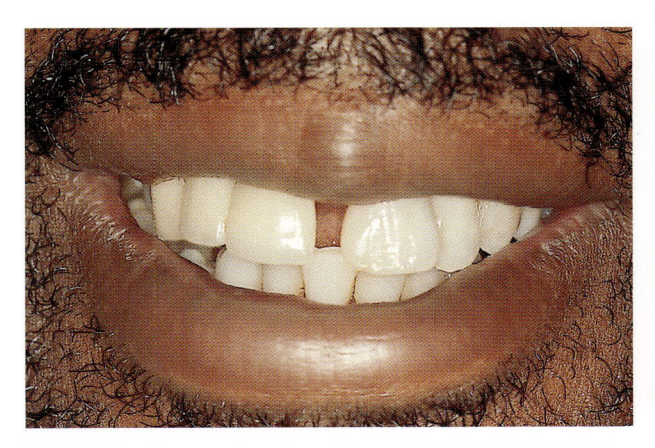

**Fig 14-15**  Preoperative view of the patient smiling, showing the displacement of the anterior teeth caused by advanced periodontal disease.

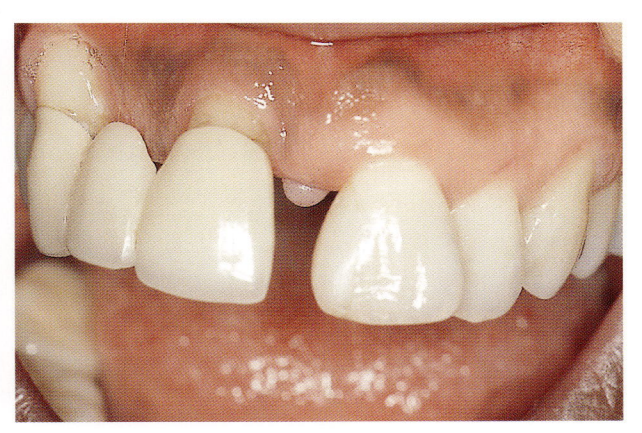

**Fig 14-16**  Labial view of the intraoral situation showing the central diastema and the exposure of the roots.

## Extensive Bone Grafts: Clinical Cases

### Case 1: Bone Graft from the Iliac Crest for Reconstruction of a Deficient Ridge

This case study demonstrates the use of bone grafts obtained from an extraoral site for the reconstruction of a ridge destroyed by extensive periodontal disease. The treatment of this patient was driven prosthetically. A provisional metal-acrylic Rochette bridge was used to establish the correct tooth form. The information gathered was then transferred to the definitive restoration in a number of stages (described in Chapter 10). The provisional restoration was used to diagnose and identify the need for a bone graft in conjunction with diagnostic imaging consisting of CT scans and conventional radiographs. This case study is also described in Chapter 8, on provisional restorations (Figs 8-37–8-41, pp. 115–116). Harvesting bone from the iliac crest requires a general anaesthetic. Assessment of the patient in terms of general health is essential and must be carried out thoroughly to ensure the patient's well-being. This is particularly necessary in view of the fact that surgery for the reconstruction of the jaws is an elective procedure. Preoperative assessment of the patient must also be carried out by the anaesthetist. Medical evaluation for this patient was carried out by Dr Michael Boscoe and included a physical examination, a blood test involving biochemistry and electrocardiography (Figs 14-15–14-42).

# III   Augmentation

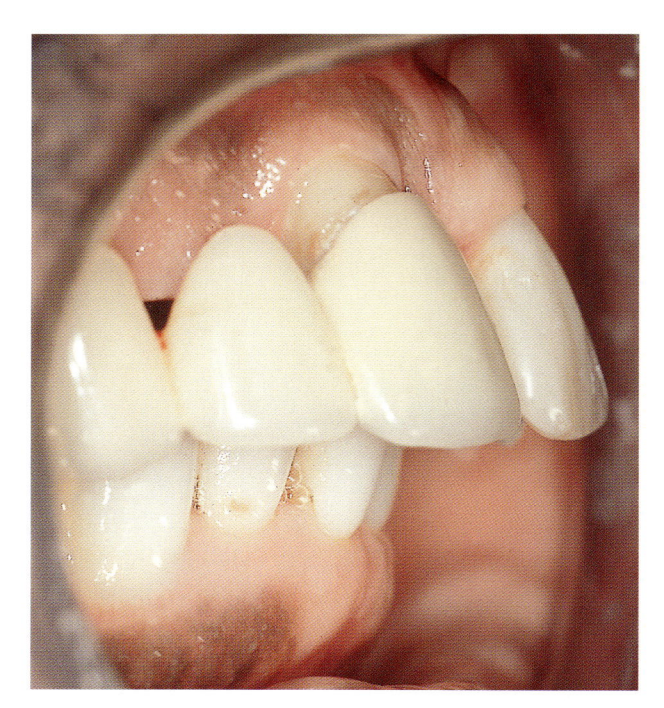

**Fig 14-17**   Lateral view of the failing dentition showing the degree of proclination that had taken place as a result of drifting caused by periodontal bone loss.

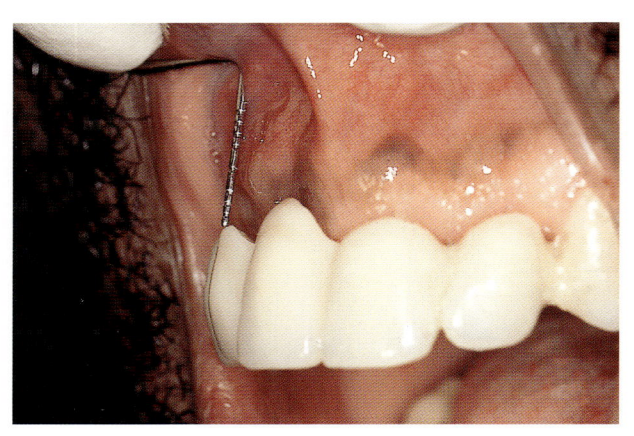

**Fig 14-18**   Lateral view of the provisional metal-acrylic Rochette bridge showing the loss of tissue on completion of soft tissue healing following tooth loss, in relation to the ideal tooth position.

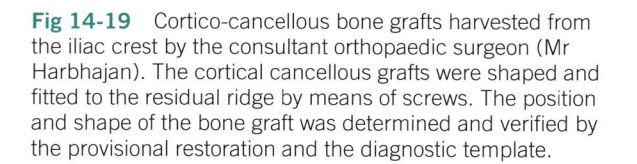

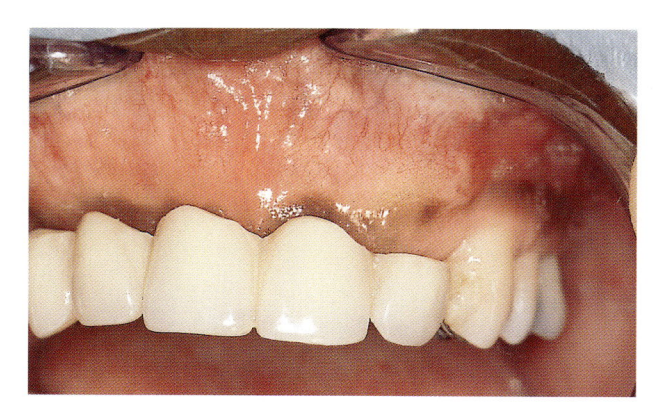

**Fig 14-19**   Cortico-cancellous bone grafts harvested from the iliac crest by the consultant orthopaedic surgeon (Mr Harbhajan). The cortical cancellous grafts were shaped and fitted to the residual ridge by means of screws. The position and shape of the bone graft was determined and verified by the provisional restoration and the diagnostic template.

**Fig 14-20**   Post-operative view on the completion of healing prior to implant placement. The ridge has been reconstructed and can be seen in relationship to the provisional restoration, which has been modified to allow for the altered ridge dimensions. The bone graft was allowed to mature for a period of 10 weeks prior to implant placement.

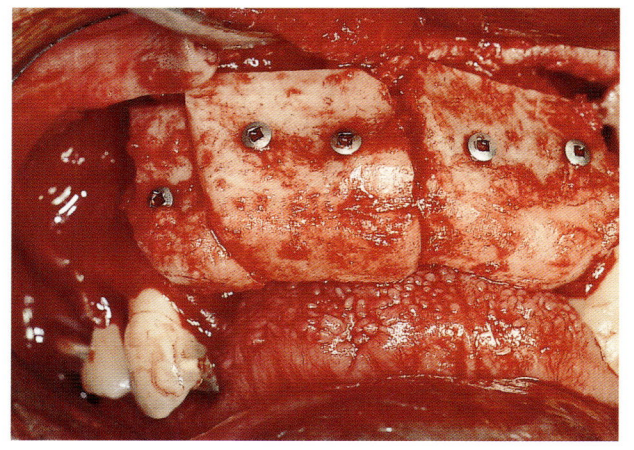

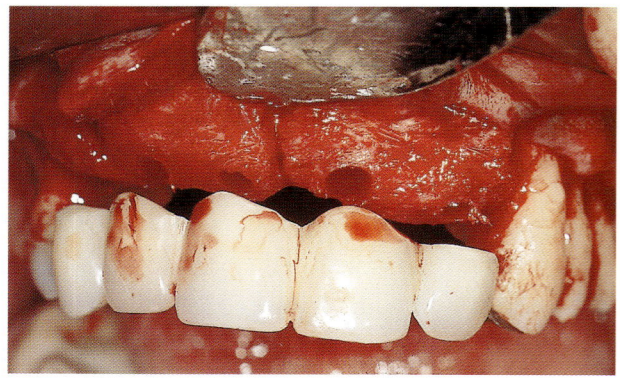

**Fig 14-21**   Intraoral operative view of the healed graft with the provisional restoration being used to select the implant positions.

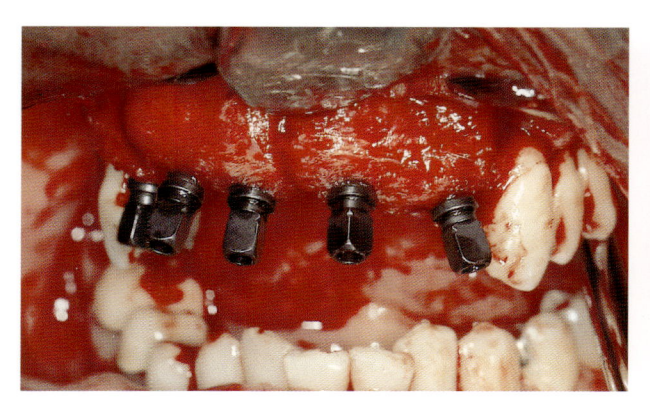

**Fig 14-22** Labial view of the implants inserted with the implant carriers visible. Note the position and angulation of the implants. The implants have been placed so that they engage both the bone graft and the residual ridge. The point of emergence of the implants is coincident with the tooth position.

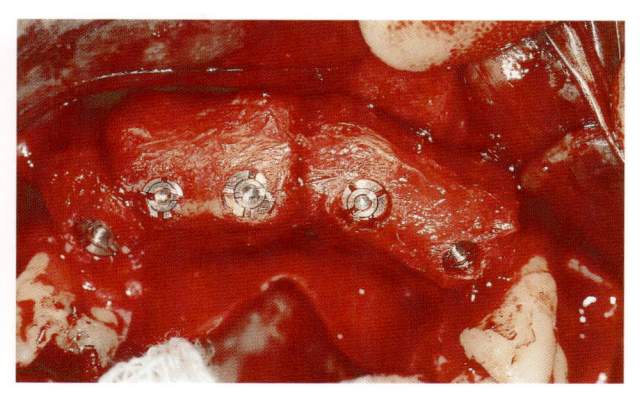

**Fig 14-23** The clinical view of the implants with the carriers removed. The implants and the cover screws (which come pre-attached) can be seen.

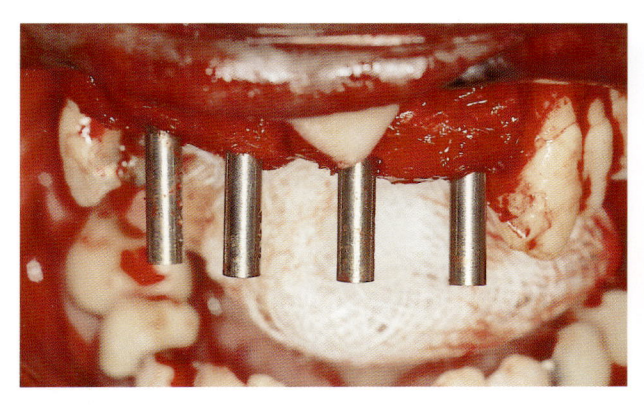

**Fig 14-24** Prototype direction indicators can be seen being used to select the abutment to provide the correct alignment in readiness for the exposure of the implants on completion of integration.

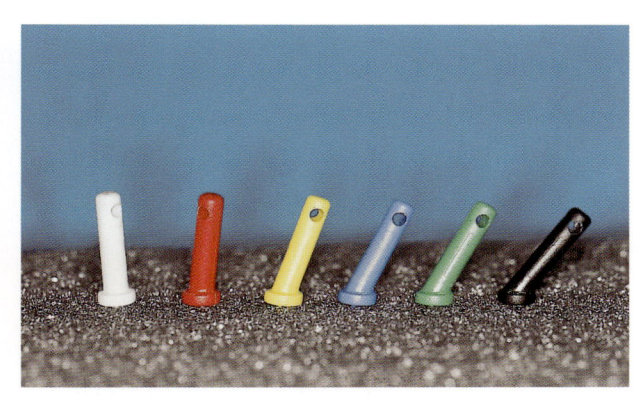

**Fig 14-25** The range of six direction indicators with corresponding angles, which are colour coded for ease of identification.

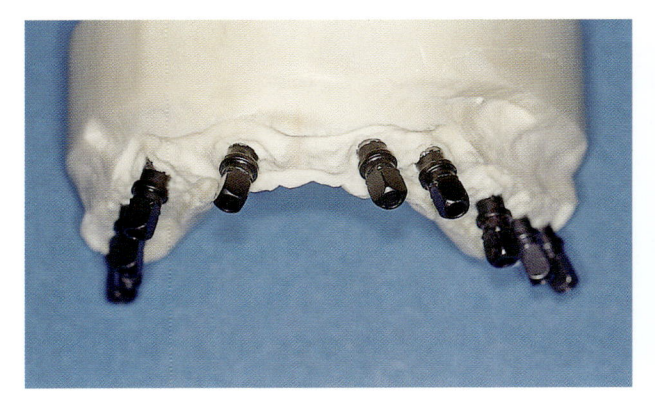

**Fig 14-26** Laboratory cast with the implant carriers attached to the implant analogues to demonstrate the range of angles at which the implants have been placed in an edentulous maxilla.

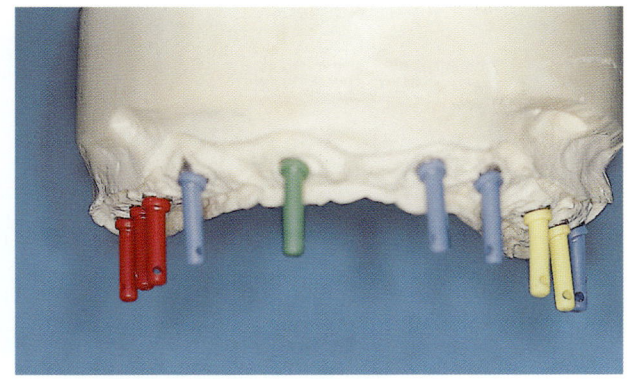

**Fig 14-27** The laboratory cast demonstrates the use of direction indicators to select abutments. Direction indicators are used to choose the angled abutment, which will fit within the prosthetic envelope and provide parallel and aligned abutments for the prosthetic phase. The direction indicators fit into the cover screw. Note the range of angles that have been used, ranging from 7.5 degrees (yellow) to 30 degrees (green).

## III  Augmentation

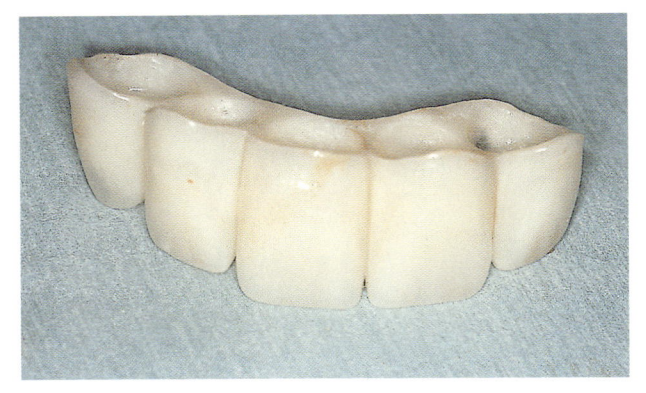

**Fig 14-28**  Hollow acrylic resin transitional restoration fabricated from information gained from the provisional metal-acrylic Rochette bridge. The transitional restoration is designed to fit over the abutments, which were selected using the diagnostic template and direction indicators.

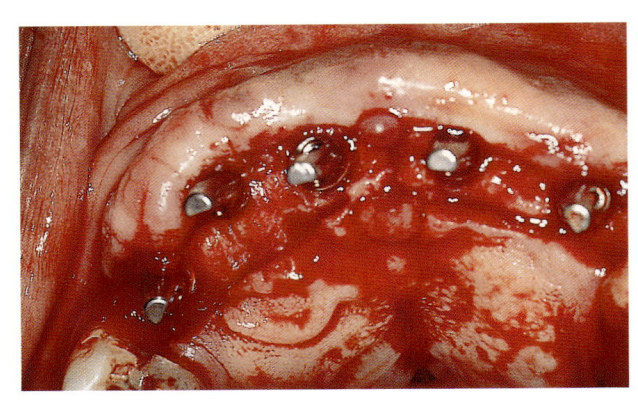

**Fig 14-29**  Maxillary ridge exposed via a full-thickness incision situated towards the palatal aspect of the ridge. The abutments selected at first-stage surgery have been attached and can be seen.

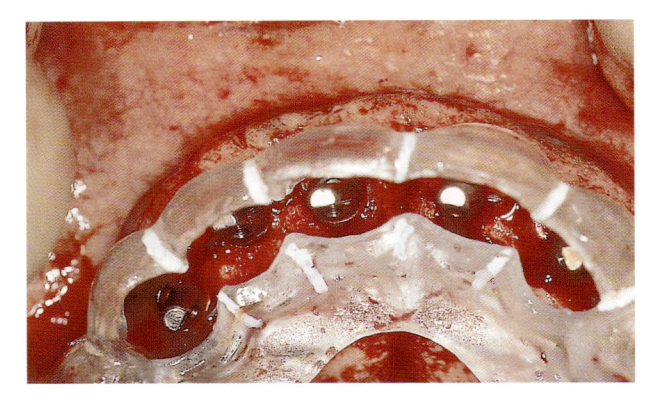

**Fig 14-30**  The diagnostic template is used to confirm the position of the abutments in relation to future tooth position. Adequate clearance on the labial and palatal aspects must be allowed. The abutments can be seen emerging in tooth position.

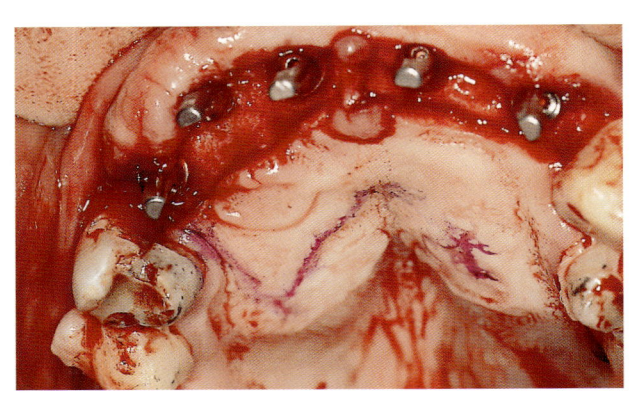

**Fig 14-31**  Occlusal view of the operative site showing a line marking the extent of the split-thickness incision that will form the sliding epithelial flap to cover the exposed bone.

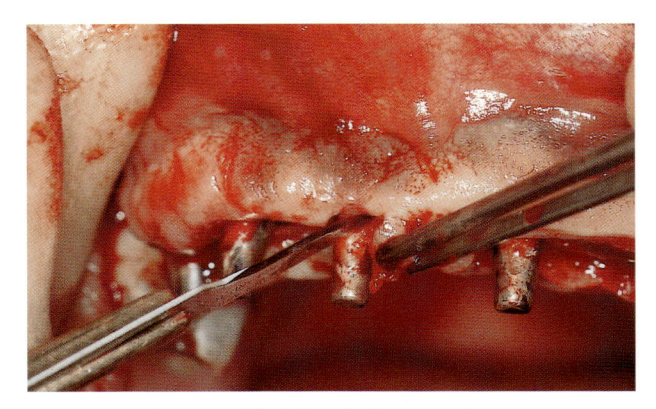

**Fig 14-32**  'S'-shaped incisions being carried out to create pedicled flaps for the reconstruction of the interdental papillae.

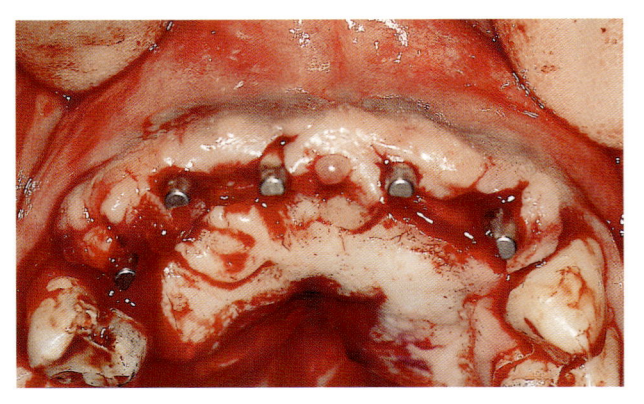

**Fig 14-33**  Clinical view showing the positioning of the pedicle flaps and the closure of the exposed bone by means of the palatal sliding split-thickness epithelial flap.

14  Extensive Bone Grafts

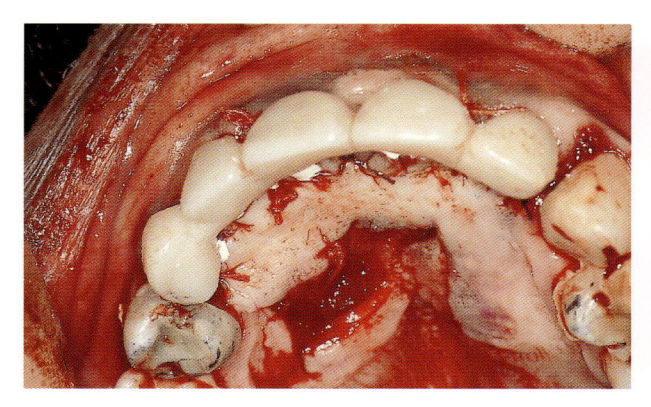

**Fig 14-34**  The transitional restoration is relined to adapt closely to the abutments and shaped to start the development of the soft tissue contours. The transitional restoration is cemented with a temporary cement. The extent to which the flap has been displaced towards the labial from the palate can be seen.

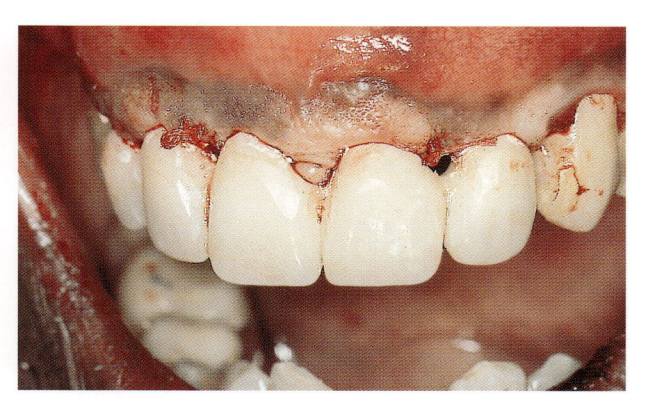

**Fig 14-35**  Labial view of the transitional restoration showing the contours, which will help to fashion the soft tissues.

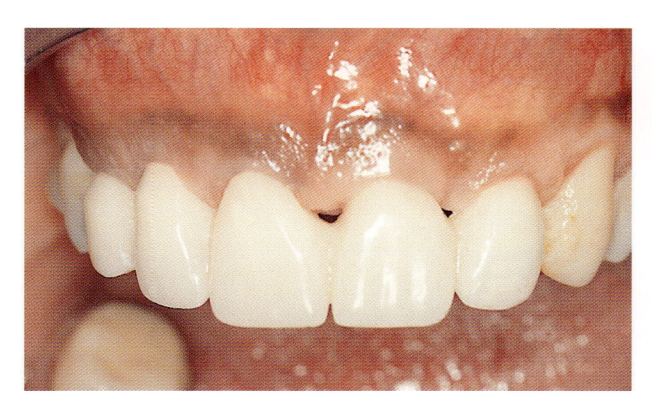

**Fig 14-36**  Labial view of the healed soft tissues in relationship to the transitional restoration, one month after the exposure of the implants.

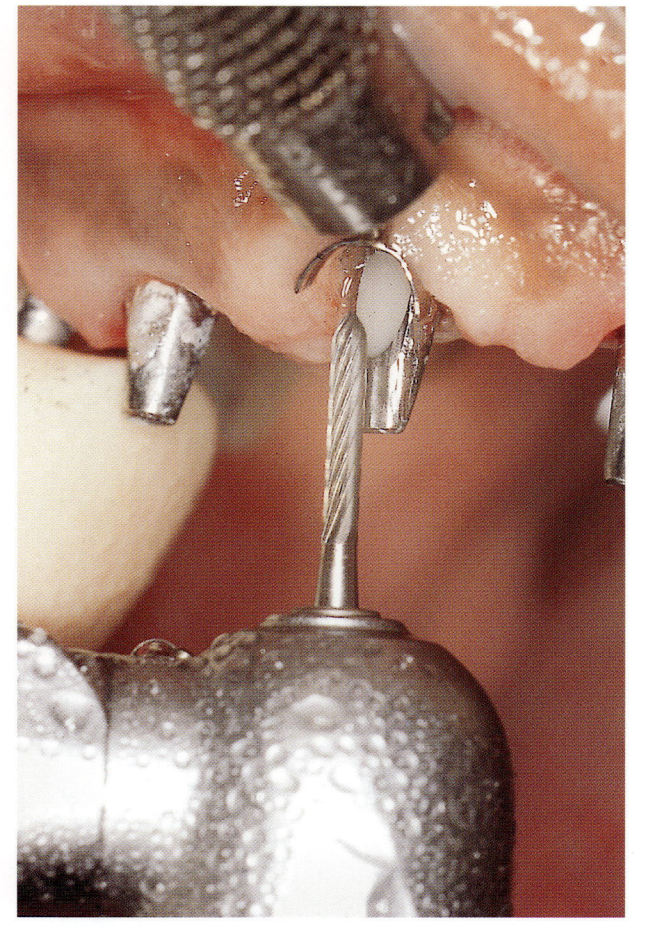

**Fig 14-37**  Labial view of the abutments emerging from the soft tissues contoured by the transitional restoration.

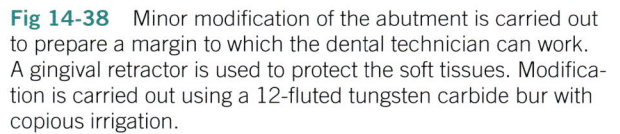

**Fig 14-38**  Minor modification of the abutment is carried out to prepare a margin to which the dental technician can work. A gingival retractor is used to protect the soft tissues. Modification is carried out using a 12-fluted tungsten carbide bur with copious irrigation.

271

III Augmentation

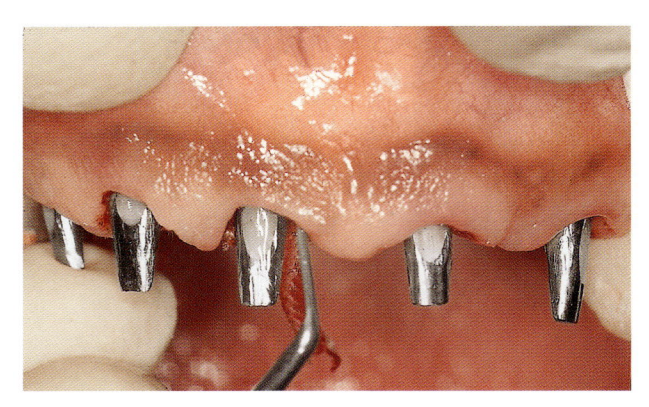

**Fig 14-39** Retraction cord is used to ensure an accurate recording of the prepared margins with the impression.

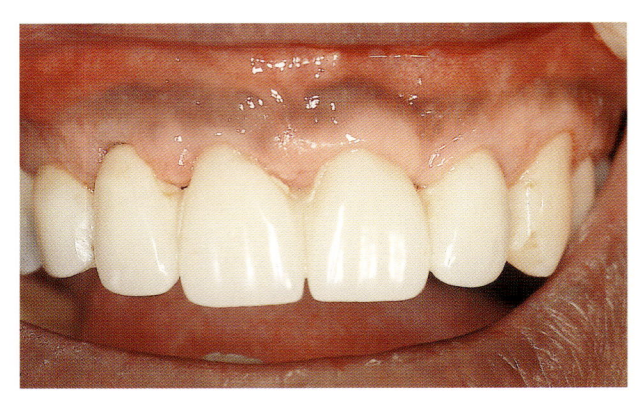

**Fig 14-40** The transitional restoration is cleaned to remove traces of temporary cement and relined using self-polymerising resin to re-adapt it to the abutments and to manipulate the soft tissues.

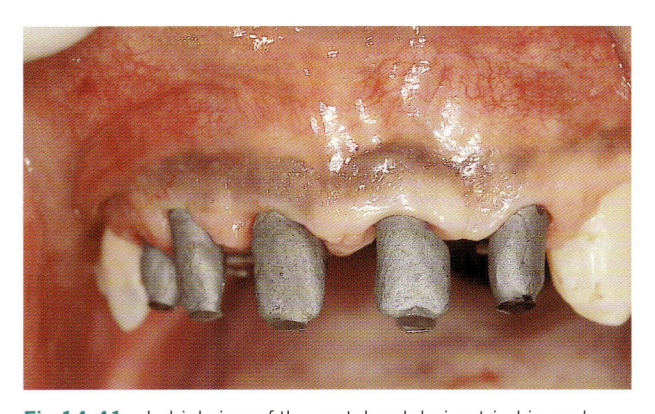

**Fig 14-41** Labial view of the metalwork being tried in and ready for a pick-up impression. The shape of the developed soft tissues is thereby recorded for the addition of porcelain to the metal copings.

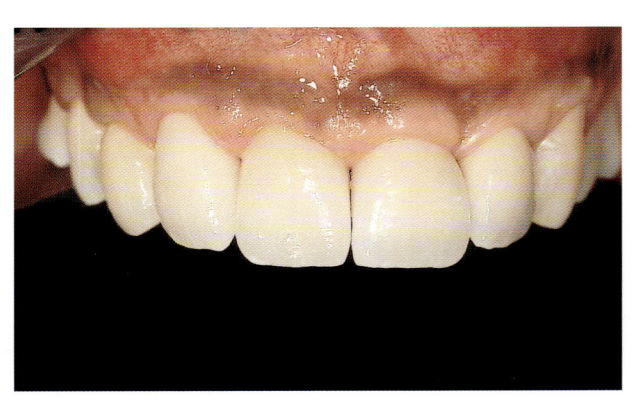

**Fig 14-42** Labial view of the definitive metal-ceramic crowns emerging from the reconstructed hard and soft tissues. The deficiency visible in the lateral view relating the provisional metal-acrylic bridge to the postextraction soft tissues has been repaired (Fig 14-18). The provisional bridge also provided information for the implants to be positioned ideally to support the teeth in an aesthetically and functionally verified position (same patient as in Figs 8-37–8-41).

## Case 2: Bone Graft from the Iliac Crest for a Class V Ridge

This case study illustrates the treatment of a 60-year-old woman who had lost her anterior maxillary teeth and posterior mandibular teeth. The destruction of the maxillary alveolar ridge may have been the result of a para-functional habit in combination with the pattern of tooth loss.

The resultant Class V ridge (Cawood and Howell[50]) required treatment with an onlay cortico-cancellous graft obtained from the iliac crest to increase the height of the ridge by 15 mm. Surgery to reconstruct the maxilla was carried out jointly with John Cawood, a consultant oral and maxillofacial surgeon. Onlay grafts were used to reconstruct the anterior maxilla, and bilateral sinus lifts were carried out to create an adequate volume of bone in the posterior quadrants.

The grafts were harvested from the anterior iliac crest by Harbhajan Plaha, a consultant orthopaedic surgeon. Preoperative assessment and perioperative care and general anaesthesia was provided by Michael Boscoe (Figs 14-43–14-49).

## 14  Extensive Bone Grafts

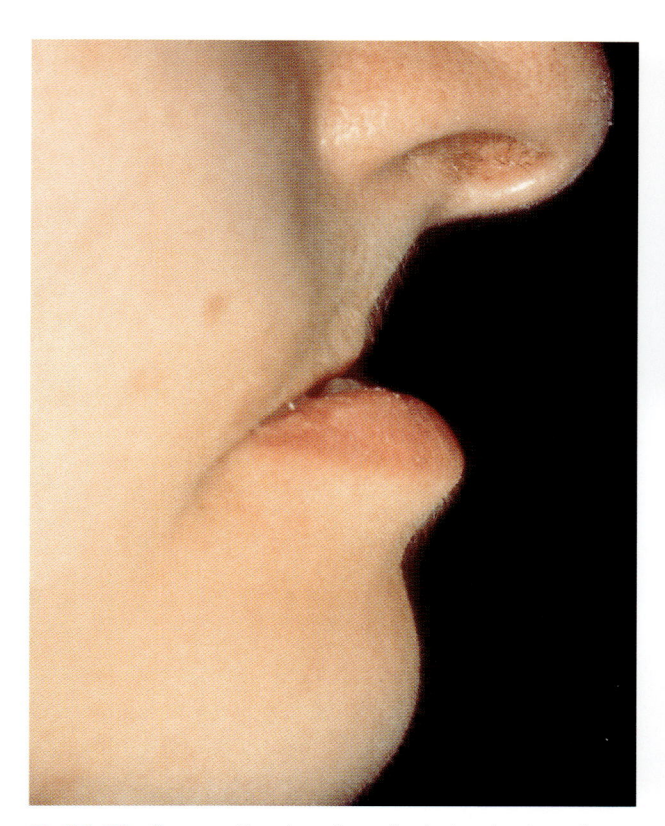

**Fig 14-43**  Preoperative view of a patient, showing loss of support for the upper lip resulting from the complete destruction of the alveolar ridge. Adequate support of the lower lip is provided by the remaining mandibular incisors.

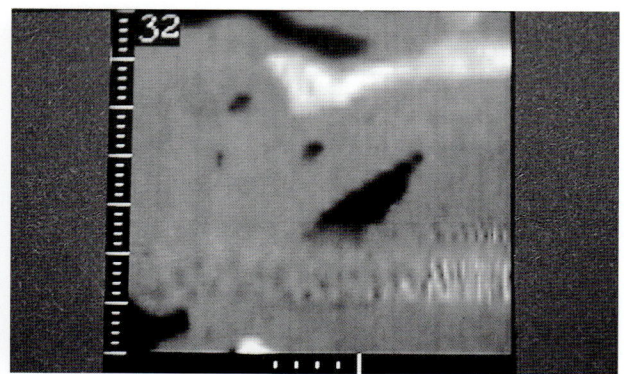

**Fig 14-44**  Oblique cross-sectional view of the CT scan of the maxilla in the central incisor region showing the complete loss of the alveolar process. The scan shows a limited amount of bone available for the fixation of the graft. The registration block, which is barely visible, and the mandibular incisor, which can be seen at the bottom of the image, give an indication of the amount of bone loss.

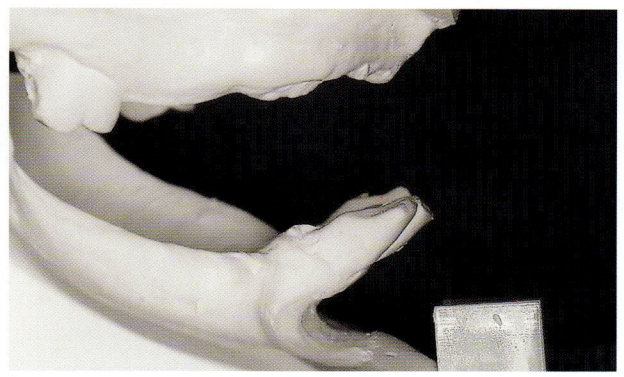

**Fig 14-46**  Articulated study casts providing information about the anterior–posterior relationship of the upper ridge to the mandibular incisors.

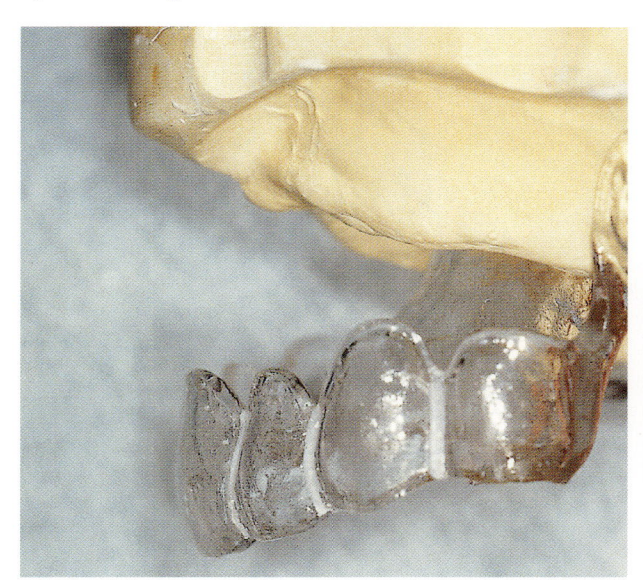

**Fig 14-45**  A laboratory cast with a diagnostic template constructed from the teeth set up and used to determine the desired end result as a part of the diagnostic preview. The dimensions of the graft are determined preoperatively by relating the tooth position to the residual ridge. Silicone templates are used to relate this information to the surgical site.

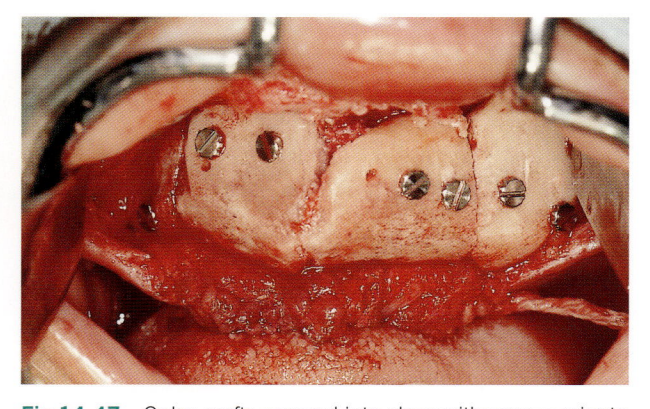

**Fig 14-47**  Onlay grafts secured into place with screws prior to closure of the surgical site. The flap created by a remote labial incision behind the vermilion border can be seen. (Surgery was carried out jointly with J. Cawood, consultant maxillofacial surgeon, Chester, UK. Bone grafts were harvested by H. Plaha; anaesthesia by M. Boscoe.)

# III   Augmentation

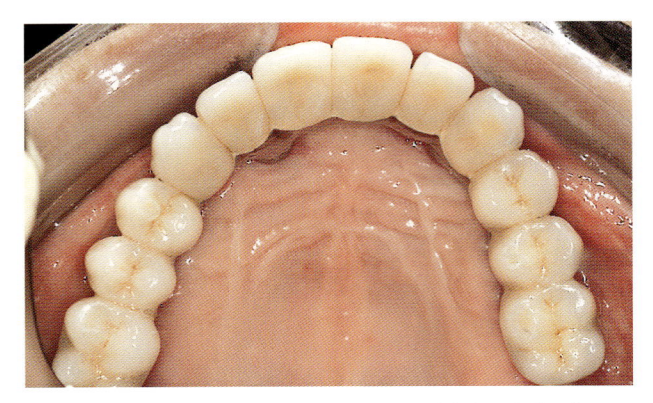

**Fig 14-48**  Occlusal view of the completed full arch fixed restoration constructed from metal and porcelain.

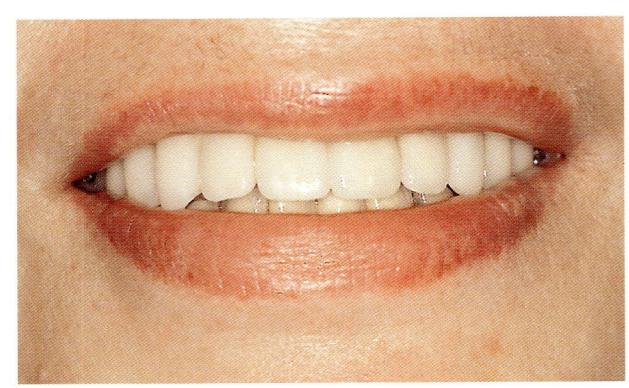

**Fig 14-49**  Anterior view of the patient showing adequate lip support. The patient has been provided with a fixed implant-supported restoration. Functional stimulation of the grafted bone will sustain it and provide the patient with function. The ongoing process of bone resorption has been arrested.

## Case 3: Aesthetic Reconstruction of the Anterior Maxilla Following Trauma

A 14-year-old girl had trauma damage to her anterior teeth (12, 11 and 21). These were treated conventionally and maintained. The high smile-line and display of the teeth and surrounding gums became increasingly unacceptable to this young girl as she progressed to womanhood. The progression of bone loss and the reoccurrence of apical pathology, as well as the development of external resorption, were monitored until skeletal growth had stabilised. At the age of 18, her teeth were removed with the immediate replacement using a metal-acrylic Rochette bridge. The deficient bone was augmented using a graft from the iliac crest followed by implant placement at two months. Three implants were placed adjacent to each other based on recent data indicating that a tight implant abutment connection would be able to sustain bone levels and, therefore, soft tissue contours (Figs 14-50–14-83).[119]

Concerns about the long-term efficacy of such treatment remain, with the knowledge that skeletal changes continue through life and it is inevitable that these will have consequences for the long-term outcome.

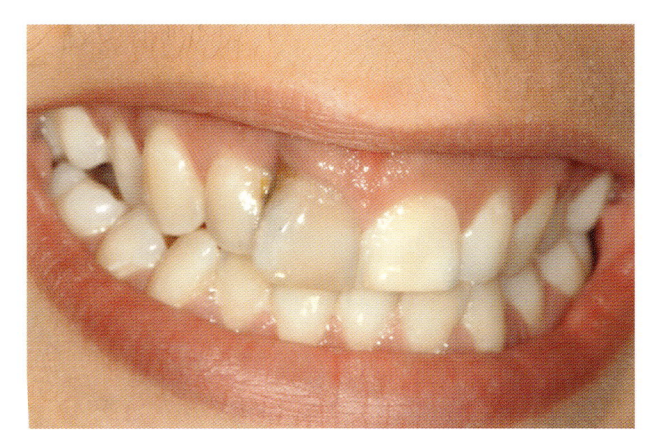

**Fig 14-50**  Extraoral overview of a young patient following trauma.

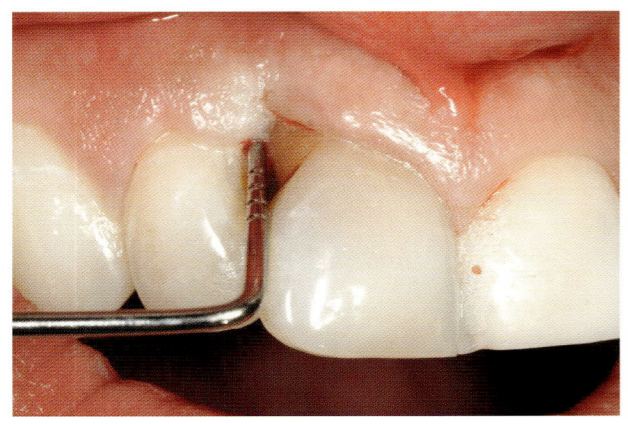

**Fig 14-51**  Intraoral view of traumatised teeth, with a periodontal probe demonstrating the loss of interdental bone.

14  Extensive Bone Grafts

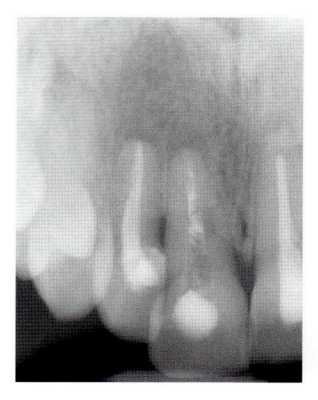

**Fig 14-52** Periapical radiograph of central and lateral incisors showing interdental bone loss and apical pathology. Signs of external resorption are also visible.

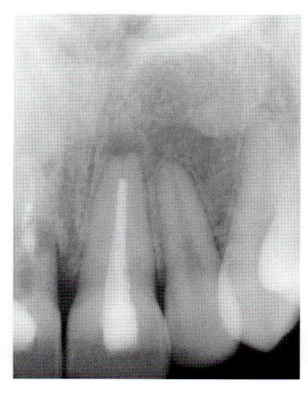

**Fig 14-53** Periapical radiograph of the left central incisor showing apical pathology. External resorption of the maxillary right central incisor is also visible.

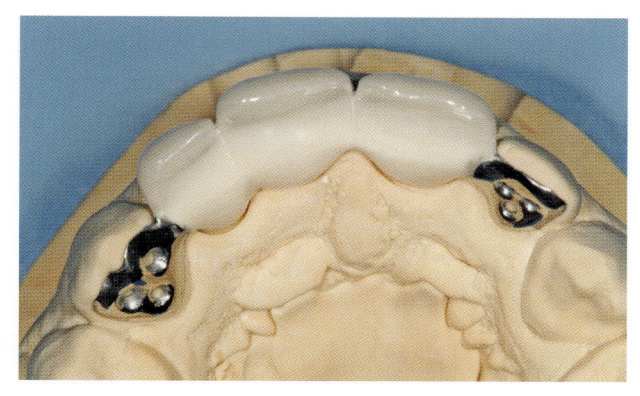

**Fig 14-54** Metal-acrylic Rochette bridge constructed to provide function during the treatment period.

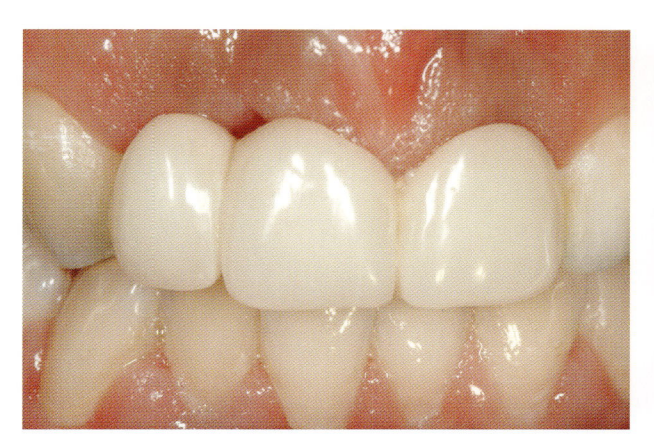

**Fig 14-55** Provisional bridge in situ showing bone remodelling.

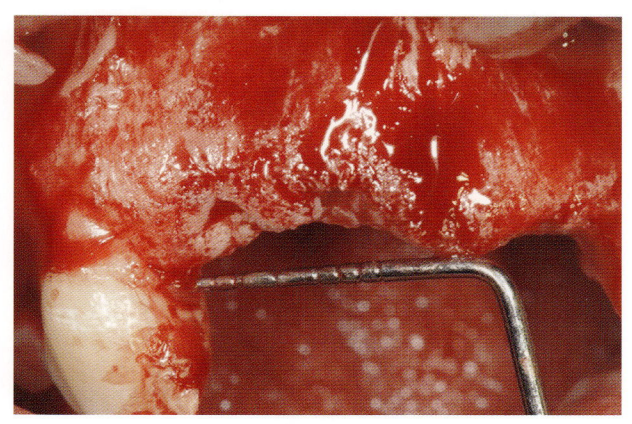

**Fig 14-56** Intraoperative view with the periodontal probe demonstrating the loss of bone.

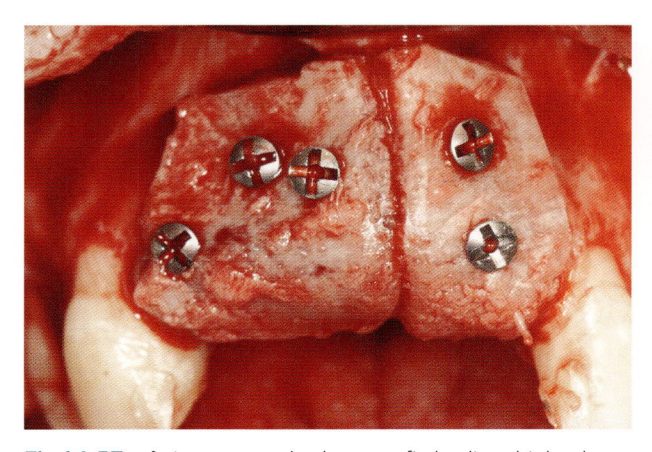

**Fig 14-57** Autogenous onlay bone grafts in situ, obtained from the iliac crest.

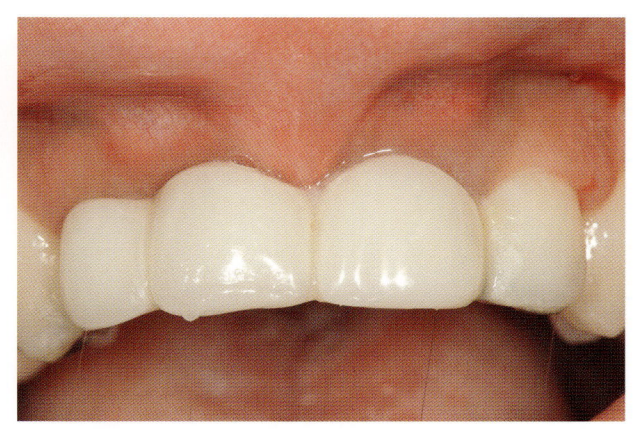

**Fig 14-58** Provisional bridge replaced. Note the relationship of the teeth to the soft tissues built up by the bone graft.

275

## III  Augmentation

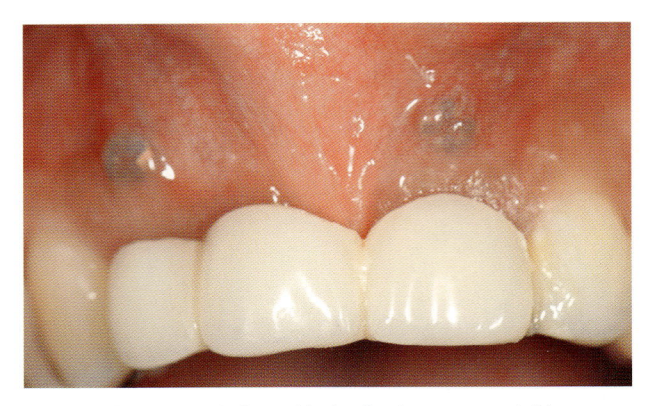

**Fig 14-59**  Intraoral view with the fixation screws visible through the soft tissues as the remodelling progresses. This indicates an increased metabolic rate in a young person, requiring implant placement at two months to prevent excessive remodelling.

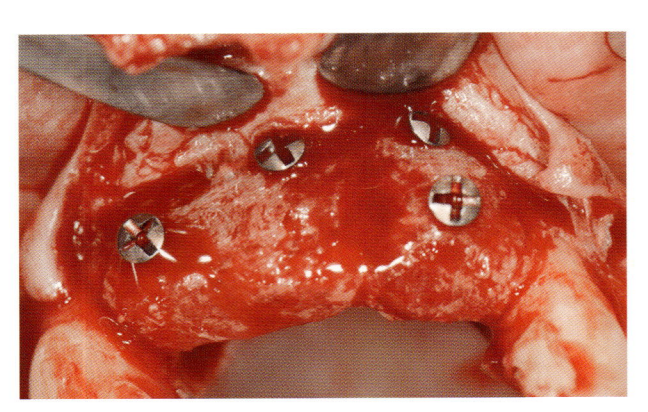

**Fig 14-60**  Intraoperative view of the bone graft with fixation screws visible. Note the bleeding surface of the graft. This is a clear sign of the viability and vascularisation of the graft.

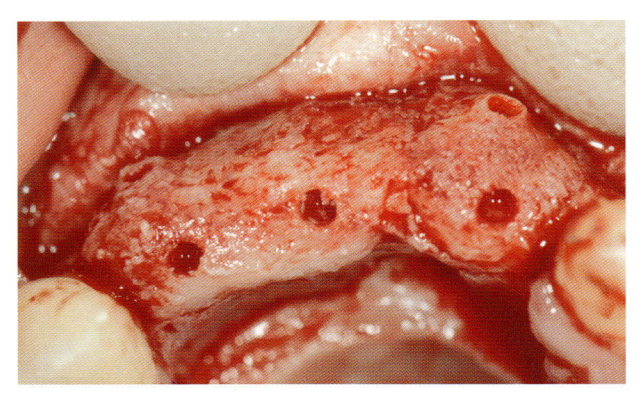

**Fig 14-61**  Occlusal overview of the graft with the implant sites marked. Note the response of the bone to the presence of the fixation screws. The presence of the screws reduces the rate of remodelling by stimulating the bone graft.

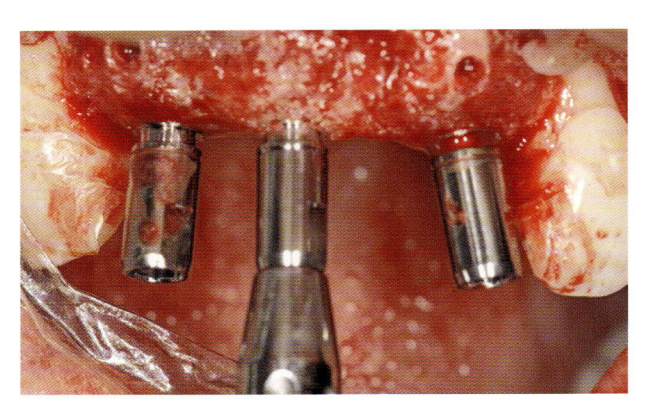

**Fig 14-62**  The implants being inserted using an insertion instrument marked with a round depression to indicate the orientation of the index within the implant. An indexed implant (Ankylos CX) has been selected and will provide an index for location of the abutment. However, the tight conical connection will provide the anti-rotation as well as a tight seal to prevent any micro-leakage. This is essential as the implant is being positioned below the crest of the bone.

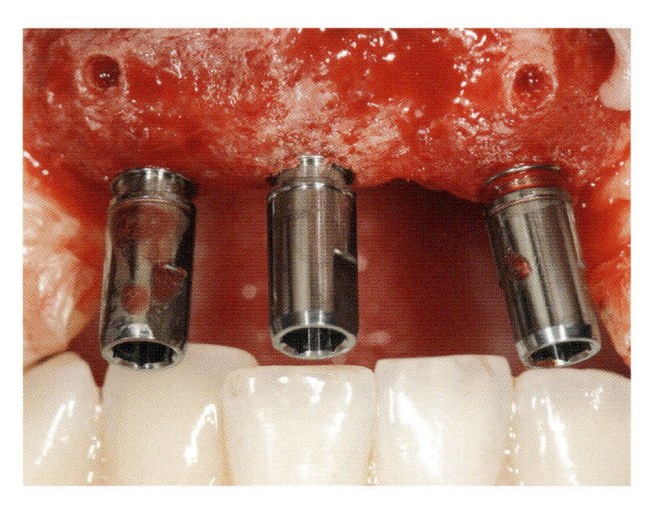

**Fig 14-63**  The implant carriers can be seen. Impressions recording the position of the implants within bone can be taken at this stage and transferred to the laboratory to enable the selection of abutments, their preparation, the fabrication of the metalwork as well as the transitional restoration.

## 14 Extensive Bone Grafts

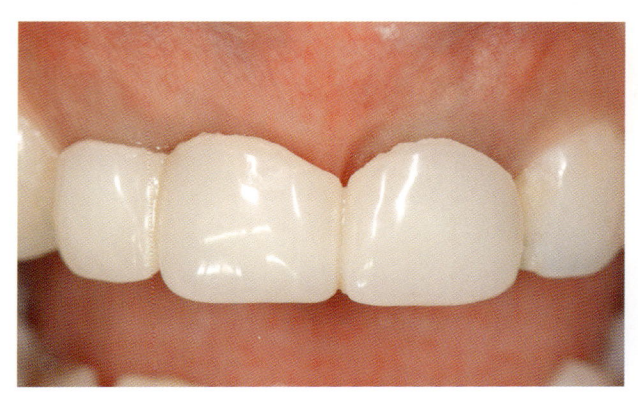

**Fig 14-64** The metal-acrylic Rochette bridge has been re-cemented following implant insertion. Please note the level of the soft tissues in relationship to the prosthetic teeth.

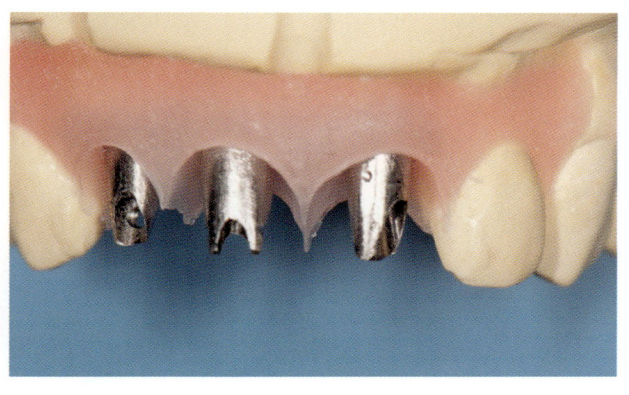

**Fig 14-65** The prefabricated abutments have been modified to ensure that they will fit within the implant without interfering with the surrounding bone. Furthermore, they have been aligned in the correct rotational orientation and modifications carried out as required.

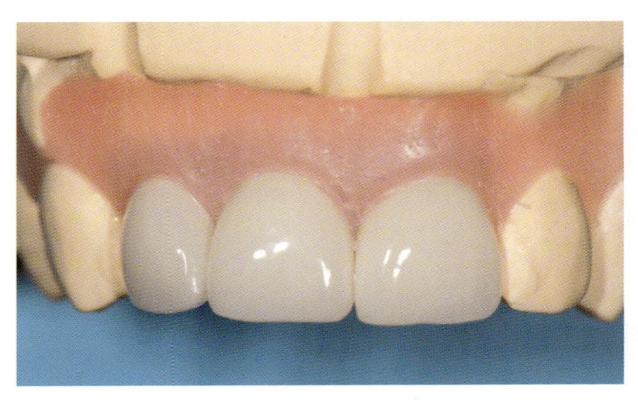

**Fig 14-66** Hollow acrylic resin transitional restorations have been constructed to fit precisely on the abutments. Pink wax has been used to recreate the ideal soft tissue contours.

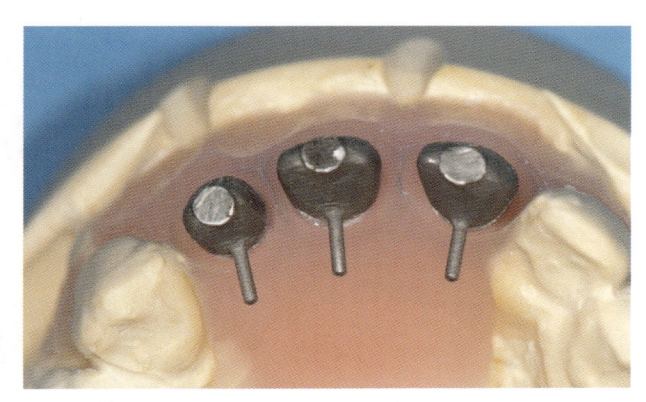

**Fig 14-67** The metalwork for individual crowns has been constructed for pick-up at the restorative phase.

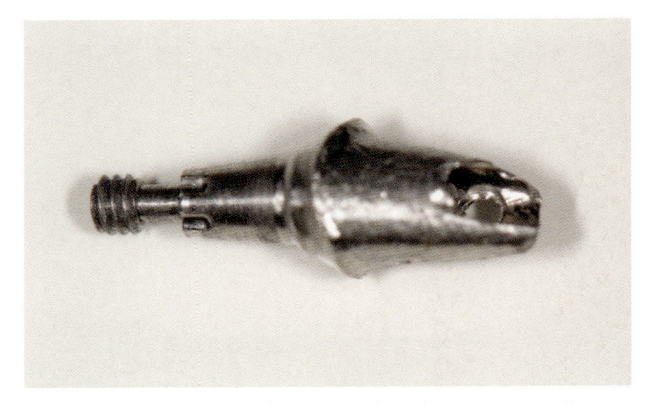

**Fig 14-68** View of the abutment, which has an index (six sided) at the bottom end of the conical connection, which will provide the seal and the anti-rotation.

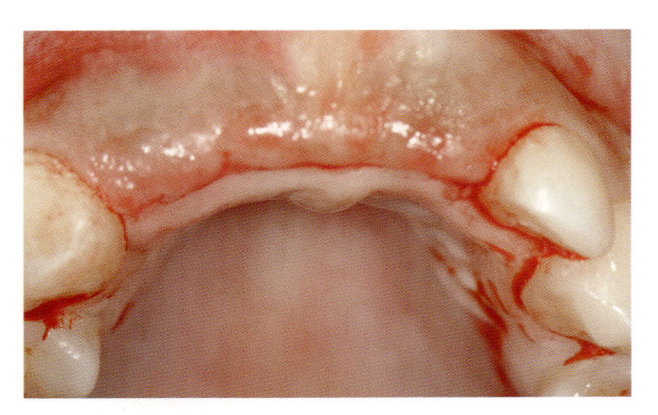

**Fig 14-69** The crestal incision is positioned towards the palatal aspect of the crest to enable keratinised tissue to be displaced towards the labial.

277

### III Augmentation

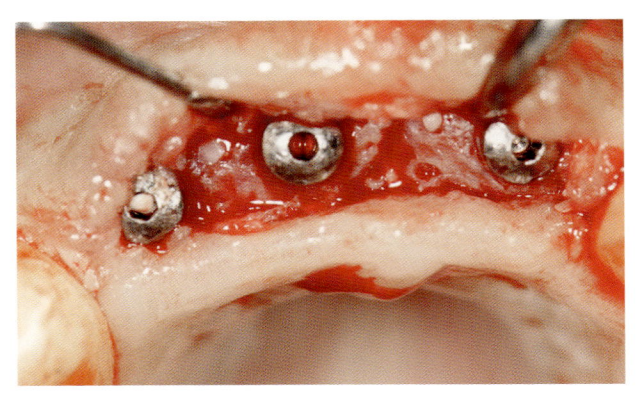

**Fig 14-70**  The keratinised tissues can be seen displaced towards the labial of the exposed implants. Sulcus formers were placed at the time of implant insertion in order to provide easy access to the subcrestally placed implants.

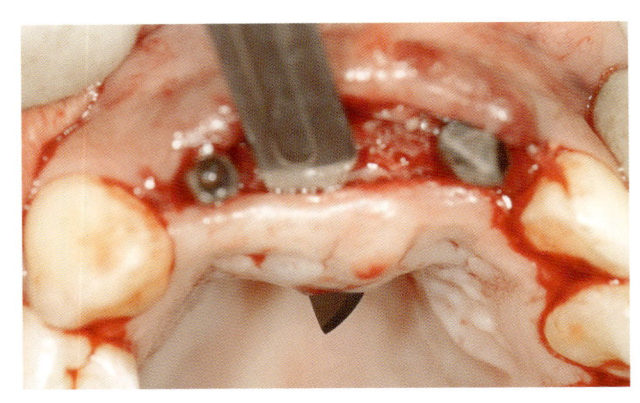

**Fig 14-71**  A relieving incision is made to slide the palatal tissue towards the labial.

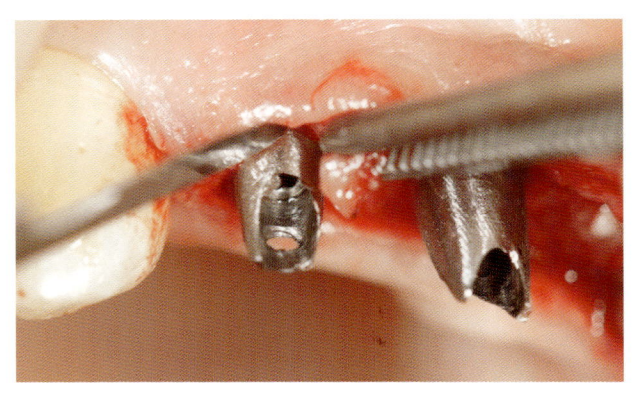

**Fig 14-72**  An 'S'-shaped incision is used to reconstruct the papilla and close over the bone graft to ensure that there is no exposure of the graft.

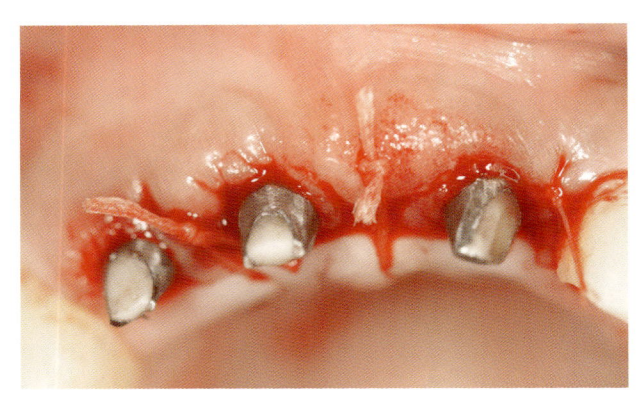

**Fig 14-73**  Occlusal view of the sutured tissues establishing closure.

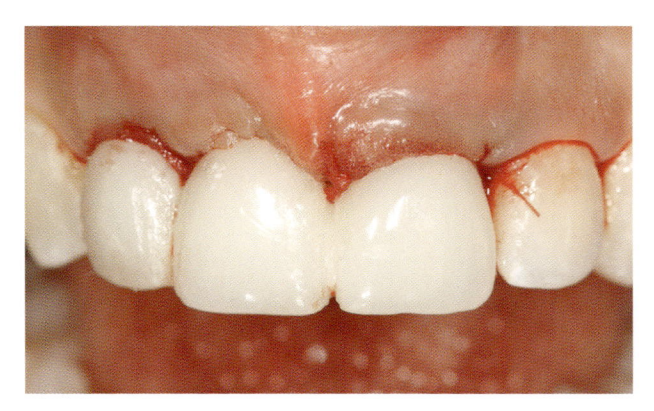

**Fig 14-74**  The transitional crowns have been fitted onto the abutments and are now used to create the emergence profile.

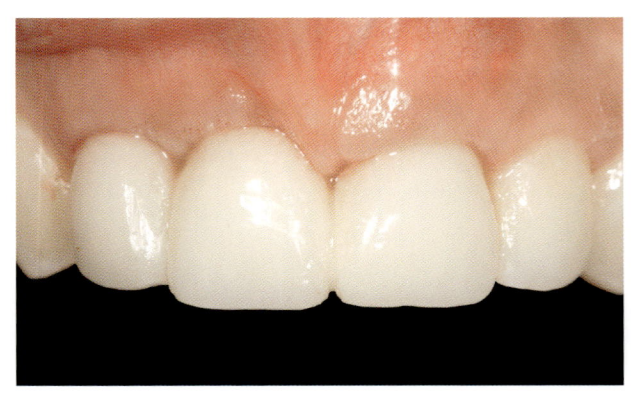

**Fig 14-75**  The development of the soft tissues by the transitional restoration can be seen.

14 Extensive Bone Grafts

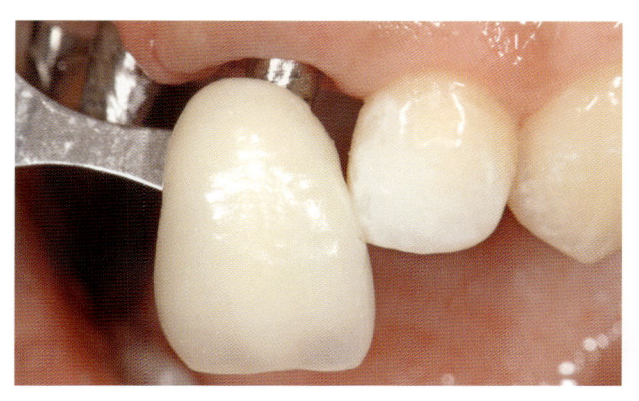

**Fig 14-76** One month following the exposure of the implants, the restorative phase may commence. A shade is taken using a custom-made porcelain shade guide fabricated by fusing porcelain onto the metal of choice. Photograph of the shade guide in situ as well as the drawing is sent to the dental technician. Alternatively the dental technician can take the shade directly.

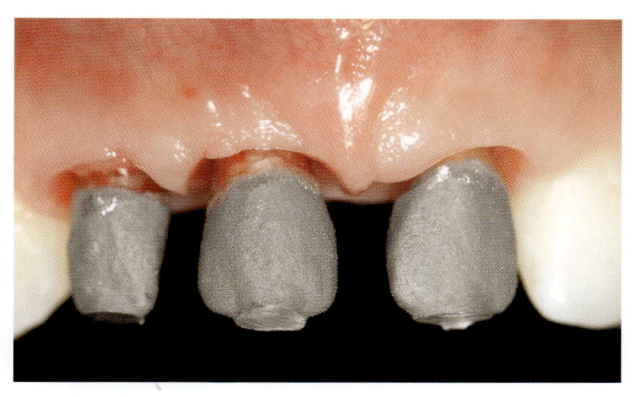

**Fig 14-77** The prefabricated metalwork seated on the abutments ready for pick-up.

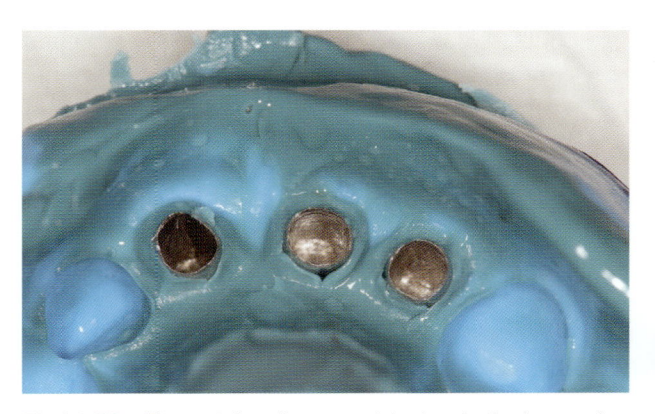

**Fig 14-78** The metal copings are picked up in the impression recording the abutment position as well as the soft tissue contours. These are transferred to the laboratory. Pattern resin is poured into the metal copings, dowel pins are inserted and the impression cast in plaster. Porcelain can now be fused to the metalwork complying with the soft tissue contours established by the transitional restorations.

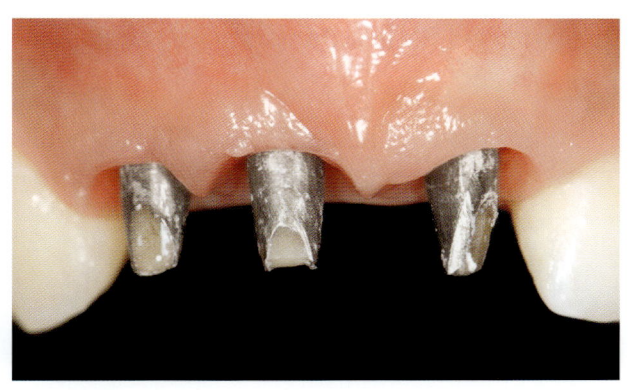

**Fig 14-79** Labial view of the abutments emerging from soft tissues contoured by the transitional restorations.

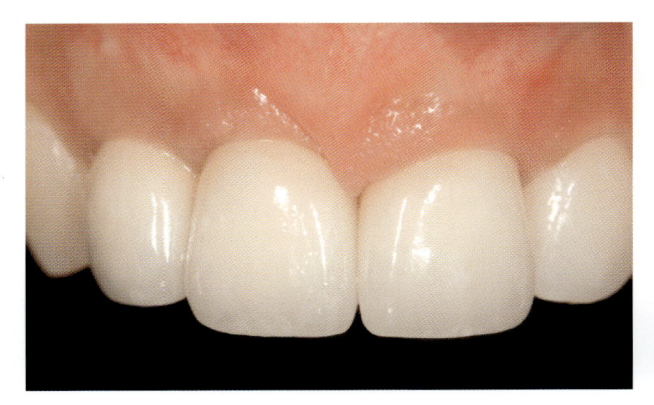

**Fig 14-80** Labial view of the definitive restorations showing naturally contoured keratinised gingival tissues.

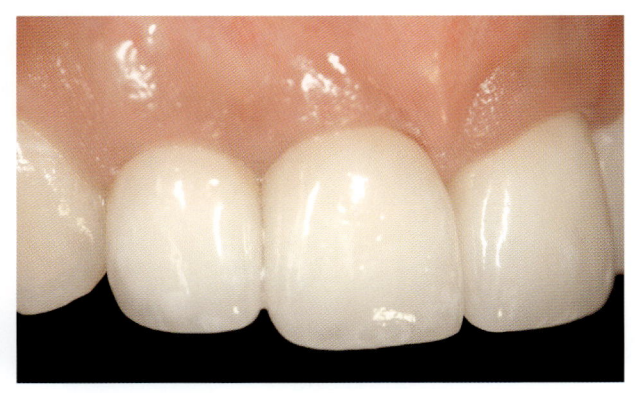

**Fig 14-81** Labial view from the right side showing the creation of the interdental papillae.

III   Augmentation

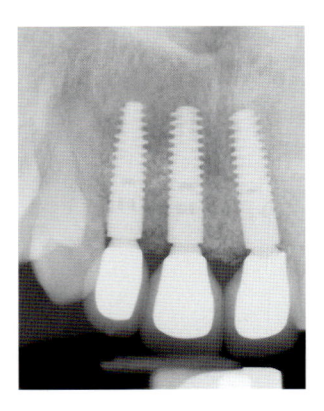

**Fig 14-82**  Post-operative periapical radiograph showing bone levels responsible for support for the papilla.

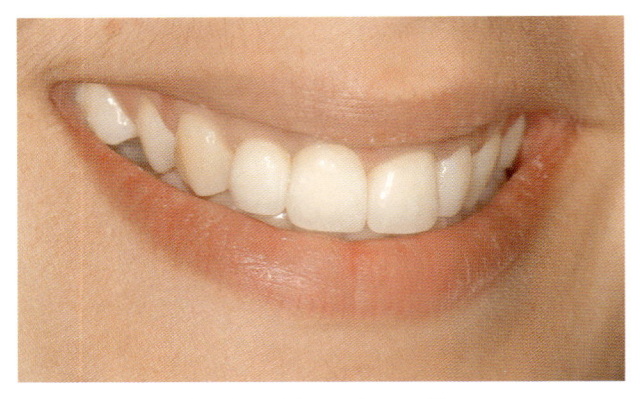

**Fig 14-83**  Anterior view of the patient smiling.

## Case 4: Management of a Periodontally Compromised Patient Requiring Augmentation

The management of this patient with failing teeth resulting from progressive periodontal disease was managed by using a metal-acrylic provisional restoration to ascertain the need for the replacement of lost hard and soft tissues. A decision was made to replace these biologically (with a bone graft from the iliac crest). Subsequently (at three months after bone grafting), implants were placed and impressions at first-stage surgery taken for the selection and modification of abutments and the fabrication of an acrylic resin transitional restoration for the development of the soft tissues. These were fitted at implant exposure and the definitive restoration constructed once soft tissues had matured. Implants adjacent to each other and positioned less than 3 mm apart have been used based on recent data, support from the inter-implant bony peaks for the gingival tissues is evident.[103,119]

The stability of the implant–abutment interface and the soft tissue development using the transitional restoration has resulted in a favourable aesthetic outcome, which is reflected in the patient's gain in self-esteem (Figs 14-84–14-115).

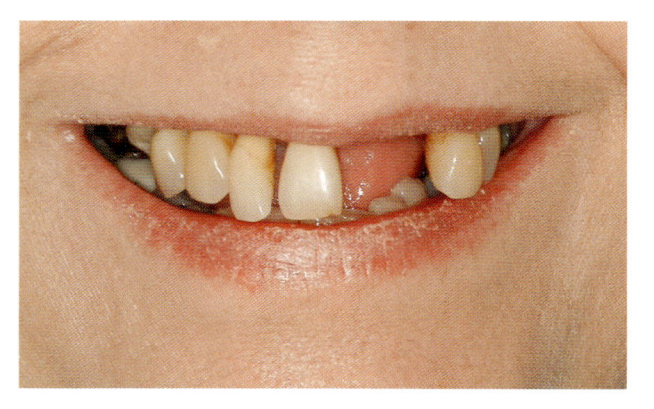

**Fig 14-84**  Preoperative view of patient with failing teeth.

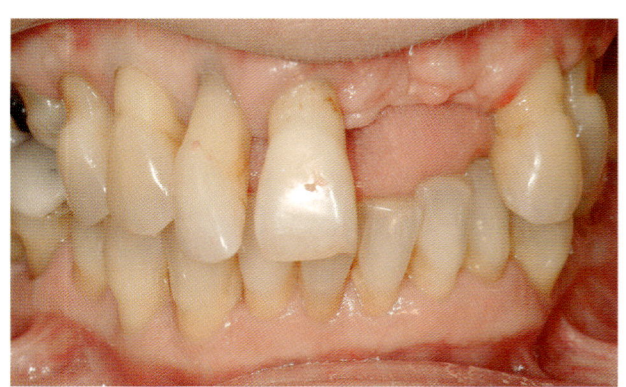

**Fig 14-85**  Intraoral view showing extensive tissue loss.

14   Extensive Bone Grafts

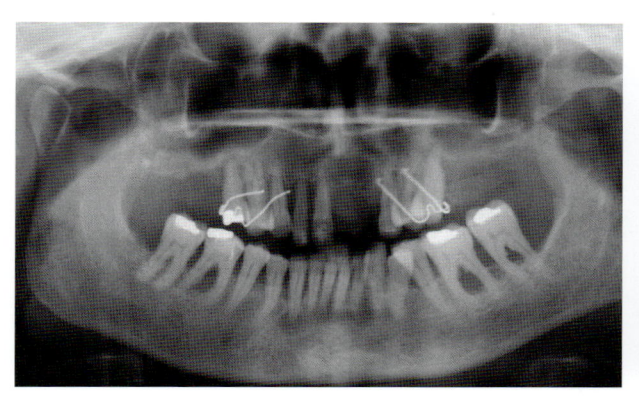

**Fig 14-86**   Panoral radiograph showing extensive bone loss in the maxilla with enlarged sinuses. Pathology in the mandible jaw is also visible.

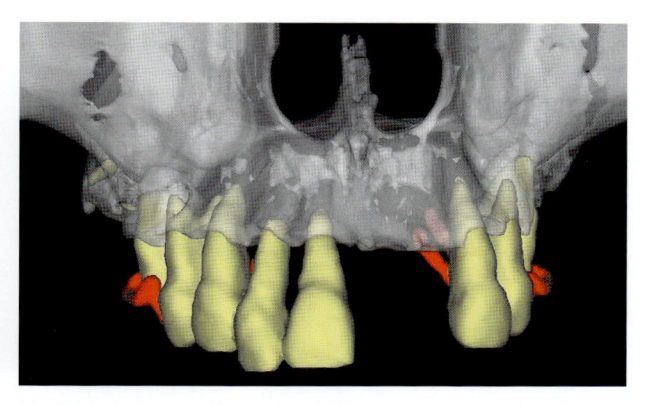

**Fig 14-87**   Three-dimensional CT scan reconstruction demonstrating the amount of bone loss.

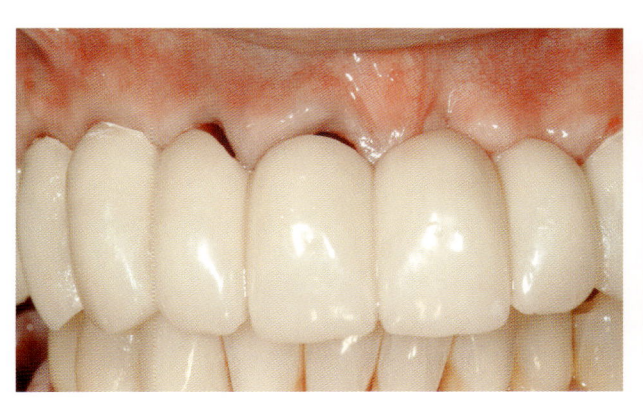

**Fig 14-88**   Labial view of the provisional bridge showing elongated teeth. Further recession will be monitored as remodelling takes place.

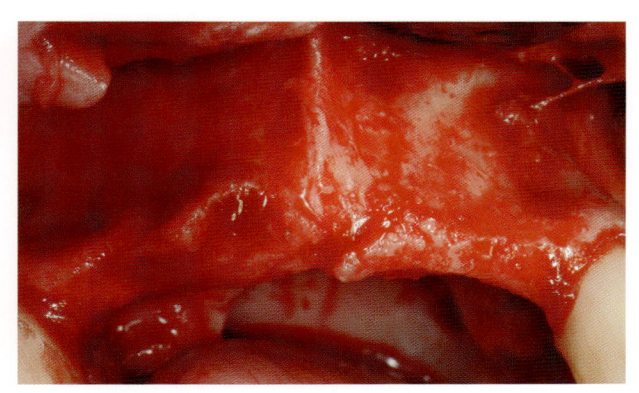

**Fig 14-89**   Exposed alveolar ridge prior to grafting.

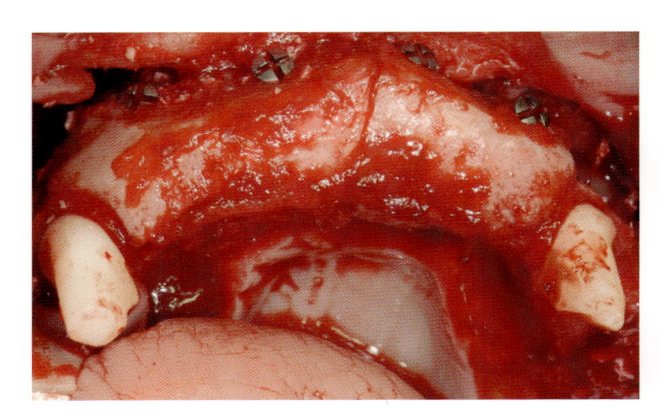

**Fig 14-90**   Bone graft from the lateral aspect of the anterior iliac crest in situ. Note the accurate adaptation of the graft with the cortical surface on the outside to provide stability and controlled remodelling.

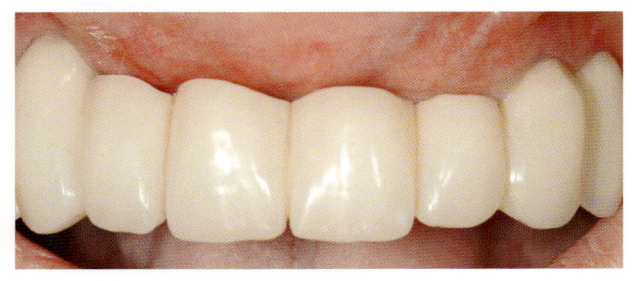

**Fig 14-91**   Appearance of provisional bridge after bone grafting. Note the reduced length of the teeth.

III Augmentation

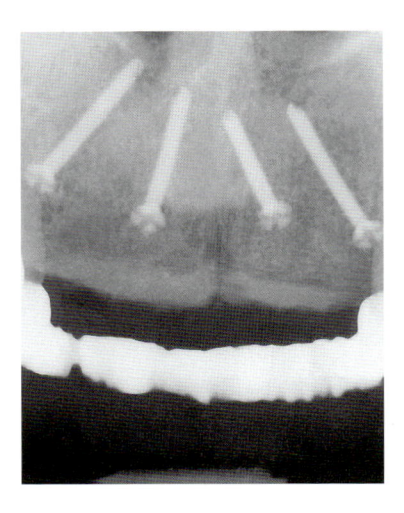

Fig 14-92 Periapical radiograph being used to monitor bone remodelling to identify the correct time for implant placement.

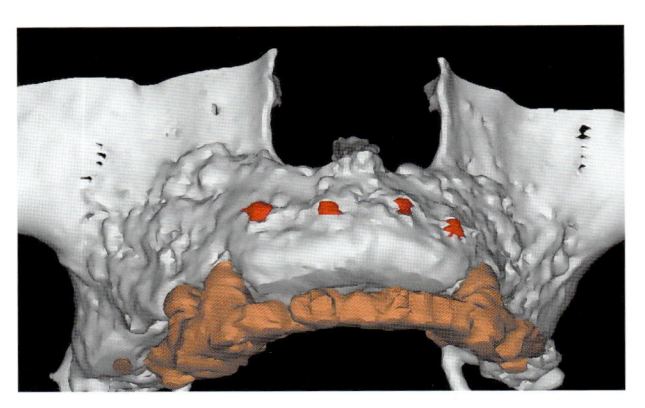

Fig 14-93 Three-dimensional reconstruction using CT scan data acquired after bone grafting for purposes of planning implant placement.

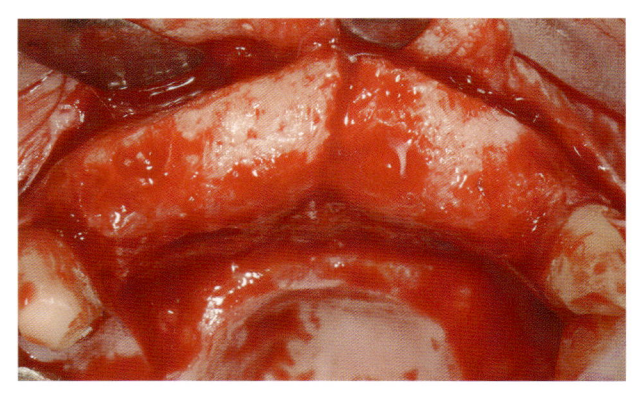

Fig 14-94 Intraoperative view of reconstructed ridge at the time of implant placement. Note the bone screws have been removed and the surface of the graft is bleeding indicating vascularisation.

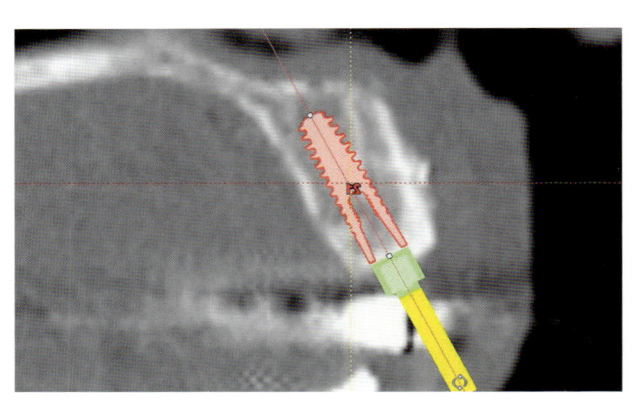

Fig 14-95 Cross-sectional view of CT scan during interactive placement of implants into reconstructed ridge. (Image was flipped horizontally for easy comparison.)

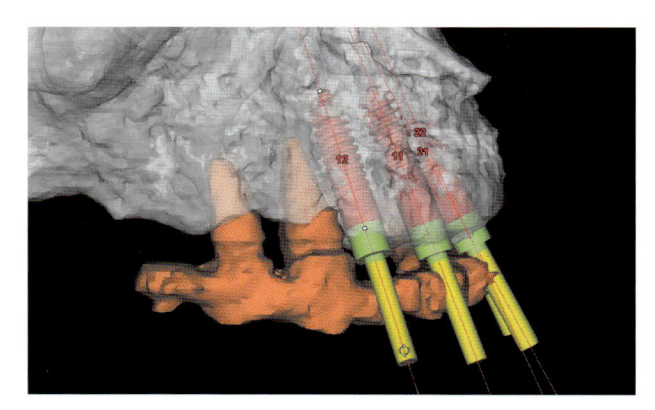

Fig 14-96 Three-dimensional reconstruction with proposed implants in situ for purposes of assessment of positioning.

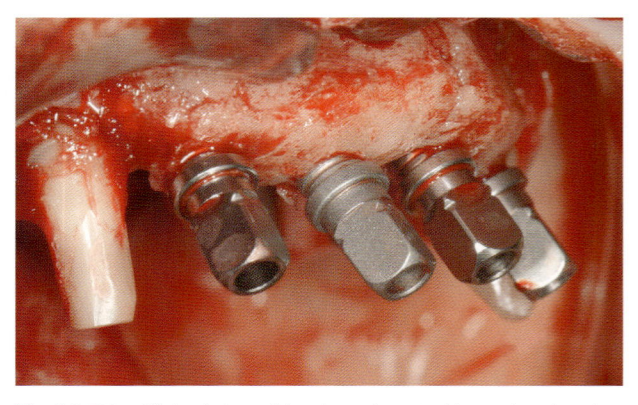

Fig 14-97 Clinical view of implants inserted by estimating the position based on CT scan data. (Guided surgery could have also been used.) Impressions of the implant carriers enable the information to be transferred to the dental technician for planning for subsequent stages.

282

14 Extensive Bone Grafts

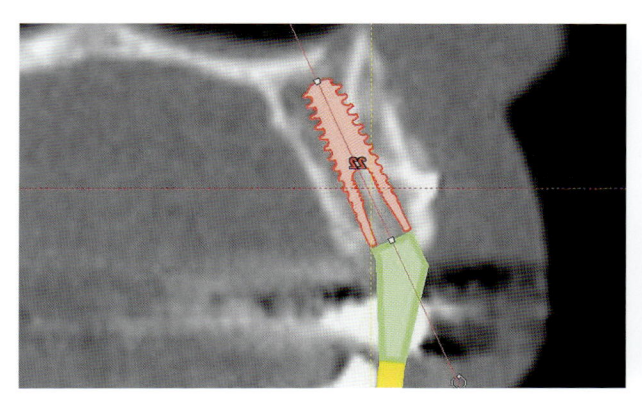

**Fig 14-98** Interactive selection of abutment visualised on a cross-sectional view in relation to the provisional restoration and mandibular incisor. (Image was flipped horizontally for easy comparison.)

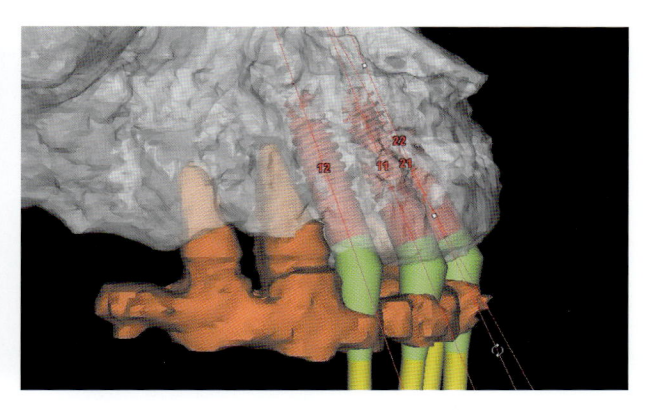

**Fig 14-99** Three-dimensional reconstruction with proposed abutments angled to fit within the prosthetic envelope as indicated by the provisional restoration.

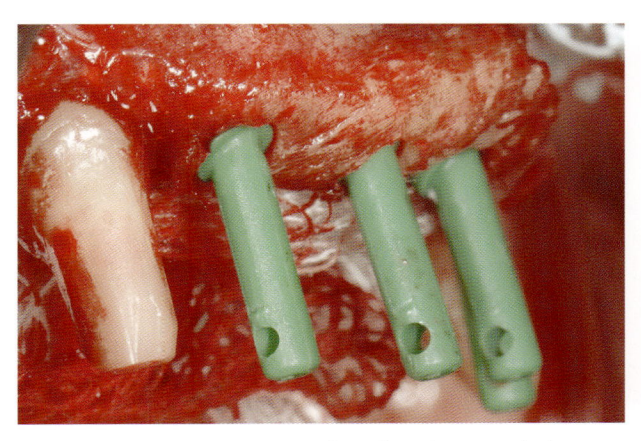

**Fig 14-100** Intraoperative confirmation of proposed abutment angulation using direction indicators.

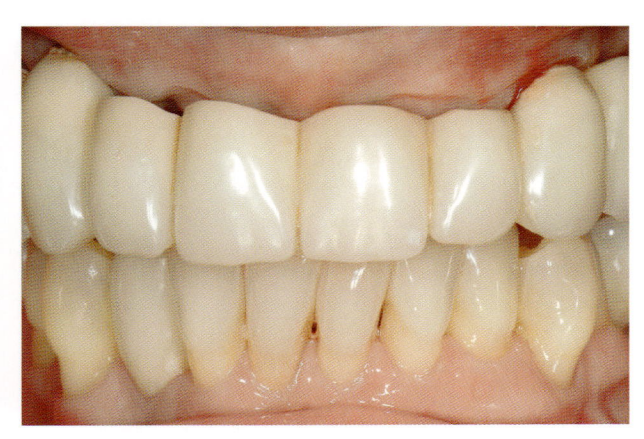

**Fig 14-101** Intraoral view of provisional restoration after implant placement.

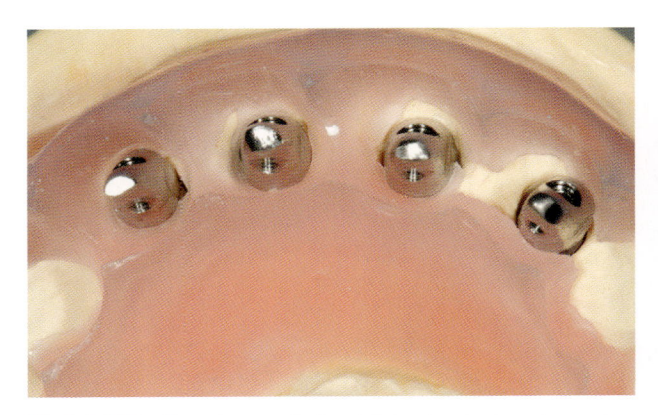

**Fig 14-102** Based on casts (containing implant analogues) made from impressions at implant placement, abutments have been selected to be parallel and in tooth position.

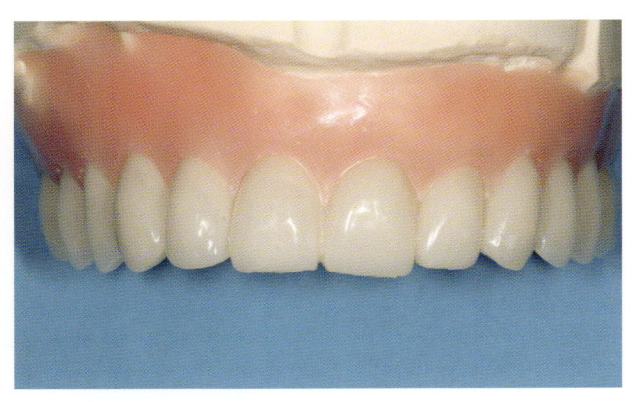

**Fig 14-103** Labial view of transitional restoration fabricated on the abutments seen in Fig 14-102.

283

III Augmentation

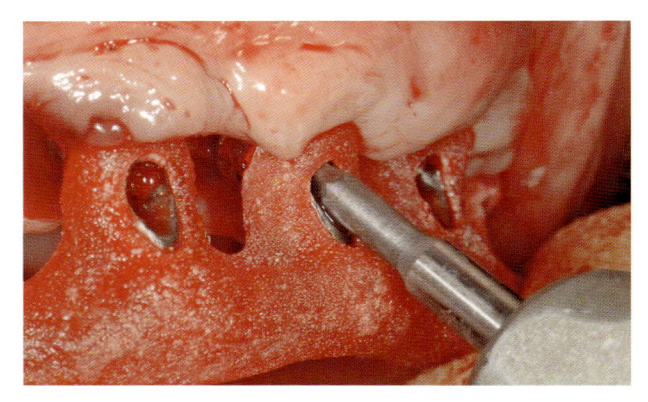

**Fig 14-104** Abutments selected and modified by the dental technician are attached to the implants using an acrylic resin index to replicate the position on the cast.

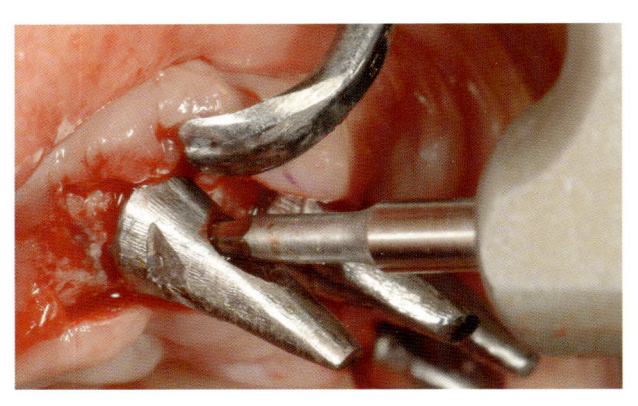

**Fig 14-105** The abutments are tightened into position, engaging the conical connection, using a torque of 15 Ncm.

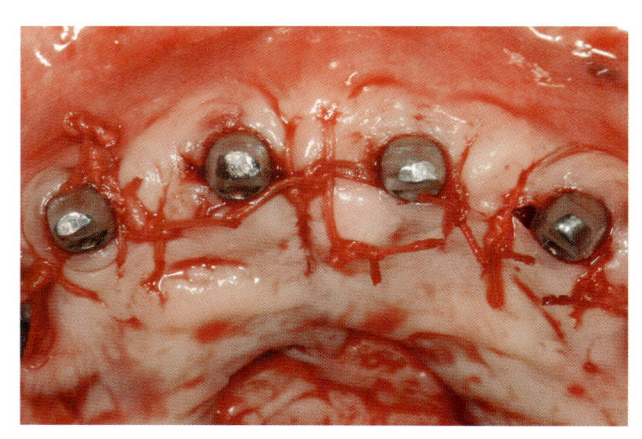

**Fig 14-106** The tissues are mobilised using 'S'-shaped incisions on the labial aspect and a split-thickness relieving incision on the palate to ensure good closure over the graft.

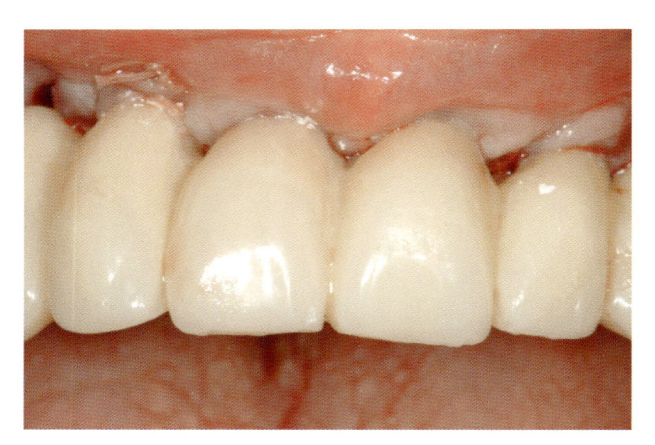

**Fig 14-107** The transitional restoration is fitted on the abutments and will provide guidance for the soft tissues during healing.

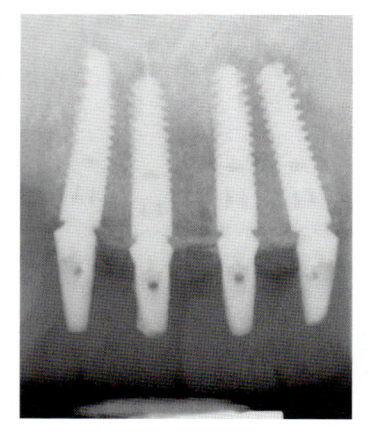

**Fig 14-108** Post-operative periapical view showing bone levels in relation to implants and abutments.

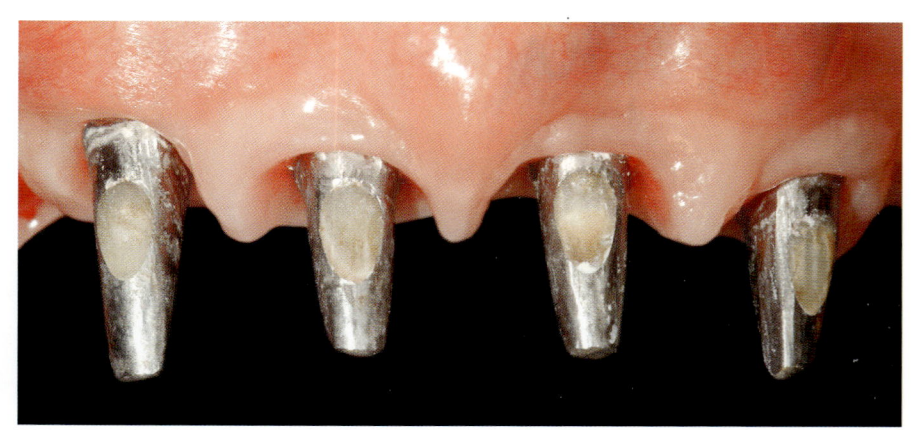

**Fig 14-109** Labial view of the abutments and soft tissue contours established by the transitional restoration approximately three months after exposure prior to fitting the definitive restoration.

14  Extensive Bone Grafts

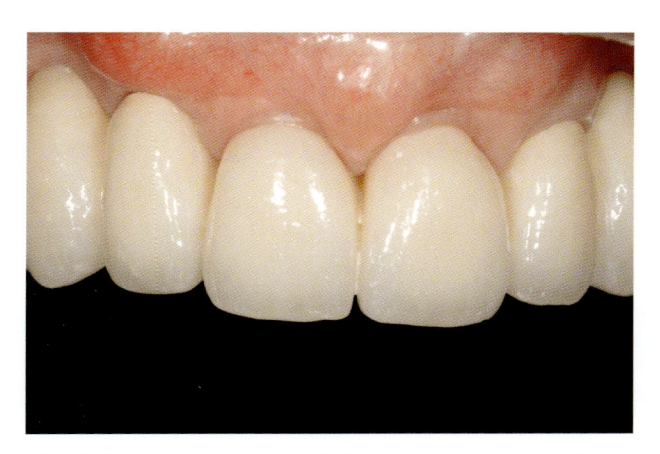

Fig 14-110  Labial view of definitive restoration showing the presence of papillae and a natural emergence profile.

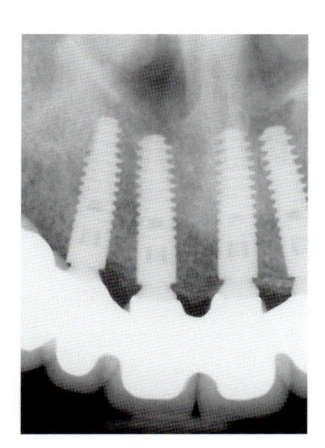

Fig 14-111  Periapical radiograph taken after insertion of the definitive restoration. No excess cement is seen and the bone levels can be noted.

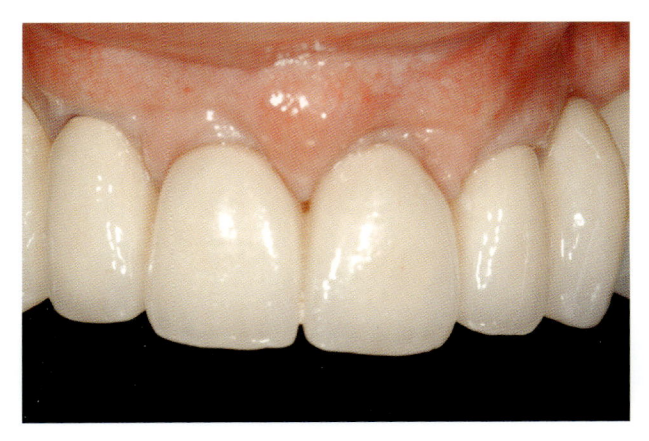

Fig 14-112  Clinical view of crowns at review one year after restoration, showing minimal changes related to tissue maturation.

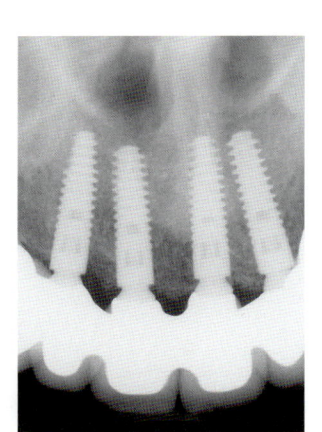

Fig 14-113  Periapical radiograph taken at the one-year review, showing stable bone levels.

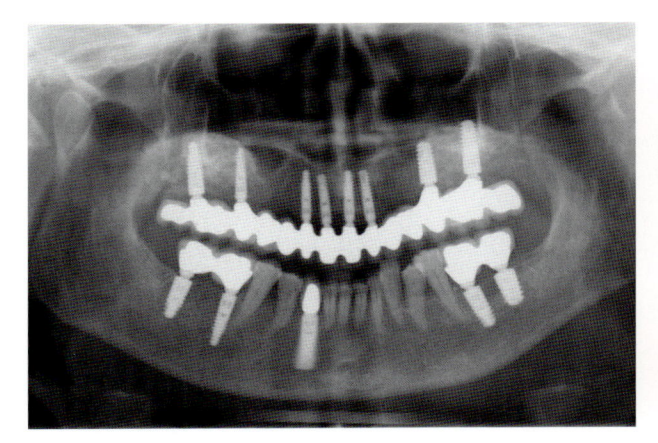

Fig 14-114  Panoral radiograph on completion of treatment showing dental and implant status.

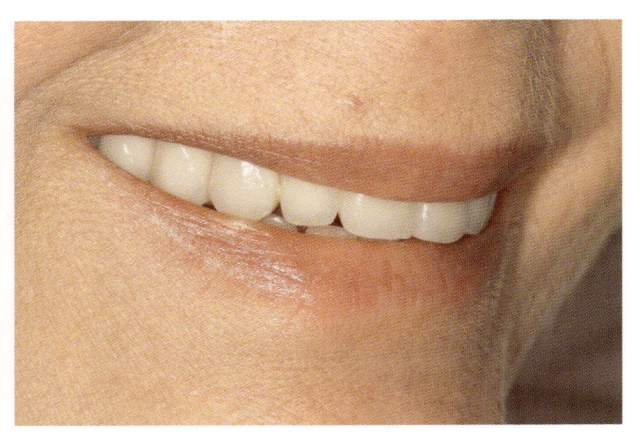

Fig 14-115  Image of the patient on completion of treatment.

285

III Augmentation

## Case 5: Replacement of Failing Teeth with Implants

For this patient, three failing teeth were replaced with three implants following an iliac crest bone grafting procedure. Long-term stability is evident, both for the soft tissues as seen from the clinical images and the hard tissues as seen from the radiographs. The radiographs show bone levels at the first thread 2 mm below the level of the implant–abutment junction. This case study demonstrates the principle of stimulation and, therefore, stabilisation of the bone graft by means of load via an implant (Figs 14-116–14-122).[217,218] Bone levels here differ from those observed in Cases 3 and 4, where a different implant–abutment connection was used to enable an infracrestal placement of the implant.

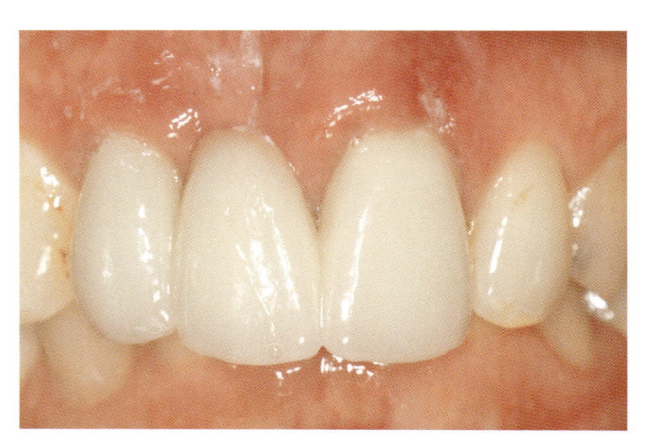

**Fig 14-116** Clinical image of failing teeth associated with bone loss and infection.

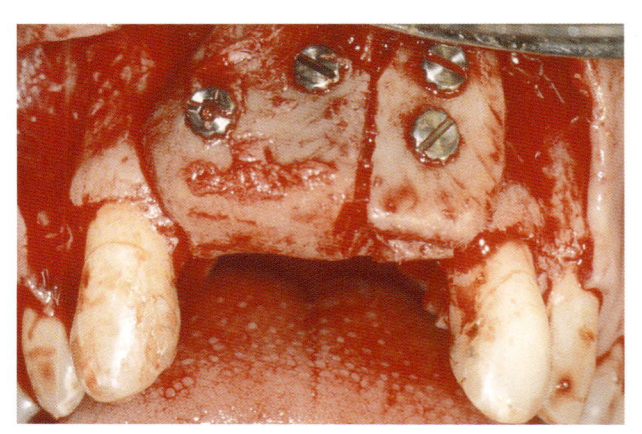

**Fig 14-117** The ridge reconstructed with 'J'-shaped cortico-cancellous grafts obtained from the iliac crest.

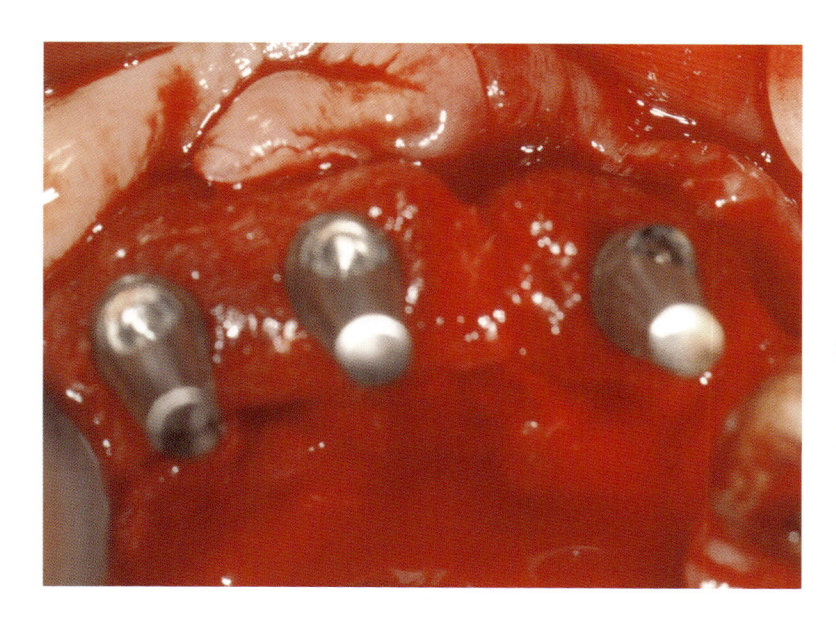

**Fig 14-118** Intraoperative view at the time of implant placement. Abutments (angled prefabricated) can be seen being tried in. Impressions taken of the abutments at this stage provide the technician with the facility to prepare for the second stage of implant exposure. In view of the fact that an implant system with an indexed connection was used in this case, the use of the abutments at this stage enables the implants to be turned into the correct rotational position.

## 14 Extensive Bone Grafts

### Case 6: Management of an Edentulous Patient with Ridge Augmentation in the Maxilla and Mandible

This case study demonstrates the management of an edentulous patient with augmentation of a class IV ridge in the maxilla and a class V ridge in the mandible. The maxilla was treated using autogenous onlay bone graft from the iliac crest to increase both width and height. The mandible was treated without bone grafts but using nerve repositioning in the posterior mandible, allowing posterior implants to be placed and thus avoiding cantilevers and their attendant disadvantages. Two sets of CT scans were used in the maxilla to assist in the placement of the graft especially subantrally as well as for the placement of the implants. The mandibular scan permitted the spatial position of the inferior dental canal to be accurately identified prior to repositioning as well as allowing implant site selection. Cement-retained porcelain-fused-to-metal restorations were constructed and have demonstrated stability over four years. The maturation of the soft tissues over the four years in developing stippling is indicative of a stable environment (Figs 14-123–14-160).

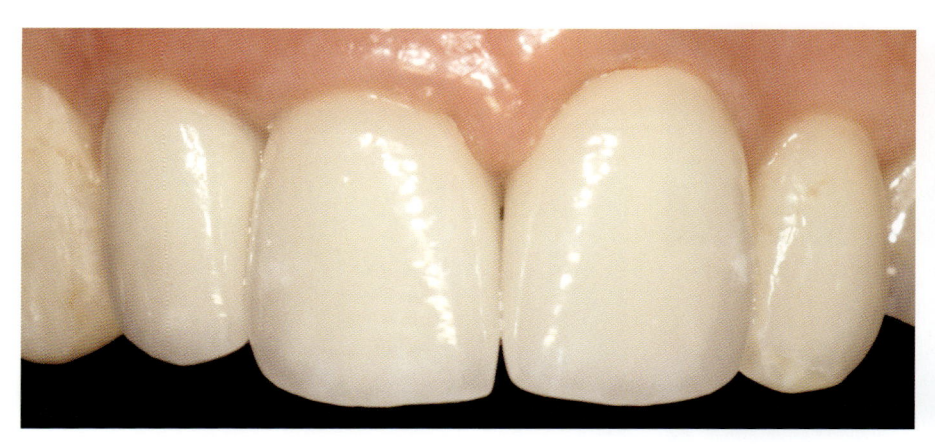

**Fig 14-119** The definitive restoration (three individual crowns) fitted in 2000. The clinical image shows well-developed soft tissue contours and emergence profile in comparison with the preoperative situation.

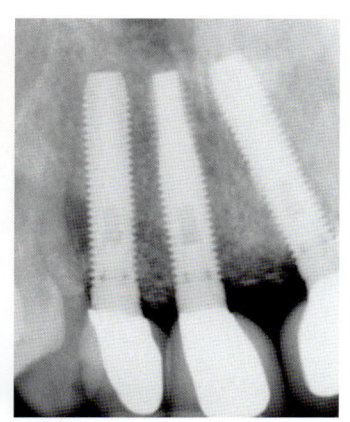

**Fig 14-120** Radiograph taken for regular monitoring in 2005 showing stable bone levels. Fragments of dense hydroxyapatite (Osteograf 70 μm) used to stabilise soft tissues are visible.

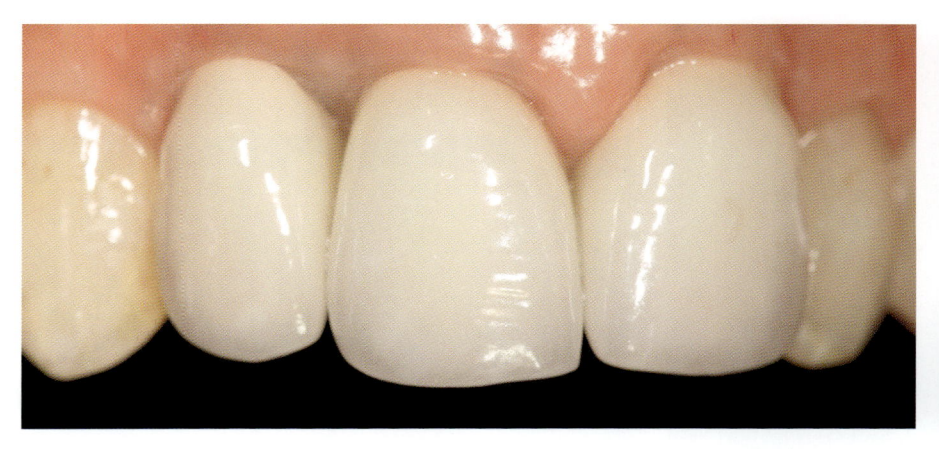

**Fig 14-121** Clinical view of the restoration taken in 2010 showing the stability of the soft tissue profile established 10 years earlier.

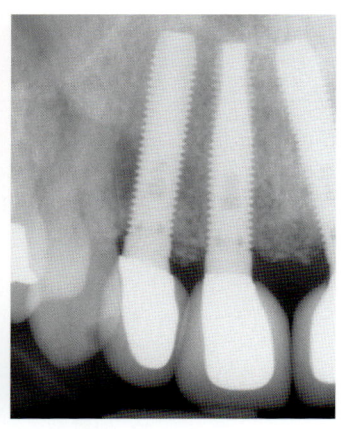

**Fig 14-122** Monitoring radiograph taken in 2010 showing stable bone levels. Bone grafts stimulated by dental implants appear to remain stable.

### III    Augmentation

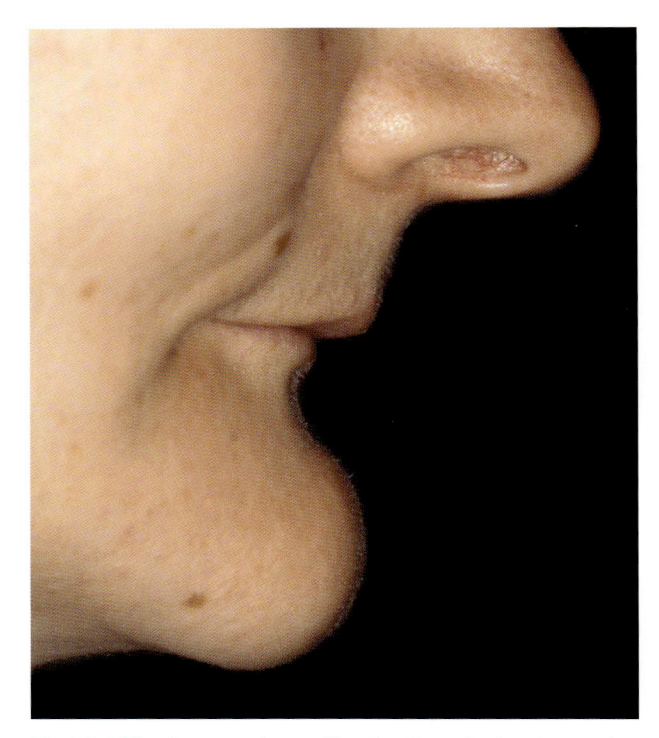

**Fig 14-123**  Preoperative profile of patient who lost her teeth at the age of 16 years. Collapse of the perioral soft tissues resulting from atrophy is apparent. A prominent chin and an increased naso-labial angle can be noted.

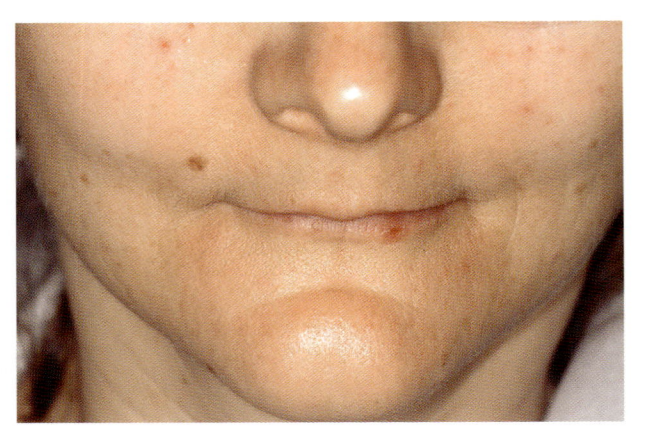

**Fig 14-124**  Anterior view.

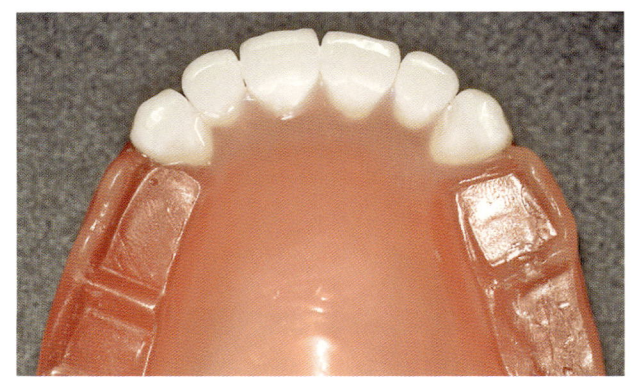

**Fig 14-125**  Registration block with radiopaque teeth set in a position that produces the desired facial profile.

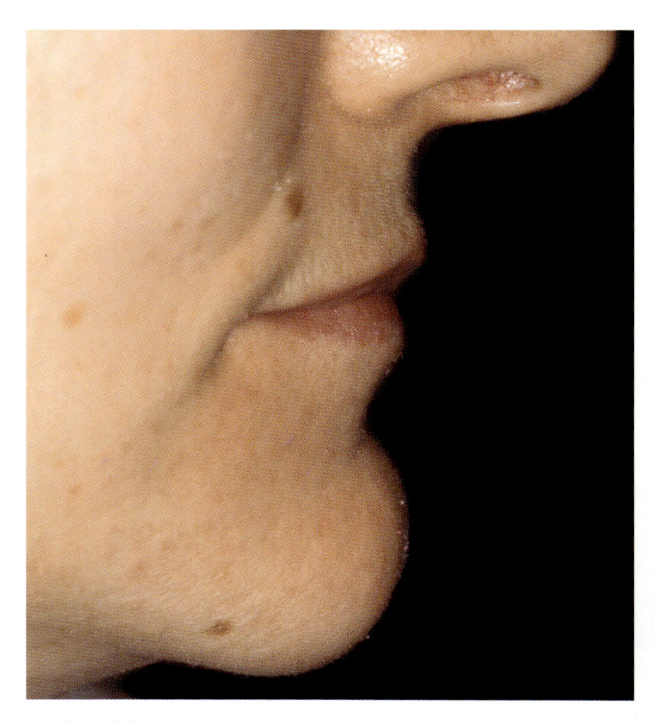

**Fig 14-126**  Profile of the patient with corrected facial contours identifying the ideal tooth position using the registration block.

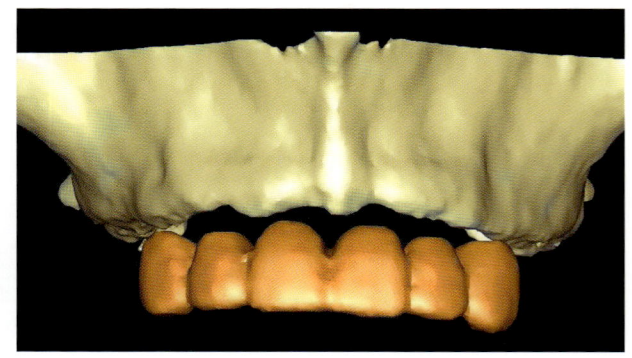

**Fig 14-127**  CT 3D view of the maxilla. The radiopaque teeth in relation to the residual bone can be seen.

14 Extensive Bone Grafts

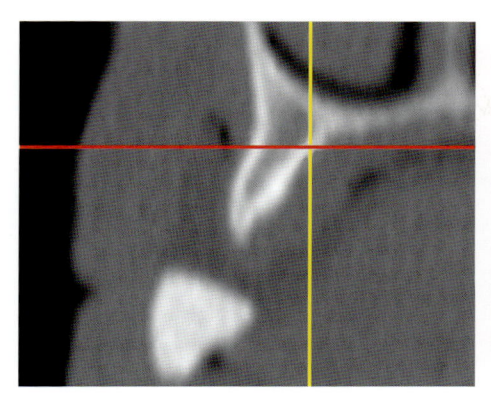

**Fig 14-128** CT cross-sectional image of the incisor region. The radiopaque teeth in relation to the residual bone can be seen.

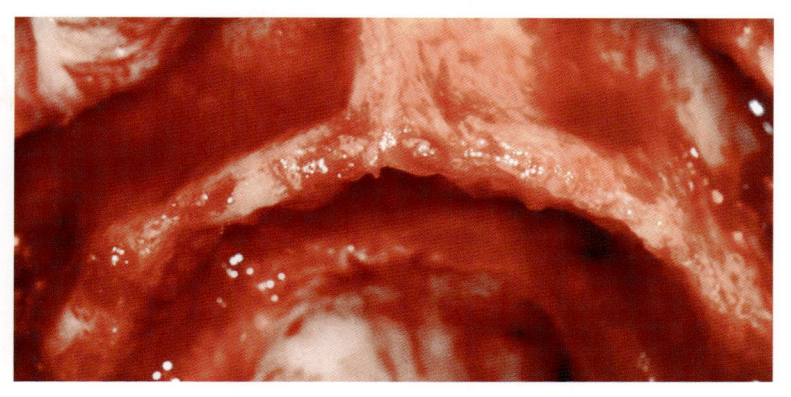

**Fig 14-129** Intraoperative view of the maxillary ridge showing the resorption that has taken place, which is consistent with the CT data.

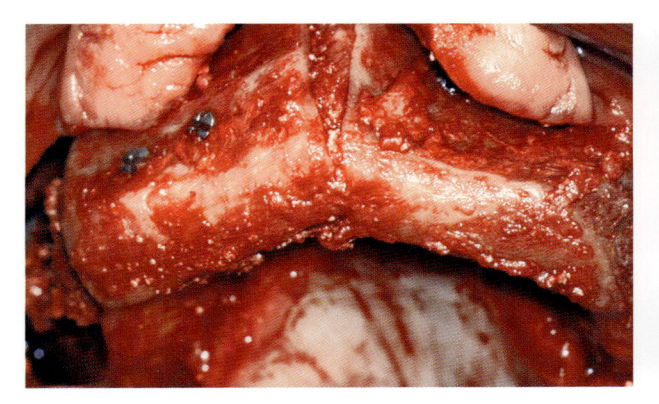

**Fig 14-130** Cortico-cancellous grafts being used to reconstruct the atrophic ridge. Bilateral subantral augmentation was carried out at the same time, using autogenous cancellous bone in conjunction with a xenograft to lend stability and reduce the rate of resorption.

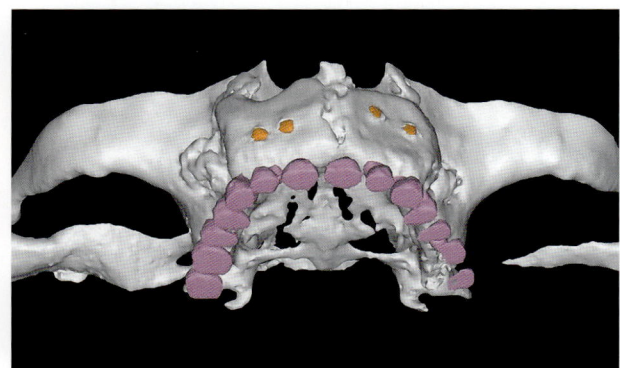

**Fig 14-131** CT 3D view taken approximately three months after the bone graft and prior to implant placement.

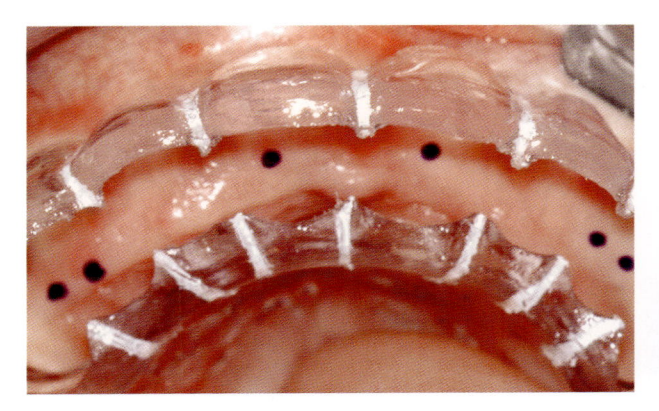

**Fig 14-132** Possible sites for implants being identified using the diagnostic template. These will aid in the design of the flap, preventing the incisior from overlying a proposed implant position.

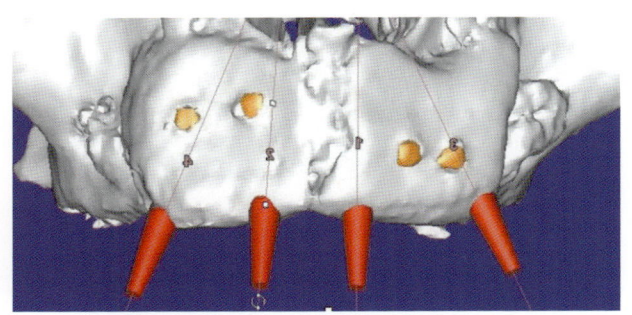

**Fig 14-133** CT 3D interactive planning showing implants sited in central incisor and canine positions.

III  Augmentation

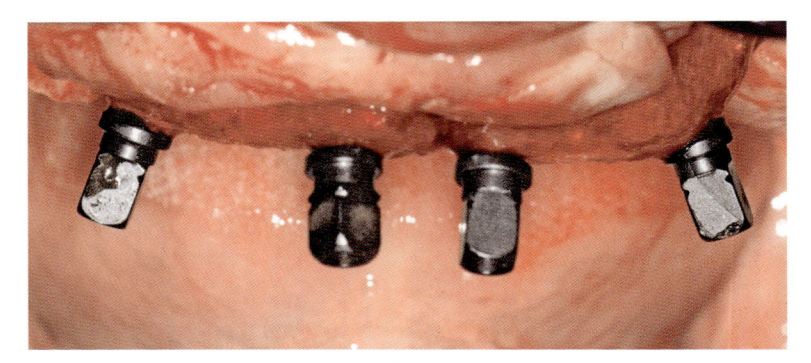

Fig 14-134  Clinical image of the implants, simulating 3D planning.

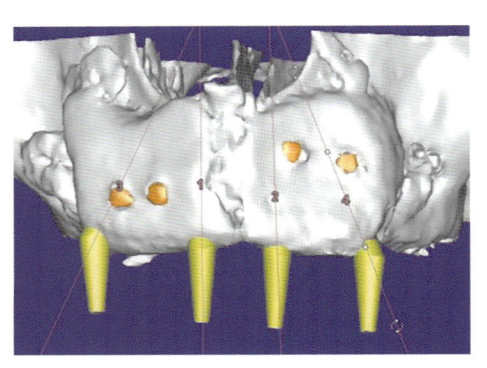

Fig 14-135  Interactive planning showing the selection of abutments on the CT 3D image.

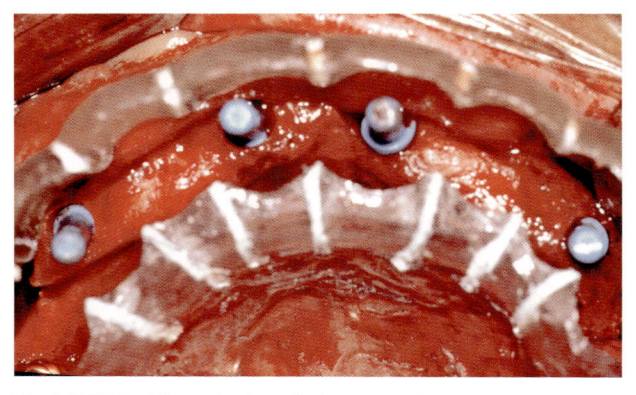

Fig 14-136  The selection of abutments being carried out intraorally using the diagnostic template and direction indicators.

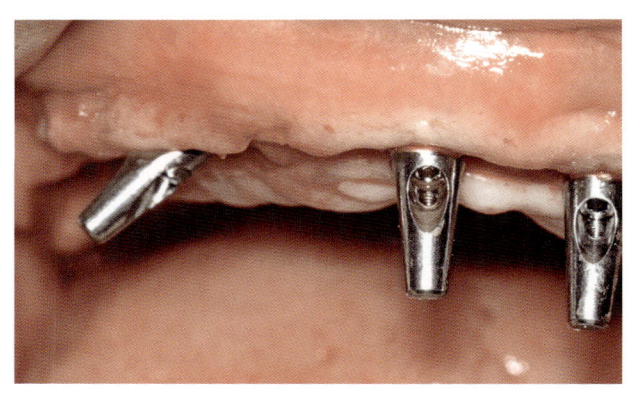

Fig 14-137  Abutments being attached at second-stage surgery following the completion of integration. The implants will be exposed and the definitive abutments attached. A non-indexed connection enables the alignment of the abutment to be carried out by merely rotating it until it is aligned, as seen in Fig 14-138.

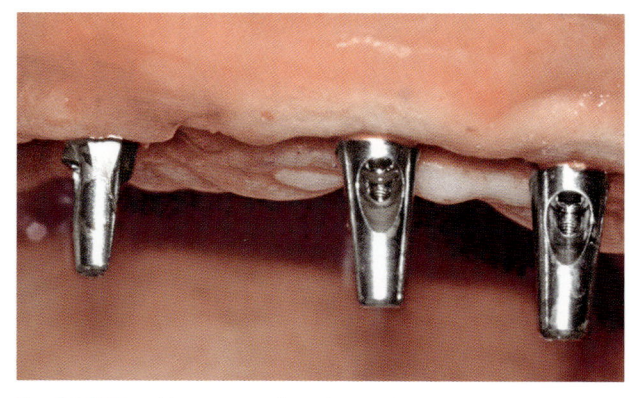

Fig 14-138  Abutments aligned to each other. These can now be tightened to 15 Ncm to engage the conical connection.

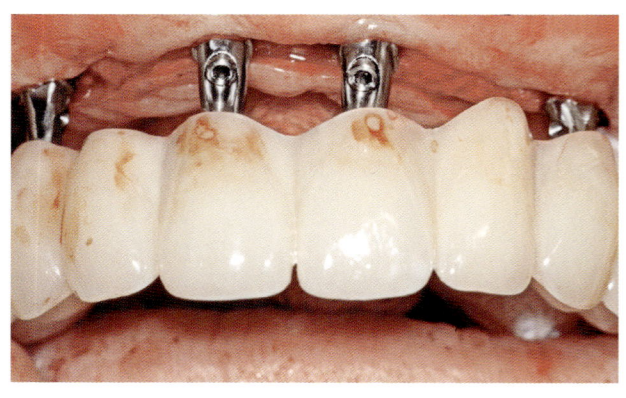

Fig 14-139  A hollow acrylic resin transitional bridge can be seen being tried in to verify accurate information transfer through the stages. The transitional denture has been constructed from data gathered during the diagnostic preview phase.

14   Extensive Bone Grafts

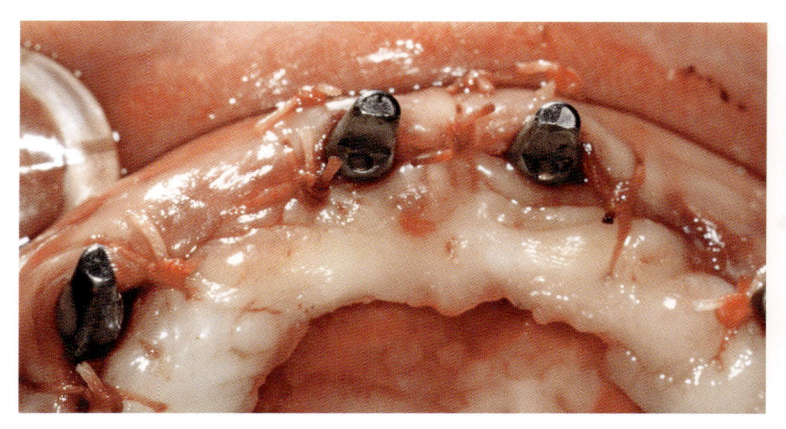

**Fig 14-140**   The wound is closed around the attached abutments. A split-thickness sliding flap from the palate is advanced to ensure closure over the graft.

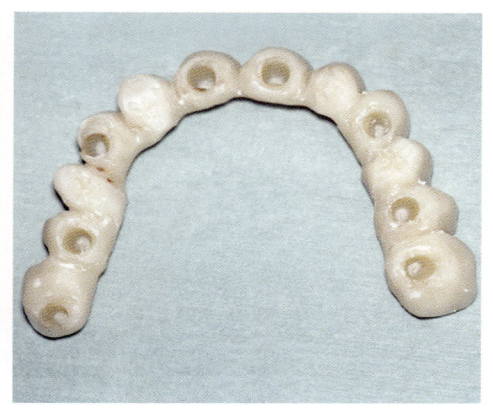

**Fig 14-141**   The hollow acrylic resin transitional bridge is relined directly over the abutments. Note the positioning of the abutments in relation to the teeth.

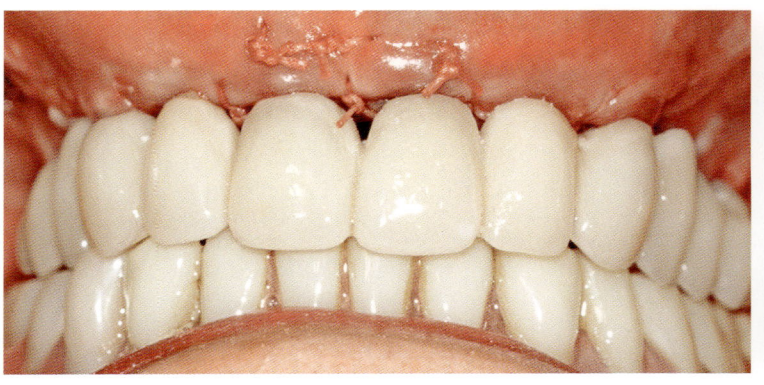

**Fig 14-142**   Transitional restoration in situ occluding against the lower denture.

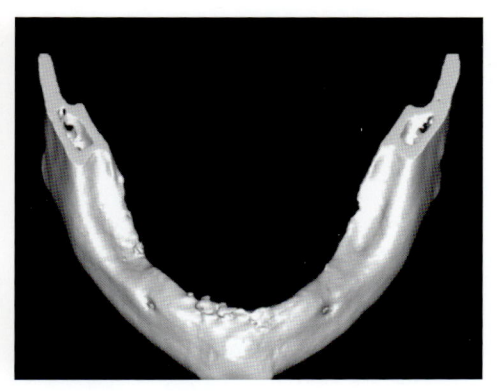

**Fig 14-143**   CT 3D view of the Class V mandible.

**Fig 14-144**   Cross-sectional view in the posterior region showing the proximity of the inferior alveolar canal to the superior surface and the residual of the alveolar ridge.

**Fig 14-145**   Clinical view of the residual ridge showing atrophy of the hard tissues as well as a reduction of keratinised attached tissue.

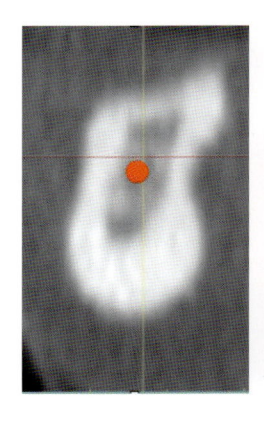

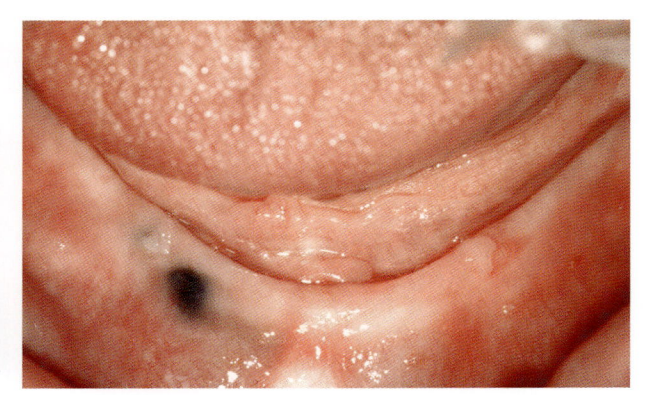

291

III  Augmentation

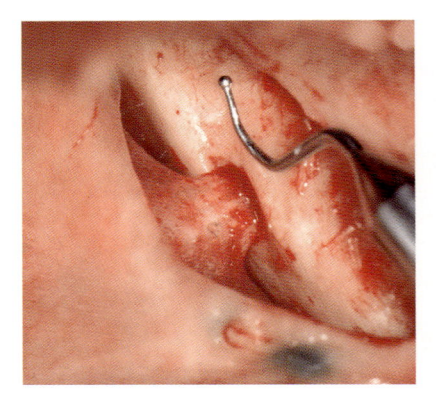

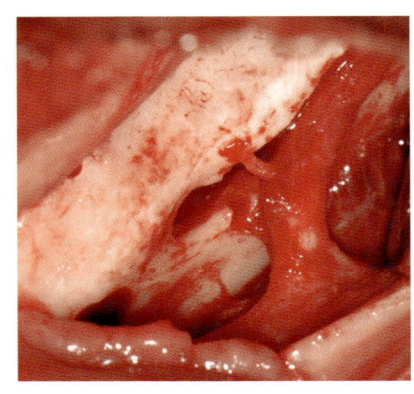

**Fig 14-146** (left) Exposure of the right mental foramen with the curved probe, which will be used to explore the canal.

**Fig 14-147** (right) Left inferior alveolar neurovascular bundle exposed and repositioned buccally. A small ancillary incisive branch is visible.

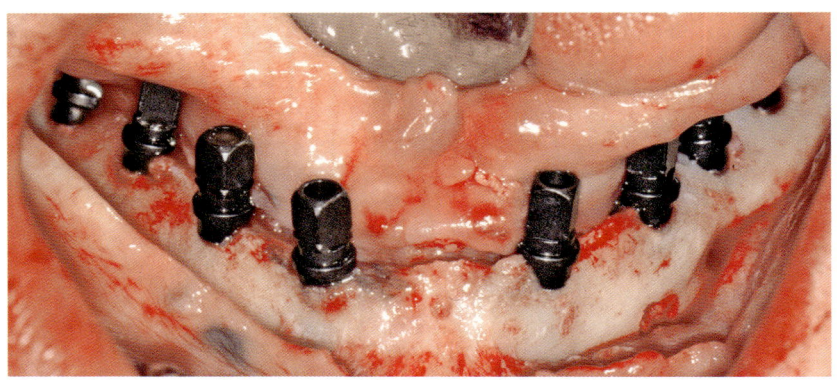

**Fig 14-148** Mandibular implants in situ following the repositioning of both inferior alveolar neurovascular bundles.

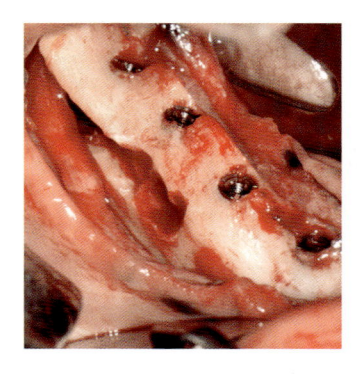

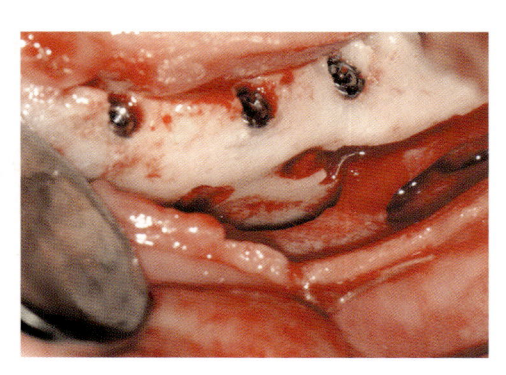

**Fig 14-149** (left) Intraoperative view of the right neurovascular bundle. The implants have been placed and the bundle can be seen intact. The incisive branch has been severed.

**Fig 14-150** (right) Left neurovascular bundle, with implants in situ, prior to being repositioned back into the groove.

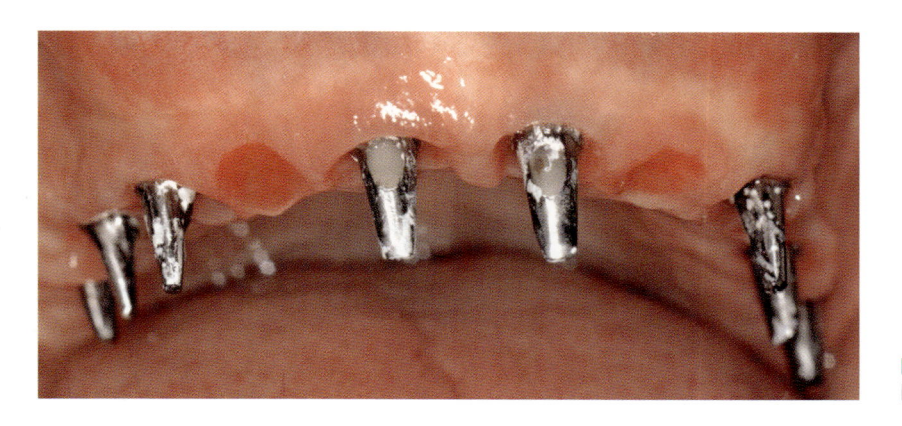

**Fig 14-151** Maxillary abutments can be seen with the healed soft tissues.

14   Extensive Bone Grafts

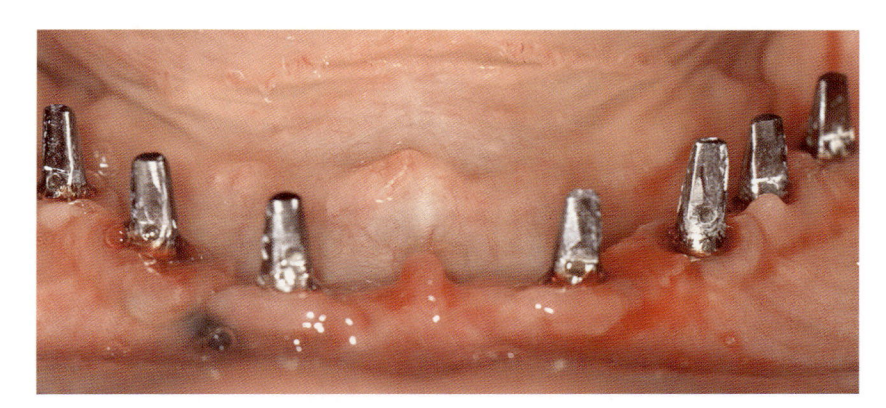

**Fig 14-152**   Mandibular abutments aligned to each other and in the position dictated by the teeth.

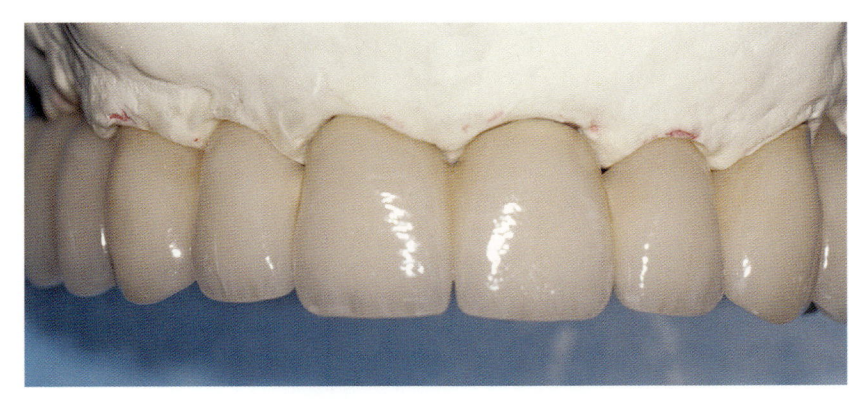

**Fig 14-153**   Porcelain-fused-to-metal bridge on a solid cast fabricated to the soft tissue contours transferred during impression taking.

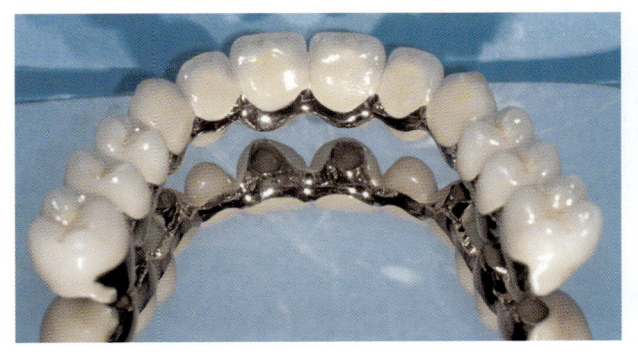

**Fig 14-154**   Definitive maxillary bridge. The positioning of the abutments is closely related to the tooth position, as seen on the fit surface in the reflection.

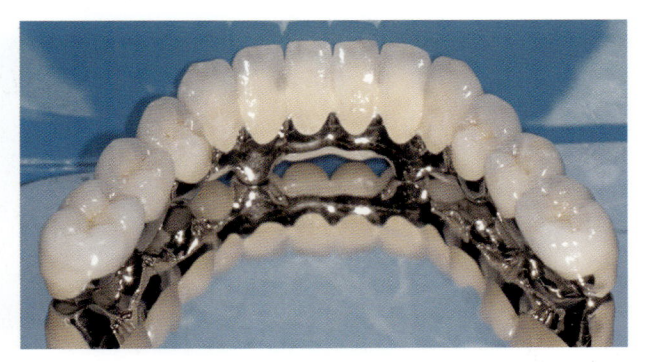

**Fig 14-155**   Definitive mandibular bridge. The positioning of the abutments is closely related to the tooth position, as seen on the fit surface in the reflection.

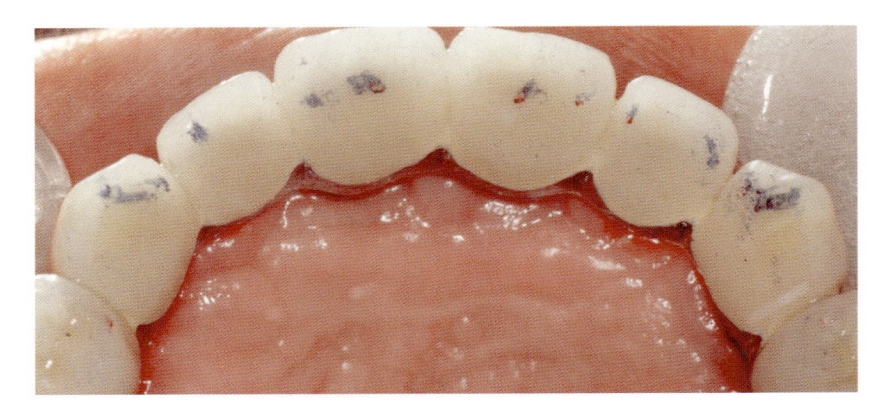

**Fig 14-156**   Occlusal surface showing articulated paper markings indicating functional contact with the mandibular bridge.

III  Augmentation

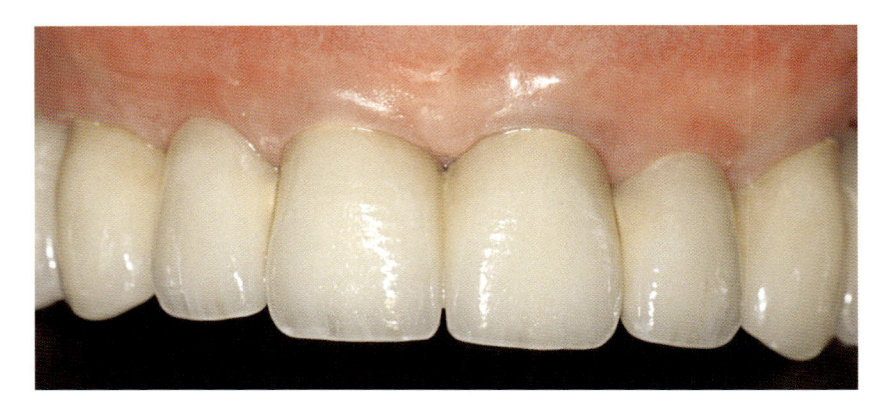

**Fig 14-157** Labial view of the bridge in situ with well-contoured soft tissues.

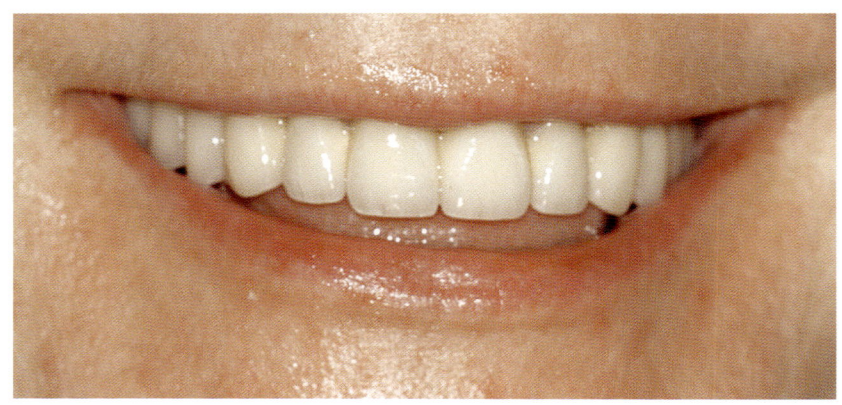

**Fig 14-158** Frontal view of the patient smiling, with well-supported circumoral tissues.

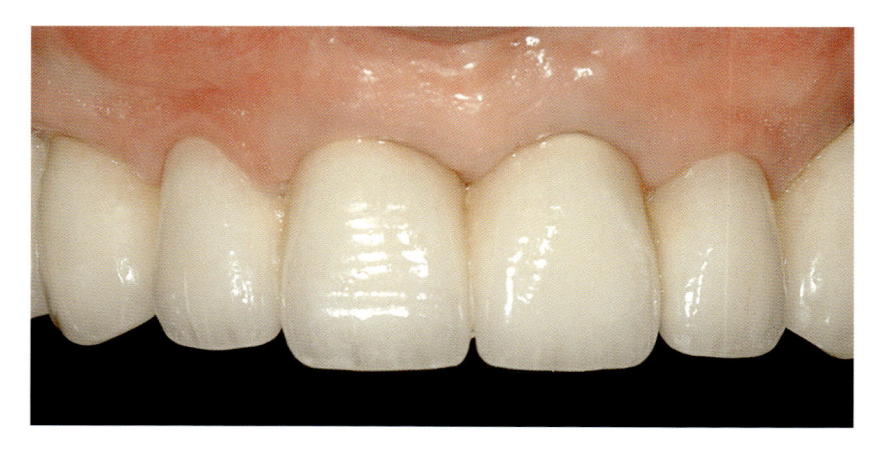

**Fig 14-159** Image shows a labial view taken four years after the fitting of the restoration. Stippling and maturation of the soft tissues is visible. This is indicative of a healthy functional status quo.

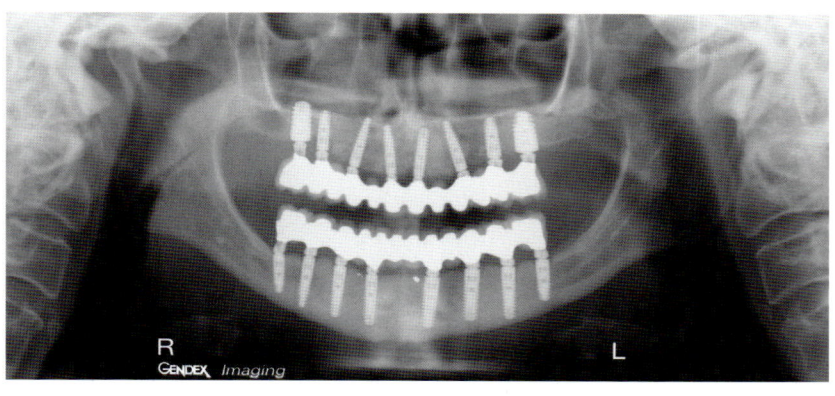

**Fig 14-160** Post-operative panoramic tomograph summarising the levels and information relating to implant position and dimensions.

14  Extensive Bone Grafts

## Case 7: Augmentation of Both Jaws

Case 7 demonstrates the treatment of a class IV maxilla and a class VI mandible. Severely resorbed jaws are often indicative of parafunctional habits and denture wear at night. The loss of bony support severely compromises function. Muscle attachment loss and soft tissue atrophy results in loss of support for the circumoral soft tissues, which can result in an unacceptable facial profile. The augmentation of the mandible becomes essential to prevent pathological fractures occurring. Augmentation of both jaws with bone grafts and subsequent restoration with metal-ceramic implant-supported restorations restored function and the facial profile for this patient. The ongoing stability of the hard and soft tissues following restoration supports the validity of the extensive treatment undertaken for this patient. Particular attention is drawn to the improvement in the soft tissue quality resulting from physiological function (Figs 14-161–14-192).

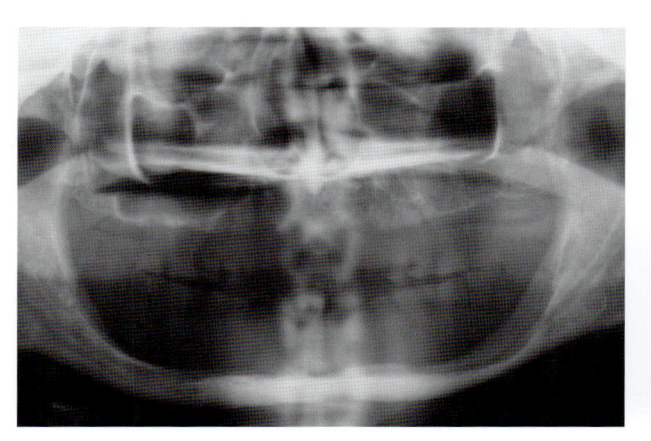

**Fig 14-161** Panoramic tomograph showing the preoperative state. Preliminary observation may show the mandible to be more substantial than that evident in the 3D imaging.

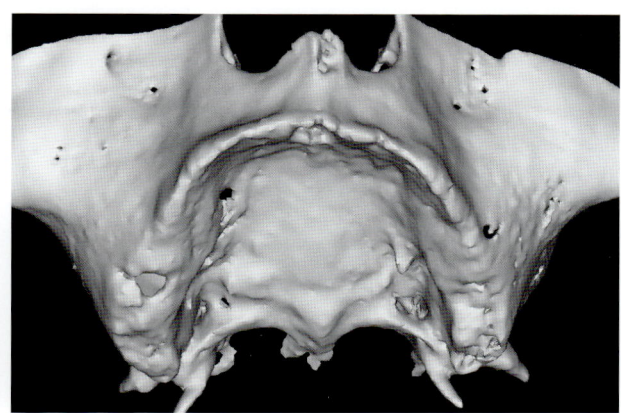

**Fig 14-162** CT 3D view of the maxilla showing a Class IV jaw with some loss of height but largely a loss of width.

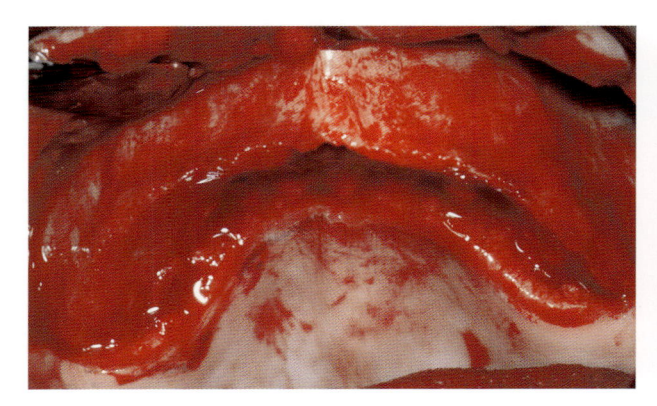

**Fig 14-163** Intraoperative view showing the narrow maxillary ridge as depicted in the CT scan.

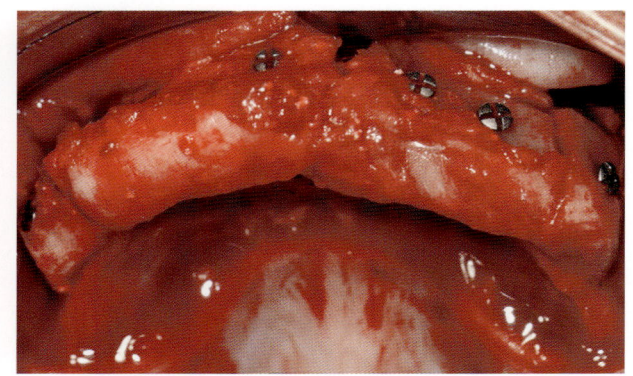

**Fig 14-164** An autogenous bone graft obtained from the iliac crest in situ restoring the dimensions of the maxilla. Overcompensation by approximately 20% is recommended to allow for remodelling. The floor of the sinus was augmented at the same time.

III   Augmentation

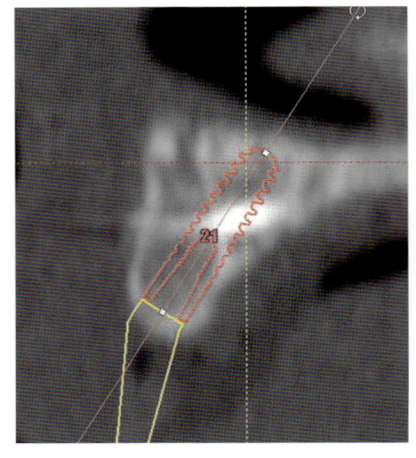

**Fig 14-165**   Cross-sectional view showing interactive planning for implant placement following the healing of the bone graft. The increase in the dimension is evident. Note that the implant is sited at an angle to engage the residual ridge.

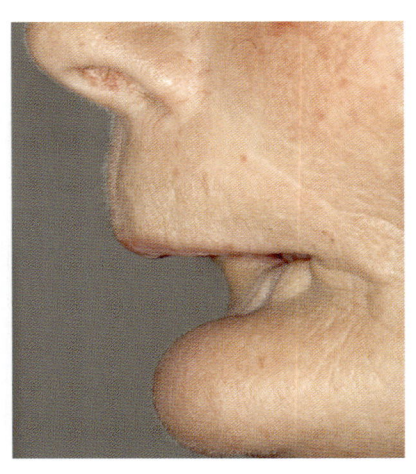

**Fig 14-166**   Profile view of the patient following the maxillary graft, demonstrating the increase in support for the upper lip. The lack of support for the lower lip is indicative of a Class VI mandible where the alveolar and basal bone has been eroded.

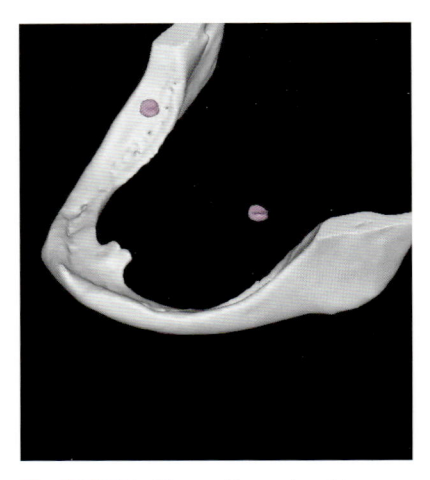

**Fig 14-167**   Three-dimensional image based on CT scan data showing the hollow superior surface of the mandible caused by a denture worn at night. Coupled with a parafunctional clenching habit, this may be considered to have caused the excessive amount of resorption that has taken place.

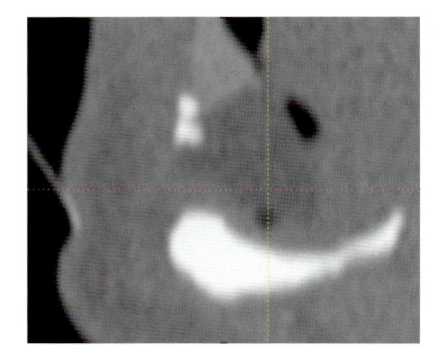

**Fig 14-168**   Cross-sectional CT image through the midline showing the very limited amount of bone available. The genial tubercle can be seen. It is also evident in Fig 14-167. The radiopaque tooth visible at the top of the image is indicative of the volume of bone loss that has taken place.

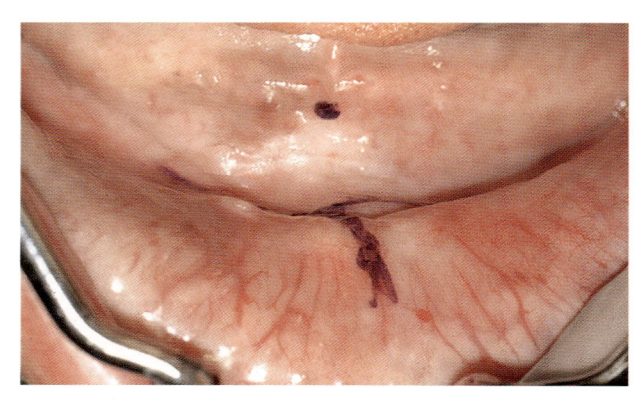

**Fig 14-169**   Intraoral view of the concave region where the alveolar ridge used to be. The marks represent the midline, the region where the crest of the ridge used to be and the genial tubercle. Note that all the keratinised tissue has atrophied.

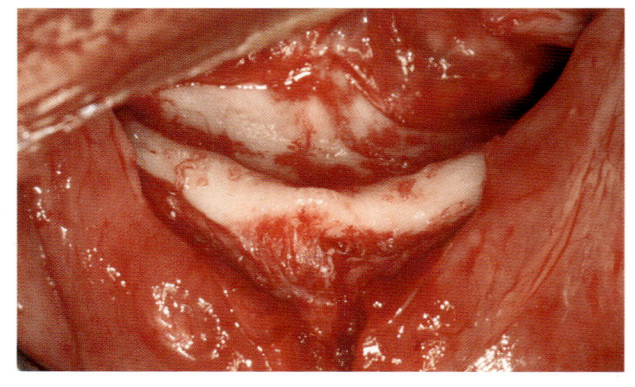

**Fig 14-170**   Intraoperative view showing the concave mandible, the inferior portion of the mental process and the genial tubercle at the top end of the image.

14  Extensive Bone Grafts

**Fig 14-171** (left) The inferior alveolar neurovascular bundle exposed from the lingual aspect of the mandible. Two notches can be seen in the remnants of the external oblique ridge, one of which will receive the repositioned neurovascular bundle.

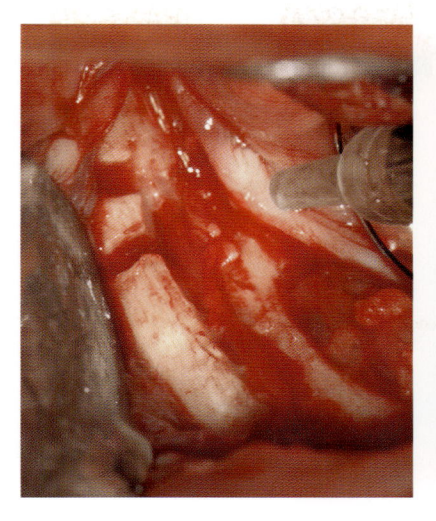

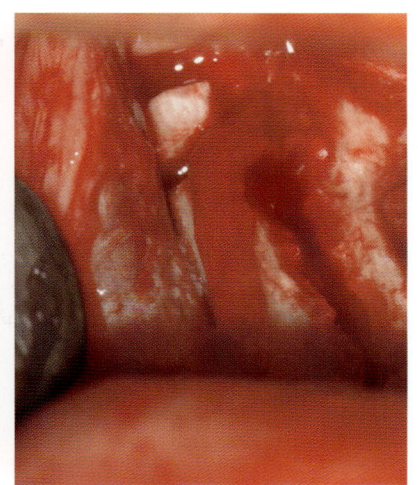

**Fig 14-172** (right) The repositioned neurovascular bundle placed in the anterior notch.

**Fig 14-173** (left) Bi-cortical corticocancellous graft 15 mm in height and 35 mm in length.

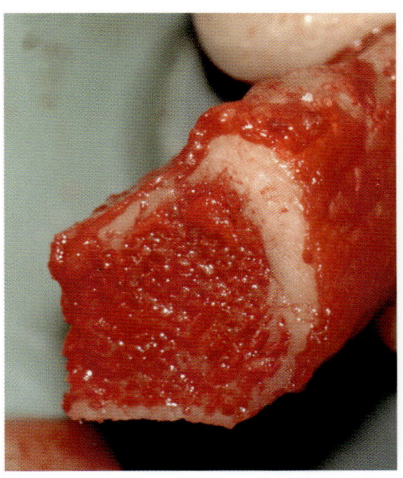

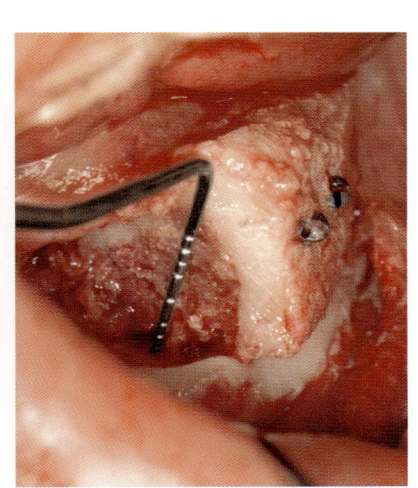

**Fig 14-174** (right) One of the grafts secured into position, demonstrating the height gained.

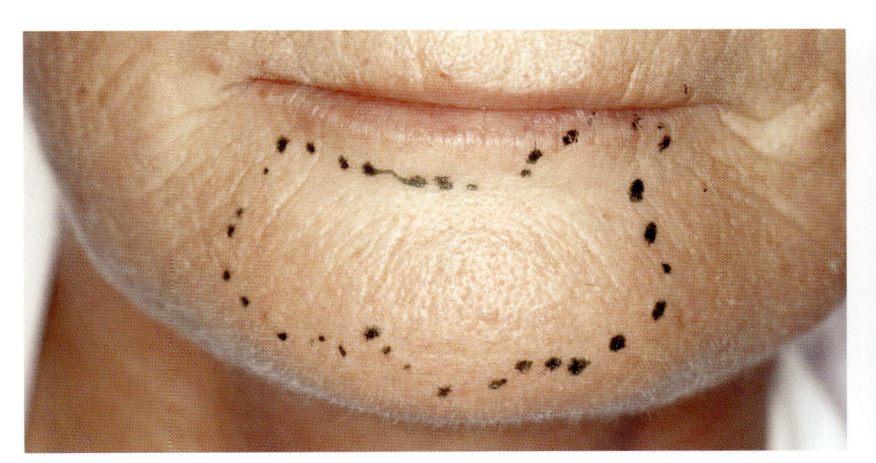

**Fig 14-175** Anterior view of patient showing the support provided by the graft for the circumoral tissues. The area of altered sensation is depicted by the green pen and will be monitored until a full recovery takes place.

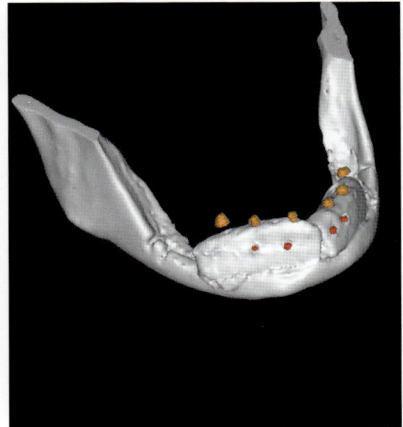

**Fig 14-176** Three-dimensional CT image of the healed bone graft showing the height gained as well as the notches created to receive the repositioned neurovascular bundle. The radiopaque markers locate the positions of the lateral incisors, first premolars and first molars.

III Augmentation

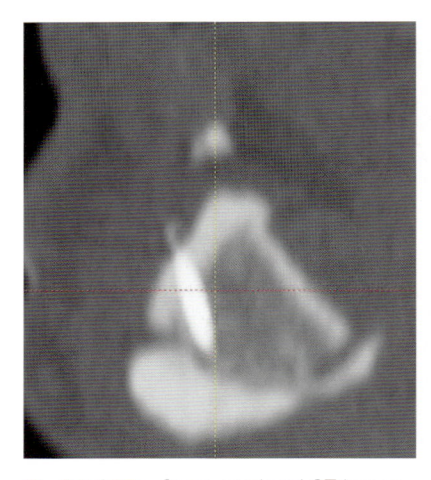

**Fig 14-177** Cross-sectional CT image showing the amount of height gained by the graft in relation to the tooth position depicted by the radiopaque marker.

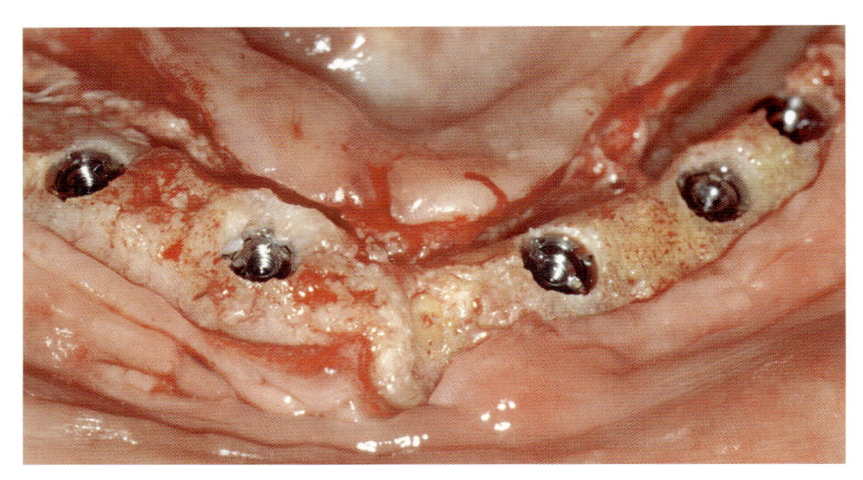

**Fig 14-178** Intraoperative view of the implants in the healed bone grafts, three months after the augmentation surgery.

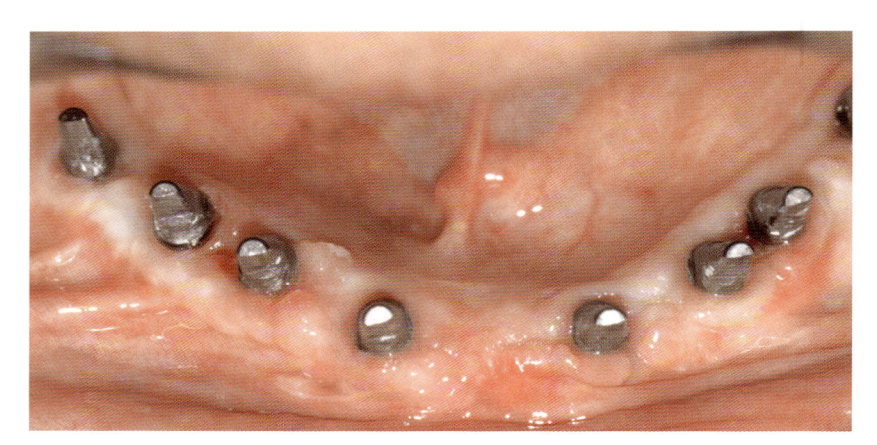

**Fig 14-179** Intraoperative view of the abutments, which were placed approximately four months after implant insertion. Note the appearance of the keratinised tissue, which is not evident in the preoperative clinical image of the mandible.

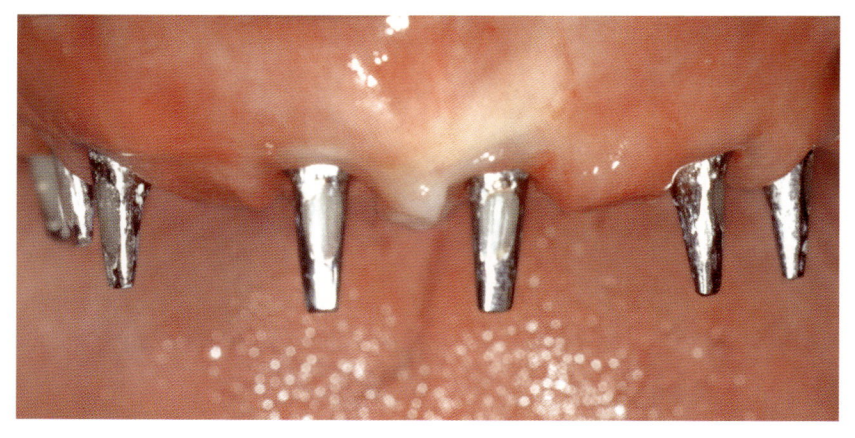

**Fig 14-180** Labial view of the maxilla showing the abutments emerging from the soft tissues. No keratinised tissue is visible.

14  Extensive Bone Grafts

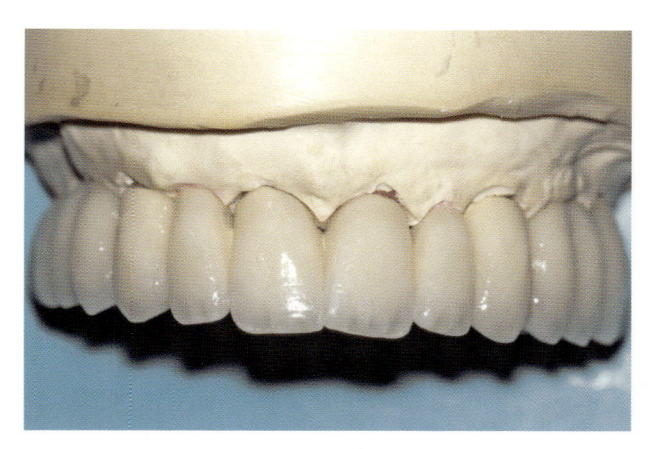

**Fig 14-181**  The definitive maxillary bridge on a solid cast with porcelain constructed to the soft tissue contours developed by the transitional restoration.

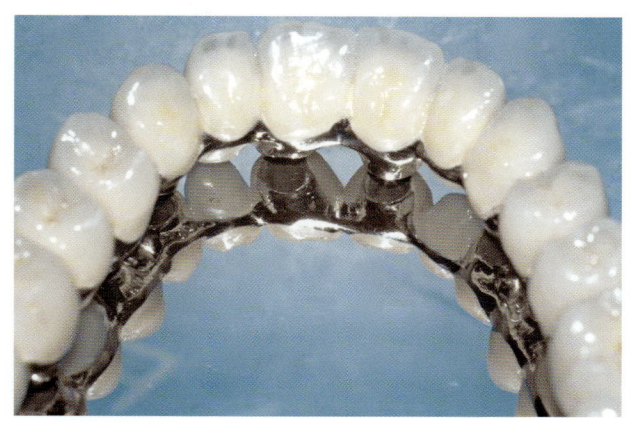

**Fig 14-182**  Occlusal view of the maxillary bridge. Note that the implant and abutment position is coincidental with tooth position as seen in the reflection in the mirror.

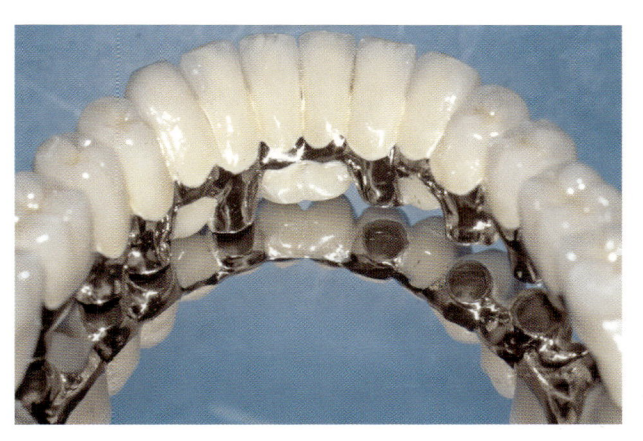

**Fig 14-183**  Occlusal view of the mandibular bridge. Note that the implant and abutment position is coincidental with tooth position as seen in the reflection in the mirror.

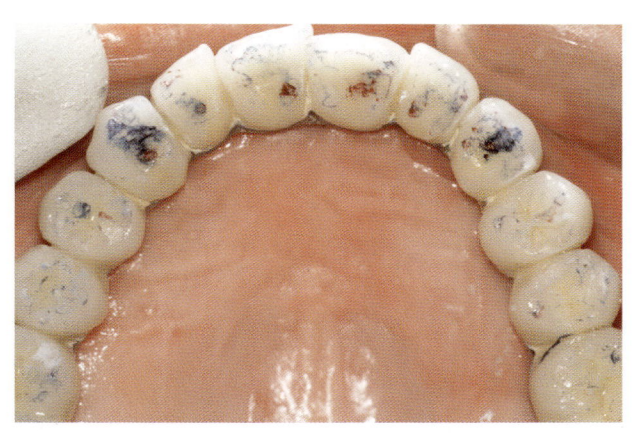

**Fig 14-184**  Occlusal view of the maxillary bridge with articulating paper markings demonstrating contact in centric relation and during lateral and protrusive excursions.

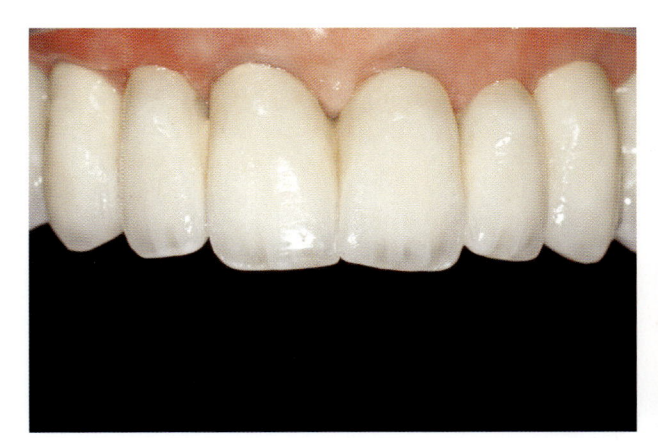

**Fig 14-185**  Labial view of the fitted restoration showing the contours established. However, no keratinised tissue or stippling is evident.

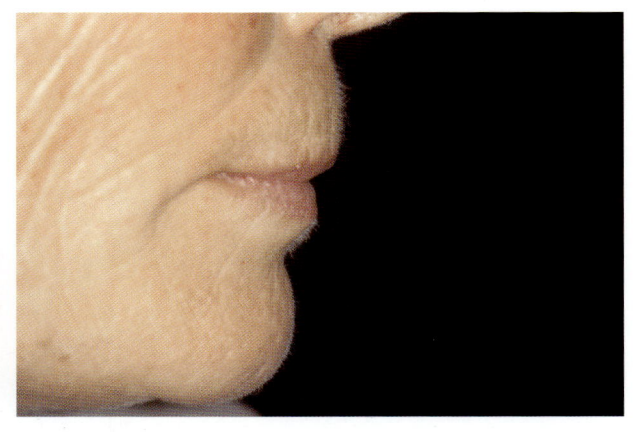

**Fig 14-186**  Profile view of the patient showing the re-established facial contours.

III Augmentation

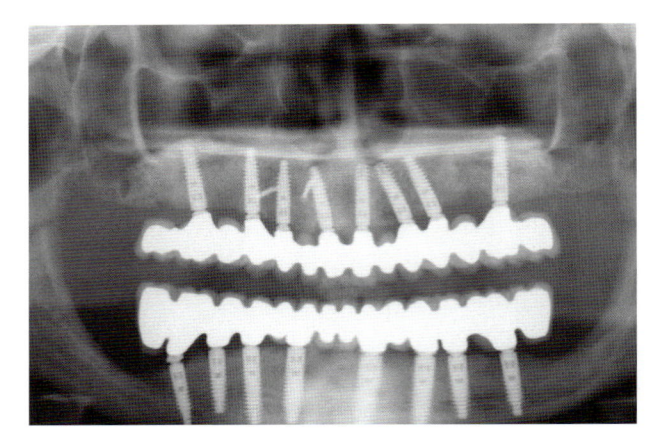

Fig 14-187 Post-operative panoramic tomograph showing the distribution and the dimensions of the implants.

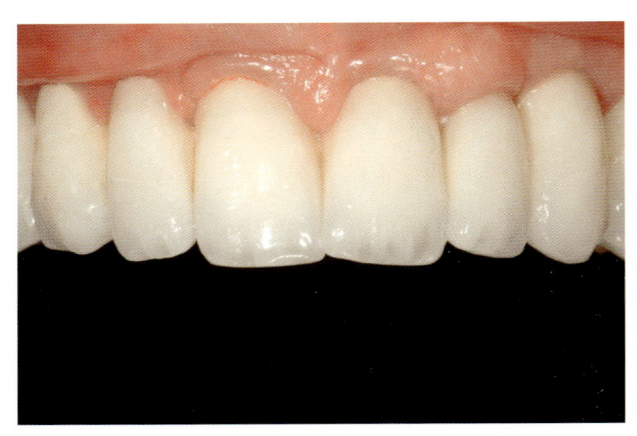

Fig 14-188 Image taken five years following the completion of the treatment. Development of keratinised tissue is evident.

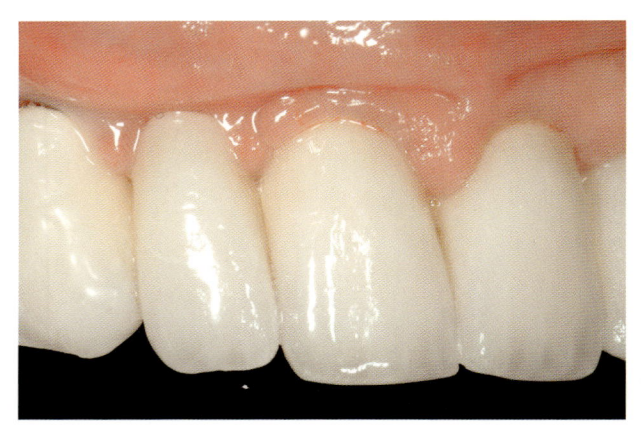

Fig 14-189 Close-up of the right lateral region.

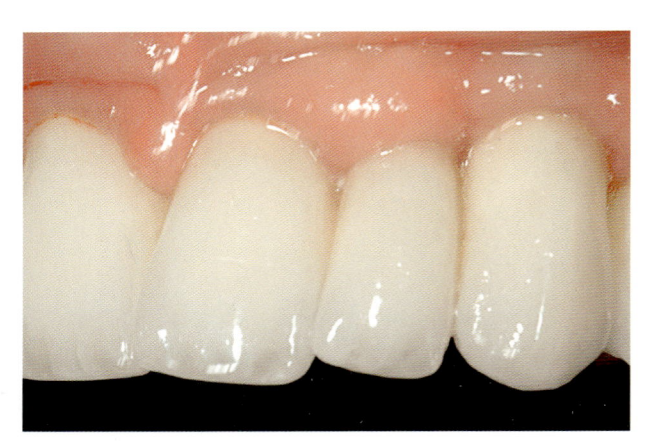

Fig 14-190 Close-up of the left lateral region.

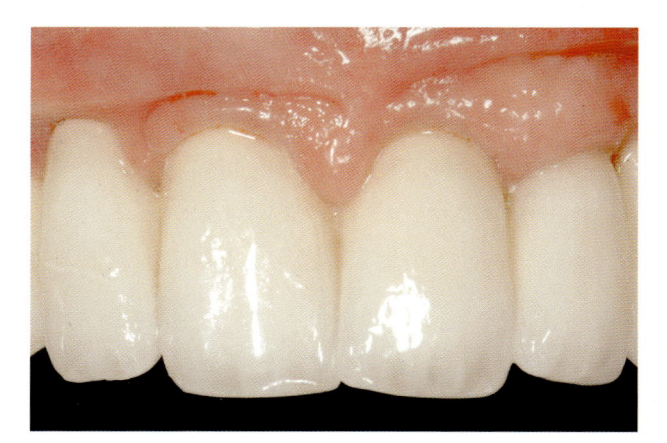

Fig 14-191 Close-up of the anterior teeth showing well-developed contours and keratinised tissue.

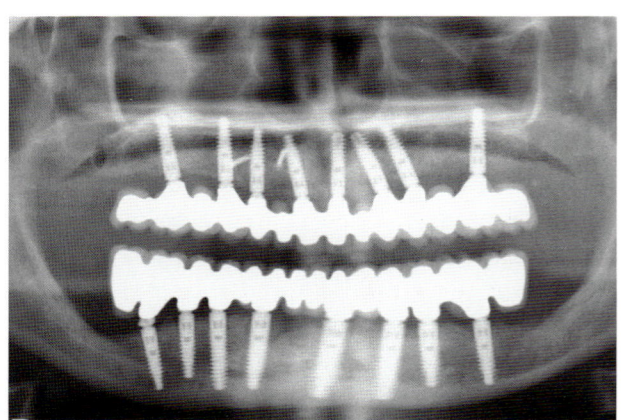

Fig 14-192 Panoramic tomograph taken five years after completion of the treatment showing stable bone levels.

# Chapter 15

# Posterior Maxilla

## Introduction

Several features characterise the posterior maxilla, namely bone quality, sinus size, ridge width and alveolar height.

- **Bone quality.** Bone in the posterior maxilla is most commonly of low density, consisting of a thin cortical bone with sparsely trabeculated cancellous bone. In the region of the premolar teeth, medium density bone may occasionally be encountered.
- **Sinus extent.** The enlargement of the maxillary sinus is the most significant factor restricting the amount of bone available in the posterior maxilla.
- **Ridge width.** The width of the ridge is usually adequate in the region of the molar teeth although some narrowing may be observed in the region of the premolar teeth.
- **Alveolar height.** Loss of alveolar height is occasionally a consequence of periodontal disease or other pathological conditions. It rarely needs correcting (Fig 15-1) because the aesthetics are not often compromised and substantial height can be gained by subantral augmentation (sinus lift). Onlay grafts are sometimes indicated to improve biomechanics, hygiene, aesthetics and function by placing the abutment more labially and coronally to allow proper positioning of teeth for occlusion (Fig 15-2).

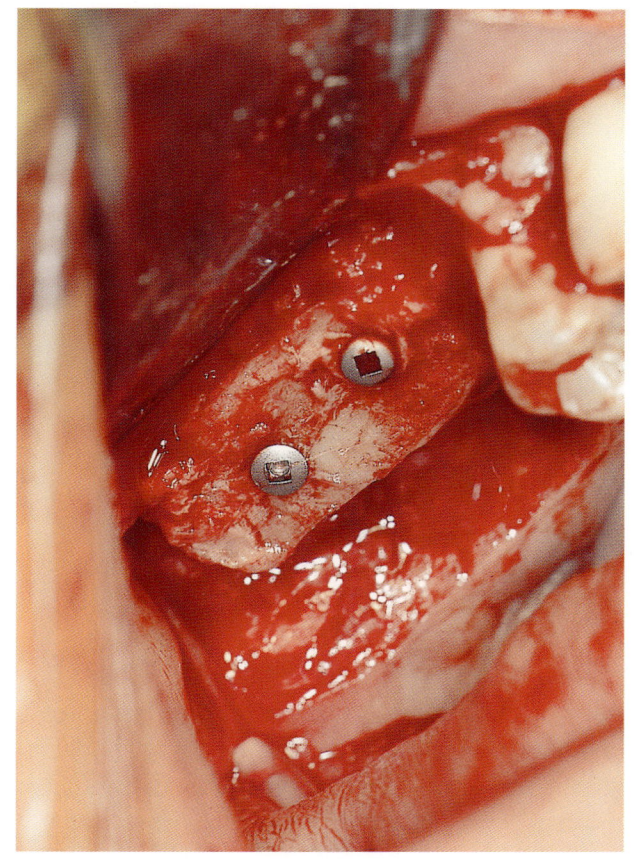

**Fig 15-1** Intraoral view of an onlay graft being used in conjunction with a sinus lift to increase the ridge height in a case where alveolar bone loss has taken place.

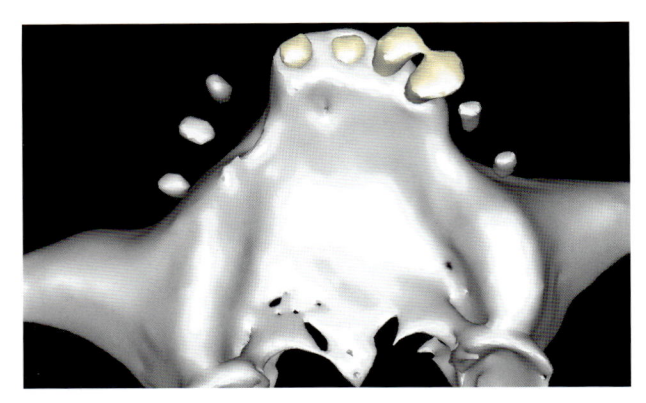

Fig 15-2 Three-dimensional view of a CT scan indicating the discrepancy between the radiopaque markers and the deficient ridge requiring augmentation to enable the implants to be positioned within the prosthetic envelope.

## Anatomy

### Development

The maxillary sinus develops in the 12th week of intrauterine life as a small bud from the middle meatus of the lateral wall of the nose. At birth, it is approximately 1 cm³ in size and develops as the mid-face height increases until adulthood. It is associated with the eruption of the permanent teeth, and progressive pneumatisation of the sinus continues throughout adulthood, supposedly as a result of the increased atmospheric pressure within the sinus.

### Physiology

The sinuses are part of the respiratory system and the lining consists of a layer of loose connective tissue, a surface layer of ciliated columnar cells, and subepithelial mucous-secreting serous cells. The sinus lining is poorly vascularised and has not been shown to have osteogenic potential, although it does contain osteoclasts, which contribute to the pneumatisation.

### Anatomical Relationship

A working knowledge of the anatomy of the sinuses is critical for the safe perioperative management of surgery in this region. Surgery must not be carried out in this region without proper training. Some salient features of the maxillary sinus are outlined below.[219,220] The maxillary sinus lies in close proximity to several midfacial structures.

The anterior wall of the sinus often coincides with the canine fossa distal to the root of the canine tooth. This is in close proximity to the neurovascular structures that emerge from the infraorbital foramen. It is in this region that the overlying bone is quite thin and from where the sinus is accessed for the traditional Caldwell–Luc procedure. The posterior wall of the sinus often coincides with the pterygoid plates, the pterygoid venous plexus and the numerous neurovascular structures that are in close proximity. The lateral extension of the sinus extends to the zygomatic arch and may excavate into the zygomatic bone. The medial wall coincides with the lateral wall of the nose, which may be very thin. The sinus may extend under the nose, creating an apex in this region. The superior border of the sinus forms the base of the orbit. The floor of the sinus may wrap itself around the roots of the teeth. The sinus may be multichambered with septa of different heights and orientations. These surface characteristics of the floor of the sinus will have a considerable influence on the manner in which any surgery designed to augment the floor of the sinus is carried out.

The maxillary sinus communicates with the nasal cavity via the ostio-meatal complex. This consists of the ostium on the medial wall of the sinus, which opens into the nasal cavity via the semilunar opening positioned under the middle concha. It is, therefore, normally positioned above the level to which any augmentation will need to be carried out. The ostio-meatal opening is close to the junction communicating with the anterior, sphenoid and ethmoid sinus cavities.

Although the sinus lining itself is poorly vascularised, the maxilla has an excellent blood supply, which is provided by several branches of the maxillary artery – the infraorbital, the superior alveolar, the paranasal and the greater palatine arteries. There is also a contribution from the transverse facial (branch of the superior temporal) and the facial arteries. There are numerous anastomoses providing excellent collateral circulation. With the pneumatisation of the sinuses, some of these blood vessels may be found lying within grooves on the surface of the bony walls of the sinus.

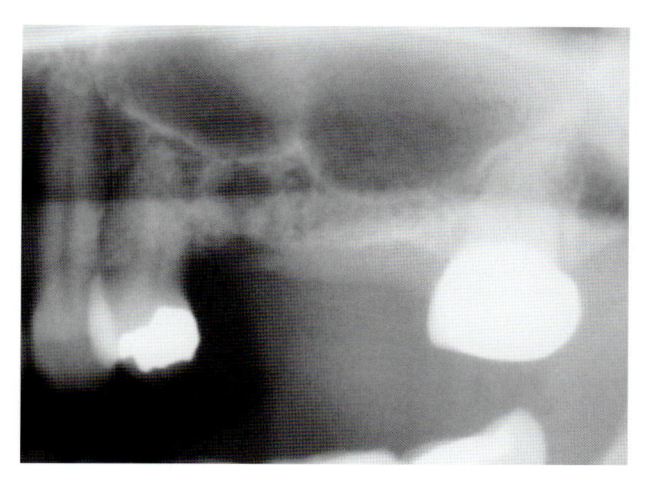

**Fig 15-3** Preoperative panoramic tomograph showing the floor of the sinus and the septum. The radiograph is taken with the Frankfurt plane at 25 degrees to the horizontal during exposure to deflect the shadow of the palate.

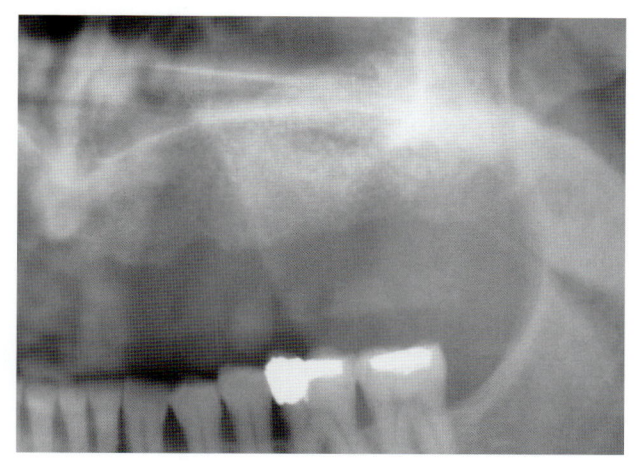

**Fig 15-4** Preoperative panoramic tomograph (taken with the Frankfurt plane at 25 degrees to the horizontal, to deflect the shadow of the palate) of the left-hand side showing an enlarged maxillary sinus and a limited amount of alveolar bone available in the posterior maxilla. The panoramic tomography is a valuable preliminary examination but a limited amount of diagnostic information can be obtained because of the superimposition of several anatomical structures.

## Assessment of Available Bone and the Maxillary Sinus

### Dental Panoramic Tomograph

The DPT taken for the diagnostic assessment of the maxillary sinus gives the best results when the head is tilted forward and the Frankfurt plane is at approximately 25 degrees to the horizontal. This will result in the dense radiopaque shadow of the hard palate to be displaced and dispersed away from the region of interest in most patients (Figs 15-3 and 15-4). This type of investigation provides an excellent overview and is valuable for planning treatment and surgery with respect to incisions and bony access to the maxillary sinus.

### Computed Tomography

CT scans taken in the axial plane using multiple panoral and cross-sectional reformations will provide the information required for the volumetric assessment of this region (Figs 15-5–15-7). Interactive programs will provide an assessment of the bone density. The information that can be gained from this investigation include:

- height of bone
- width of bone
- orientation and position of alveolar ridge
- nature of the cortical and cancellous bone
- density of bone in Hounsfield units
- thickness of the sinus lining
- pathology within the alveolar bone and within the sinus
- surface topography of sinus floor
- size, position and orientation of septa
- sinus floor contours in proximity to tooth roots
- blood vessels within the lateral wall of the maxilla
- proximity of the greater palatine foramen
- extensions of sinus: subnasal, anterior and zygomatic
- thickness of the walls of the sinus.

The considerable information that can be gathered from these investigations must be used to the maximum in planning and executing treatment. It is clear that the information gained from CT is crucial for both planning surgery and minimising the risks during the surgical procedures. The information gained from CT is, therefore, considered to be of vital importance, particularly for sinus lift procedures.[221]

III   Augmentation

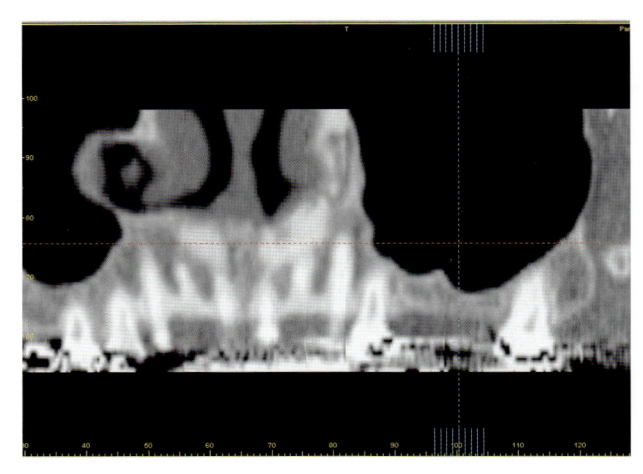

**Fig 15-5**   Panoramic reconstruction of the maxilla. The plane selected for the reconstruction passes through the roots of the maxillary teeth, the conchi of the nose and the sinus showing the septum (same patient as in Fig 15-3).

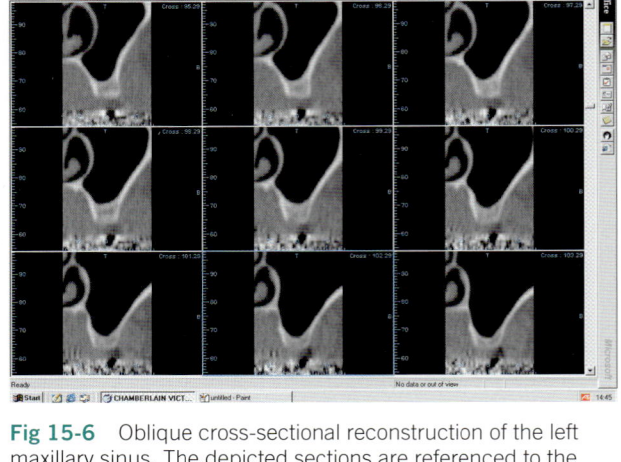

**Fig 15-6**   Oblique cross-sectional reconstruction of the left maxillary sinus. The depicted sections are referenced to the lines on the panoramic section (Fig 15-5). The lateral wall of the sinus is visible on the right-hand side of the image, and the thickness of the wall can be assessed. The medial wall coincides with the lateral wall of the nose, and the contours of this region are valuable landmarks during elevation of the sinus lining. The varying amount of remaining alveolar bone is also visible.

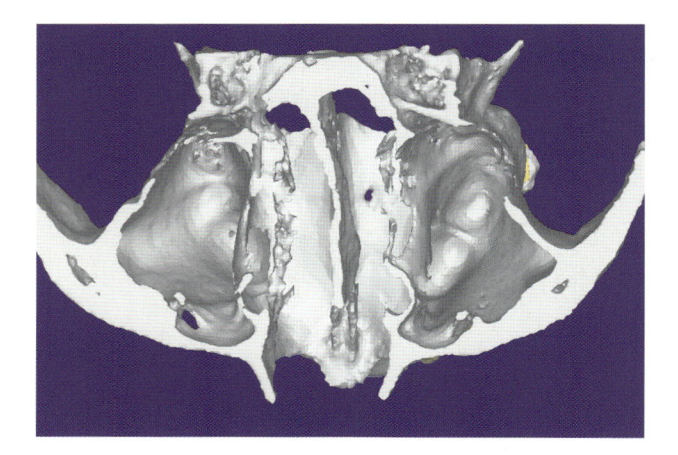

**Fig 15-7**   Three-dimensional reconstruction of CT scan viewed from the superior aspect, showing the internal anatomy of the floor of the nose and the sinus. The vomer, the pterygoid plates and the zygomatic process are also visible. A small septum can be observed in the left sinus (same patient as Fig 15-5).

Additional imaging techniques, such as MRI and conventional tomography, can also be used. CT scans taken in the coronal plane are used for investigation of sinus pathology, as it enables other sinuses to be investigated. Specific views using conventional radiography (Waters view) are used for investigating fluid levels.

## Assessment of Pathology

Acute sinusitis should be treated prior to augmentation. No elective procedure should be carried out in the presence of any acute pathological process. Appropriate therapy (antibiotic, anti-inflammatory and decongestant) should be implemented to treat the condition, and augmentation of the sinus should be undertaken only once the symptoms have resolved.

A CT scan is very valuable for determining the nature of the hard and soft tissues in the maxilla and the sinuses (Figs 15-8–15-10). Although MRI may be used for soft tissue imaging, the range of software available for CT provides an excellent ability to visualise any pathology of dental or respiratory system origin. Other findings discovered using modern imaging techniques should be addressed according to the guidelines outlined below. Consultation with ENT surgeons regarding the pathology of the sinuses is recommended.

### Assessment of Sinus Lining: Pathology
### Thin Lining

Thin linings are healthy and are not visible on a CT scan.

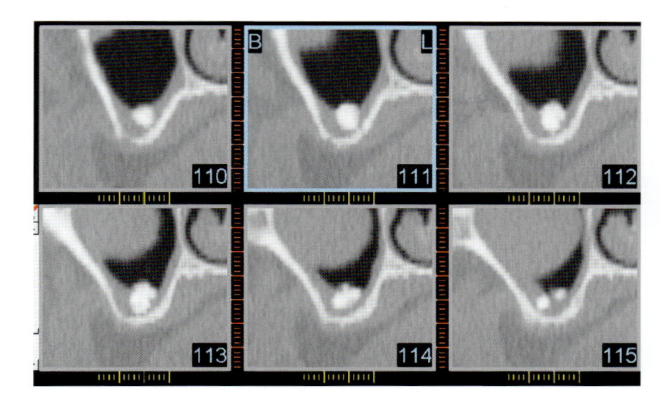

**Fig 15-8**  Oblique cross-sectional reconstruction of maxillary sinus. An object of high radiopacity can be seen within the thickened sinus lining. In addition, the edge of a rounded object with a density corresponding to soft tissues can be seen. These were unrelated and were discovered to be an odontome and a mucocele, respectively, on histopathological examination.

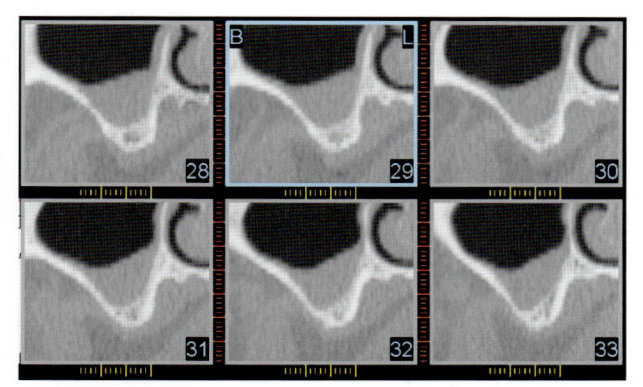

**Fig 15-9**  Cross-sectional CT scan reconstruction of the left maxillary sinus, showing a thickened sinus lining and a limited amount of residual alveolar bone. The lateral wall of the maxilla and the thickness of the cortical bone can be seen. This will assist in the design of the window. The buccal side is on the left of each image, and the palate and the nasal structures can be seen on the right. A greater amount of information can be obtained by this imaging technique than with the panoramic tomography (Fig 15-4).

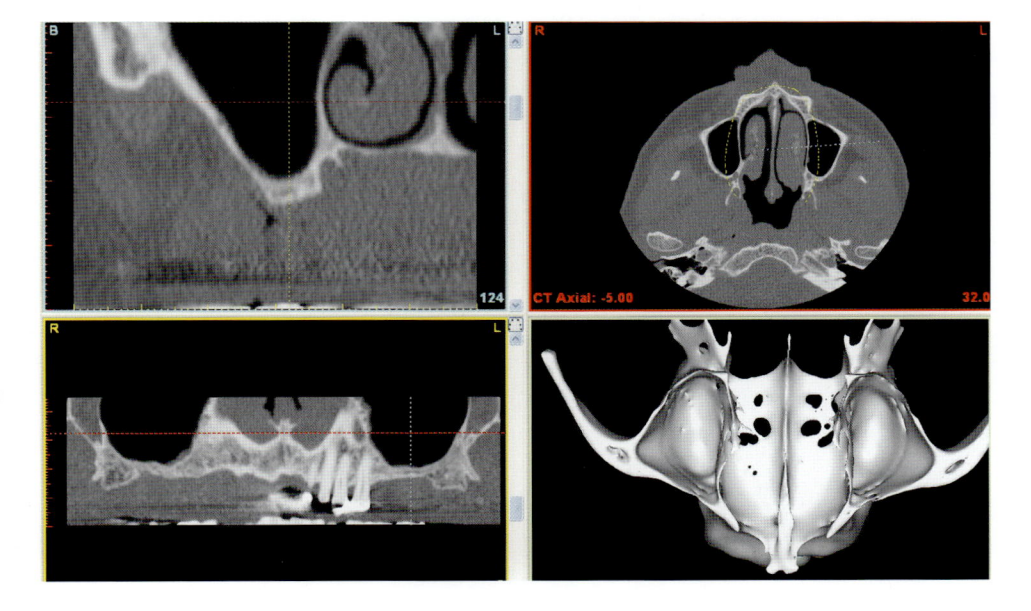

**Fig 15-10**  The four panels of the Simplant program are essential for planning. The top left panel shows the branch of the maxillary artery in the lateral wall, which can also be seen in the bottom right panel as a groove.

## Thick Lining

A thick lining is visible on the CT scan but does not contraindicate treatment. A thickened lining may have several causes, for example allergy, smoking or other conditions that lead to a generalised inflammatory response.

A localised thickening of the lining may be of dental origin, which will need to be addressed prior to proceeding.

## Polyp or Mucocele

A polyp or mucocele has a distinct appearance. Differential diagnosis based on a CT scan is difficult and treatment will depend upon the size of the polyp or mucocele. Large obstructive lesions are generally better removed prior to or during augmentation. Mucoceles can be drained during the grafting operation. Polyps, however, will need to be removed and the augmentation carried out at a later stage.

## III  Augmentation

### Generalised Obstructive Radiopacity in the Sinus

A generalised radiopacity requires investigation to determine the cause, which is most effectively carried out by an ENT surgeon. CT scans using coronal sections enable the other sinuses to be visualised for the diagnosis of pansinusitis.

Endoscopic examination of the sinuses may be coupled with endoscopic removal of pathology and greatly facilitates healing. The Caldwell–Luc procedure coupled with a nasal antrostomy should be avoided if possible to facilitate access for the sinus lift procedure at a later stage.

### Removal of Diseased Tissues and Foreign Bodies

Should an intraoral approach to the removal of pathology or foreign bodies be decided upon, the Caldwell–Luc approach with a high access should be used. The position of the access window should be accurately noted on the charts to facilitate re-entry, which may be carried out three months later.

## Assessment of Load

The potential load on the implants should be assessed by considering:
- occlusal wear
- parafunctional activity
- opposing dentition
- hypertrophy of masticatory muscles
- dietary habits.

It would be advisable to consider implants of larger dimensions both in length and diameter for patients with higher functional and parafunctional loads. Consideration should also be given to the implant surface and design of the implant. This will clearly influence the planning and timing of treatment as well as the type of augmentation that will be required. This will be discussed in a later section.

## Planning Treatment

Flowchart 15-1 (see pp. 308–309) provides the clinician with a guide to selecting a procedure that might be suitable for the patient. The focus must be the thorough assessment of the patient and the selection of a procedure that will produce a predictable outcome with a minimal risk of complications.

The aim is to deliver an implant of minimum length of 11 mm, under ideal conditions of good bone density and low occlusal loads, and preferably 15 mm in length, particularly when adverse conditions, such as high load and poor-quality bone, are present.

### Informed Consent

The patient will need to be involved in the discussions regarding the biomaterials that may be used for augmentation. The clinician needs to be aware of the efficacy and safety of the material proposed for use. The patient should be informed of the type of material, its origin and efficacy. Consent should be obtained from the patient before proceeding. A pragmatic and practical approach addressing benefits, risks, costs and severity of the surgery should be considered. The overall treatment plan should be borne in mind as well as the health of the patient. For example, patients requiring general anaesthesia for augmentation of the premaxilla with autogenous bone from the iliac crest are obviously better treated with autogenous bone harvested for the sinuses at the same time (preferably in combination with stabilising biomaterial). By comparison, the augmentation of a sinus for the replacement for a single tooth may not warrant a general anaesthesia for procurement of bone from the iliac crest.

## Clinical Protocols

The clinical protocols for managing the posterior maxilla and the specific morphological and anatomical features of this region are described in the sections below. They address the management of structural deficiencies of the maxillary bone as well as volumetric deficiencies.

## Using Available Bone

The protocol for the use of the available bone must follow sound guidelines to enable a functional restoration to be constructed.

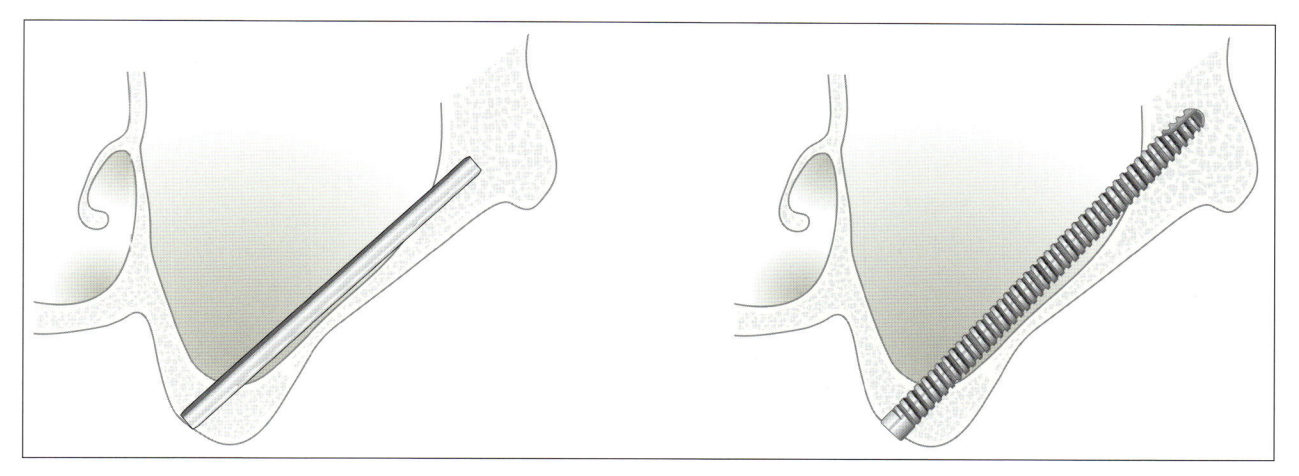

**Fig 15-11** Insertion of a zygomatic implant, which traverses from the ridge to the zygomatic bone, gaining anchorage at both ends. Long implants specifically manufactured for this application are required.

The tooth position must be identified where the abutment must emerge to enable a restoration to be constructed, meeting aesthetic and functional needs. The available bone must be identified, ensuring that the implant can be placed within this bone without any surgical compromises. Three techniques have been described: pterygoid implants, zygomatic implants and angled implants.

## Pterygoid Implants

Pterygoid implants are designed to use the plates of the pterygoid bone to anchor implants placed in the posterior maxilla.[133,222–225] Clinicians must be aware of the likelihood of the poor position of the abutment and the risks associated with the insertion of implants in this region.

## Zygomatic Implants

The procedure for inserting zygomatic implants has been described and is designed to engage the zygomatic bone traversing the maxillary sinus from the region of the first molar.[226–230] Clinicians should be aware of the possible palatal malpositioning of the abutments and the risk to the normal anatomical structures in this region (Fig 15-11).[231–233]

Furthermore, a minimal bone loss at the permucosal site (opening into the maxillary sinus) would lead to an oroantral communication, which would prove to be very difficult to manage. To minimise this risk, a procedure to avoid perforating the sinus has been advocated.[234]

## Angled Implants

Implants may be placed to avoid the maxillary sinus, which invades the alveolar bone locally in a particular area. The implants may be inclined mesially or distally, or towards the palate, to avoid perforation of the maxillary sinus (Figs 15-12 and 15-13).[7,134] The use of bone condensers reduces the risk of perforating the floor of the sinus.

The technique involves selecting the implant site using a radiopaque marker to transfer the ideal future tooth position to the CT scan or radiographic image. The trajectory of the implant is planned to avoid sinus and any associated structures. The use of an angulated abutment becomes necessary to be able to restore the implant.

## Manipulating Bone of Low Density

Maxillary bone in the posterior area is particularly sparsely trabeculated. Techniques for osteotomy preparation that involve the removal of what little bone is present have poor success rates.[235,236] Osteotomy preparation using instruments to increase the trabecular density is recommended.[237]

### Manual Manipulation
#### Bone Spreaders
Bone spreaders are sharp-tipped rounded blades available in incrementally increasing diameter (Dentsply Friadent). They are recommended for use following the initial preparation of the osteotomy with a pilot bur to

III   Augmentation

```
                          ┌─────────────────────┐
                          │  Sinus enlargement  │
                          └──────────┬──────────┘
                    ┌────────────────┴────────────────┐
          ┌─────────┴──────────┐              ┌───────┴────────────┐
          │ Residual bone height│              │Residual bone height│
          │       >7 mm         │              │       <7 mm        │
          └─────────┬──────────┘              └───────┬────────────┘
          ┌─────────┴──────────┐                      │
          │   Decision based on │                      │
          │  · Occlusal load    │                      │
          │  · Bone quality     │                      │
          │  · Number of implants│                     │
          └─────────┬──────────┘                      │
         ┌─────────┴─────────┐                        │
┌────────┴────────┐  ┌───────┴────────┐     ┌─────────┴────────┐
│ 1 stage sinus lift│  │  Sinus floor   │     │ 2 stage sinus lift│
│ · Implant length  │  │  manipulation  │     │ · implant length  │
│   ≥ 15 mm         │  │ · Implant length│    │   ≥ 15 mm         │
│                   │  │   ≈ 11 mm      │     │                   │
└──────────────────┘  └───────────────┘     └──────────────────┘
```

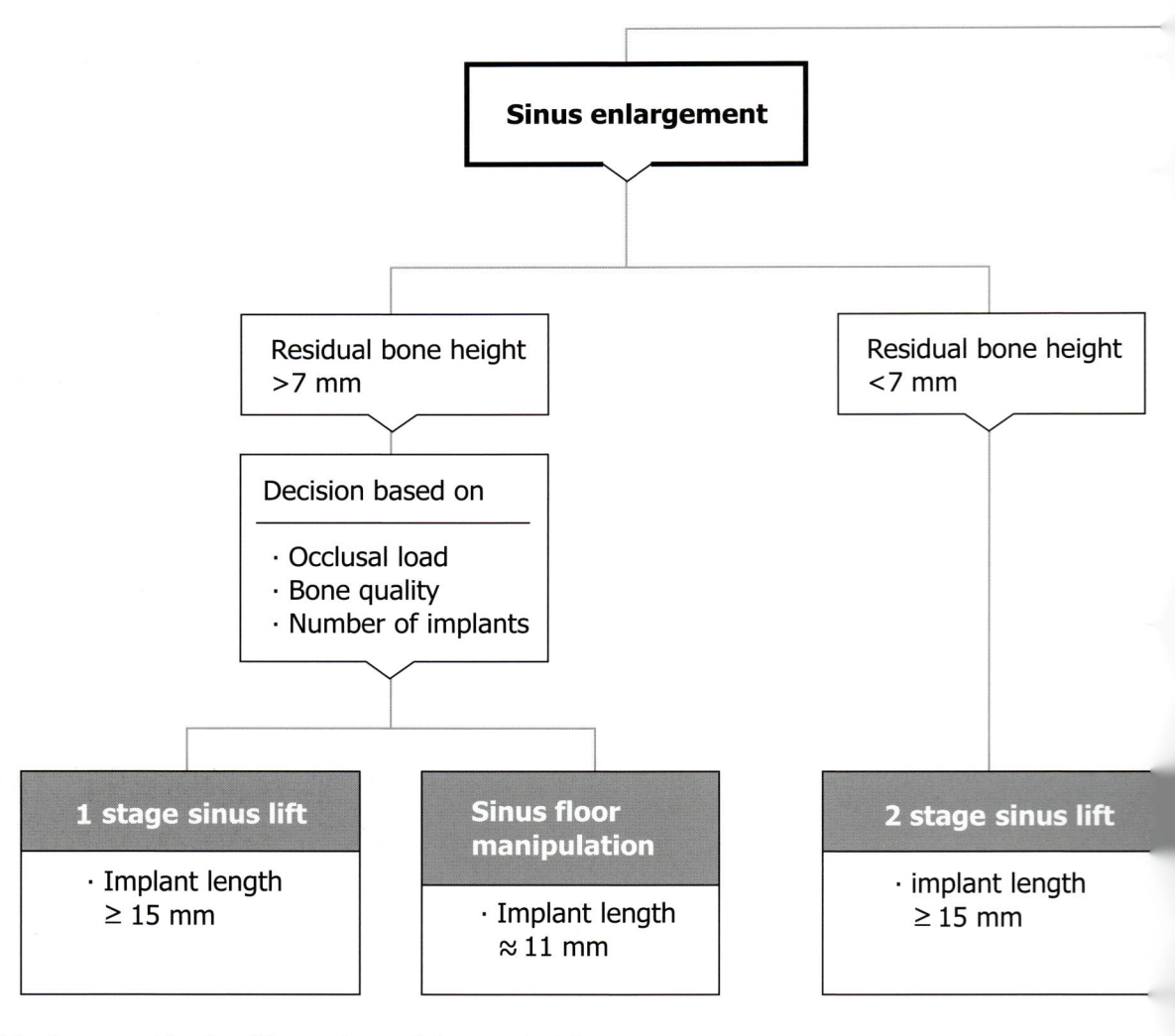

**Flowchart 15-1**   Assessment for sinus lift procedure and sinus manipulation.

15  Posterior Maxilla

**Insufficient bone**

Main decision criteria based on

- DPT
- CT scan
- Absence of sinus pathology
- Favourable internal sinus anatomy
- Interocclusal distance

**Combination of sinus enlargement and alveolar bone loss**

Treatment decision based on:

- Soft tissue availability for wound closure
- Interocclusal distance
- Availability of donor site
- Residual bone height < 5 mm
- Occlusal load
- Bone quality
- Number of implants
- Aesthetic needs

**Alveolar bone loss**

Decision based on:

- Soft tissue availability for wound closure
- Interocclusal distance
- Availability of donor site
- Residual bone height ≥ 7 mm

**2 stage sinus lift combined with onlay bone graft**

- Implant length ≥ 15 mm

**Onlay bone graft**

- Implant length ≥ 11 mm

# III  Augmentation

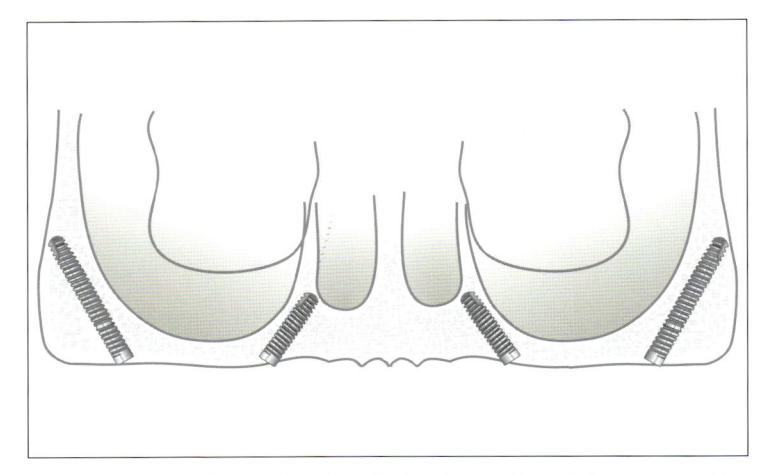

**Fig 15-12** Use of angled implants inclined mesially and distally to avoid the sinus. Care should be taken not to extend the implant beyond the pterygoid plates.

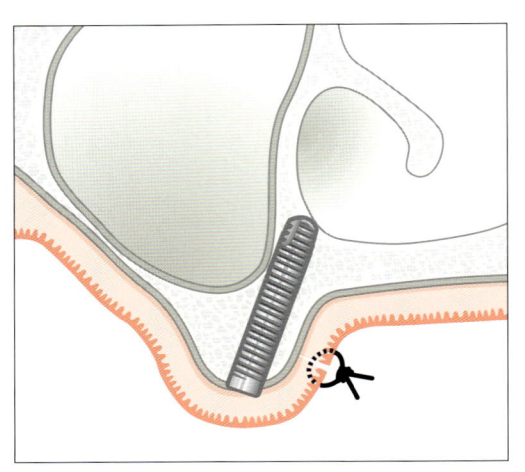

**Fig 15-13** Inclination of an implant towards the palate to make use of available bone in this region. The use of angled abutments is obviously necessary to bring implants placed at angles into function.

establish the direction and depth. The instruments are inserted into the osteotomy and rotated clockwise and anti-clockwise through 180 degrees along the long axis of the instrument. Bone spreaders are not designed to increase the depth of the osteotomy and are, therefore, inserted only to the predetermined depth. Subsequent instruments increase the diameter of the osteotomy to enable the implant to be inserted.[9,238]

## Percussion
### Bone Condensers

Bone condensers are a series of instruments that are round in cross-section and designed to incrementally increase the osteotomy until the implant can be inserted (Dentsply Friadent). The series consists of a site marker, which enables a site to be selected and the direction of the osteotomy to be established. The pilot bone condenser is used to enlarge the osteotomy to enable the first bone condenser to be inserted. Subsequent bone condensers are matched to implant diameter and length. They enable the entire osteotomy to be prepared to enable the implant to be inserted.

These instruments may be used by hand, using a rotational motion along the long axis of the instrument or with the use of a mallet, which offers more control during insertion of the instruments. The condensers matched to implant diameter may be used to increase the depth to which the osteotomy is prepared by manipulating the nasal or sinus floors.

## Increasing the Available Bone
### Sinus Floor Manipulation

Sinus floor manipulation is designed to increase the height of available bone by manipulating the sinus floor through the osteotomy.[239] A 4 mm increase in height can predictably be achieved by the technique outlined below. The minimum level of bone that should be available is 7 mm below the sinus floor to allow an 11 mm implant to be inserted. Ideally sufficient width should be available for at least a 4.5 mm diameter implant, although an implant with a diameter of 3.5 mm is acceptable if favourable conditions prevail.

### Surgical Technique

- **Incision.** A remote or crestal incision may be used, depending on whether loading is going to be immediate or delayed. The criteria used for making this decision have been described in Chapter 7.
- **Osteotomy.** The osteotomy is prepared to a point 1 mm short of the sinus (Fig 15-14). Conventional osteotomy burs are used in bone of medium density, while bone condensers are used in poor-density bone.

15  Posterior Maxilla

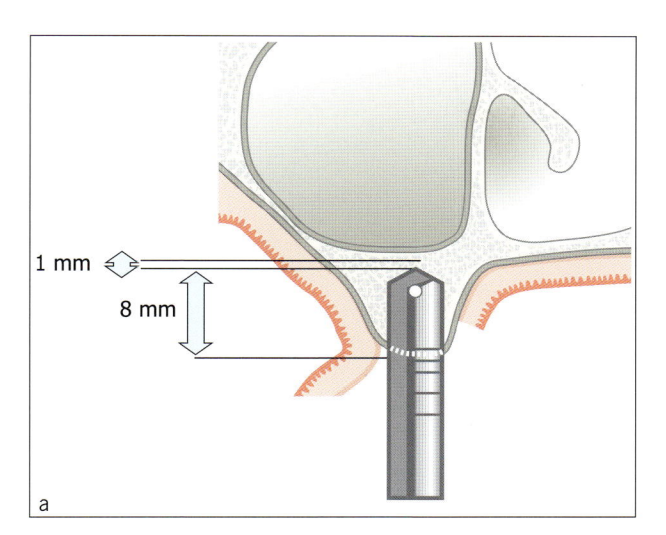

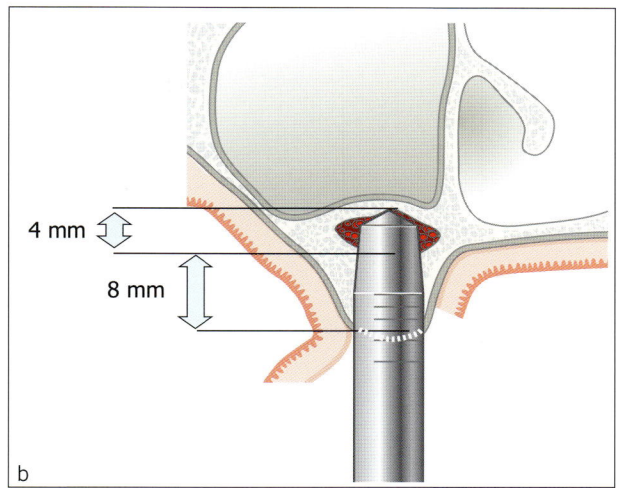

**Fig 15-14**  The principles behind sinus floor manipulation. (a) Exposure of a maxillary ridge via a remote palatal incision for delayed loading. An osteotomy is prepared using an internally irrigated osteotomy bur to a point 1 mm short of the cortical plate. In bone of poor density, the opening through the cortical plate is made with an osteotomy bur and the rest of the osteotomy is prepared using bone condensers.
(b) The sinus floor, consisting of the intact sinus lining, the cortical bone and the cancellous bone, which has been compacted, are manipulated superiorly by 4 mm. A blood clot, some displaced cancellous bone and some particulate material contained within the cutting flutes of the implant fills the void created by the manipulation. Additional particulate biomaterials are not used in order to reduce the perceived risk of perforation of the lining and displacement of the particles into the sinus.

- **Bone condensers.** The bone condenser of the correct diameter is then inserted into the base of the osteotomy (Figs 15-15 and 15-16). A mallet is used to insert the condenser, using controlled force until a fracture to the sinus floor takes place. Careful observation of the markings on the condenser is used to detect the fracture of the sinus floor. This is coupled with acoustic feedback, which results in a duller sound when the instrument fractures the bone.
- **Assessment of sinus floor.** The bone condenser is removed and the patient is asked to exhale through the nose with the nares pinched. Any perforations can be detected by the expiration of air through the osteotomy. The instrument is reinserted and the sinus floor manipulated to the desired height (Fig 15-17). The integrity of the sinus floor is reconfirmed at this stage. A bone tap may be used in denser bone, particularly when wide-diameter implants are to be used.
- **Implant insertion.** Assuming that no perforations have been made in the sinus the implant is then inserted to the required depth (Figs 15-18 and 15-19). Biomaterials are not used because of the

**Fig 15-15**  An osteotomy bur and a corresponding bone condenser. The angle at the tip of the osteotomy bur and the bone condenser correspond to 120 degrees. The bone condenser, therefore, fits perfectly into the floor of the osteotomy created with the bur. This enables even pressure to be transmitted to the floor enabling it to be manipulated.

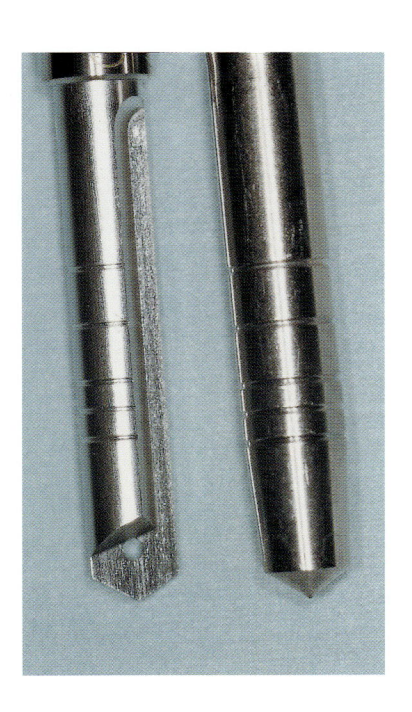

risk of perforation during the insertion of the implant and the difficulty in ascertaining the integrity of the sinus lining at this stage.

III  Augmentation

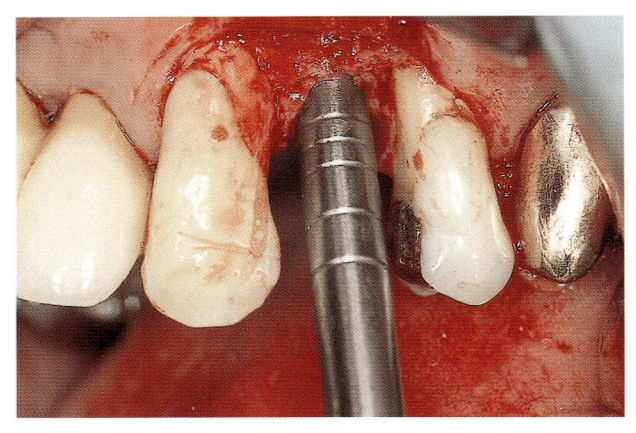

**Fig 15-16** Clinical view of the bone condenser, which has been inserted to the floor of the osteotomy at approximately 7 mm.

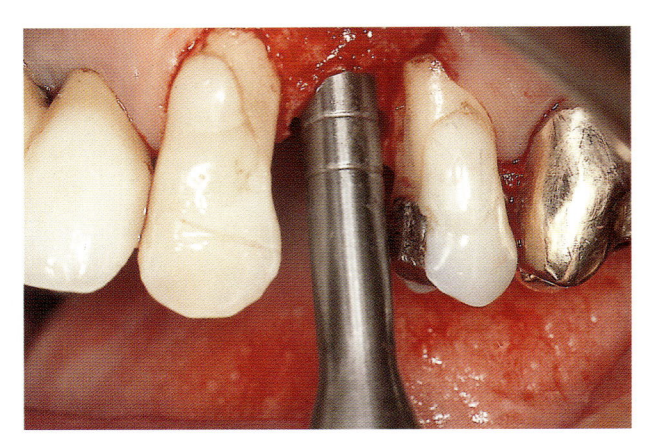

**Fig 15-17** The bone condenser can be seen inserted to 11 mm. The sinus floor is manipulated with the aid of a mallet until an increase in depth of 4 mm is achieved (see Fig 15-14).

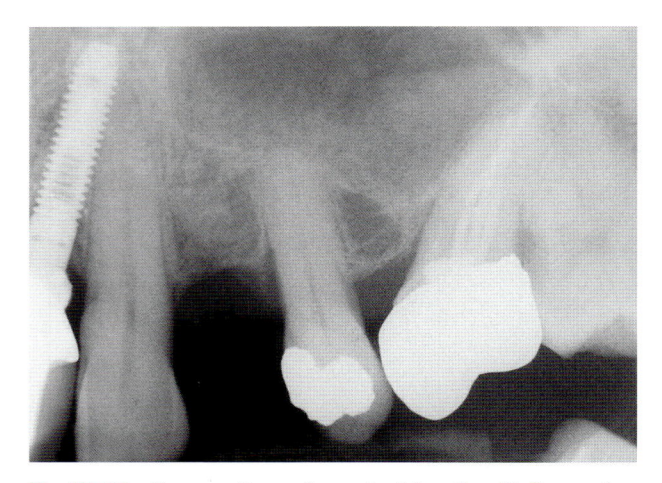

**Fig 15-18** Preoperative radiograph of the site with 7 mm of bone available beneath the sinus.

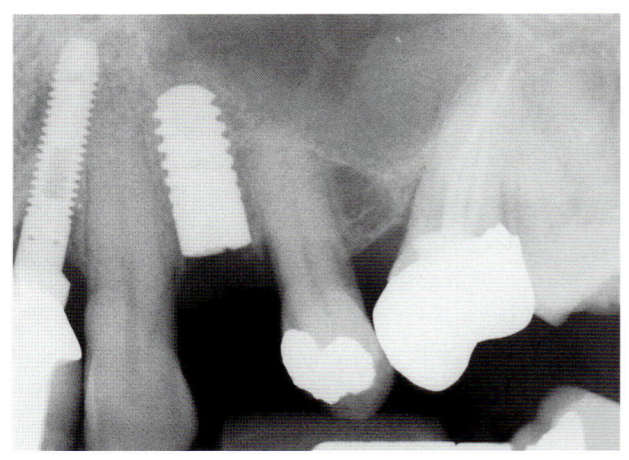

**Fig 15-19** Post-operative radiograph with an 11-mm implant inserted following sinus floor manipulation. The raised floor of the sinus can be seen above the implant tip.

- **Perforation.** In the event of a perforation being detected where it is not possible to place an implant of an adequate length, the procedure is aborted. Subsequent treatment may be carried out three months later, and a formal sinus lift can be undertaken.

### Sinus Lift: Lateral Approach

The maxillary sinus is a predictable site for bone augmentation procedures. The technique was developed by Tatum and first published by Boyne.[206,240,241] The form of the sinus, essentially a cavity within bone with four bony walls, is predisposed to form bone once the lining has been successfully elevated from the floor and the walls surrounding the floor. Regeneration of bone into the cavity that has been created can take place from the surrounding bony walls as long as they have the regenerative capacity and the space can be maintained. A variety of biocompatible and resorbable materials are available and these can be used as space maintainers while the bone regenerates to replace them. Where the bone surrounding the floor of the maxillary sinus is thin (less than 2 mm) and considered to possess little regenerative capacity, autogenous bone with osteogenic and osteoinductive capacities should be used as a graft. Additional osteoconductive materials may be used to supplement this.

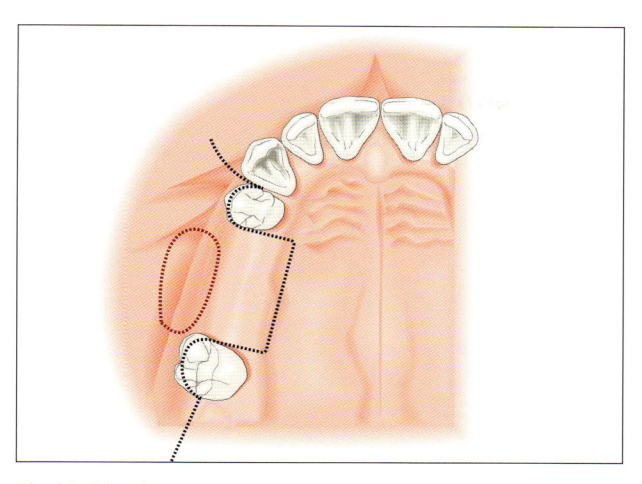

**Fig 15-20** Remote palatal incision with a vertical release at least one tooth distant from the mesial or distal extent of the bony window, which minimises the risk of complications arising from wound breakdown. The vertical release incision is not extended beyond reflection of the mucosa in the sulcus in order to prevent damage to branches of the infraorbital nerve.

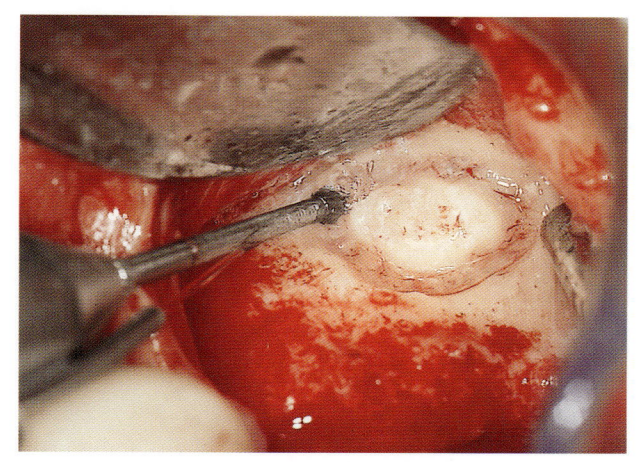

**Fig 15-21** Intraoperative image of a window being created in the lateral wall of the sinus. A large round bur is used in a straight handpiece to remove the bone, with a light brushing motion until the increasing translucency of the remaining bone takes on a grey appearance.

This procedure should be carried out under conditions of strict asepsis and prophylactic antibiotic cover because a large biomass will be placed into a bony cavity that is at the ideal temperature for bacterial proliferation. The blood supply to the graft will not develop for some time and during this period the graft will be at risk from colonisation by microorganisms. Therefore, during the surgical procedure an environment that will minimise the risk of contamination has to be created by adequate infection control.

## Surgical Technique

- **Incision.** A remote incision, preferably palatal, with a vertical release incision at least one tooth-width away from the planned margin of the bony window is considered to be the safest (Fig 15-20). During completion of the vertical release incision in the region of the canine tooth, care should be taken to avoid any damage to the branches of the inferior orbital nerve. The incision should not be extended beyond the vestibular sulcus, particularly in patients with short mid-face height. Adequate reflection of the muco-periosteum will expose the lateral wall of the maxilla from the canine fossa over the zygomatic process of the maxillary bone to the tuberosity.
- **Access to the sinus cavity.** A bony window is designed using clinical landmarks with assistance from the radiographic information. The window should be designed to stay clear of root apices. The inferior margin of the window should be positioned approximately 5 mm above the floor of the sinus, particularly where there is a limited amount of residual bone. Where there is a significant amount of bone present (more than 7 mm), the window can be created at the same level as the sinus floor as long as one bears in mind that the lateral wall of the maxilla may be quite thick at this level. The presence of blood vessels that traverse the maxilla and the septa extending from the lateral wall of the sinus should also be taken into account when planning access to the sinus cavity.
- **Formation of the sinus window.** Extension beyond the maximum curvature of the zygomatic process will make the elevation of the sinus lining more difficult because of the limited access. The variable thickness of the cortical plate should also be taken into account. The bony window should be created with a large round bur in a straight handpiece used at a speed of 20,000 rpm or more to provide precise control; copious irrigation with sterile saline should be used throughout the procedure. The outline for the window is inscribed with the bur, using a light brushing motion, until the thickness of the bone is reduced and the bony incision starts to appear translucent, as characterised by a bluish-grey colour (Fig 15-21).

III   Augmentation

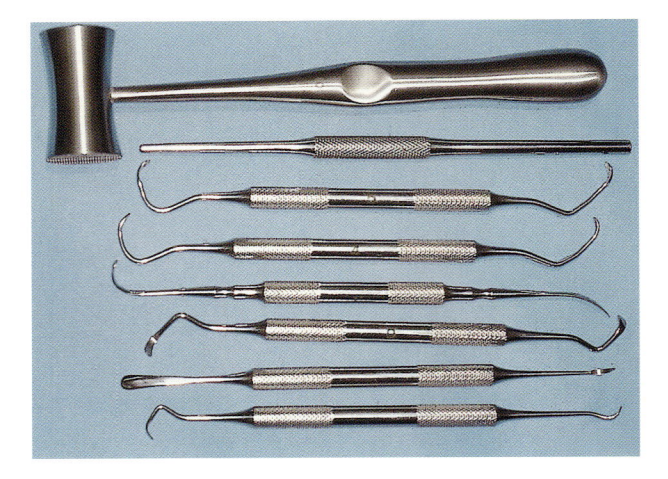

Fig 15-22  Instrument kit for sinus floor elevation. From top to bottom:
- surgical mallet (300 g) to ensure the delivery of the correct force for the infracture of the window
- metal punch with serrated edges to prevent sliding during infracture
- two instruments (wide and narrow) for distal and mesial extension of the sinus floor elevation procedure
- instrument for access to the medial wall of the sinus
- multipurpose instrument for commencing and extending the elevation in all directions
- periosteal elevator with tip for elevating papillae
- periosteal elevator for elevating the remote palatal flap.

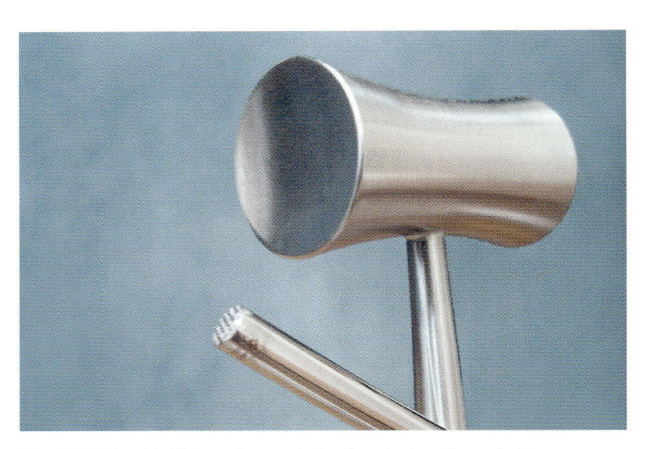

Fig 15-23  Mallet and punch for fracturing the window.

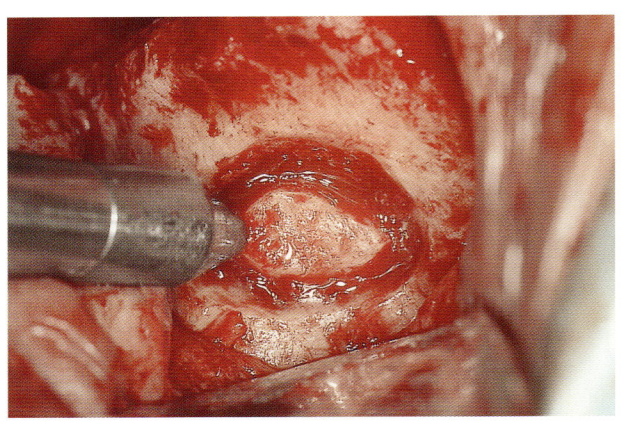

Fig 15-24  The window is carefully fractured using a punch with a light tap from a mallet. The bony window is freed from the surrounding bone until it is mobile prior to elevating the lining.

- **Instrumentation for sinus lift.** The following steps are best undertaken with a selection of specially designed instruments (Fig 15-22). These instruments, which are available as a kit, are used to carry out the range of tasks required for the execution of this very delicate procedure. The use of specially designed instruments is recommended to maximise the chances of completing the procedure without complications. The instruments have been designed with round handles, the diameter of which provides the ideal grip for the control required during the manipulation of the delicate sinus lining. The handles are hollow, and this not only makes the instruments lightweight but also provides a certain degree of tactile feedback (available from Dentsply Friadent).

- **Accessing the sinus lining.** The area selected for the window is fractured inwards with controlled force, using a metal punch and a mallet (Figs 15-23 and 15-24). Fracture of the bone at the window margin can be confirmed visually and aurally by the change from a sharp to a dull sound (Figs 15-25 and 15-26). There should be free movement of the window around the entire margin. However, in the event that the window is still attached to the surrounding bone at any point, careful elevation, using a hand instrument (excavator) to separate the bone, should be performed prior to elevation of the sinus lining.
- **Other approaches for preparing the access window.** A number of other approaches have been developed.

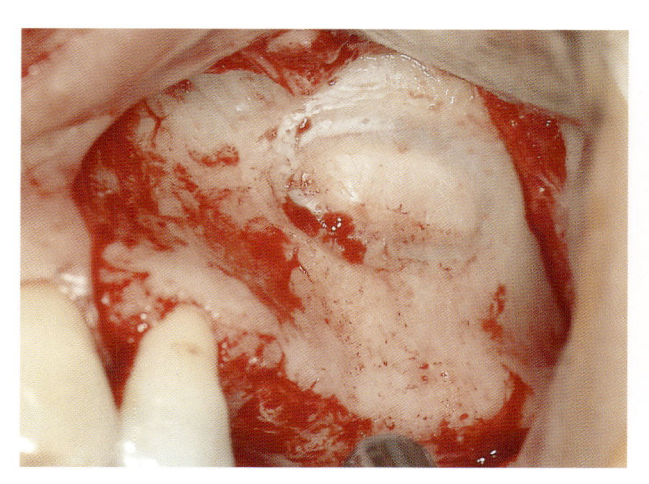

**Fig 15-25** A window created in the lateral wall of the sinus prior to fracturing showing the grey appearance within the groove and bleeding from an intraosseous blood vessel.

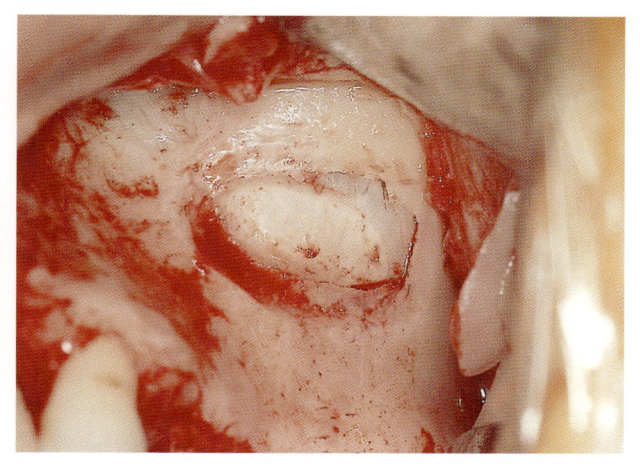

**Fig 15-26** Fractured window (same patient as in Fig 14-23), with the fracture line clearly visible.

**Piezosurgery.** This enables the bone to be removed entirely from a circular groove using tips that do not perforate the lining. This removes the need to fracture the bony window. Elevation of the sinus lining and the attached bony portion of the lateral wall can be carried out as described above.

**Dentium Advanced Sinus Kit** (DASK; Dentium, Cypress, USA). This essentially consists of a large internally irrigated semi-circular bur that removes a large amount of bone from the lateral surface, creating a bony hole. Damage to the sinus lining is avoided by hydraulic pressure generated by the flow of the saline solution. This is not suitable for larger windows and suffers the disadvantage of removing bone that would otherwise form the floor of the sinus. Elevation of the sinus lining is commenced by the rotary internally irrigated instrument and completed as described above (Figs 15-27–15-32).

- **Elevation of the sinus lining.** The sinus lining should be elevated evenly by approximately 5 mm from the edge of the window to create some mobility (Figs 15-33–15-35). The elevation is extended towards the floor of the sinus and simultaneously towards the anterior and posteriorly towards the tuberosity. The clinician's fingers should be well supported to maximise control so that the sharp edge of the instrument remains in contact with the underlying bone. Small motions of the instrument enable the lining to be lifted evenly. The lining of the sinus is elevated first from the floor and then from the medial wall of the sinus. The choice of instruments will depend on access and should ensure that the tip of the instrument can easily contact the bony wall. The opening may be widened to enable better access. Special care should to be taken when elevating the sinus lining over any irregularly contoured surface (Figs 15-36 and 15-37). Other regions that demand care are the medial wall where the sinus has been excavated under the nose, and the anterior portion, which may become very narrow. The elevation of the lining over sharp septa requires particular attention, and the possibility of using two separate windows should not be excluded (Fig 15-38). Adequate access to the septum should be established from the coronal (superior) aspect, if at all possible. In situations where the septum has a high labial attachment, consideration to two separate areas of augmentation should be given. The movement of the sinus lining in response to the patient's breathing will give a clear indication of whether the integrity of the lining has been maintained (Figs 15-39 and 15-40). This is not possible under general anaesthesia.

III   Augmentation

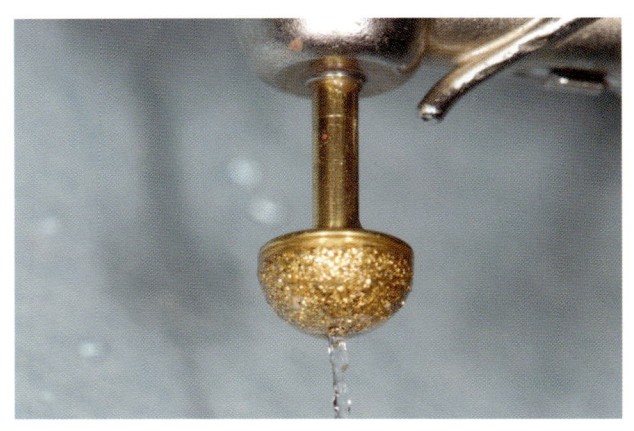

**Fig 15-27**   A large hemispherical diamond bur with internal irrigation is used to remove the bone overlying the sinus. The constant flow of sterile saline forms a cushion protecting the sinus lining. It provides a safe way of accessing the sinus, particularly in single teeth. It suffers the disadvantage of the bone being removed and not being available to form the new floor of the sinus.

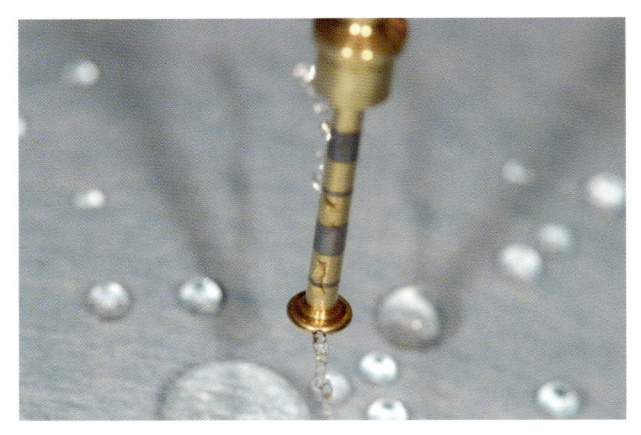

**Fig 15-28**   A disc-shaped smooth bur, which is also internally irrigated, may be used to commence the procedure of separating the sinus lining from the edge of the osteotomy.

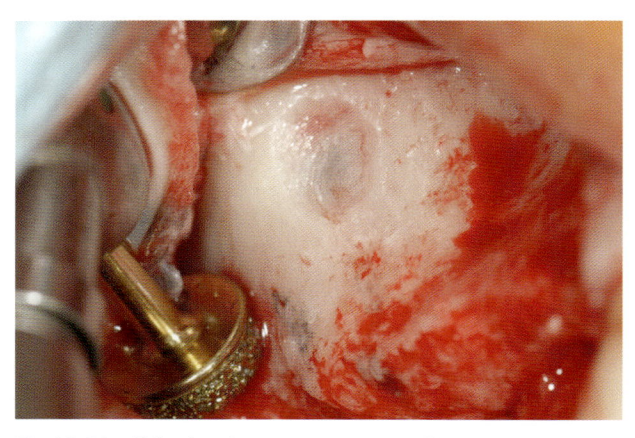

**Fig 15-29**   Following the commencement of the osteotomy, the thinning of the bone and exposure of the membrane can be seen.

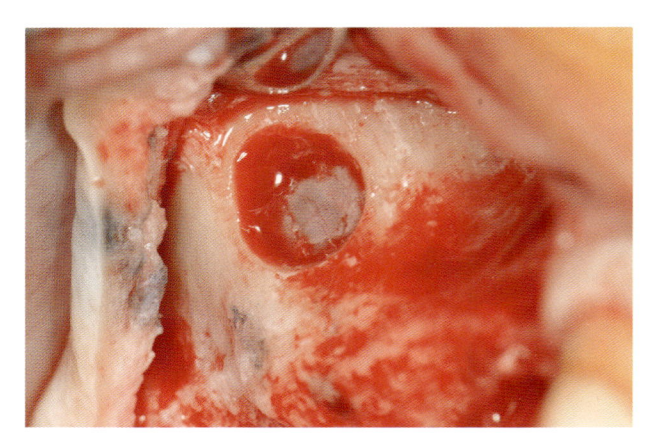

**Fig 15-30**   The window has been successfully prepared without tearing the sinus lining.

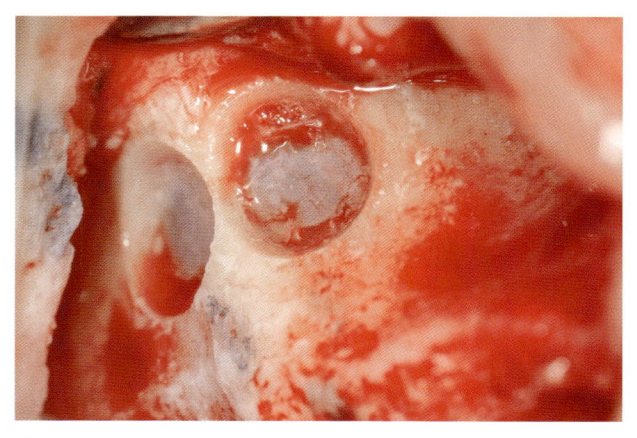

**Fig 15-31**   A second window has been prepared on the distal aspect of the zygomatic process to give better access to the large sinus.

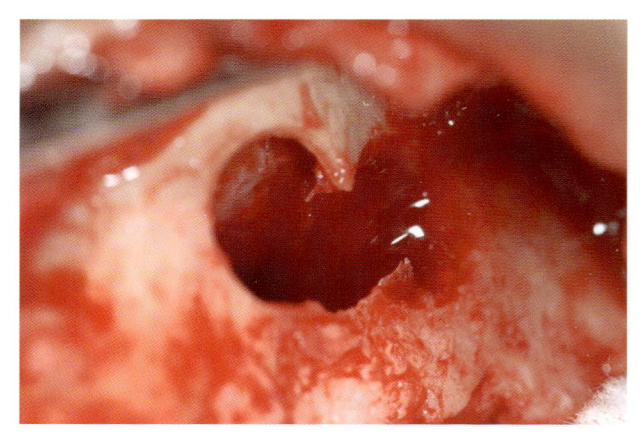

**Fig 15-32**   The two windows connected.

316

15  Posterior Maxilla

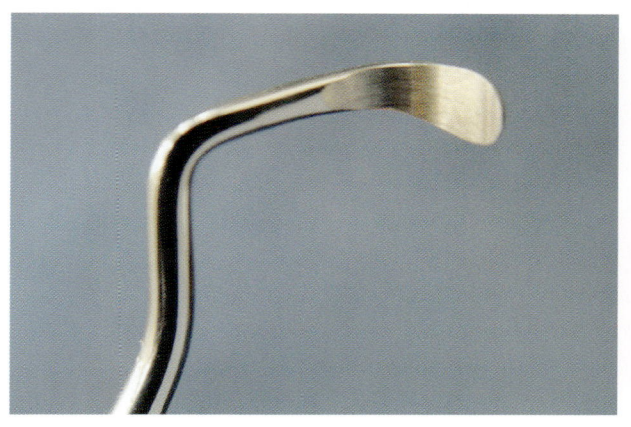

**Fig 15-33** Access to the walls adjacent to the window is easily gained by using the instrument depicted here.

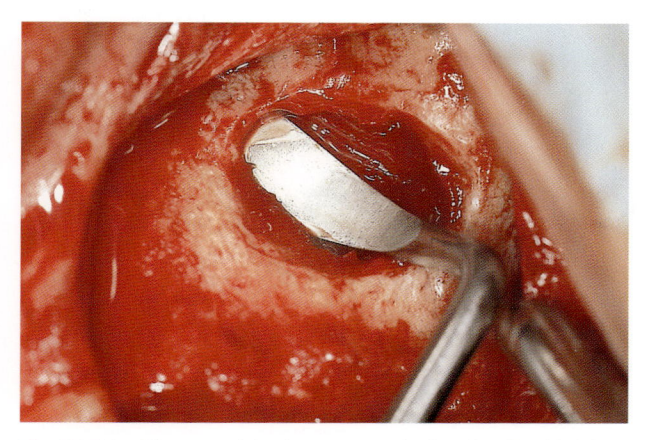

**Fig 15-34** The use of the instrument depicted in Fig 15-33 gaining access to the mesial aspect of the sinus.

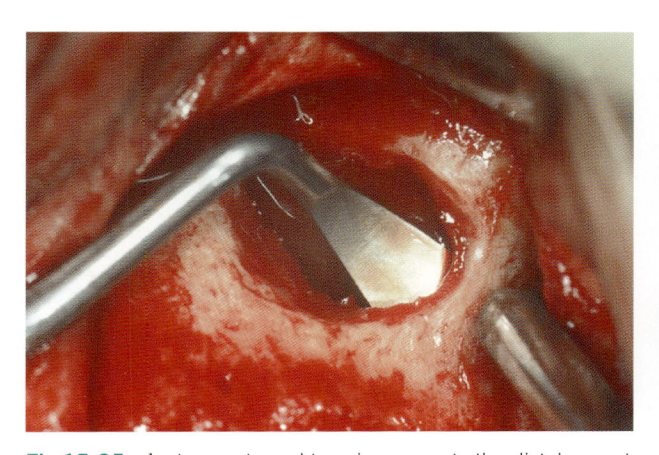

**Fig 15-35** Instrument used to gain access to the distal aspect of the sinus, ensuring that the sharp tip is kept on the bony floor all the time.

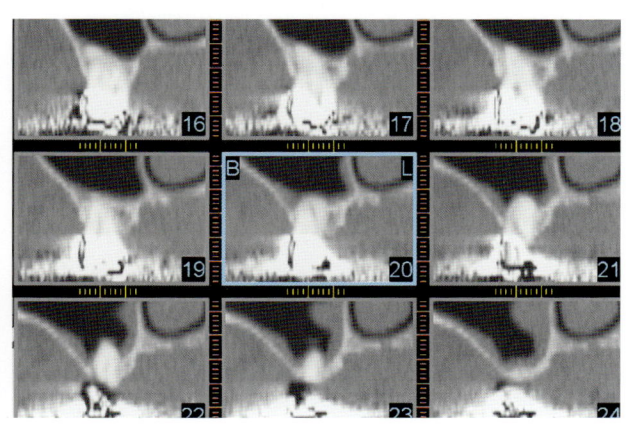

**Fig 15-36** Cross-sectional CT scan reconstruction showing the root of a molar tooth protruding into the maxillary sinus. This provides valuable information for the elevation of the sinus lining around the root.

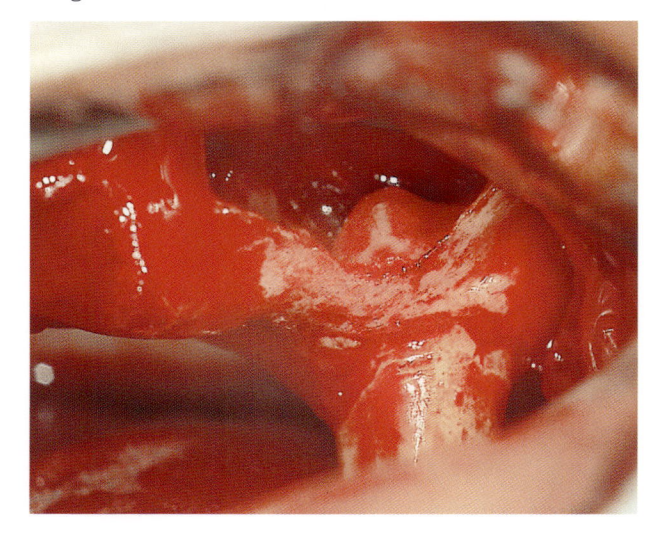

**Fig 15-37** A root is clearly visible after reflection of the sinus lining (same patient as in Fig 15-36).

# III Augmentation

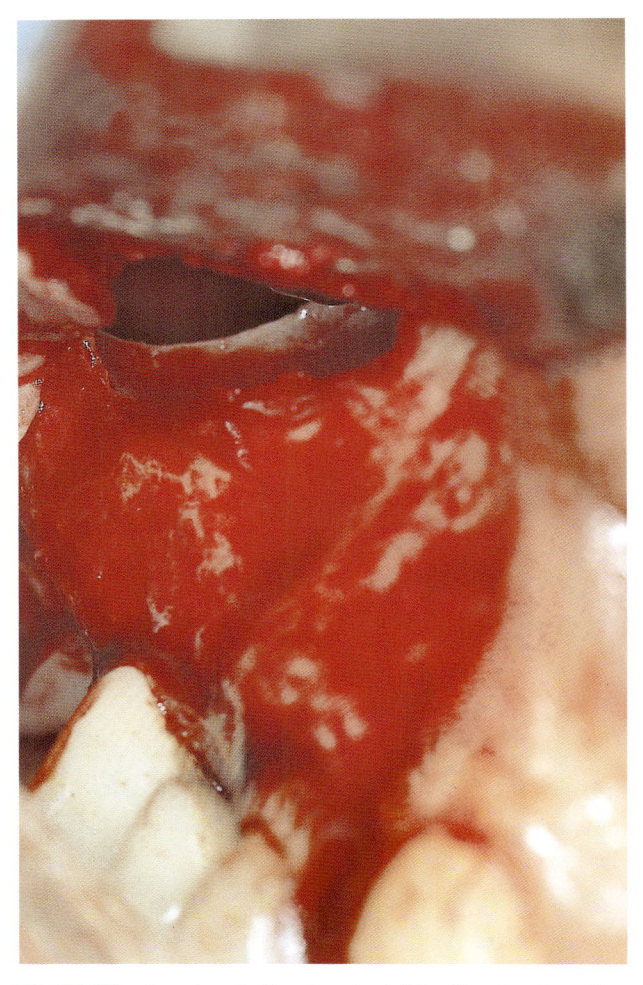

**Fig 15-38** A septum in the sinus is visible after elevation of the sinus lining. Great care needs to be taken to avoid perforation.

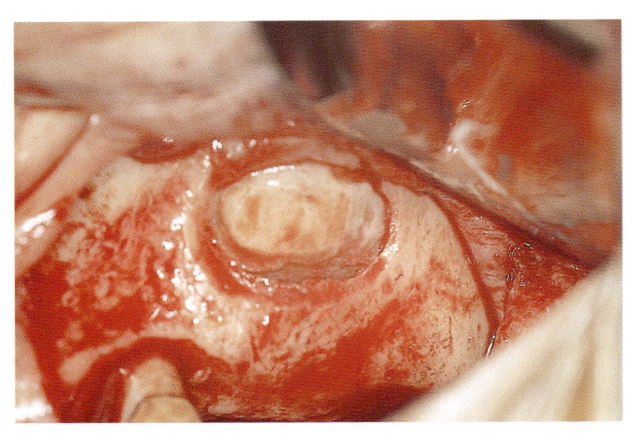

**Fig 15-39** Once the sinus lining has been elevated, the absence of perforations is indicated by the free movement of the lining during breathing. The image shows the position of the lining during exhalation.

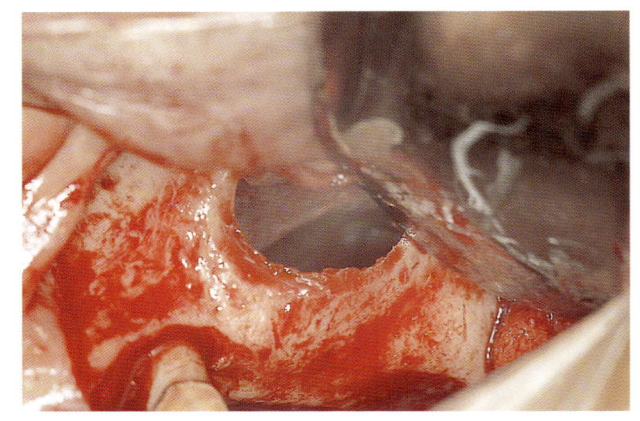

**Fig 15-40** On inhalation, the lining and the window move inwards as shown in this figure.

## Sequence for Implant Insertion and Sinus Lift

The ideal site into which an implant should be placed is vital vascularised bone. Therefore, a period of healing to allow the graft to establish a blood supply and become viable is preferable before the insertion of implants. Furthermore, inserting the implant at the same time as carrying out grafting procedures will increase the complexity of the procedure as well as the risk.

Increasing the complexity of the procedure may result in greater difficulty in positioning the implant precisely for prosthetic needs and may lead to an increased risk of infection and the risk of tearing the lining. The risk of implant failure will also be increased. In the event of an infection the implant as well as the graft may be lost, which may lead to an oro-antral fistula.

### Sinus Lift: Two-stage Approach
### First stage: Particulate Graft

Placement of a particulate graft is facilitated by means of a syringe, which enables the material to be introduced underneath the instrument protecting the elevated sinus lining (Fig 14-41). The material is distributed within the space created without any pressure being applied against the sinus lining, which is extremely frag-

15   Posterior Maxilla

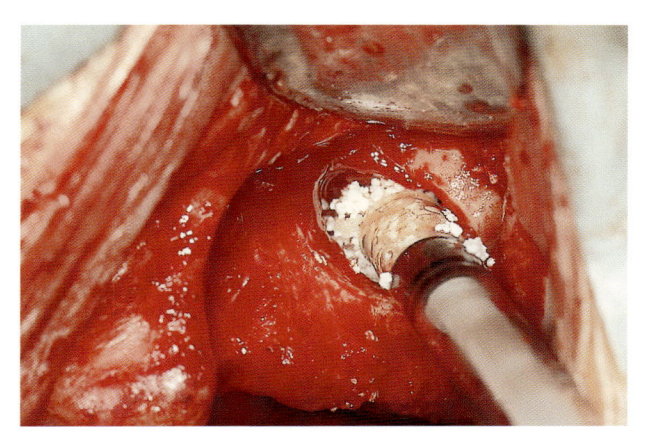

**Fig 15-41**  Particulate graft material is inserted with a syringe during the inhalation phase.

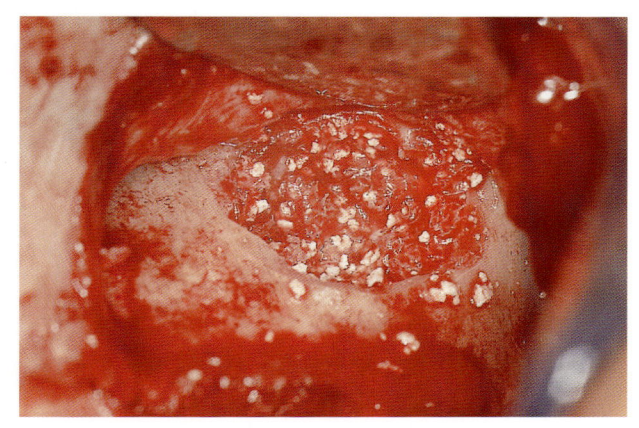

**Fig 15-42**  The particulate material is inserted with gentle pressure being applied towards the walls of the sinus in order to eliminate any voids. Pressure must never be applied towards the sinus lining in order to avoid perforation.

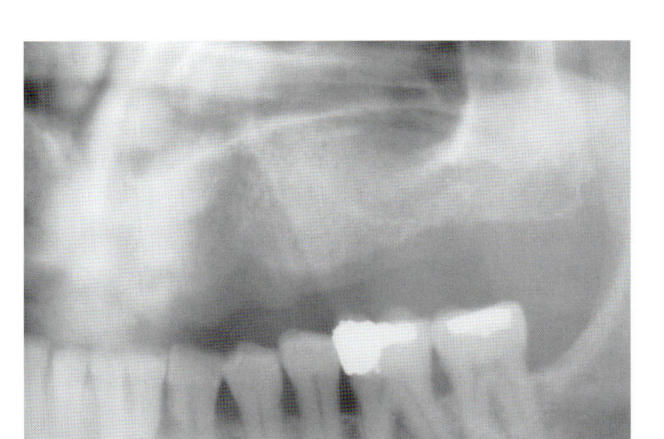

**Fig 15-43**  Post-operative panoramic tomograph showing the particulate graft material well defined within the sinus, indicating an intact sinus lining.

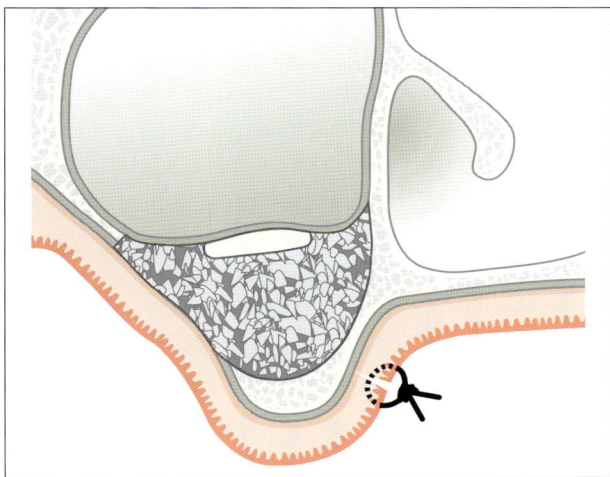

**Fig 15-44**  A two-stage sinus lift using particulate bone graft material. The window is visible on the left of the diagram; the lining has been lifted from the floor of the sinus and the bony window has been displaced superiorly. This technique enables the graft to be placed and, following a period of maturation, an implant can be inserted into the vascularised bone. Typically, when a patient has less than 7 mm of residual bone below the sinus, bone can be augmented to receive implants ranging in length from 14 to 17 mm.

ile. The material may be gently packed towards the floor of the sinus to eliminate voids. The cavity is filled until the material is level with the opening (Figs 15-42 and 15-43). The window will be positioned superiorly to create the new floor of the sinus. The wound is closed without the use of a membrane and the flap is repositioned and sutured to ensure a seal at the level of the incisions, which are remote from the grafted site (Fig 15-44).

A wide range of materials is now available and reasonably documented, providing a range of outcomes and healing times. Biomaterials, in general, have been covered in Chapter 11. Those biomaterials relevant to use in the sinus are listed below. This list is by no means exhaustive. A broad range of materials is now commercially available for the purposes of augmentation. The available documentation for these materials varies in detail, and it is beyond the scope of this book to address this issue. The clinician may choose to use any of the biomaterials that have been developed after careful assessment of their properties and the clinical evidence.[199–202]

## III  Augmentation

- **Autogenous bone.** Autogenous cancellous bone is most readily available from the iliac crest; harvesting has an associated morbidity and requires a general anaesthesia. The rapid healing and remodelling rate of autogenous bone necessitate the use of an adjunctive biomaterial to stabilise it. Autogenous bone may also be harvested from an intraoral site. A bone mill is required to particulate the material.
- **Allogeneic irradiated cancellous bone.** The mineral structure is close to autogenous bone and it may be mixed with other materials. It is solely osteoconductive and, therefore, relies on the osteogenic capacity of the surrounding bone. It suffers the perceived disadvantage of being biologically derived.
- **Allogeneic demineralised freeze-dried bone.** This creates a collagen matrix that retains its proteins and can be used for potential osteoinduction, although this ability has not been verified. It also suffers the perceived disadvantage of being biologically derived.
- **Xenogeneic material.** Preparations such as bovine bone matrix are available as particulate sponges. Data relating to resorption and remodelling demonstrate its stability and gradual turnover over periods in excess of 10 years. It suffers the perceived disadvantage of being biologically derived.
- **Synthetic materials (alloplastic materials).** Bioglass and beta-tricalcium phosphate ($\beta$-TCP) are commonly used. Beta-TCP is intimately incorporated into lamellar bone and resorbed by chemical dissolution over approximately 1 year.[242]

The development of materials containing proteins to induce certain tissue reactions (e.g. cell differentiation) is quite promising and awaits documentation of clinical applications. Factors to modulate cell proliferation and vascularisation may be derived from the patient's own blood (e.g. platelet-rich plasma). However, at present, the main reason for using such materials is the enhanced handling properties in combination with particulate material.

### First Stage: Autogenous Block Grafts

Autogenous block grafts may be harvested from an intraoral or extraoral donor site (Fig 15-45). Block grafts are harvested based on recipient site needs as already described and are inserted and placed in close contact with the surface of the floor of the sinus. The sinus lining is protected with an instrument such as an elevator while this procedure is carried out. A bone clamp may be used to hold the graft securely while it is rigidly fixed with a screw (Figs 15-46 and 15-47). Any remaining voids can be filled with particulate material (Fig 15-48).

The wound is closed without the use of a membrane and the flap is repositioned and sutured to ensure a seal at the level of the incisions, which are remote from the grafted site.

Healing times will vary depending on the source of the graft. Intraoral grafts require four months to ensure that adequate integration has taken place to withstand instrumentation during osteotomy preparation and implant insertion. The osteotomy must be completed conventionally and the threads cut with a bone tap. Bone condensers are not indicated. Assessment of the incorporation of the bone graft must be carried out preoperatively.

Autogenous cortico-cancellous bone grafts from extraoral donor sites may be used and secured in place with the cortical portion forming the new floor of the sinus. A shorter healing time of three months is normally adequate.

### Record Keeping

Records of all biomaterials should be kept with the patient's chart as well as on a central register to facilitate tracking. Batch numbers should also be noted. The quantity and positioning of the graft should be recorded to facilitate implant placement.

### Second Stage: Osteotomy Preparation

Osteotomy preparation may be carried out after the healing phase, which is dependent on the type of biomaterial used. A remote incision is used to establish access to the site selected for the prosthetic reconstruction. Osteotomy preparation may be carried out using conventional osteotomy burs or bone condensers for particulate materials to a depth that is 2–3 mm short of the new floor of the sinus. Bone condensers may be used to manipulate the tissues in order to gain additional height, if necessary. Care must be taken not to perforate the sinus with any of the instruments in order to prevent the dislodgement of particulate graft material

15  Posterior Maxilla

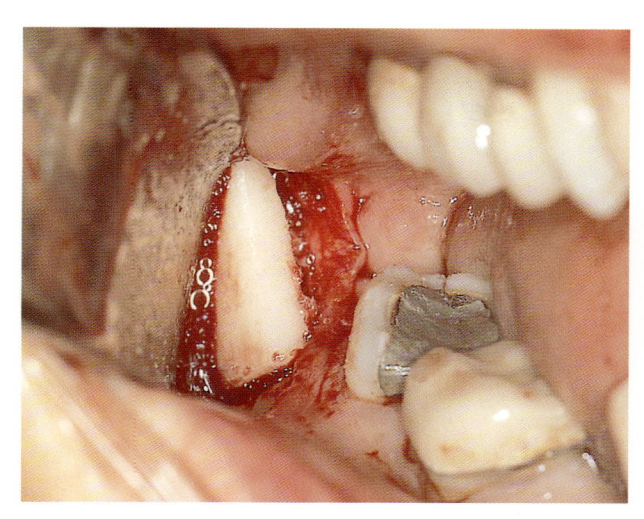

**Fig 15-45**  Bone graft being harvested from the right retromolar area.

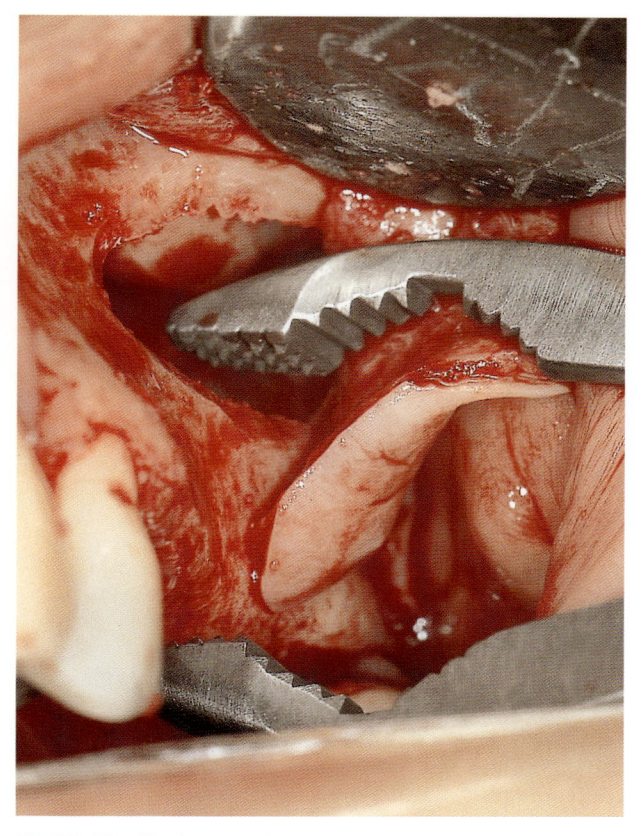

**Fig 15-46**  The bone graft in situ being held with bone fixation tongs to stabilise the graft during fixing with either a screw or an implant.

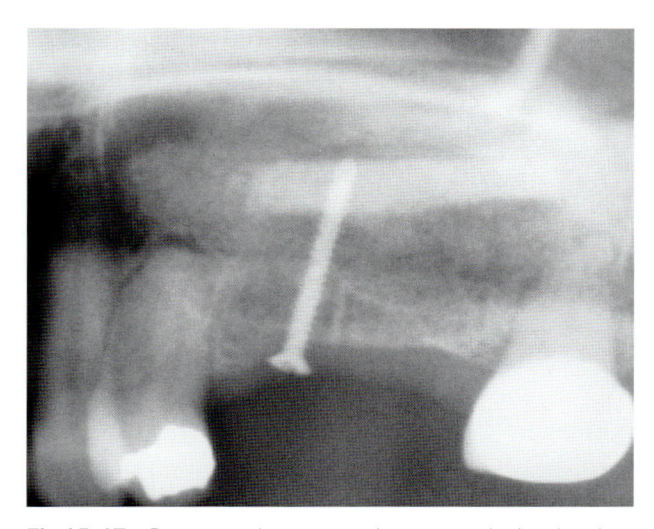

**Fig 15-47**  Post-operative panoramic tomograph showing the autogenous block graft secured by means of a screw.

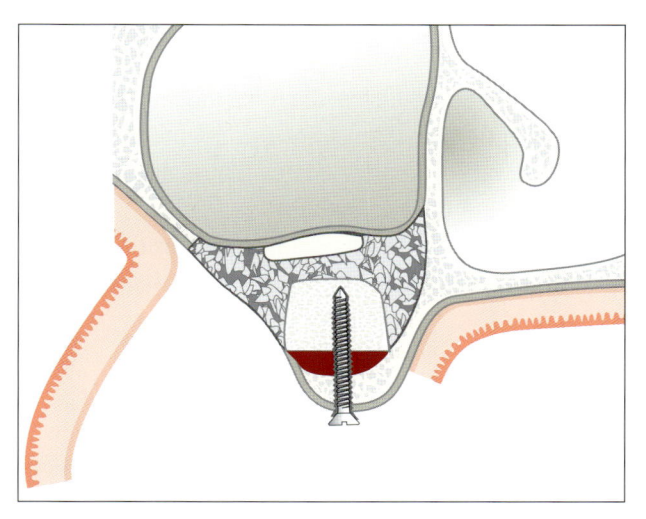

**Fig 15-48**  A two-stage sinus lift with the use of a block autogenous bone graft. The graft is harvested from the donor site and positioned, with the cancellous part facing the floor of the sinus. A fixation screw is used to secure the graft. Additional particulate material may be placed above the graft, which will facilitate implant placement. The length of implant that can be placed following graft maturation will depend on the size of the block graft.

III   Augmentation

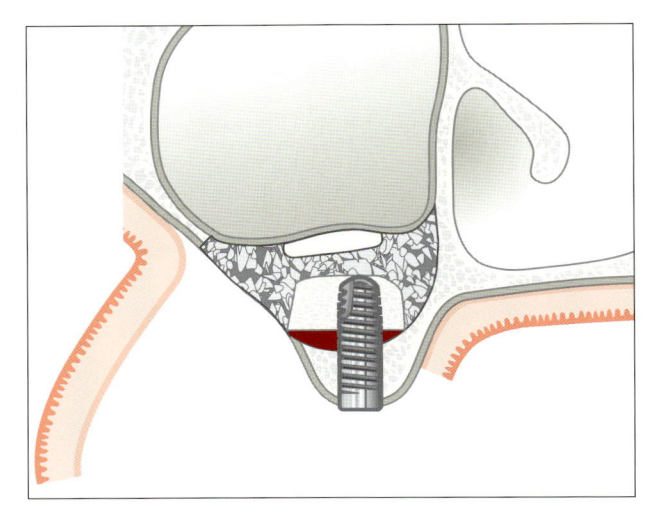

**Fig 15-49**  A one-stage sinus lift using an autogenous block bone graft secured in place with the implant. The 7–8 mm of residual bone permits the placement of an implant of 14 mm in length. The level of elevation of the sinus lining and the size of the block graft serves as a limit. It is possible to use a particulate material above the block graft.

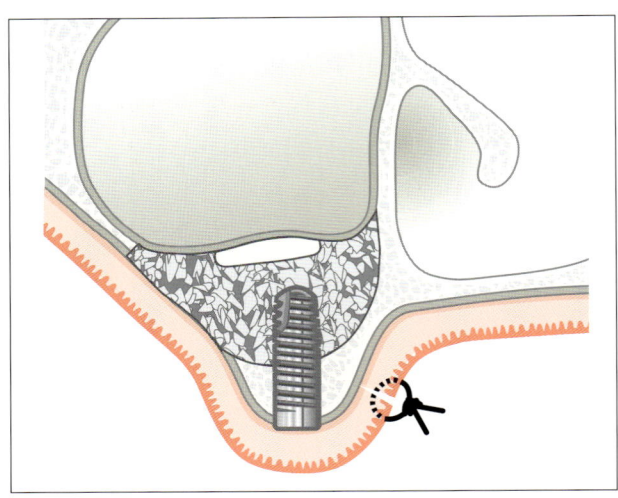

**Fig 15-50**  A one-stage sinus lift procedure with the particulate graft inserted at the same time as the implant. Residual bone of 7–8 mm at the base of the sinus enables an implant of length 14 mm to be placed simultaneously. The residual bone provides adequate primary stability.

into the sinus cavity. A healing period of up to six months (depending on the material used) is recommended to ensure that adequate osseointegration has taken place prior to the implants being brought into function.

### Sinus Lift: One-stage Approach

There are certain advantages to a single-stage approach. These are:

- **reduced treatment time:** inserting the implants at the same time as undertaking the augmentation procedure will eliminate the need for the healing period to allow the bone to mature
- **reduced number of surgical interventions:** if implants are inserted at the same time as the augmentation process is carried out, a separate surgical procedure for the insertion of implants can be avoided.

The one-stage approach can be undertaken only if there is sufficient bone available to establish good primary stability, and a depth of 7 mm is usually considered to be sufficient. Bone attachment to the portion of the implant that is positioned within the non-vascularised graft is more demanding in terms of the biological burden on the body and results in reduced bone-to-implant contact.

### Autogenous Block Bone Graft

Elevation of the sinus lining is carried out in the manner described above. The block of bone is harvested and seated within the sinus. It is essential to stabilise the graft during osteotomy preparation, and implant insertion and special clamps are used for this purpose. The implant site is selected according to the required position of the prosthetic tooth.

The implant should be introduced so that it can engage both the residual bone and the graft (Fig 15-49). The graft therefore needs to be positioned accurately with this in mind. The implant is then carefully seated into the graft, which has been secured and will thus provide stability for the graft. An implant with a progressive thread design is particularly suited for this purpose, as it improves stability of the graft (e.g. Ankylos system).

### Particulate Material

On completion of the sinus-lining elevation, osteotomy for the implant is carried out until the bur perforates the sinus floor. The sinus lining must be protected while the osteotomy is being prepared. The implant is inserted to a predetermined depth which will provide support for the sinus lining until the graft has been introduced. The particulate graft material is then placed into the space

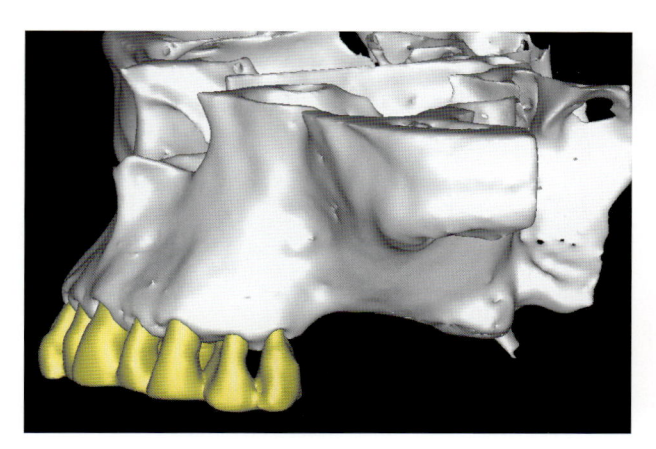

**Fig 15-51** A CT 3D image showing the loss of height distal to the second premolar. In addition, the sinuses were excessively pneumatised. This requires a combined approach to reconstruct the ridge as well as augment the sinuses.

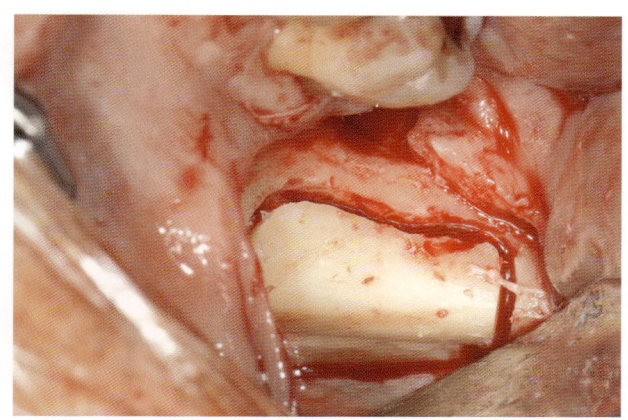

**Fig 15-52** The donor site preferred for the reconstruction of the ridge is the external oblique ridge of the ramus. Such a graft can be shaped and adapted accurately onto the ridge.

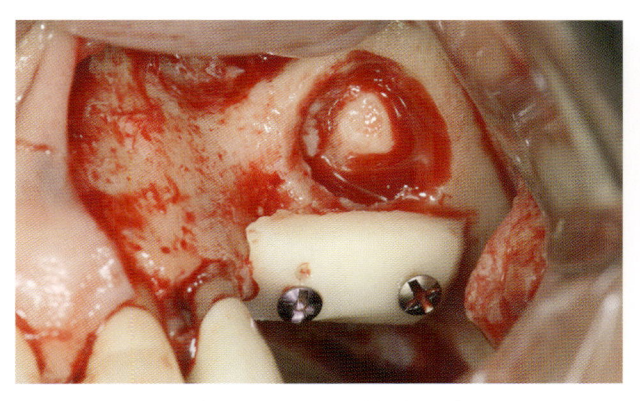

**Fig 15-53** View of the autogenous block graft in situ, correcting the deficiency in height. This sinus lining has been elevated. The window to the maxillary sinus is visible with the access hole closed on exhalation.

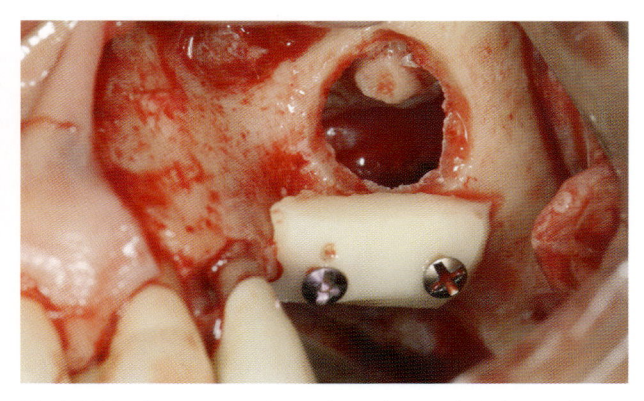

**Fig 15-54** The sinus lining is drawn in on inhalation and is indicative of an intact lining with no perforations. The space created by elevating the sinus lining was filled with a xenograft, which was mixed with particles of autogenous bone obtained from shaping the block graft.

created by the sinus lift. It is important to ensure that the graft eliminates dead spaces, particularly palatal to the implant (Fig 15-50). The graft is packed gently towards the floor of the sinus, ensuring that a perforation of the lining does not take place.

## Subantral Augmentation plus Ridge Augmentation: Clinical Cases

Substantial loss of ridge height in combination with an enlarged maxillary sinus may require a combined approach that builds up the ridge at the same time as subantral grafting. This approach reduces the crown–implant ratio favourably. Furthermore oral hygiene can be facilitated in many cases. Patients who have an excessive display of the buccal corridor may also benefit from an aesthetic improvement. Cases 1 and 2 demonstrate these benefits.

### Case 1: Subantral Augmentation in Combination with Intraoral Block Graft

An intraoral graft from the ramus was used to augment the deficient ridge. At the same time a xenograft was used to augment the sinus. This approach enabled the reduction of the considerable crown–implant ratio. Intraoral donor sites provide a limited volume of bone but have the benefit of avoiding an extraoral donor site (Figs 15-51–15-57).

III Augmentation

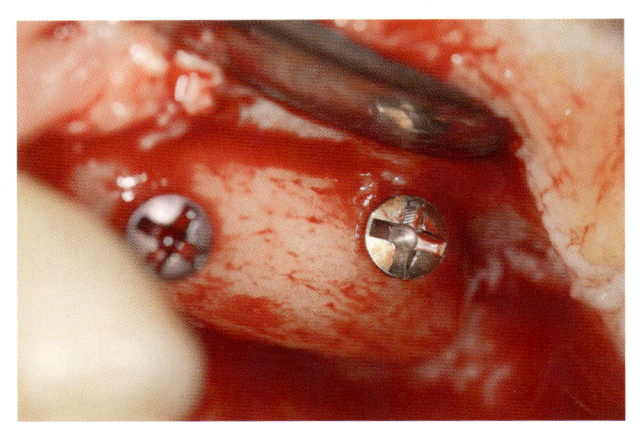

**Fig 15-55** Clinical review of the graft three months after insertion, showing the bleeding surface indicative of revascularisation of the graft.

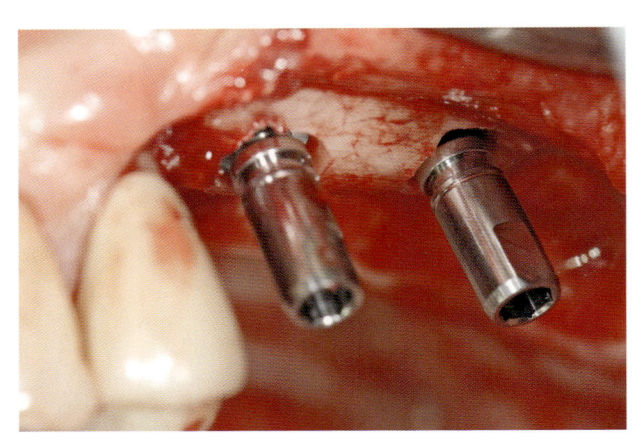

**Fig 15-56** The implants inserted following the removal of the fixation screws.

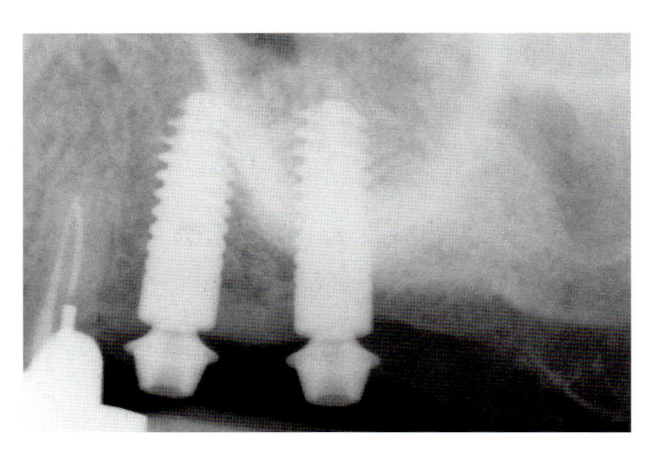

**Fig 15-57** Radiograph of the implants exposed four months later with abutments for screw retention attached (balance base abutments, Ankylos implant system).

## Case 2: Subantral Augmentation Combined with an Onlay Bone Graft from the Iliac Crest

This case study demonstrates the improvement in biomechanical as well as aesthetic outcomes. Use of a larger amount of bone enabled ridge reconstruction to a level that is harmonious with the adjacent sides (Figs 15-58–15-74).

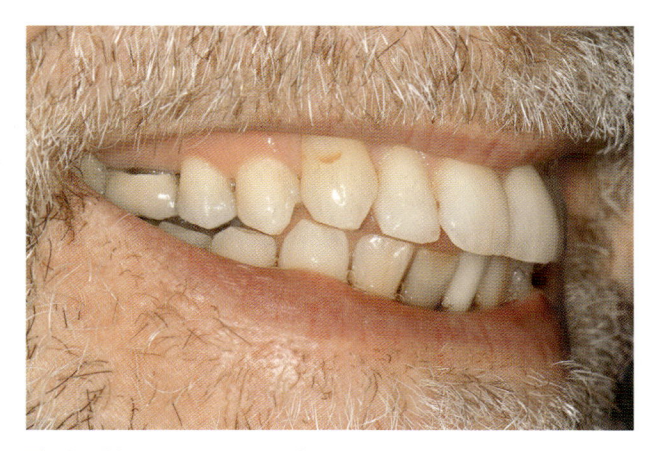

**Fig 15-58** Extraoral view of the right side of the patient, showing the smile line.

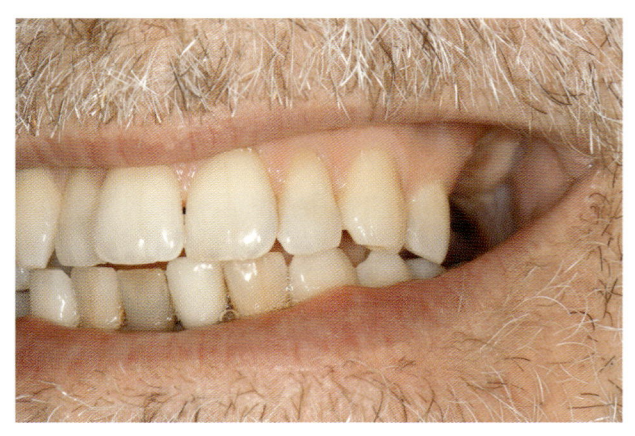

**Fig 15-59** Anterior left view showing the patient smiling, with missing teeth evident.

15 Posterior Maxilla

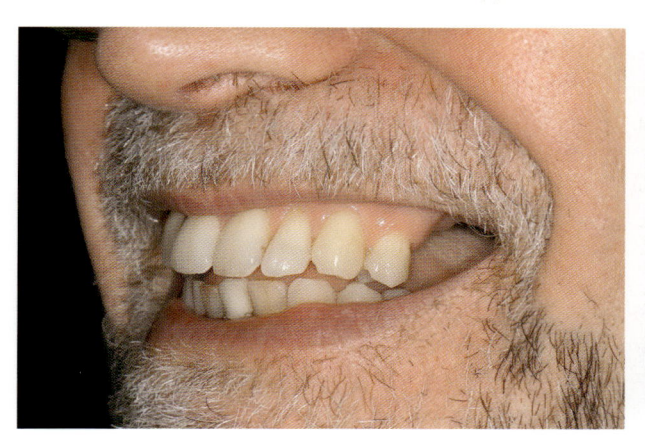

**Fig 15-60** View of the left side showing the missing teeth as well as the bone deficiency caused by periodontal disease and tooth loss. The extent of the smile line and the prospect of long teeth were not acceptable to the patient. Augmentation of the lost ridge height was indicated.

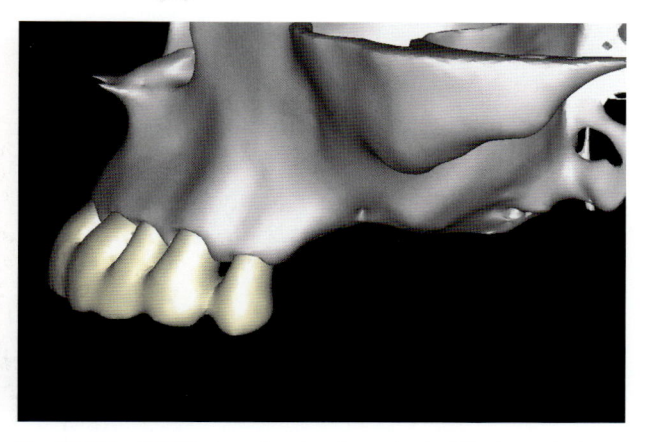

**Fig 15-61** CT 3D view showing the extent of the bone lost.

**Fig 15-62** Cross-sectional view in the molar region showing the thickness of the lateral wall and the residual bone in the floor of the sinus.

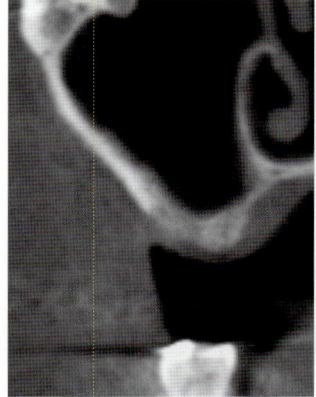

**Fig 15-63** Panoral image based on CT scan data showing a very irregular sinus floor and confirming the loss of height.

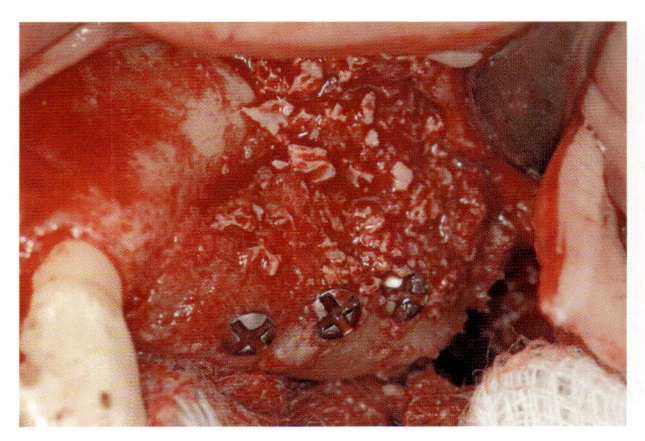

**Fig 15-64** A cortico-cancellous block graft obtained from the iliac crest is used to build up the deficient ridge at the same time as creating bone under the sinus lining, with cancellous bone mixed with xenograft.

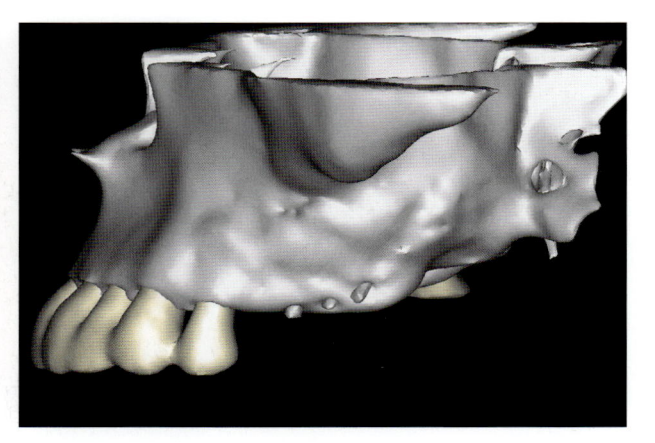

**Fig 15-65** Three-dimensional view of the reconstructed ridge based on CT scan data.

325

III   Augmentation

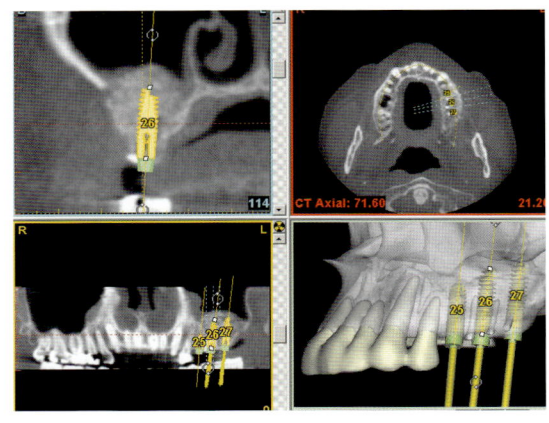

Fig 15-66   Interactive planning for implant placement in the regenerated bone.

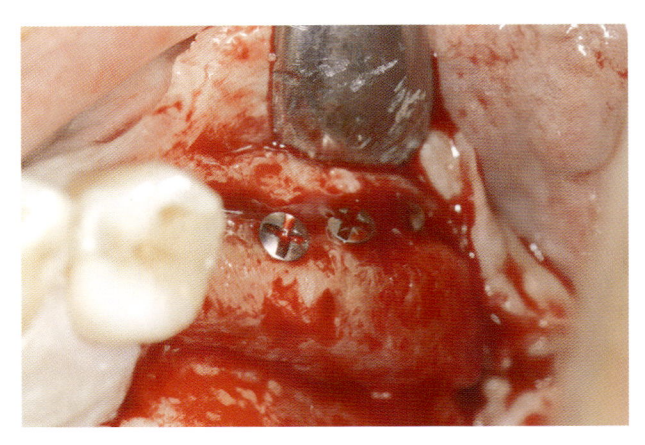

Fig 15-67   Healed graft, confluent with the recipient site, exposed for the placement.

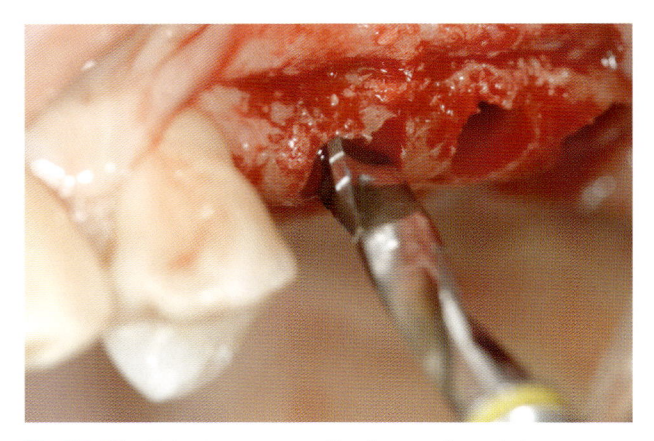

Fig 15-68   Osteotomy preparation in preselected sites.

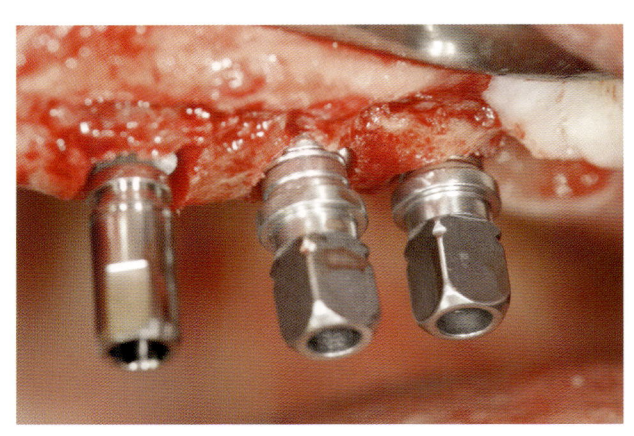

Fig 15-69   Three implants inserted into the revascularisation graft three months after augmentation.

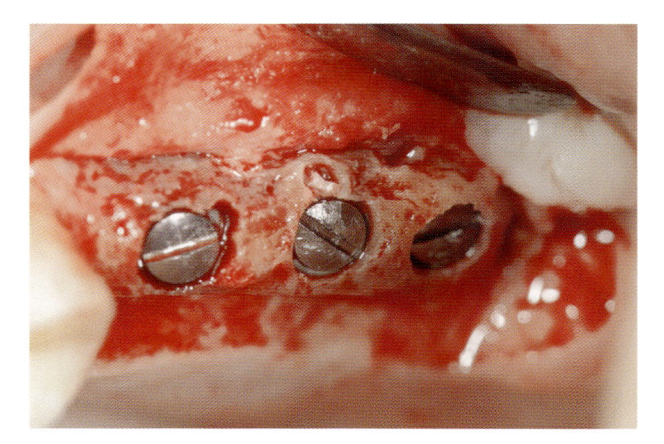

Fig 15-70   The implants can be seen placed below the bony crest, with membrane screws to provide easy access to the implant at the time of exposure.

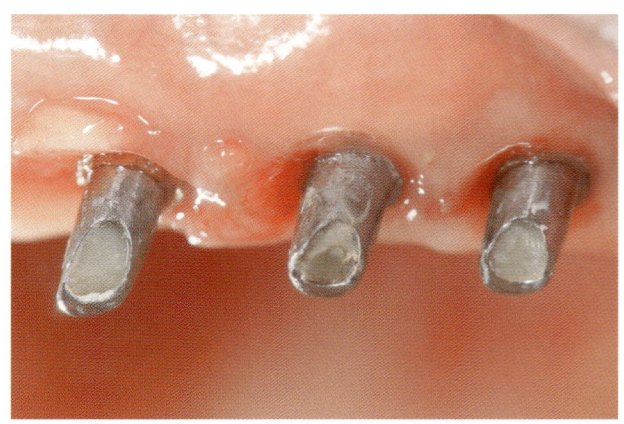

Fig 15-71   Abutments emerging from soft tissues.

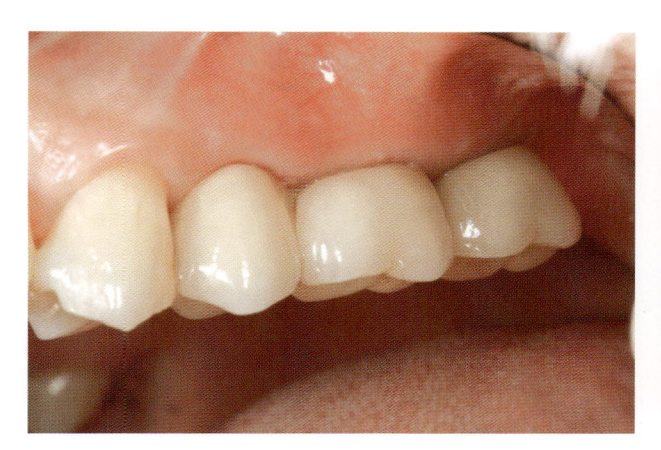

**Fig 15-72** Intraoral view of the restoration supported by the implants.

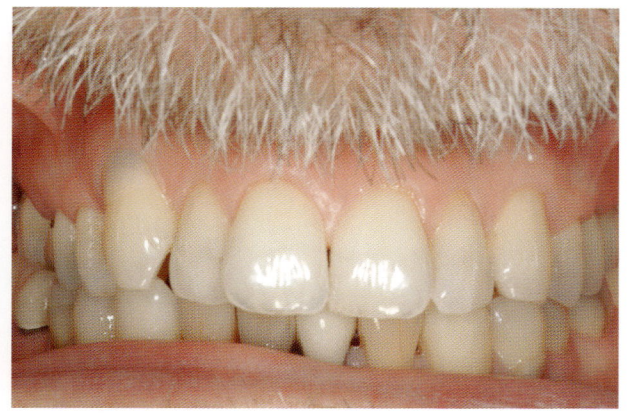

**Fig 15-73** Anterior view showing gingival levels of both sides. Compare with the preoperative view (Fig 15-60).

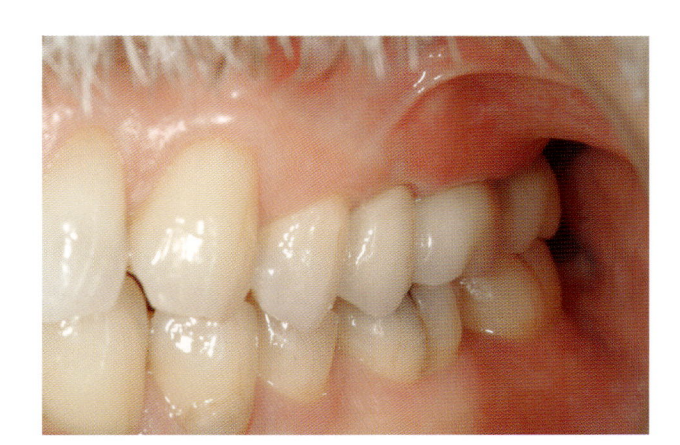

**Fig 15-74** Buccal view of the definitive restoration showing the re-contoured soft tissue levels. Compare with the preoperative view (Fig 15-60). (Restorative work completed by Dr Gus Ghani.)

## Complications

### Intraoperative Complications

Complications may arise during surgery, and certain guidelines should be followed.

### Haemorrhage

Bleeding during surgery often emanates from a blood vessel within the wall of the sinus and can be controlled by applying pressure, if possible, or waiting for a natural haemostasis to take place. Electro-cauterisation may be used if the bleeding persists, provided that the procedure does not create a perforation in the sinus lining.

### Tears in the Lining

The management of a tear will depend very much on its size.

- **Perforation.** A perforation of approximately 3 mm in diameter does not need to be sutured. Elevation of the sinus lining enables sufficient surplus tissue to be generated to close the perforation within the folds of the lining spontaneously. A collagen-based membrane may be used to cover the area in order to prevent any particulate material from escaping (Fig 15-75).
- **Small tear.** A small tear of approximately 5–10 mm may be sutured to the bony wall at the edge of the window. The suturing is carried out using a fine

# III Augmentation

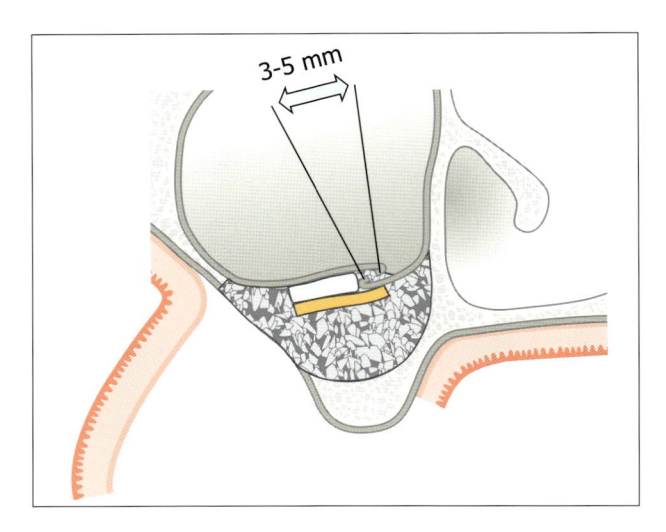

**Fig 15-75** Management of small perforation ranging from 3 to 5 mm. Careful elevation of the membrane around the perforation enables the lining to be folded to spontaneously close the defect. A supplementary collagen membrane (Bio-Gide or CollaTape [Centerpulse Dental, Carlsbad, CA, USA]) is used to prevent migration of particles into the sinus.

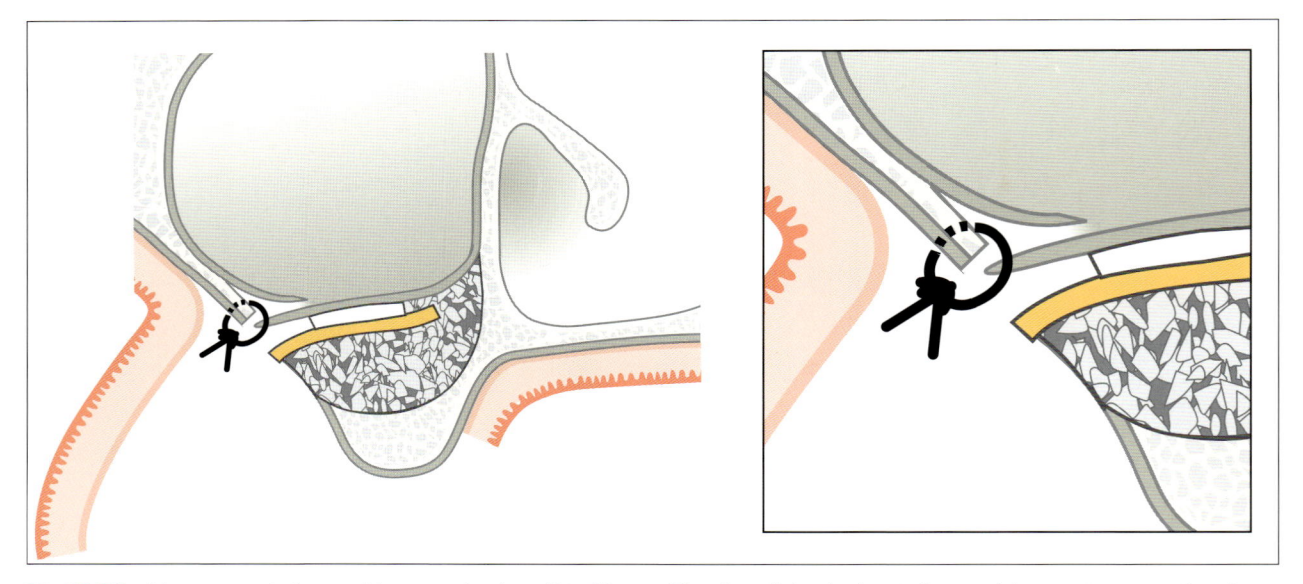

**Fig 15-76** Management of a small tear ranging from 5 to 10 mm. The sinus lining is elevated around the tear to ensure that the tear does not enlarge. A small perforation at the edge of the bony window is made to which the sinus lining is carefully sutured using a resorbable material. A supplementary collagen membrane (Bio-Gide or CollaTape) is used to prevent migration of particles into the sinus.

resorbable suture after the sinus lining has been elevated. The use of a collagen membrane over the area is also recommended (Fig 15-76).

- **Large tear.** Tears larger than 10 mm are difficult to repair and the procedure should be aborted. Prior to wound closure any predisposing structures, such as a septum, should be removed and the area smoothed with a hand curette. Re-entry may be attempted approximately three months later when the sinus lining has matured. Access to the sinus is through the original window; however, care should be taken while dissecting the soft tissues in this area from the sinus lining in order not to create a perforation.

The clinical case illustrated in Figs 15-77–15-84 demonstrates the management of septa in the maxillary sinus. Bilateral septa were present; the right septum was negotiated without a tear using the techniques described above. The left-hand side, unfortunately,

## 15 Posterior Maxilla

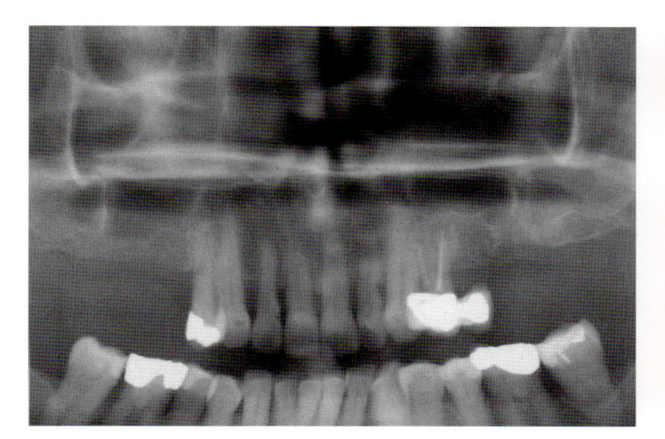

**Fig 15-77** Panoral panoramic tomograph showing the presence of septa bilaterally in the maxillary sinus.

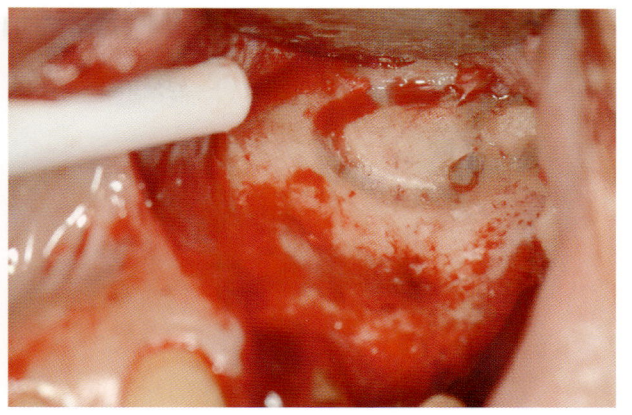

**Fig 15-78** Access being gained to the maxillary sinus using two separate windows.

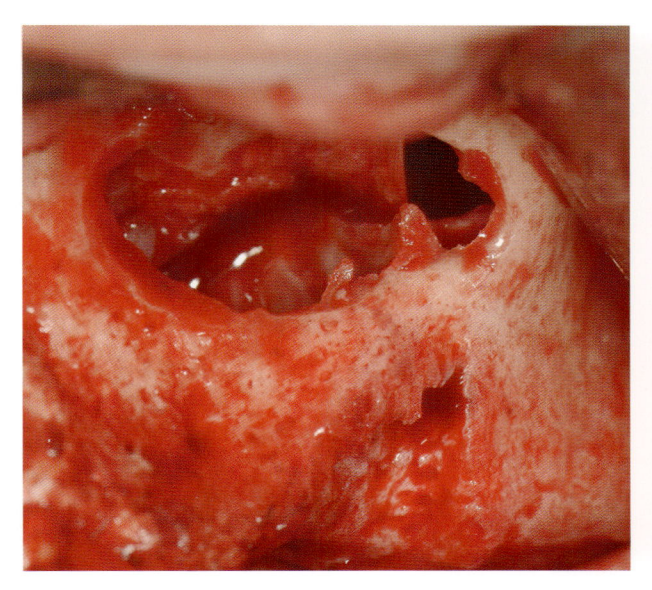

**Fig 15-79** Intraoperative image showing the septum and the tear in the lining, which is approximately 5 mm in diameter.

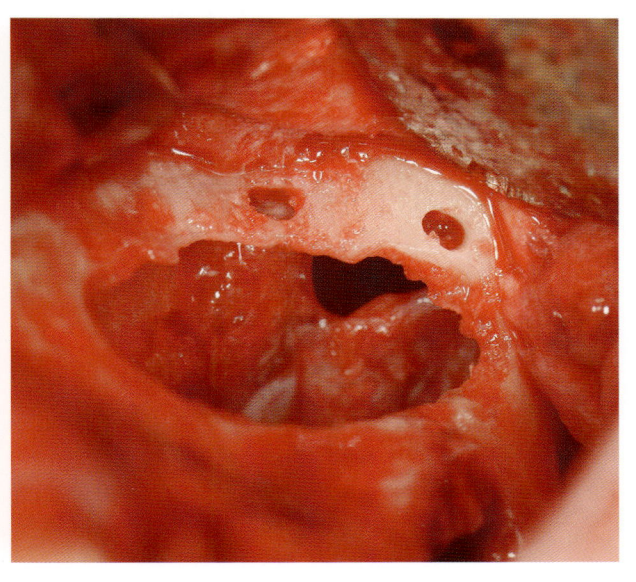

**Fig 15-80** Two small holes have been drilled through the superior aspect of the maxillary sinus bony wall. The sinus lining has been elevated without enlarging the tear by approaching the tear remotely. It is important for substantial elevation to be carried out to ensure sufficient play for tension-free closure.

became torn. The small tear was managed by limiting its size and suturing it to perforations created in the maxillary sinus wall. Following the use of a membrane (Bio-Gide) to further protect the fragile lining, both sides were grafted using a xenograft (Bio-Oss). This was followed by a post-operative radiograph to ensure containment of the graft.

### Contamination

Contamination of the area by a local source of pathology requires careful consideration. Purulent exudates (e.g. from an apical cyst) require the procedure to be aborted because of the increased risk of infection of the graft. The procedure may, however, be completed if there is a non-purulent exudate (e.g. clear serous fluid from a mucocele). However, if any doubt exists, it is considered safer to abandon the procedure and return after removal of the pathology.

III  Augmentation

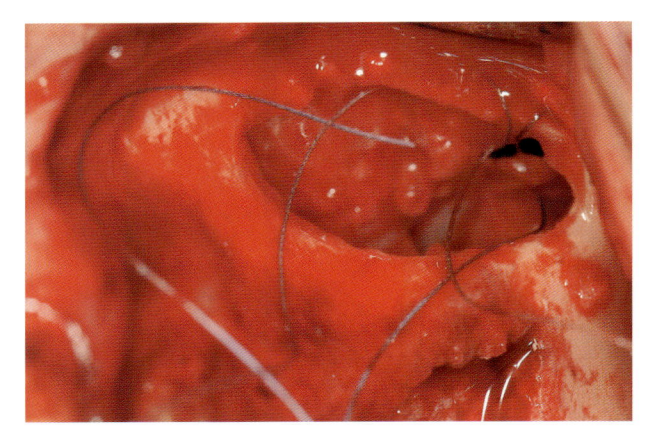

Fig 15-81  A resorbable suture (4-0 Vicryl) is used. The suture is inserted through one of the holes in the maxillary wall; the sinus lining at the lower border of the tear is picked up and the suture threaded through the second hole.

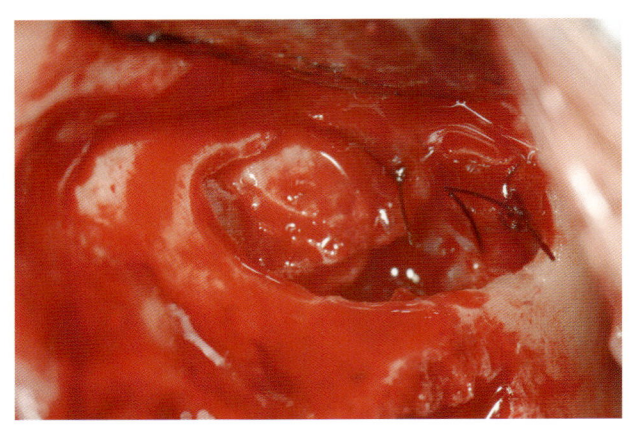

Fig 15-82  The suture is drawn and tightened, attaching the sinus lining to the superior aspect of the bony window.

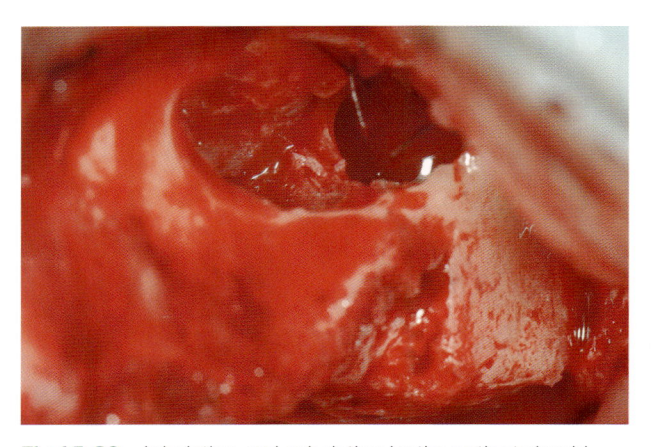

Fig 15-83  Inhalation and exhalation by the patient should result in movement of the sinus lining without leakage. The image depicts inhalation.

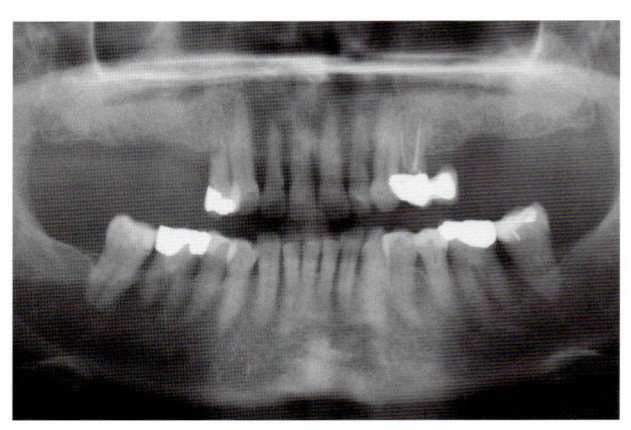

Fig 15-84  Post-operative radiograph showing well-contained graft material in both sinuses. This is indicative of an absence of residual perforation, which would result in escape of the material into the sinus beyond the lining.

## Immediate Post-operative Complications

The management of post-operative complications is based on the cause and is influenced by the level of consolidation that has taken place postsurgically.

### Haemorrhage

Ensuring that specific instructions are given for the avoidance of bleeding is the best way to prevent post-operative haemorrhage.

This includes the medical management of patients who are predisposed to bleeding either as a result of a disorder or because of any medication they may be taking.

- **Oral bleeding.** Management of the patient and the anxiety related to the incident are fundamental to controlling the haemorrhage. Oral haemorrhage is effectively managed by applying pressure to the area of bleeding. Local anaesthetic containing a vasoconstrictor may be used to supplement the application of direct pressure.
- **Nasal bleeding.** This may occur and is best treated by the use of cold compresses in conjunction with ensuring that the patient maintains an upright posture in order to reduce the blood pressure in the maxilla. Once again, the management of the patient is central to the control of bleeding.

- **Persistent bleeding.** If bleeding persists, either from the oral cavity or the nose, it may be treated with an anti-fibrinolytic agent such as tranexamic acid, which can be administered orally or intravenously.

### Infection

The risk of infection should be minimised by the use of appropriate aseptic techniques and the elimination of foci of infection within the mouth. In the event of an infection, which will be characterised by increased discomfort, swelling and rubor leading to the formation of an exudate, treatment should be immediate and decisive. Any antibiotic regimen in place should be continued and a swab should be taken for culture and to establish the sensitivity of the infecting organisms to the antibiotic(s) being administered. It may be necessary to change the antibiotic and, if the infection cannot be brought under control within 14 days, the graft should be evacuated.

## Intermediate Post-operative Complications

Complications that occur between two weeks and two months after surgery are considered to be intermediate post-operative complications.

### Infection

Infection characterised by swelling, pain and a possible exudate should be treated with a prescription for an antibiotic regimen that is effective against both aerobic and anaerobic microorganisms. A sample should be taken for culture and to establish the sensitivity of the infecting organisms to the antibiotics prescribed. The antibiotic regimen should be changed if organisms resistant to the prescribed antibiotics are discovered. The absence of foci of infection should be confirmed, and if no resolution of the infection takes place the graft should be evacuated within 7 to 21 days.

## Delayed Post-operative Complications

Complications that occur more than six months after surgery are often related to or noted during subsequent treatment.

### Absence of Bone Formation

The absence of bone formation in the graft material may become evident during implant insertion and is based on the observation of unaltered particulate material, which readily appears during osteotomy preparation. The absence of bone formation is also characterised by minimal bleeding and the texture of the implant site. Fortunately this is a rare occurrence, provided the guidelines for the use of biomaterials are followed.

### Implant Failure

Failure of an implant may arise through a failure to integrate or through the absence of bone formation. Implant failure occurs at or after the time of exposure, approximately 12 months after the grafting procedure. If evidence of bone formation exists in the form of other implants that have integrated, the failed implant may be replaced. This should not be carried out at the same visit. Care should also be taken not to curette the implant site to avoid creating an oro-antral fistula. The implant should be replaced at a subsequent visit after reassessing the site for hard and soft tissue healing. In the event that all the implants in the grafted site have failed, consideration should be given to the diagnosis that the graft has not been converted to bone.

### Oro-antral Fistula

An oro-antral fistula may be caused by a failed implant or an infection (Fig 15-85). The fistula should only be closed if there is no infection in the sinus. Closure can be achieved with a variety of techniques. Traditionally, a buccal advanced flap is used, but this technique often results in a reduced vestibular sulcus and loss of attached keratinised tissue. Other methods of closure will depend on the size of the fistula and are described in Chapter 17.

### Sinusitis

Sinusitis following a sinus lift operation is uncommon. It may, however, be a consequence of a complication or inadequate technique. Infection of the sinus graft may result in an infection extending to the maxillary sinus and may spread to the other sinuses and beyond. Sinusitis may also arise from particulate material that has entered the sinus through a perforation. There is a risk that the material may block the ostium, causing infection and further complications.

III  Augmentation

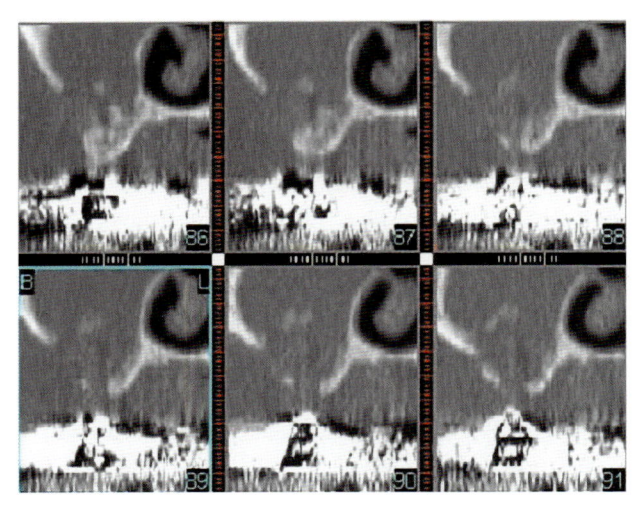

**Fig 15-85** Cross-sectional reconstruction of the maxilla showing an infected sinus with an associated oro-antral fistula resulting from a failed implant in a grafted sinus.

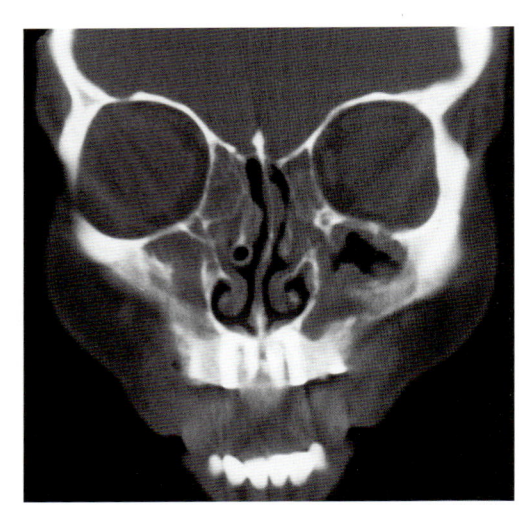

**Fig 15-86** CT scan, coronal plane, showing infected maxillary and ethmoidal sinuses. Treatment requires the management of all the sinuses to prevent reinfection. Previous nasal antrostomy is visible.

An infection of the maxillary sinus may be totally unrelated to any procedure that has been carried out and may be a cross-infection from other sinuses. Examination of the other sinuses should be carried out whenever a sinus infection is present (Fig 15-86).

## Discussion

The sinus lift procedure is a very predictable method for creating bone height in the posterior maxilla, with a very high potential for bone formation from the bony walls of the sinus floor within which the graft materials are placed. The predictability of the procedure depends on the prevention of complications, which in some cases may have a serious deleterious effect on the patient's well-being. The internal anatomy of the sinus floor should be accurately assessed, in terms of both surface irregularities and the nature of the sinus lining and any pathology associated with it.

It is essential to eliminate all pathology originating from either the lining of the sinus or from within the bony structure of the maxilla prior to the procedure of placing a biomaterial into the site. Immaculate surgical technique and a thorough understanding of the principles underlying the procedure are essential in order to prevent inadvertent perforation or tearing of the sinus lining, which may be very fragile.

Appropriate asepsis is fundamental to the exclusion of pathogens. The biomaterial selected should at least be biocompatible and resorbable at a rate that permits stable bone formation. The timescale for the incorporation of grafts into the body varies extensively among different types of material. In considering the timescale of treatment and the sequence of each stage, the nature of the biomaterial and other factors such as implant stability should be taken into account.

# Chapter 16

# Posterior Mandible

## Introduction

The posterior mandible will be considered to be the region extending distal to the mental foramina through which the inferior alveolar nerve runs. This nerve enters the mandible on the lingual aspect of the ramus through the mandibular foramen and runs through the body of the mandible, emerging through the mental foramen on the buccal aspect of the mandible with a varying pattern of emergence.[243–245]

The intraosseous course of the inferior alveolar neurovascular bundle varies both in its superior/inferior position and in its bucco-lingual position along its course.[246] The accurate location of this nerve at any given point is important if damage to the structure is to be avoided. The radiographic image will depend on the density of the trabecular bone, which enables the differential density to be detected by the imaging technique. The magnification associated with the imaging technique must be known and accurately calculated for each region to allow for variation from one site to the other.

The amount of available bone, both in terms of height and ridge width, needs to be assessed. The nature of the bone with respect to the cortical thickness and trabecular density provides valuable additional information to enable the timescales to be determined. The inclination of the jaw and the space available for the prosthetic restoration form a part of the assessment process, which is outlined below.

During the assessment, a number of additional considerations need to be taken into account. These relate to the functional and parafunctional load, the nature of the implant surface, the design and surface area of the implant and the moment of force.

Ideally a minimum length of 11 mm or more should be used. However, where the conditions are favourable, implants as short as 8 mm may be used, particularly where multiple implants are splinted, a wider diameter implant is used, good quality bone is present and occlusal load is favourable. The clinician should bear in mind the poor survival rate of implants of smaller dimensions, as these tend to fail in the short and medium term (approximately five to eight years).[247–249]

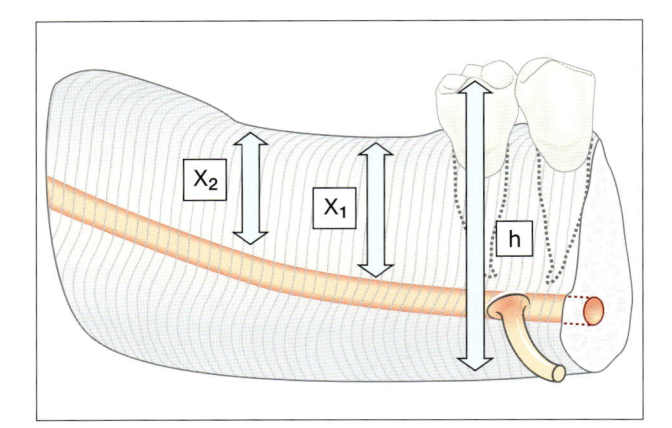

**Fig 16-1** The ratio between the mandibular height (h), measured clinically and on the radiograph, provides the magnification, which can be applied to the height of available bone measured on the radiograph. The mesial distal positioning of the site should also be addressed because of the variation in the height of available bone, as depicted by $X_1$ and $X_2$. The following formula can be used to calculate the length of implant required:

$$X_{real} = \frac{h_{real} \times X_{radiograph}}{h_{radiograph}}$$

The bone height calculated less 2 mm provides the working depth that will allow sufficient clearance above the inferior alveolar canal.

## Assessment

### Radiographic Assessment

#### Dental Panoramic Tomograph

The DPT varies in its magnification considerably depending upon the machine and the position of the patient with respect to tube and film. The magnification may be calculated by means of radiopaque objects inserted into a template worn during the examination. However, the objects (e.g. a 5-mm ball) are relatively small, and any error in measurement results in a significantly increased deviation from reality. It is considered more accurate to measure the height of the mandible on each side using specific landmarks, such as adjacent teeth. Measurements should be made in the same plane as the tooth, both clinically and on the radiograph. A Vernier caliper may be used in the patient's mouth and on the radiograph to record the height of the mandible. A simple calculation to estimate the ratios can then be easily carried out (Fig 16-1).

Care should also be taken to relate the mesiodistal position of the site accurately, as the height of available bone may vary considerably from one site to another. The horizontal magnification should, therefore, also be taken into consideration.

The mandibular canal may be difficult to visualise where there is very little difference in the density between the surrounding tissues and the nerve. Visualisation of the nerve may not be improved with other forms of imaging. Where there is a significant difference in density between the cortical plate and the trabecular bone, a similar effect may be noted.

#### Conventional and Cone Beam Computerised Tomography

Both cone beam CT and CT scans based on axial slices and their related cross-sectional, panoral and 3D reconstructions provide excellent diagnostic information. Using these methods, accurate ridge measurements and ridge orientation can be obtained and the thickness of the cortical plate can be easily determined.

Interactive CT scans enable bone density to be measured in Hounsfield units. Furthermore, it is possible to trace an elusive alveolar canal on a reformatted panoral section, enabling its position to be transferred to the oblique cross-sections where it would otherwise be difficult to visualise the canal. This also assists in differentiating between the canal and other radiolucencies (Figs 16-2 to 16-17).

In conjunction with a radiodistinct (radiopaque or radiolucent) diagnostic template outlining the prosthetic envelope, the angle of the required abutment can also be measured as the implant dimensions are calculated on the interactive program.

#### Periapical Radiography

Periapical radiographs provide additional useful information about a specific site, indicating whether there might be residual roots or pathology present. Using a long-cone paralleling technique, a minimally distorted image can be obtained for verification of available bone height. Intraoperative imaging using guide pins within the osteotomy will provide useful confirmation of the progress of the osteotomy.

#### Laboratory: Study Casts

Mounted study casts can assist in determining the tooth position and the amount of space available. Overeruption of the opposing arch can be estimated more accurately using study casts. Construction of templates for

16   Posterior Mandible

Fig 16-2 (left) Cross-sectional CT image showing multiple translucent areas without any clear indication of the position of the inferior alveolar nerve, requiring the inferior dental canal to be identified in the panoramic view.

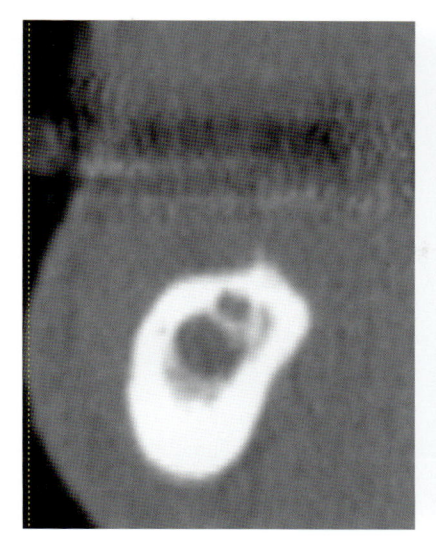

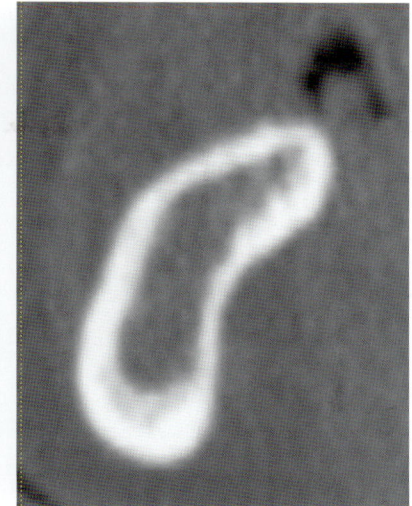

Fig 16-3 (right) Cross-sectional CT image of the posterior mandible with low trabecular density and no indication of the position of the inferior alveolar canal.

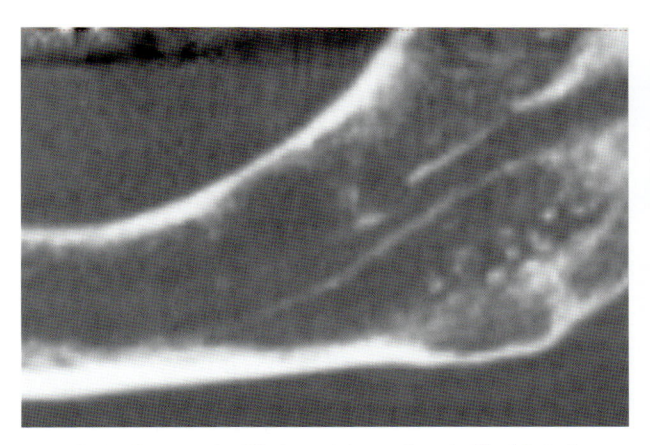

Fig 16-4   Panoramic CT view of the patient in Fig 16-3 showing a faint indication of the position of the inferior alveolar canal.

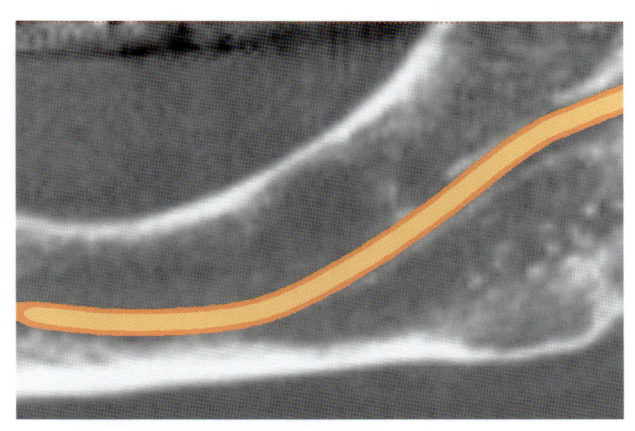

Fig 16-5   The inferior alveolar canal has been traced in the panoramic image using the Simplant software.

Fig 16-6   The inferior alveolar canal can be identified clearly in the cross-sectional image. The low trabecular density will need to be addressed during surgery by judiciously preparing the osteotomy in order to establish adequate primary stability.

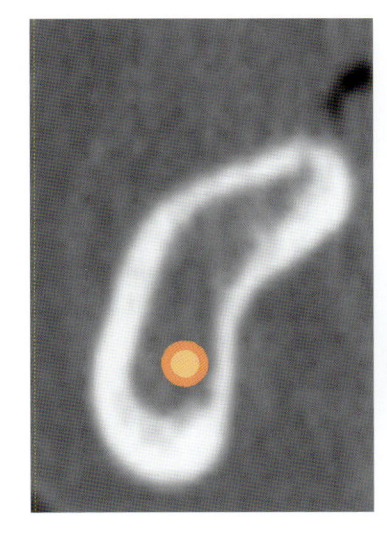

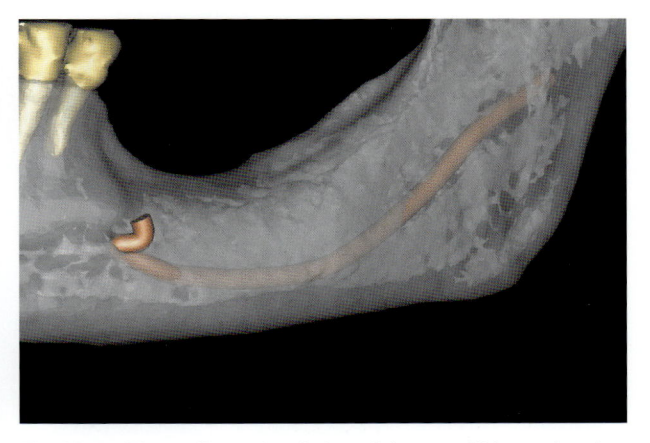

Fig 16-7   Three-dimensional view of the mandible rendered translucent, with the position of the inferior alveolar canal visible.

335

# III  Augmentation

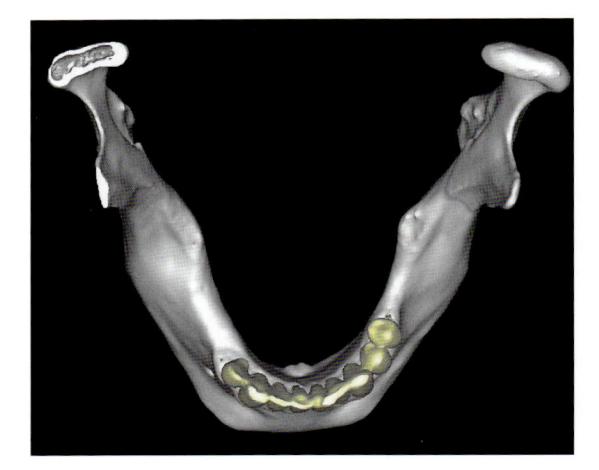

**Fig 16-8**  CT image of the mandible in occlusal view showing the resorption that has taken place on the labial aspect. This is typical and will result in the implants being positioned lingually, with the potential for food collection on the labial aspect that patients should be informed about.

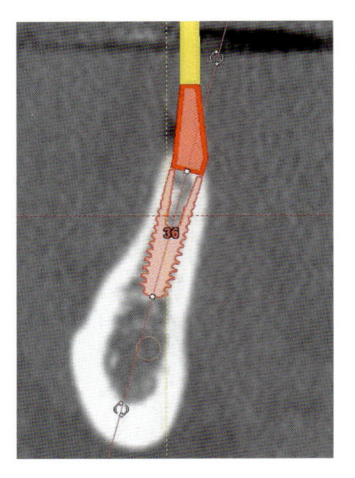

**Fig 16-9**  Cross-sectional CT image in the premolar region with an implant positioned interactively with the abutment selected (7.5 degrees). Note the orientation of the ridge in the premolar region has a minimal inclination.

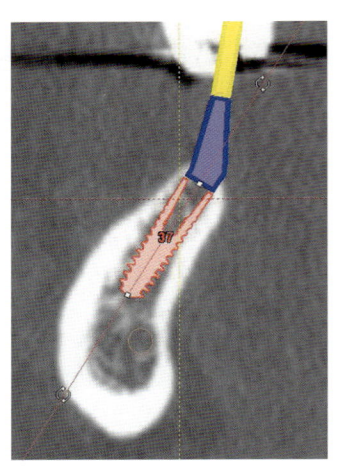

**Fig 16-10**  Cross-sectional CT image of an implant inserted in the molar region at a greater angle because of the inclination of the ridge, requiring a greater angular correction for the abutment (22.5 degrees).

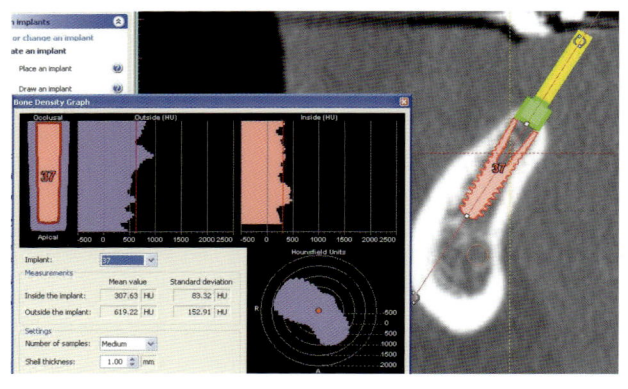

**Fig 16-11**  The bone density is calculated to assist in refining the osteotomy preparation to establish adequate primary stability for the implant.

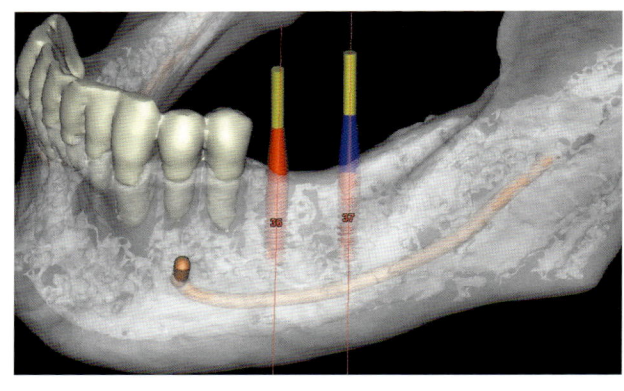

**Fig 16-12**  Three-dimensional CT image (with the mandible translucent) permitting the visualisation of the implants and abutments, as well as the inferior alveolar canal.

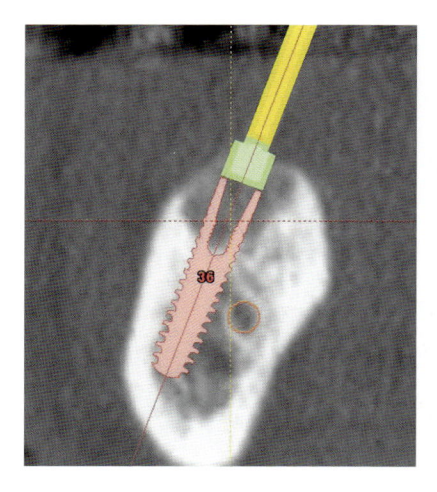

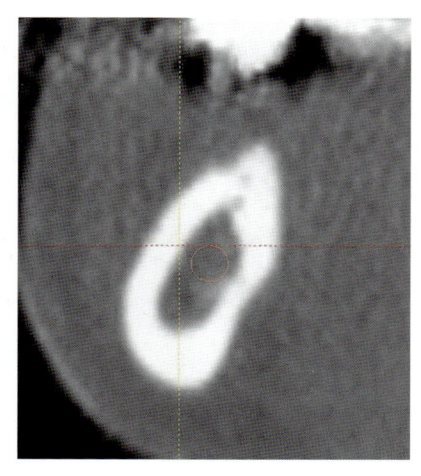

**Fig 16-13**  (left) Cross-sectional CT image of the posterior mandible showing insufficient height above the inferior alveolar canal but adequate mandibular width. The planning for the positioning of an implant beside the nerve can be seen. Care must be taken while executing such a procedure to ensure that the osteotomy bur is not deflected off the labial cortical plate of the mandible. Alternatively, computer-guided surgery may be indicated if there is adequate access.

**Fig 16-14**  (right) Cross-sectional CT image of the posterior mandible with the inferior alveolar canal not visible; it will require tracing in the panoramic view to permit visualisation.

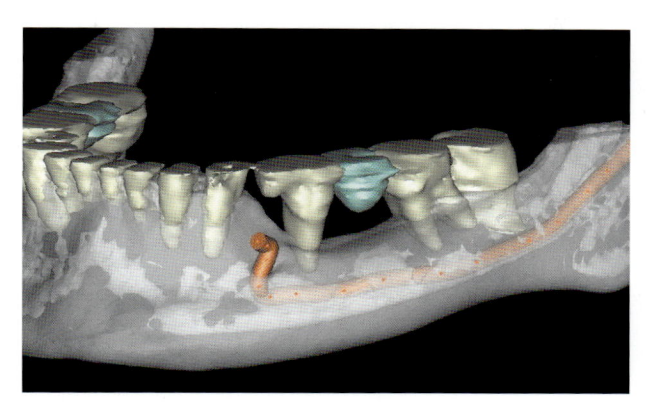

16   Posterior Mandible

**Fig 16-15** Three-dimensional CT image (rendered translucent) showing the inferior alveolar canal clearly. Its proximity to the superior surface of the mandible is indicative of a need to reposition the inferior alveolar nerve. The management of patients with low trabecular density is generally easier and requires the position to be identified by tracing back from the mental foramen.

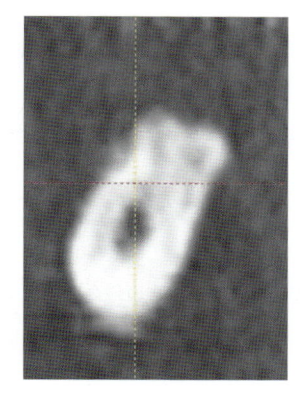

**Fig 16-16** Cross-sectional image of the posterior mandible showing very dense bone and clearly identifiable inferior alveolar canal. The management of such cases for repositioning the neurovascular bundle is more exacting.

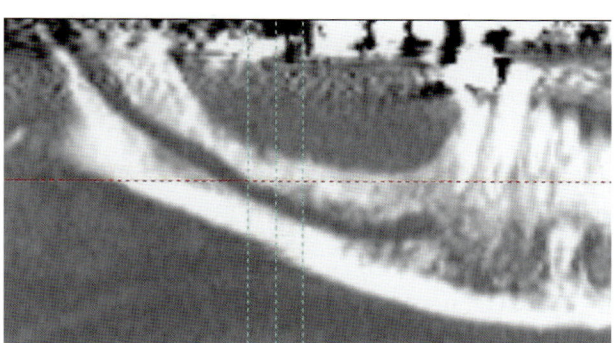

**Fig 16-17** Panoramic CT image with very clearly identifiable inferior alveolar canal.

assistance during the surgical phase or for transfer of information to the diagnostic image may also be carried out.

## Clinical Assessment

Assessment of the nature of the soft tissues provides an indication about the peri-implant tissues and the ability to close the wound. Access to the operative site can be assessed based on the space available on opening, the tightness of the circumoral tissues as well as the activity of the tongue. Care should be taken where the patient has previously undergone plastic surgery.

## Surgical Protocol: Adequate Bone

Access to the posterior mandible is the most difficult to achieve and is compounded by the lingual inclination of the ridge and the presence of the tongue. A crestal incision is most commonly advised, particularly when immediate loading or a transmucosal approach are being considered. A remote buccal incision may be used when adequate attached tissues are present, in the absence of muscle attachments, for a two-stage approach (Fig 16-18).

Reflection of the periosteum to expose the mental foramen may be carried out to assist in the precise location of the neurovascular bundle.

### Bone of Normal Density

Site selection is most effectively carried out using a small round bur in a speed-increasing handpiece. The pilot bur is used to specific predetermined depth and serves the additional purposes of determining bone density and direction of osteotomy. The depth of the osteotomy is estimated to allow a 2 mm clearance above the inferior alveolar canal, and all drilling is carried out using accurately calibrated drills to the predetermined depth. Measurements must be performed from the edge of the ridge crest, preferably from the mesial aspect, to guarantee good visibility. Measurements should not be made from the buccal aspect as scalloping of the osteotomy will result from curved or paraboloid ridge forms. This would lead to miscalculation and osteotomy preparation

III  Augmentation

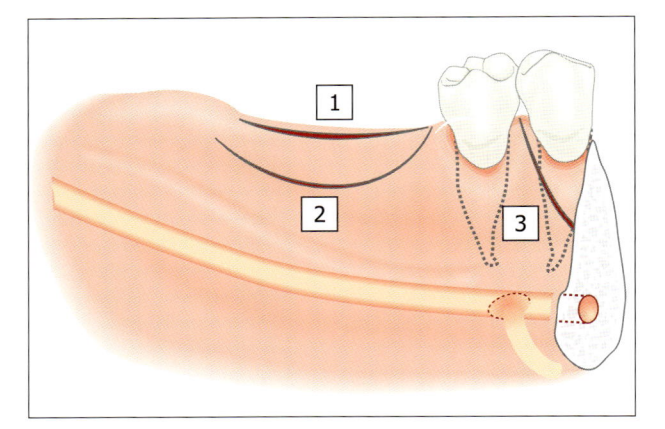

**Fig 16-18** Access to the alveolar ridge can be gained by either a crestal (1) or a remote buccal incision (2). A crestal incision (bisecting the attached tissue) may be used in situations where immediate loading is contemplated or where there is a limited amount of attached tissue with muscle attachments in the region of the planned incision. Remote incisions are indicated where delayed loading is planned and where adequate non-mobile attached tissue is present. Vertical release incisions (3) may be used in situations where the mental foramen needs to be exposed. Care needs to be taken to ensure that none of the fibres of the mental nerve is severed.

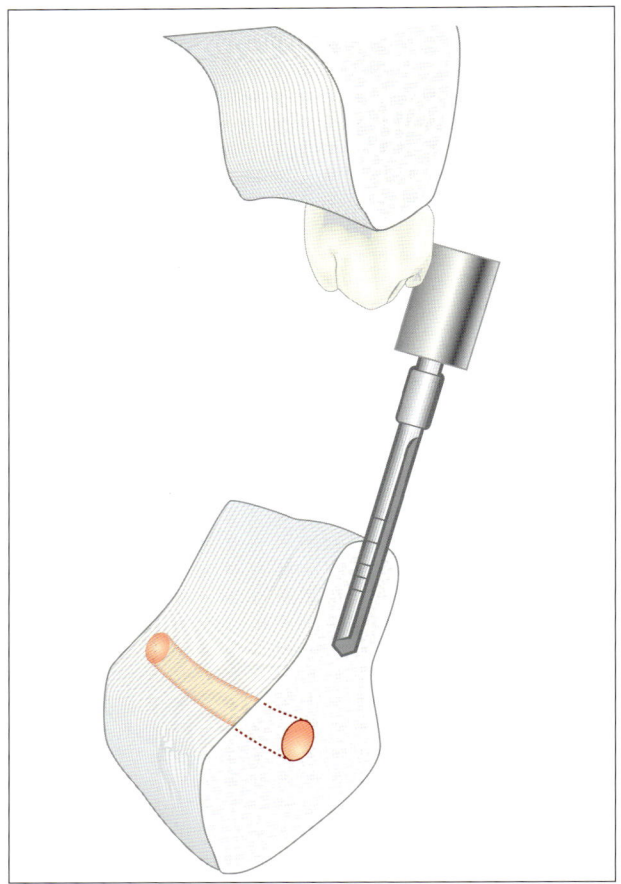

**Fig 16-19** Inclination of a drill from the palatal aspect of an maxillary molar to overcome the problem of access and ridge angulation.

to an excessive depth, resulting in possible damage to the inferior alveolar canal.

The osteotomy is enlarged in diameter to utilise the entire width of available bone. It, therefore, often engages the labial and lingual cortical plates. Consequently, it is advisable to use the full sequence of instruments, including bone taps, prior to insertion of the implant. This cautionary note is relevant because the clinician may initially assess the bone density to be low in poorly trabeculated bone as assessed from the pilot osteotomy. The incremental enlargement of the osteotomy may not provide feedback relating to the lateral engagement of the cortical plates.

Access is often gained from the palatal aspect of the opposing maxillary teeth (Fig 16-19). Consistency of the angulation of the drill can be achieved by noting the position of the handpiece in relation to the opposing maxillary teeth when the mouth is propped open at a particular height. The same angle can then be used for subsequent instrumentation.

### Immediate Loading
The definitive abutment may be attached and an acrylic resin transitional restoration fitted for immediate loading where conditions are suitable.

### Transmucosal Approach
A transmucosal approach can be achieved by the attachment of a sulcus former, which eliminates the need for second-stage surgery. This approach is particularly suitable when the patient does not wear a removable prosthesis.

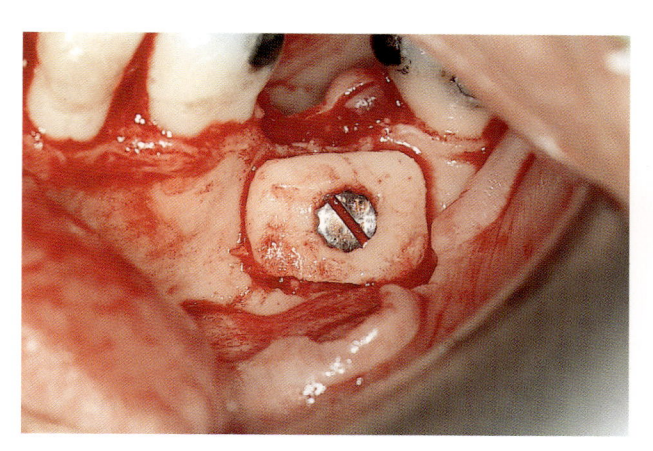

**Fig 16-20** Buccal view of an onlay graft from the symphysis being used to increase width. Note the proximity of the mental foramen to the graft site and the manner in which the recipient site has been modified to receive the graft.

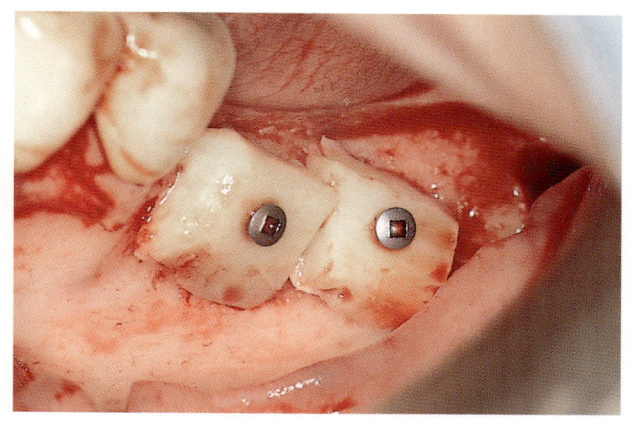

**Fig 16-21** Bone graft from the ramus being used to increase width. Note that the graft has been sectioned in order to get good adaptation to the residual mandibular ridge.

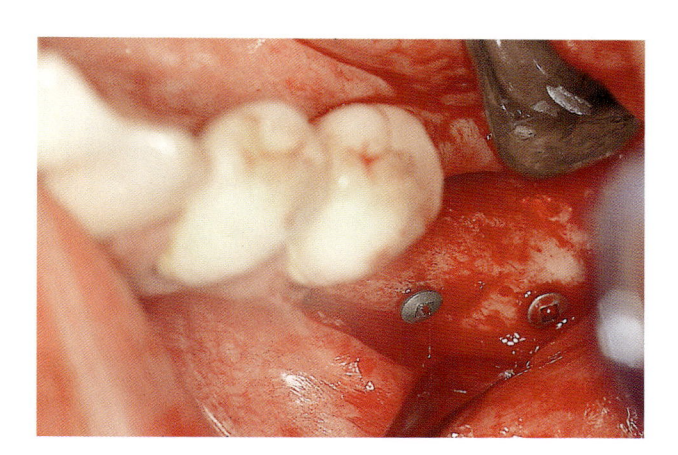

**Fig 16-22** Clinical view of the healed graft prior to implant placement. Note the increase of width that has been achieved and the manner in which the graft has incorporated. Further note the bleeding surface of the graft.

### Bone of Low Density

In low-density bone, procedures to carry out bone condensation using a range of instruments may be utilised when access permits. Some ridge widening may also be carried out, using bone spreaders. Self-tapping protocols for implants may be suitable, and a transmucosal approach or early incremental loading (bone training) rather than immediate loading is advisable.

## Insufficient Bone: Treatment Options

Assessment of the amount of bone available should be carried out using the diagnostic tools described above. Based on the type of deficiency, a treatment protocol specific to that deficiency should be employed. This is summarised in Flowchart 16-1 at the end of this chapter.

### Bone Graft: Insufficient Bone Width

A lack of bone width is ideally treated using onlay bone grafts, provided that the bone height is adequate (greater than 10 mm). The grafts can be harvested from the symphysis, ramus or an extraoral donor site (Figs 16-20–16-22). A limited increase in bone height can also be achieved using this technique (Figs 16-23 and 16-24). Sufficient interocclusal space should be available, as well as adequate soft tissues, to allow closure over the graft. A crestal incision is used, which bisects the attached tissue. The periosteum is reflected on the lingual aspect but not beyond the mylohyoid ridge. The clinican should be mindful of the risk to the lingual nerve, which may be in contact with the periosteum. On the buccal aspect, the mental foramen is exposed. Vertical release incisions anterior to the mental foramen

# III   Augmentation

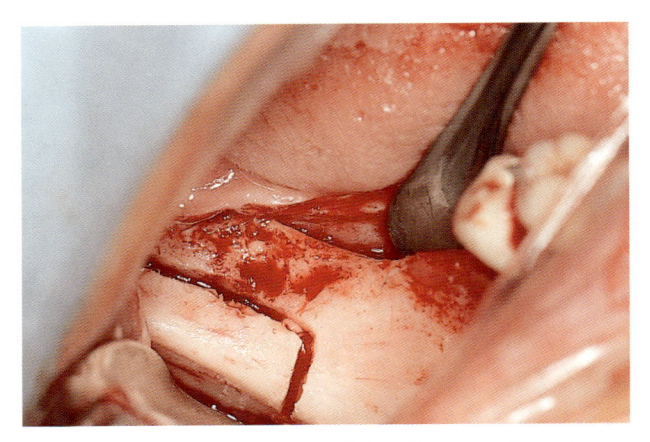

**Fig 16-23**   Bone being harvested from the ramus for grafting to correct width and height. The ramus is particularly well suited for the reconstruction of ridge form.

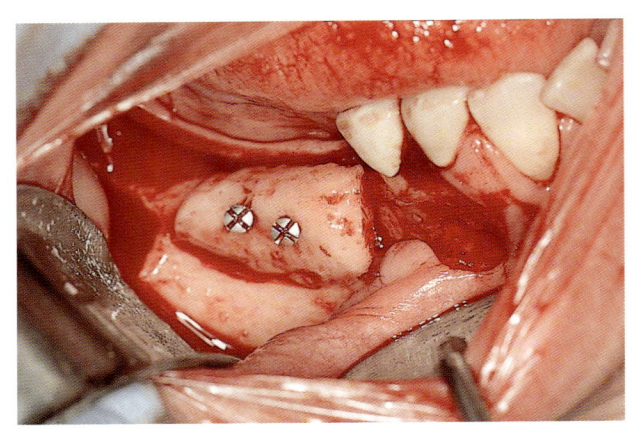

**Fig 16-24**   The bone graft secured anterior to the donor site, increasing ridge height and width.

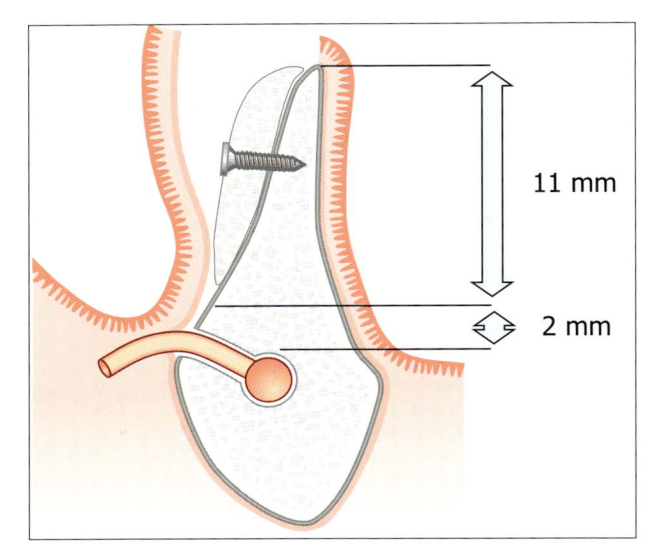

**Fig 16-25**   Diagram of an onlay graft in the posterior mandible, with the mental foramen visible. The presence of the mental nerve makes the closure of the soft tissues over the graft more difficult. Because of the hazards of nerve damage, a periosteal release incision should be avoided in the region of the mental foramen.

may be used to provide some mobility and access to the region requiring augmentation, which is often on the buccal aspect as a result of the pattern of resorption.

There is a limitation to the soft tissues available to close over a graft. The mental nerve and foramen, as well as the facial artery, restrict the amount of tissue that can be advanced on the labial aspect (Fig 16-25). On the lingual aspect, the fragility of the mucosa and the risk of damage to the lingual nerve, vessels and salivary glands and ducts also limit the advancement of tissue. The amount of augmentation (particularly height) that can be carried out on a ridge is severely limited by the presence of teeth positioned distal to the ridge that requires augmentation.

With free-end saddle, distal reflection of the soft tissues facilitates the advancement of the muco-periosteum for closure.

Adapting the bone graft to the hard cortical bone and the contours of the mandible requires considerable skill in situations where a limited amount of bone is available for adaptation. Modification of the recipient site to permit engagement of the graft greatly facilitates its positioning for fixation.

The graft is fixed firmly to the recipient site using screws to ensure that no micro-movement takes place. Any minor spaces between the graft and the recipient site should be packed with particulate material. Guided tissue regeneration may be used, if necessary. Closure of the wound following graft placement must be carried out to achieve a hermetic seal, using horizontal or vertical mattress sutures without any tension. Implant placement can be carried out as described in earlier sections based on adequate healing prior to excessive remodelling of the graft.

## Bone Graft: Insufficient Bone Height

The height of bone can only be increased by a limited amount using a bone graft because of the difficulties associated with the closure of the soft tissues over

## 16  Posterior Mandible

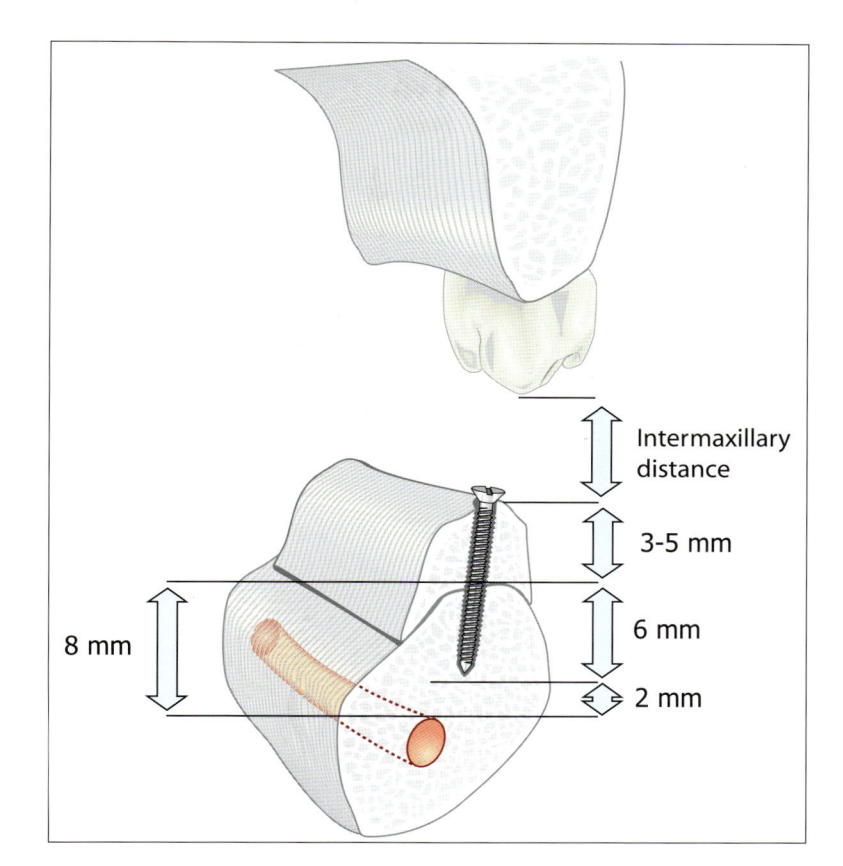

**Fig 16-26** The use of an onlay graft in the posterior mandible. Increase in bone height in the posterior mandible must take into account the following points:
- the soft tissues required for closure and access to this region
- the 2 mm clearance above the inferior alveolar canal
- the intermaxillary distance for prosthetic restoration
- the remodelling of the graft
- the length of implant that may finally be placed.

the graft. A significant increase in height can only be achieved in those cases where a free-end saddle is present and where there is an adequate interocclusal distance (Fig 16-26). An increase in ridge height of more than 3 to 5 mm often necessitates procurement of the graft from an extraoral site (Fig 16-27). Practically, up to 10 mm of bone height can be obtained from the iliac crest.

The benefits of an onlay graft to increase height should be carefully assessed by the clinician. Consideration must be given to the total length of the implant that can be inserted following the grafting procedure and the remodelling that is related to the healing process. Placement of the implant requires a specific amount of bone above the inferior alveolar canal. In addition to this there should also be a clearance distance of 2 mm. A minimum of 5 mm of bone above the canal is therefore considered necessary before grafting can be considered without repositioning the inferior alveolar nerve bundle.

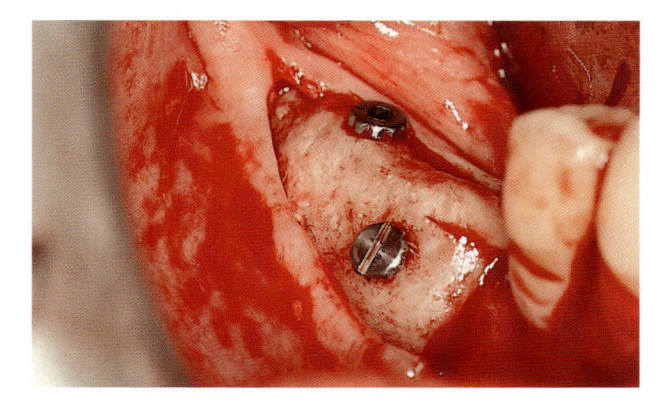

**Fig 16-27** Clinical view of a bone graft from the iliac crest being used to increase ridge height.

The following examples illustrate the possible outcomes of using onlay bone grafts in the posterior mandible. In studying these examples the interocclusal space available as well as the remodelling (which may vary from approximately 20 to 40%) of the graft must be taken into account.

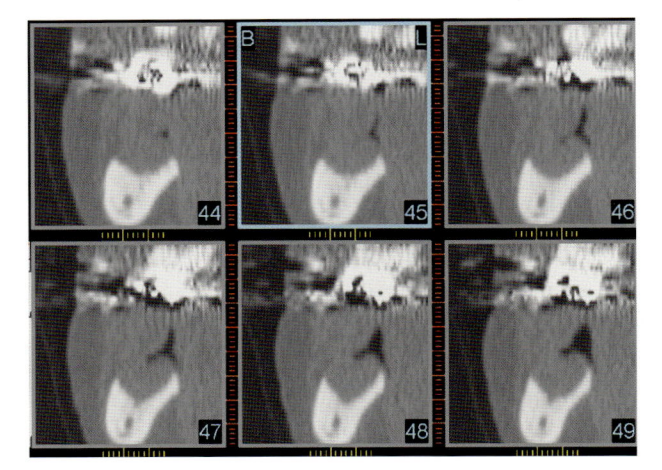

**Fig 16-28** Cross-section reformation of posterior mandible showing a deficient alveolar ridge with 3 mm of bone available above the canal for implant placement. The deficiency was caused by extensive periodontal disease and prolonged periodontal treatment. There is adequate intermaxillary space for bone augmentation to increase ridge height.

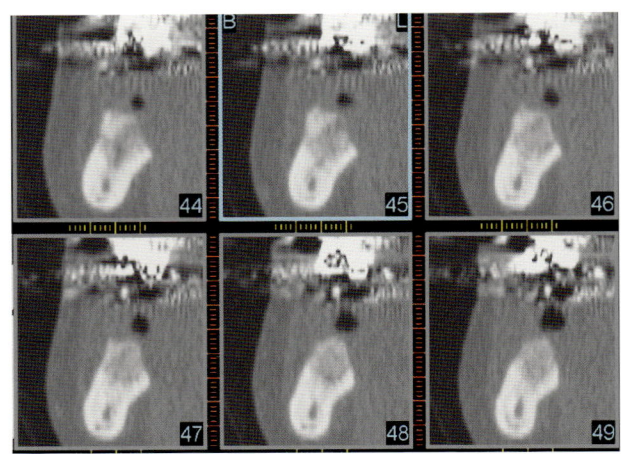

**Fig 16-29** Post-operative image of reconstructed mandibular ridge using autogenous bone from the iliac crest. A total of 13 mm of bone is now available for placement of an implant of 11-mm length (same patient as in Fig 16-28).

If an intraoral bone graft is going to be used to gain height, a minimum of 8 mm of bone must be present preoperatively. An increase of 5 mm will, therefore, result in 11 mm of available bone, taking into account the required 2 mm minimum clearance above the inferior alveolar canal. If an extraoral bone graft is used, an increase of 8 mm in height will enable an 11-mm implant to be used, provided that the preoperative height of the available bone is 5 mm above the inferior alveolar canal (Figs 16-28 and 16-29).

## Nerve Repositioning with Simultaneous Implant Placement

The presence of the inferior alveolar nerve prevents the entire height of the mandible from being used for implant placement (Fig 16-30). Where a limited amount of bone is present above the inferior alveolar canal (10 mm or less), repositioning of the inferior alveolar neurovascular bundle would make the entire height of the mandible available for implant placement. This would permit the insertion of implants of 14 mm or more in size into bone of good quality where bicortical fixation can be achieved (Fig 16-31). Implants inserted in this way have very high stability and are able to resist occlusal loads.[250–256]

Repositioning the nerve requires its manipulation and, therefore, there will invariably be a certain amount of altered sensation, which normally recovers after a certain amount of time, how long being dependent on the trauma resulting from the manipulation.[257] Compression and tension result in transient states of altered sensation, with tension causing the greater effect.[258] Permanent sensory changes may result from physical trauma that causes organic damage to the multifascicular nerve structure.[259,260] The benefits of the procedure need to be assessed against the risks and the patient must be informed accordingly. Although patients respond differently to the treatment because of the numerous endogenous factors, modern imaging techniques facilitate the assessment process with regard to the ease of access and any difficulties that may be encountered during surgery.

### Assessment

DPTs provide good initial assessment and must be viewed with the clinical observations in mind. CT, however, provides the most valuable information. The course of the nerve and its 3D relationship within the mandible, as well as the density of the cortical and trabecular bone, provide valuable information with regard to the complexity of surgery. The width of the mental

# 16 Posterior Mandible

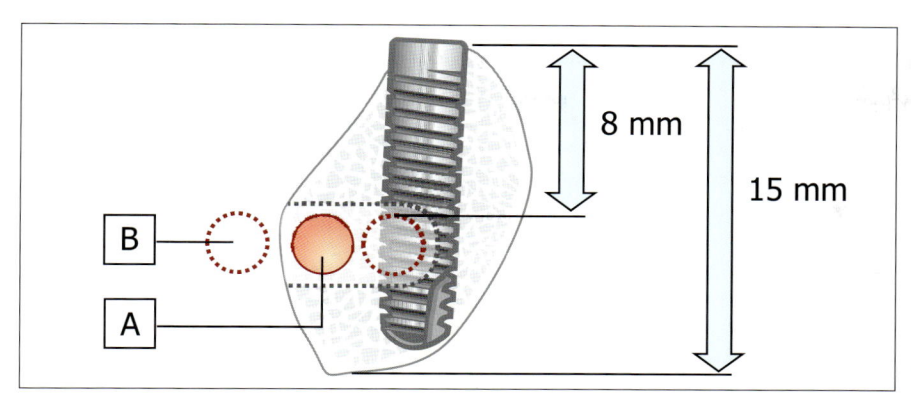

**Fig 16-30** Cross-sectional view illustrating nerve repositioning with simultaneous insertion of an implant. Repositioning the inferior alveolar neurovascular bundle makes available the entire height of the posterior mandible. This permits the use of implants of up to 14 mm in length, or more. The bundle is replaced into the groove to recreate normal anatomy (A). With narrow mandibles the neurovascular bundle may need to remain outside the mandible (B). In these cases, the altered anatomy must be recorded and relevant health professionals as well as the patient informed.

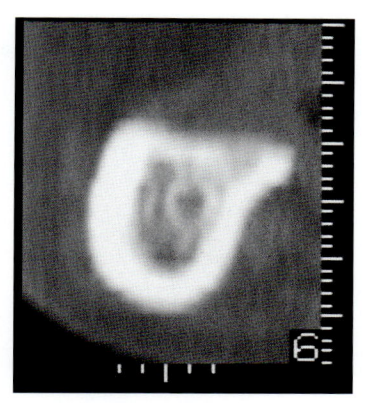

**Fig 16-31** Cross-sectional CT image of a posterior mandible, where the inferior alveolar canal can clearly be seen. Note the lack of bone above the canal and its bucco-lingual position within the mandible. Repositioning the inferior alveolar nerve will provide approximately 15 mm of bone for implant placement.

**Table 16-1** Anatomical variations and their possible influence on the nerve repositioning procedure

| Feature | Foramen | Cortical bone | Trabecular bone | Bucco-lingual position | Inferior position | Difficulty |
|---|---|---|---|---|---|---|
| **Favourable** | Shallow | Thin | Sparse | Buccal | Superficial | Easy |
| | * | * | * | * | * | |
| | ** | ** | ** | ** | ** | |
| | *** | *** | *** | *** | *** | |
| **Unfavourable** | Deep | Thick | Dense | Lingual | Low | Difficult |

foramen and its exact path as it exits the cortical plate provides crucial information relating to the ease with which access to the deeper portions can be gained. A range of variations has been observed, which affects the ease with which surgery can be carried out and influencing the amount of possible trauma to the nerve (Table 16-1).

The most favourable features are that the foramen is wide and connected to an inferior alveolar canal that runs a short distance lingual (approximately 2 mm) to a thin buccal cortical plate. The width of the canal is ideally approximately 3 to 4 mm in diameter and surrounded by very sparse trabecular bone. Ideally, it should not lie close to the inferior border of the mandible.

The most difficult nerves to deal with are those that emerge through narrow mental canals transversing a thick cortical plate over a distance of at least 7 mm. Typically, the position of the neurovascular bundle would be close to the inferior border and on the lingual aspect of a relatively wide mandible. The neurovascular canal wall is dense, as is the trabecular bone. Additional foramina or a neurovascular bundle that divides into more than one branch may also compound this (Figs 16-32 and 16-33).

## Surgical Technique

The technique described is designed to minimise the trauma to the nerve. It is also intends to avoid sectioning the incisive branch, as long as the mental branch is not

III Augmentation

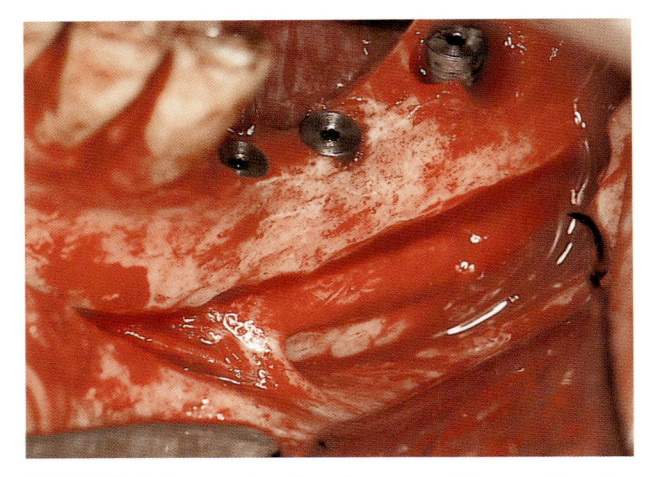

Fig 16-32 Intraoperative view of a successfully repositioned nerve, showing a variation in anatomy. The implants have been inserted. Two branches of the incisive nerve are visible.

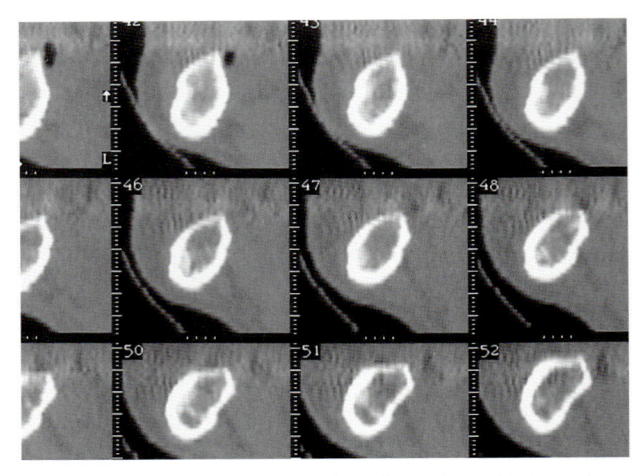

Fig 16-33 The intraoperative view of a patient with two adjacent mental foramina.

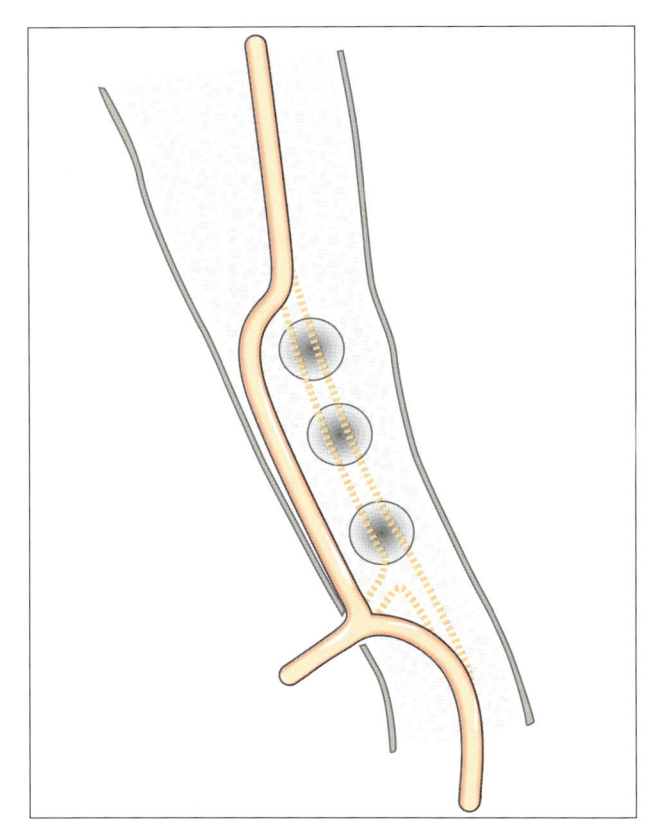

Fig 16-34 Axial view of the mandible with the implants in place after the nerve has been repositioned. When implants are placed simultaneously and where the anterior teeth are present, the incisive branch is retained. The nerve is replaced lateral to the implants within the groove created in the mandible if the cross-sectional width permits it. Mobilisation of the bundle distally as well as mesially (exposing the incisive branch) reduces the stretching of the nerve.

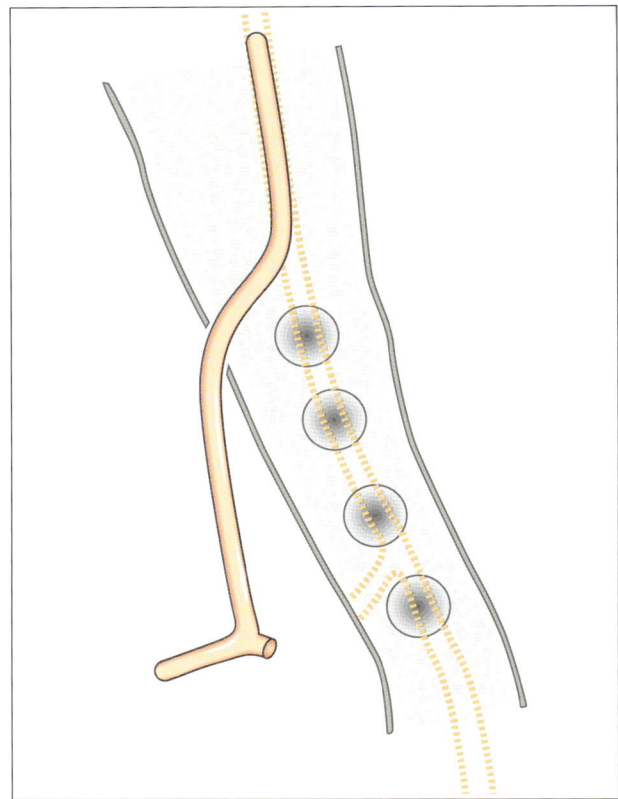

Fig 16-35 Axial view of the mandible with the implants in place after the nerve has been repositioned. When the incisive branch is severed, a new mental foramen is created at the point where the nerve exits through the lateral wall of the mandible. This occurs most commonly with patients with edentulous jaws where bone grafts are placed simultaneously or at a subsequent visit.

**16** Posterior Mandible

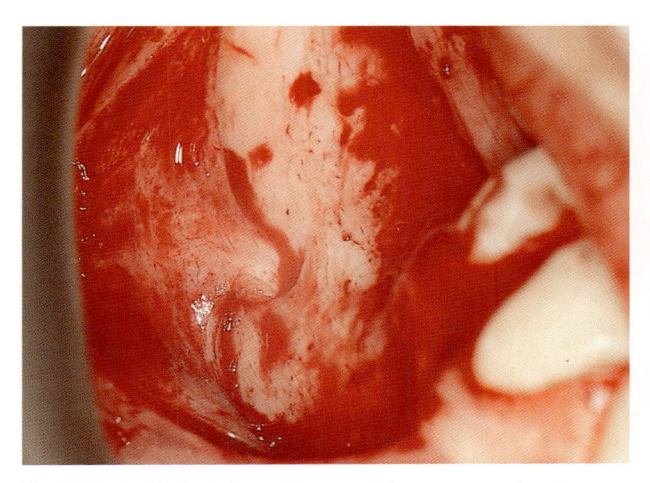

**Fig 16-36** Clinical view of the mental nerve emerging from the mental foramen. Two of the fascicles are visible through the periosteum.

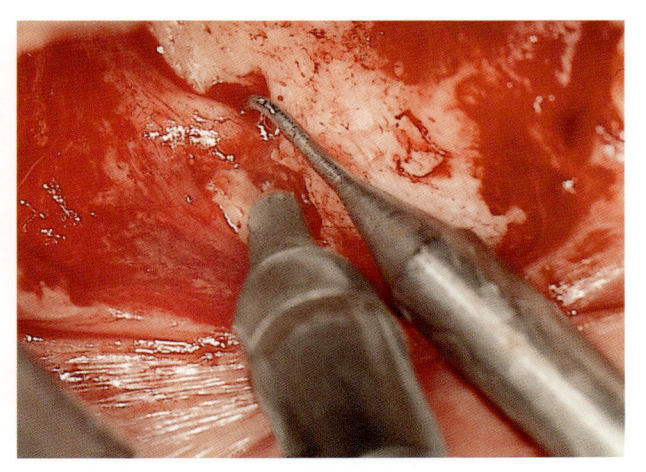

**Fig 16-37** Curved probe being introduced into the foramen in order to explore the inferior alveolar canal. The bone overlying the incisive canal has been removed to facilitate atraumatic introduction of the probe.

compromised. It is also considered advantageous not to alter the normal anatomical course of the inferior alveolar nerve, by returning it into the body of the mandible after the insertion of the implants (Fig 16-34). This is easily achieved with a wide mandible; however, in a narrow mandible the nerve may come to lie on the surface in the groove created for access to the inferior alveolar canal (Fig 16-35). Two variations of the technique are considered to be sufficient to address most clinical situations.

### Incision

A crestal incision bisecting the attached tissue will provide access to the alveolar crest, and a vertical-release incision anterior to the mental foramen will provide adequate periosteal reflection to expose the foramen. The distal extension of the incision is carried to the retromolar pad and then buccally in the direction of the coronoid process. Reflection of the periosteum is extended inferior to the mental foramen, freeing the neurovascular bundle (Fig 16-36). Implant sites are selected prior to the repositioning of the nerve because the extent to which the nerve needs to be repositioned can then be determined. Implant sites are selected based on prosthetic need.

### Access to the Inferior Alveolar Nerve

Access to the nerve is obtained starting at the mental foramen. A fine curved ball-ended probe is used to

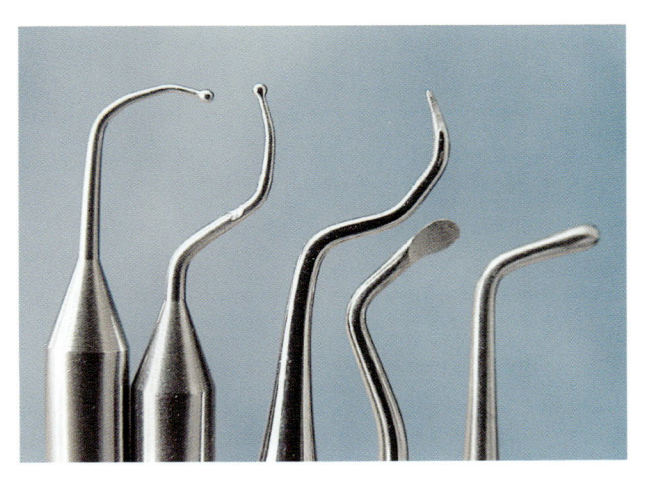

**Fig 16-38** Customised instruments consisting of fine curved probes and excavators for nerve repositioning.

explore the bony walls of the foramen to confirm the observations made from the CT image regarding the direction and depth of the foramen.

Where the foramen is narrow or if access to the inferior alveolar canal is difficult, it becomes pertinent to explore the incisive canal for the purpose of exposing the incisive branch of the nerve. The bone overlying the incisive canal may be removed using the probe as an indicator (Figs 16-37 and 16-38). This serves the purpose of increasing the mobility of the neurovascular bundle to provide better access. The amount of exposure of the incisive branch will vary depending on

345

# III Augmentation

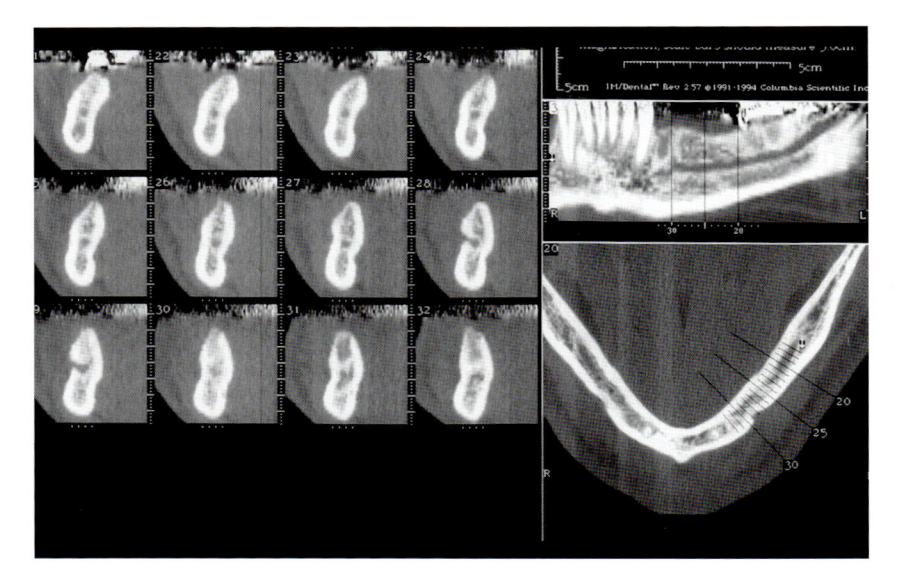

**Fig 16-39** CT scan reconstructions showing oblique sections on the left-hand side, panoramic reconstruction at top right and axial section at bottom right. A narrow ridge with the inferior alveolar neurovascular canal positioned high within the mandible leaves very little bone for implant placement. The position of the neurovascular canal can be verified and cross-referenced to each type of reconstruction. This type of anatomy is not suited for access to the canal by the window technique because of the close proximity of the nerve to the buccal cortical plate. Access to the canal is best achieved using a probe within the canal to guide the removal of the overlying bone. The morphology of the mental foramen can also be seen and is valuable for planning access to the inferior alveolar canal.

the need and the presence of tooth roots. The probe is inserted distally into the inferior alveolar canal, and the overlying bone is removed carefully until the probe starts to become visible through the bone surrounding the canal. The instrument used for the removal of the bone is a speed-increasing contra-angled or straight handpiece with copious sterile saline irrigation and tungsten carbide burs of the appropriate size. The speed-increasing handpiece allows a brushing motion to be used, minimising the risk of damage caused by a loss of control using slow handpieces. Support for the handpiece during the procedure is essential for the precise removal of bone in close proximity to these critical structures. During all procedures where rotary instruments are used, great care must be taken to ensure that the nerve is protected.

Once the probe is visible, the thin layer of remaining bone may be elevated manually and the probe inserted further into the canal for this step to be repeated. The entire inferior alveolar nerve may be exposed in this way, particularly when the nerve lies adjacent to the buccal cortical plate (Fig 16-39). The inferior alveolar nerve is exposed to a point approximately 1 cm distal to the last planned implant site.

Alternatively, a window in the buccal bone may be created once the position of the nerve in relation to the mental foramen has been determined. The formation of a buccal window greatly improves access to the nerve (Fig 16-40). This is particularly useful where the neurovascular bundle is positioned further towards the lingual and inferior aspect of the mandible (Fig 16-41).

Where there is dense trabecular bone, it is advisable to trace the nerve distally, as described above, following the removal of bone to create the buccal window. Where the trabeculae are sparse, the nerve becomes very easy to locate, as there is very little bone obstructing access.

The most significant advance in the safety of surgical technique is the advent of piezosurgery. This permits relatively safe removal of bone in close proximity to the inferior alveolar canal. The protection of the neurovascular bundle is maintained in the same way during the surgical procedure. Access via a window is also facilitated by use of the piezosurgery instruments. Although safety is improved, duration of the procedure is not greatly decreased through use of piezosurgery because of the relatively slow removal of bone. The two tips that we find most useful are the scraper and the diamond ball.

## Mobilisation of the Neurovascular Bundle

The narrow groove created in the surface of the canal is widened using the flat end of a fine periosteal elevator. Care must be taken to position the edge of the elevator against the edge of the canal and to avoid impingement of the neurovascular bundle. Leverage

16   Posterior Mandible

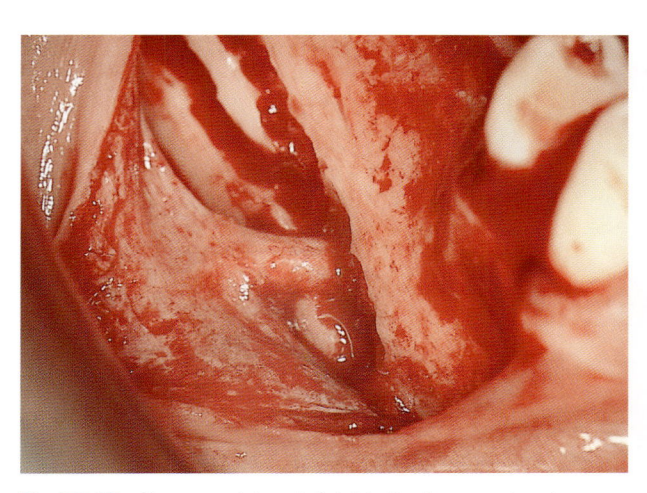

**Fig 16-40**  Bone mesial and distal to the foramen has been carefully removed until the probe is visible. Distally, a window has been outlined prior to its removal to gain access to the canal. There must be some clearance between the buccal cortical plate and the inferior alveolar canal to enable this method to be used with safety.

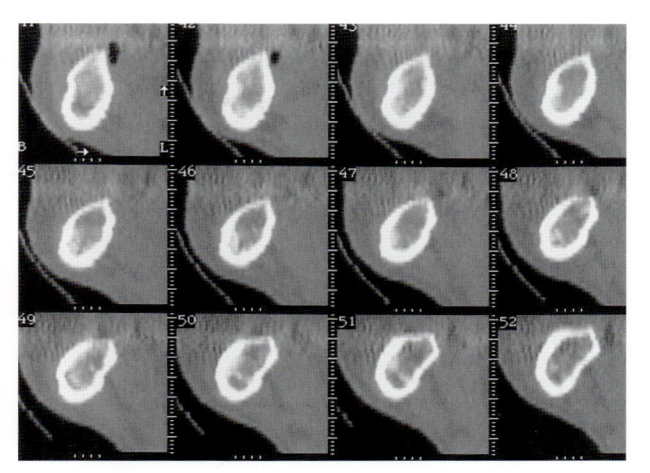

**Fig 16-41**  Oblique sections of the posterior mandible (buccal side on the left of each image) showing the inferior alveolar canal barely visible on the lingual inferior part of the mandible. Precise location can only be achieved by cross-referencing from other reconstructions, preferably interactively. Only 8 mm of bone is present above the canal. Repositioning the nerve will provide 15 mm of available bone. This sort of mandibular morphology is ideally suited for the window technique to gain access to the inferior alveolar canal.

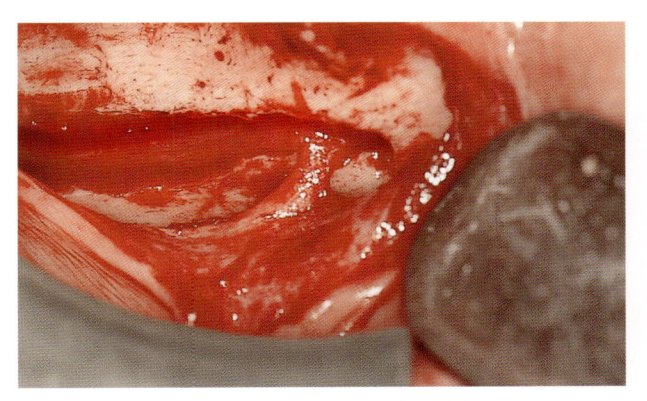

**Fig 16-42**  The inferior alveolar neurovascular bundle is visible and has been mobilised prior to implant placement. There is no breach evident in the continuity of the neurovascular sheath, indicating that complete recovery is likely. Photographs, therefore, form a crucial part of the clinical records.

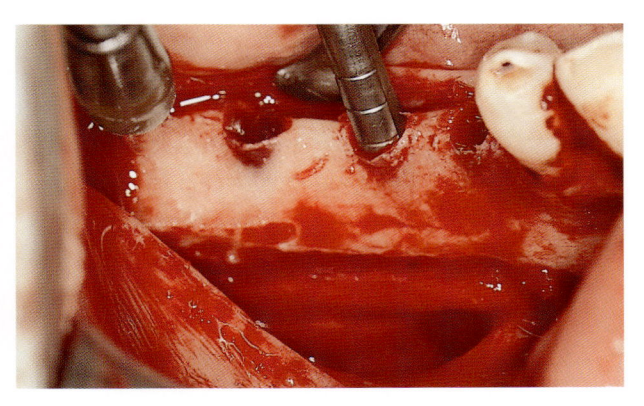

**Fig 16-43**  The osteotomy being prepared with the bundle carefully retracted away from the osteotomy bur. Care must be taken while using all instruments for osteotomy preparation and implant insertion.

is gained from the wall of the groove, and the fragile bone surrounding the canal is carefully displaced, first superiorly and then inferiorly, as depicted in Fig 16-42. The bundle is then carefully mobilised, using an excavator and ensuring that the sharp edge remains in contact with the canal walls (Fig 16-42). Once mobilised, the structure is bodily moved buccally along the entire length of the exposed canal, using the excavator.

## Insertion of Implants

The repositioned nerve is retracted, ensuring that it is kept clear of the osteotomy site. The osteotomy is prepared using rotary instruments (Fig 16-43), and in the majority of cases all the steps, including bone tapping, are required to ensure precise positioning and engagement within the inferior cortical plate of the mandible (Fig 16-44). Because good implant lengths can be achieved, the need to use wider implants is less criti-

### III   Augmentation

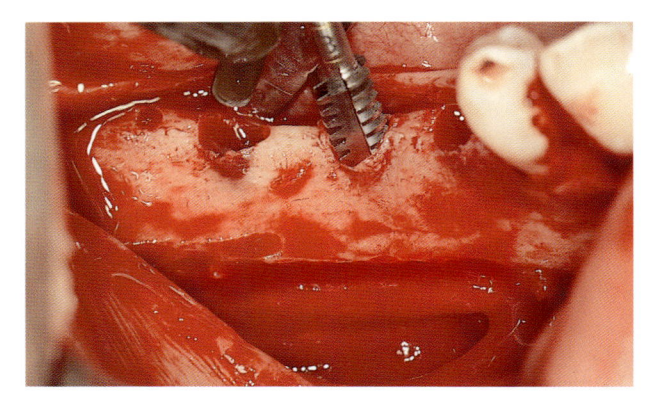

**Fig 16-44**   Bone tap being used. These are often necessary to prepare the threads for ease of insertion of the implants into dense cortical bone. The neurovascular bundle can be seen safely retracted.

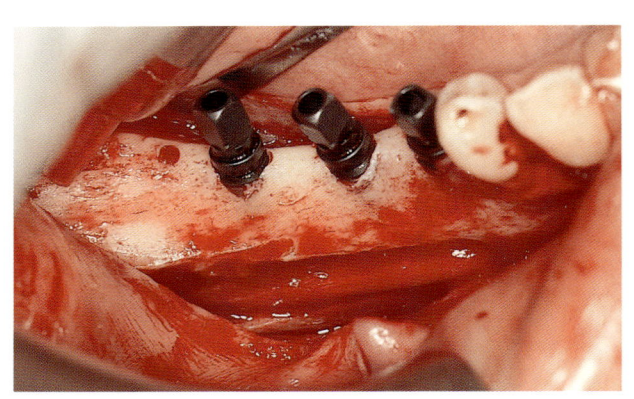

**Fig 16-45**   The implants can be seen in situ with the neurovascular bundle adjacent to them.

cal. This also leaves a greater amount of space for the nerve to be replaced within the body of the mandible after implant placement (Fig 16-45).

Once the implants have been inserted and the angles required for the abutments measured, the nerve can be replaced within the body of the mandible. Space between the implant and the neurovascular bundle may be maintained by using a particulate resorbable biomaterial, such as beta-tricalcium phosphate. Additional material may be used within the groove before wound closure to ensure the complete healing of the cortical plate.

### Wound Closure

Careful closure of the wound to produce a hermetic seal should be carried out. Horizontal mattress sutures interspaced with interrupted sutures provide excellent closure. The implants are normally allowed to heal for six months to ensure that integration has taken place prior to exposure and restoration, as described above.

### Monitoring

Recovery of sensation is monitored using sensory tests for a range of nerve fibres representing full sensory function:

- *Sharp test*. A sharp probe is used to elicit a pain response. Hyper- and hyporesponses are recorded and mapped using different coloured pens. Hypersensitivity is taken as a sign of recovery, while dullness of the response signifies a slow rate of recovery.

- *Wisp test*. A wisp of cotton wool is lightly brushed over the lip and chin to monitor the recovery of the sense of touch.
- *Heat test*. A cotton roll dipped in a water bath at 55°C can be used to monitor sensitivity to heat.
- *Cold test*. Ethyl chloride sprayed on cotton wool may be used to elicit a response to cold.
- *Discriminatory test*. This is a measure of the minimum distance between two points of a divider that can be felt as two separate points. For each patient, calibration of the discriminatory distance is carried out by testing a non-affected site. The upper lip is ideal, as it has a similar distribution of sensory innervation. The distance between the divider points when the two points can be discriminated is recorded and used to test the affected site by comparing the discriminatory distances.

These tests are carried out after surgery at two weeks, one, three and six months to monitor the rate of recovery (Fig 16-46).

### Nerve Repositioning in Combination with Onlay Bone Graft

Combining an onlay bone graft with repositioning of the nerve becomes necessary where severe resorption of the mandible has taken place and there is a risk of fracture of the weakened jaw (Fig 16-47).

**16   Posterior Mandible**

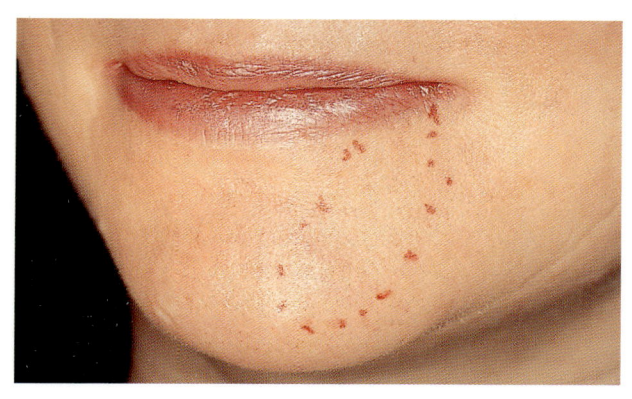

**Fig 16-46**   Post-operative monitoring using a series of sensory tests depicting altered sensation. Areas that are hypersensitive have been marked in red. Areas that are hyposensitive would be marked in green for ease of documentation. The hypersensitive areas represent the progression of sensory recovery.

**Fig 16-47**   Cross-sectional CT scan of a patient with an extremely resorbed posterior mandible. The neurovascular bundle is lying superficially within the groove that is visible. Some idea of the amount of bone loss can be obtained from the wax jaw registration block, which is visible as the radiolucent area above the ridge.

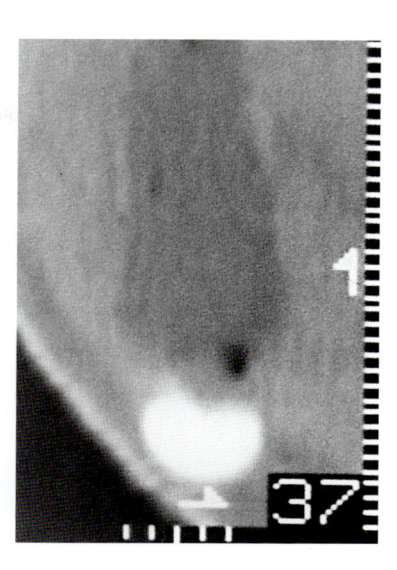

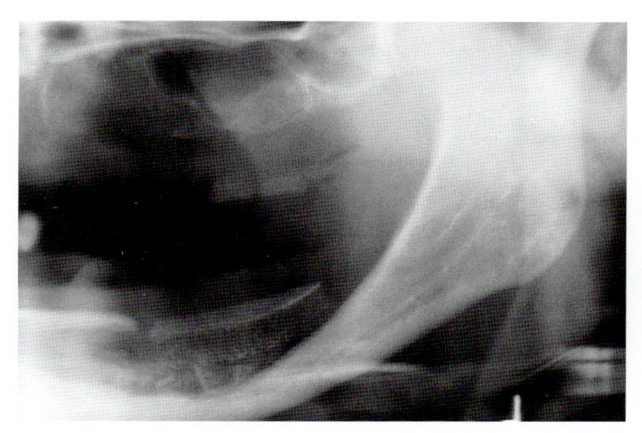

**Fig 16-48**   A panoral panoramic tomograph of the left side of the jaw after the placement of the graft. The nerve can be seen emerging through its new foramen distal to the position of the graft. The neurovascular bundle can be seen. Note that the graft has been secured and is in two pieces. (Graft placed by B. O'Riordan, London, UK.)

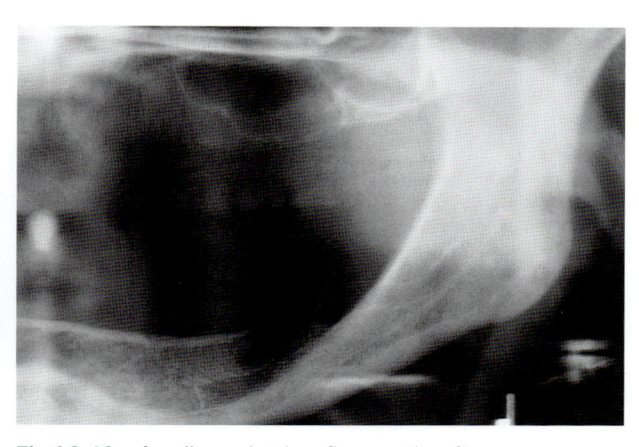

**Fig 16-49**   A radiograph taken five months after surgery, showing that the two pieces of graft have become confluent with each other and the residual bone.

Nerve repositioning is carried out with the graft being placed at the same time or at a subsequent visit (Fig 16-48). It is preferable to place the graft at the same time, as this eliminates the need to locate the nerve, which lies within the soft tissues, during a second stage. In this procedure, it is necessary to sever the incisive branch, which has minimal significance. The anatomical course of the inferior alveolar nerve will, therefore, be changed and will require to be recorded on the patient's notes. Implants are not inserted at the same time as the bone graft but at a subsequent visit, once remodelling has taken place and the graft has vascularised (Figs 16-49–16-52).

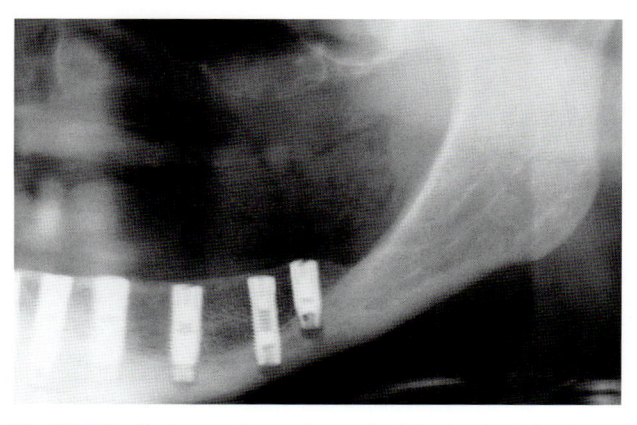

**Fig 16-50**   Post-operative radiograph of the implants in place.

349

III   Augmentation

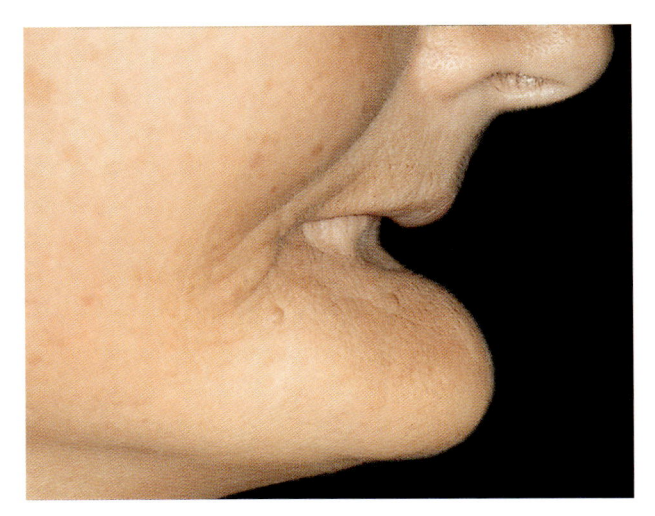

**Fig 16-51**   Lateral view of the patient showing the preoperative profile. Note the increased naso-labial angle depicting the loss of maxillary bone in height. The protrusion of the chin is a clear sign of overclosure (same patient as in Fig 16-47).

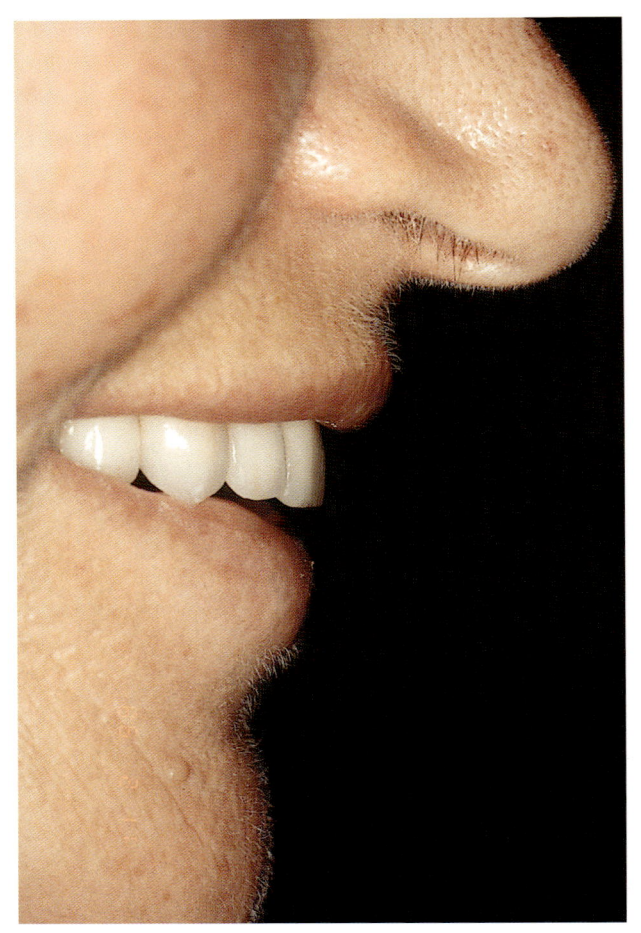

**Fig 16-52**   Lateral view of the same patient showing the re-establishment of facial features, which had been lost through atrophy. The fixed definitive restoration can also be seen.

## Surgical Technique

### Incisions

The incision is made on the crest bisecting the attached tissue (Fig 16-53). It must be borne in mind that the nerve may be dehiscent in areas and damage must be avoided by placing the incision judiciously. The incision is extended from the midline to the retromolar area. The reflection of the periosteum is carried out to provide adequate exposure, particularly with respect to the bone graft, which will need to be covered.

### Access to the Inferior Alveolar Canal

Access to the inferior alveolar canal is gained via the mental foramen, which may lie on the superior surface of the mandible (Fig 16-54). The incisive branch is

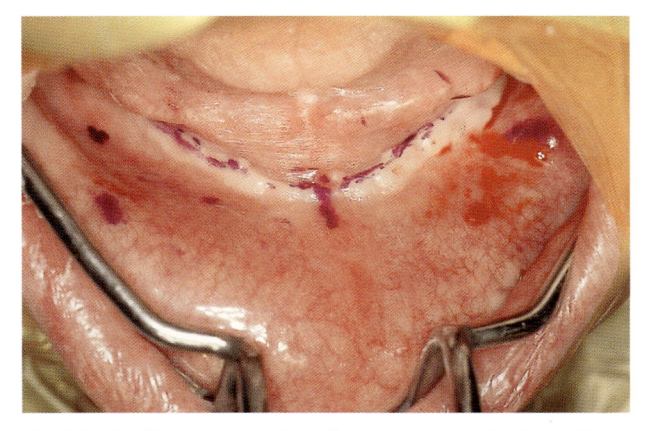

**Fig 16-53**   Preoperative view of a severely resorbed mandible prior to nerve repositioning and bone grafting. The genial tubercle is visible above the keratinised tissue identifying the ridge crest. The position of the incision along the crest of the ridge as well as the position of the mental foramina can be seen marked.

16 Posterior Mandible

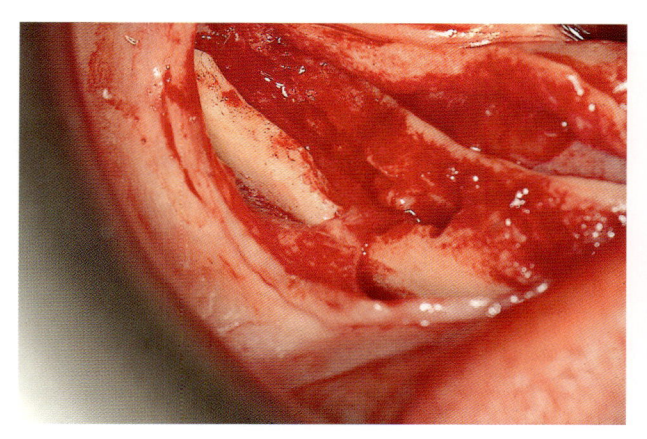

**Fig 16-54** Intraoperative view of the right side with the mental foramen and inferior alveolar neurovascular bundle exposed. Note the position of the foramen and the access to the inferior alveolar canal via the superior surface of the mandible.

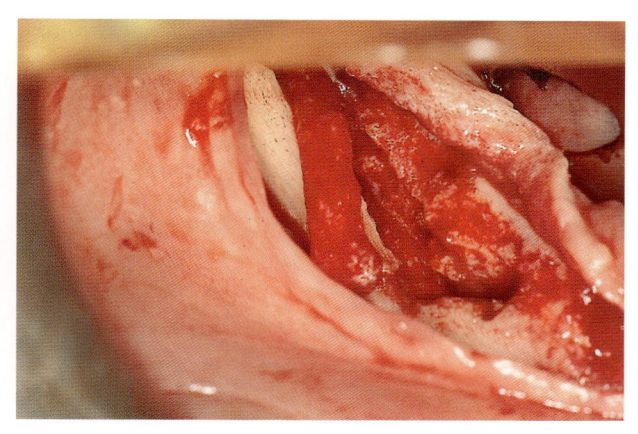

**Fig 16-55** The neurovascular bundle being repositioned. The incisive branch has been severed.

traced anteriorly by approximately 5 mm and severed (Fig 16-55). The inferior alveolar canal is approached from the crestal aspect of the mandible and is exposed and repositioned, creating a foramen for its exit in the region of the second molar.

### Bone Graft

Bone grafts are harvested simultaneously from the iliac crest and secured into place using ligatures, sutures or screws, as indicated (Fig 16-56). Under certain circumstances bone grafting may need to be carried out at a later stage.

### Implant Insertion

Implants should be inserted on completion of remodelling and vascularisation of the graft. The positioning of the implants is ideally to traverse from the grafted bone and to gain anchorage within the residual mandibular bone. They are allowed to integrate for three to six months prior to exposure and restoration.

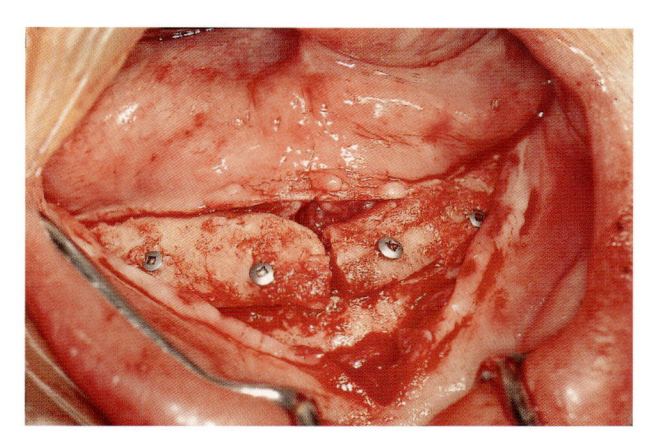

**Fig 16-56** Autogenous onlay bone grafts, harvested from the iliac crest, are secured in place prior to closure. Implants will be placed approximately three months after grafting to allow sufficient time for healing. (Grafts harvested by Mr H. Plaha.)

## Summary

Flowchart 16-1 gives an overview of the assessment of the posterior mandible.

## III  Augmentation

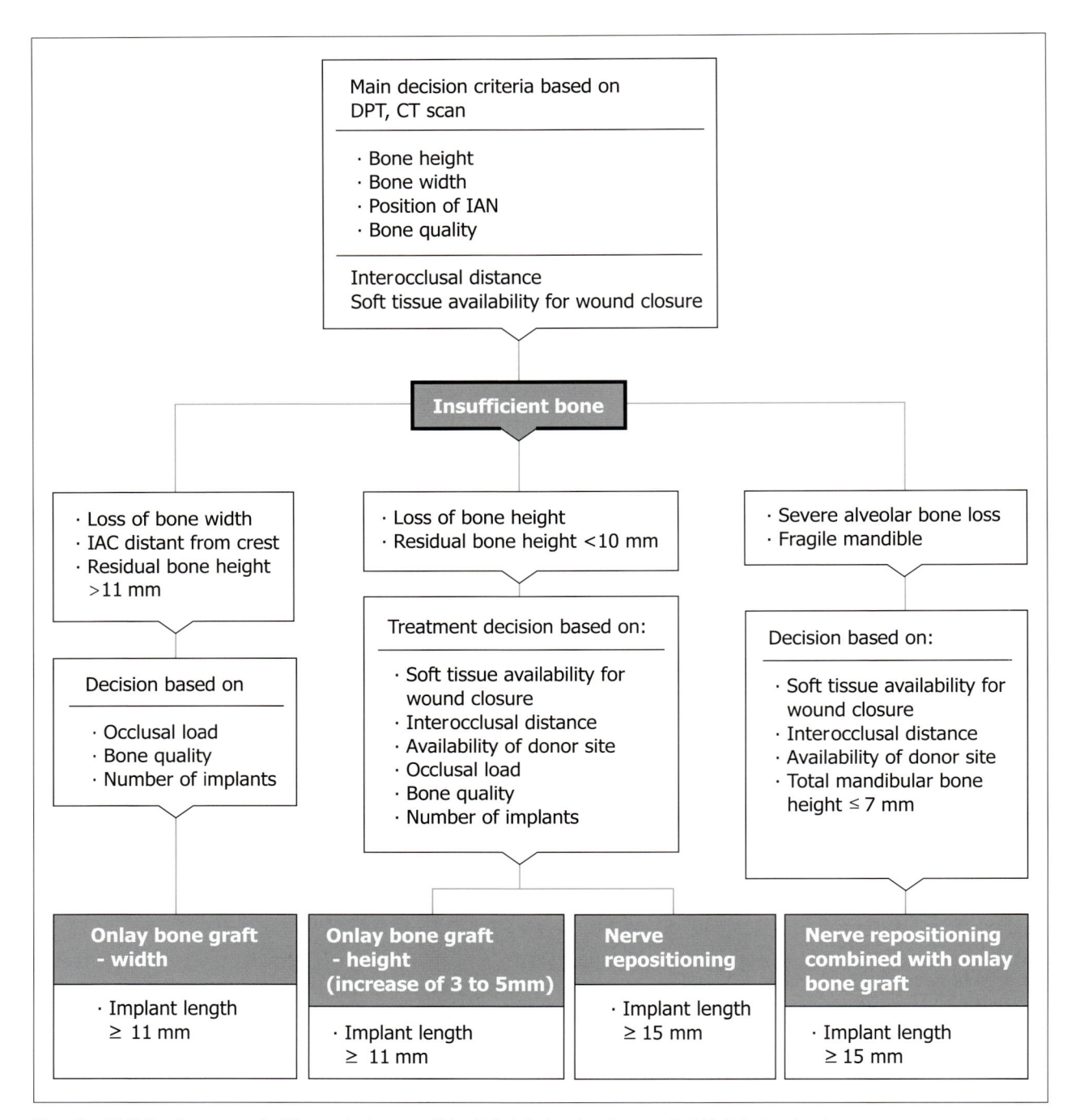

```
                    ┌─────────────────────────────────────┐
                    │ Main decision criteria based on     │
                    │ DPT, CT scan                        │
                    ├─────────────────────────────────────┤
                    │  · Bone height                      │
                    │  · Bone width                       │
                    │  · Position of IAN                  │
                    │  · Bone quality                     │
                    ├─────────────────────────────────────┤
                    │ Interocclusal distance              │
                    │ Soft tissue availability for wound  │
                    │ closure                             │
                    └─────────────────────────────────────┘
                                      │
                           ▼ **Insufficient bone** ▼
```

| · Loss of bone width<br>· IAC distant from crest<br>· Residual bone height >11 mm | · Loss of bone height<br>· Residual bone height <10 mm | · Severe alveolar bone loss<br>· Fragile mandible |
|---|---|---|
| **Decision based on**<br>· Occlusal load<br>· Bone quality<br>· Number of implants | **Treatment decision based on:**<br>· Soft tissue availability for wound closure<br>· Interocclusal distance<br>· Availability of donor site<br>· Occlusal load<br>· Bone quality<br>· Number of implants | **Decision based on:**<br>· Soft tissue availability for wound closure<br>· Interocclusal distance<br>· Availability of donor site<br>· Total mandibular bone height ≤ 7 mm |
| **Onlay bone graft - width**<br>· Implant length ≥ 11 mm | **Onlay bone graft - height (increase of 3 to 5mm)**<br>· Implant length ≥ 11 mm | **Nerve repositioning**<br>· Implant length ≥ 15 mm | **Nerve repositioning combined with onlay bone graft**<br>· Implant length ≥ 15 mm |

**Flowchart 16-1**  Assessment of the posterior mandible. IAC, inferior alveolar canal; IAN, inferior alveolar nerve.

# Chapter 17

# Corrective Soft Tissue Surgery

## Introduction

The aim of the protocols that have been outlined in this book is to establish clear outcomes and to base them on predictable procedures. Human variation in terms of host response might lead to unplanned outcomes requiring corrective surgery. Corrective soft tissue surgery is designed to improve the functional and aesthetic outcome in situations where compromise has taken place.

This chapter will deal with some of the surgical procedures available for the manipulation of soft tissues and provide examples of situations where they may be used.

It is essential that a clinician understands the principles underlying successful soft tissue surgery so that the techniques can be applied to a greater range of situations than those outlined here. Flowchart 17-1 provides the reader with guidance during the decision-making process with regard to the most suitable procedure. However, for the sake of convenience specific procedures will be outlined, with possible applications listed.

The periodontal literature is replete with procedures designed to correct soft tissue deficiencies associated with the teeth. It is not the intention to cover these here. However, the reader should become familiar with these as they outline certain principles. Some of the procedures described in the periodontal and preprosthetic surgical literature will also be covered here because of their relevance to implant dentistry.

## Vestibuloplasty

A large area of mobile non-keratinised peri-implant mucosa may result in a number of problems for the patient. These may be of an aesthetic nature where poor-quality tissue is inconsistent with the adjacent areas. A broad band of mobile tissue may also result in functional problems that relate to considerable difficulties in hygiene; these, in turn, may cause inflammation. It goes without saying that inflammation with its associated pain and swelling will result in poorer oral hygiene, which, in turn, will compound the situation.

Mobile, non-keratinised peri-implant mucosa can often be found where there is advanced atrophy and the keratinised tissue is essentially non-existent and muscle attachments are present at the level of the ridge crest. Following implant exposure, the inability of the patient to maintain normal hygiene procedures for these areas may require intervention.

## III Augmentation

**Deficien**

- Muscle attachment or mobile non-keratinised peri-implant mucosa
- Fistula

- Localised muscle attachment (frenum)
- Wide area (due to atrophy) of mobile non-keratinised peri-implant mucosa
- · Premature exposure of implant
  · Perforation of flap during surgery (e.g. during bone graft procedure)

- Frenectomy
- Vestibuloplasty
- Free gingival graft

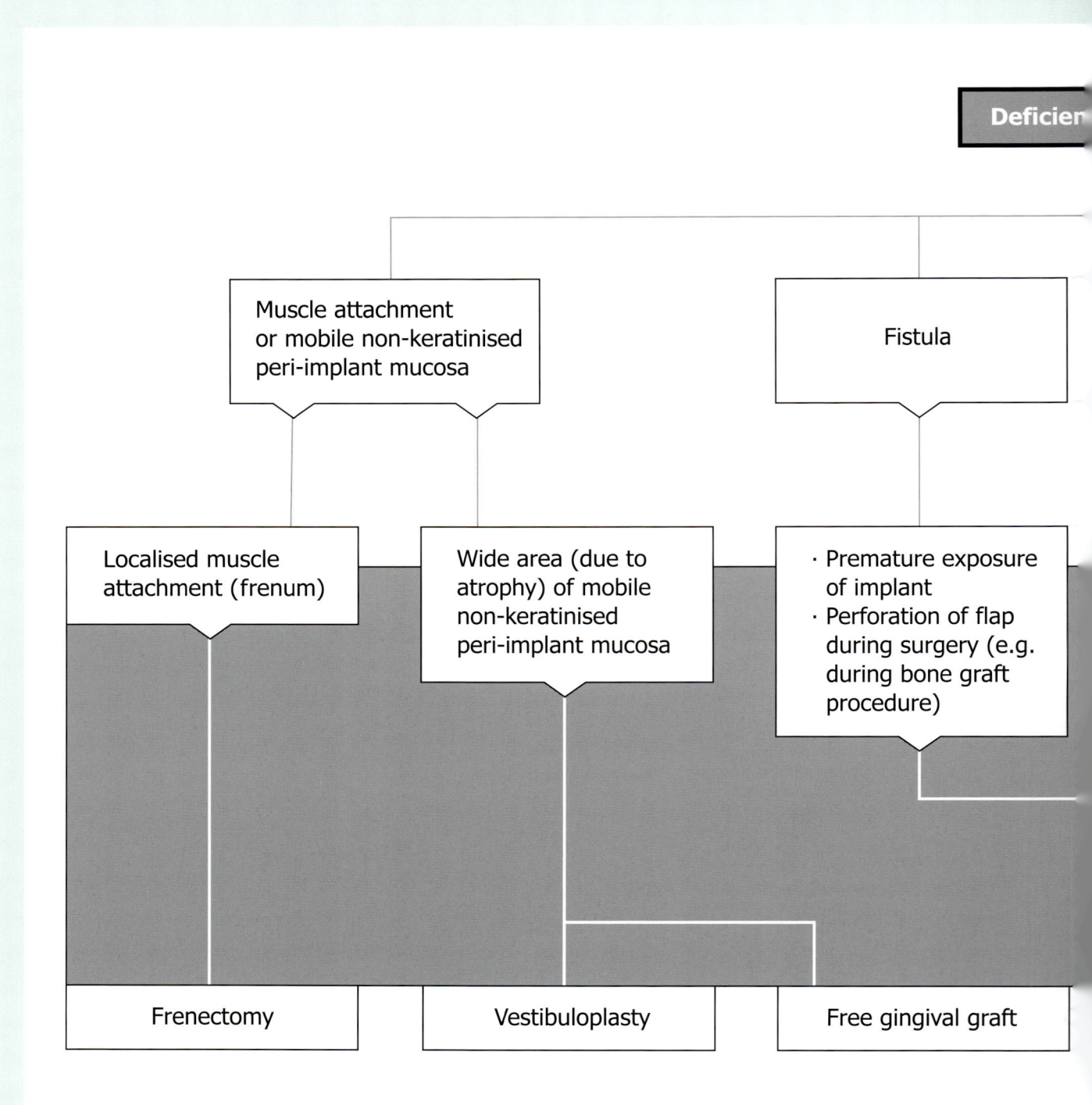

**Flowchart 17-1** Corrective soft tissue surgery. OAF, oro-antral fistula.

**17  Corrective Soft Tissue Surgery**

roblem

| Socket | Inadequate thickness or height of peri-implant soft-tissue | Absent interdental papilla |

- Extraction socket (immediate implant)
- Communicating fistula (e.g. OAF)

- Peri-implant recession
- No keratinised tissue

Adequate hard tissue support

| Connective tissue graft | Pedicle graft | Composite (keratinised and connective tissue) graft |

The situation may also be found after bone grafting of atrophic ridges with atrophic mucosa. The situation is often made worse by advancing tissues to effect closure over the graft, which may be quite substantial in size.

### Surgical Principles

A vestibuloplasty is designed to recreate a vestibule and does so by reattaching muscle insertions apically and producing non-mobile peri-implant soft tissues. The reattachment of the muscles may be enhanced by the creation of attached keratinised mucosa, using a free gingival graft. This will improve the stability of the soft tissues around implant abutments and superstructures.[261-264]

The surgical technique involves a partial-thickness incision around the implant abutment, which does not incise the periosteum. Care should be taken to ensure that the muscle attachments are dissected, leaving the periosteum attached to the bone. Scissors or a scalpel may be used for this procedure. The muscles are elevated with the flap and sutured to the periosteum more apically. The clinician must bear in mind that reattachment of the muscles in a more apical position may affect the facial features.

The raw exposed periosteum may be allowed to epithelialise. A dressing may be used to protect the periosteum. Alternatively, a free gingival graft can be sutured onto the periosteum, which is still attached and, therefore, ensures stability of the graft for predictable revascularisation. A free gingival graft will provide a greater thickness of attached mucosa, which is keratinised and will, therefore, enhance aesthetics and hygiene due to its greater robustness (Figs 17-1 and 17-2; see Case 1 below).

## Frenectomy

Localised muscle attachments that may result in a compromised outcome, such as gingival recession or marginal inflammation around an implant, should be addressed in the same manner as that outlined in the periodontal literature. Sectioning of the muscle attachment and its reattachment to an apical position is an effective way of eliminating a potential or actual problem.

## Free Gingival Graft

Tissue for a free gingival graft is harvested from the palate and can be used to cover the exposed periosteum. Since the graft is non-vascularised, its blood supply is obtained from the underlying periosteum; the graft must, therefore, be completely stable and free from any movement in order to enable vascularisation to take place. It should be borne in mind that the surface texture and colour of the graft is determined by the donor site and may differ from that of the recipient site. This has some consequences for small grafts that are limited to one or two teeth.

### Surgical Technique
#### Preparation of the Recipient Site

The preparation of the recipient site has already been outlined above for vestibuloplasty. The size of the required graft may either be measured directly or a template can be cut to fit over the area to be grafted. This will enable the graft outline to be marked at the donor site to ensure that the correct size of tissue is harvested.

#### Preparation of the Donor Site

Keratinised tissue is most commonly found in the palate. The amount required should be marked prior to the incision. This will ensure that the correct size is obtained. The graft is obtained using a scalpel to section an approximately 1 to 2 mm thickness of epithelial tissue. This will regenerate and re-establish the sensory innervation at both the donor and recipient sites. The donor site may be left to epithelialise or may be protected by a periodontal dressing or an acrylic resin splint.

#### Securing the Graft

The graft is best secured by means of sutures that will immobilise it. Vicryl 3-0 sutures may be used as locating sutures, and 6-0 sutures are most suitable for securing the graft to the periosteum. Additional stabilisation of the graft can be achieved with acrylic resin templates secured by means of a periodontal dressing.

17   Corrective Soft Tissue Surgery

**Fig 17-1** Incisions at the recipient and donor sites for vestibuloplasty and free gingival graft. (1) A split-thickness labial incision is made to reposition the muscle attachments apically. The periosteum is not elevated to ensure that the blood supply to the bone graft is maintained. (2) An incision is made for harvesting palatal keratinised tissue graft of 2-mm thickness. The superficial layer is harvested without interrupting the subepithelial mucosa, the nerve or the blood supply to the marginal tissues. This enables relatively large areas to be harvested.

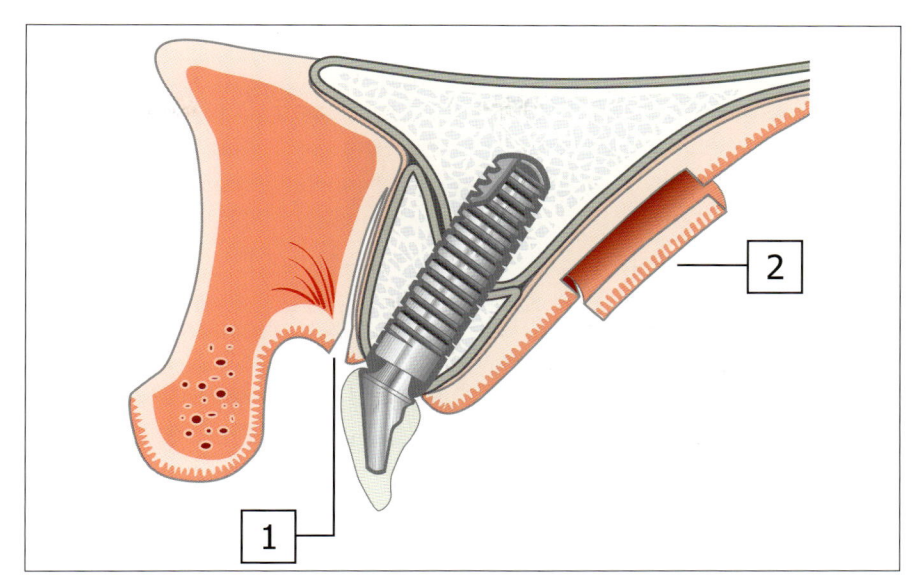

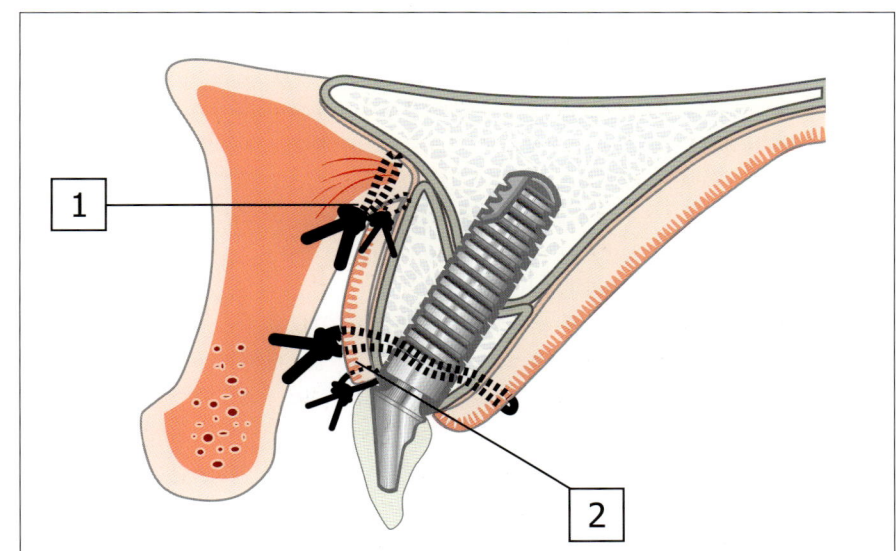

**Fig 17-2** Diagram of the completed procedure. (1) The vestibuloplasty has been completed, with the muscle attachments repositioned and sutured in a more apical position using resorbable sutures (3-0 Vicryl Rapide). (2) The free gingival graft is located in place with 3-0 Vicryl sutures. The edges are secured with 6-0 Vicryl sutures to stabilise and accurately position all the margins.

## Subepithelial Connective Tissue Grafts

Connective tissue grafts are non-vascularised and have no epithelium. They are designed to obtain their blood supply via one or both of their non-epithelialised surfaces. They are obtained from the palate and are very versatile. They have numerous applications for the closure of fistulas and the increase in soft tissue thickness.[265–273]

### Applications

Two examples of the application of connective tissue grafts are given.

### Closure of Fistulas

Connective tissue grafts lend themselves extremely well to the closure of fistulas and perforations before, during or after surgical procedures. A connective tissue graft may be used as an underlay to close a perforation in a flap made during surgery, such as a bone graft procedure. Small oro-antral fistulas can also be repaired. The principles behind these procedures are the creation of a barrier beneath the fistula or defect with a connective tissue graft, which will predictably become vascularised by the surrounding tissues through both the surfaces. The size of the area in contact with a potential blood supply increases the potential for successful revascularisation of the graft. Larger defects, such as immediate implants requiring delayed loading, will be viable only if a large connective tissue graft underlies the surrounding tissues. They may also be used to eliminate tattoos caused by amalgam used in conventional or endodontic restorations.

### Increasing soft tissue bulk

Connective tissue grafts may be used in situations where compromised healing has led to a deficiency in the soft tissue. Gingival recession around the neck of an implant or the loss of an interdental papilla can be repaired with the minimum of disruption, but with only a limited degree of predictability. A connective tissue graft can be added to increase the tissue bulk by creating a pocket into which the graft can be secured. A graft of this type can also be used to create keratinised tissue, with the advantage that the connective tissue graft will attain the colour and texture of the surrounding epithelium as it epithelialises.

### Surgical Techniques
#### Preparation of the Recipient Site

The recipient site is prepared by first creating a pocket within the tissues between the periosteum and the epithelium into which the connective tissue graft will be inserted. The size of the required graft is measured and the data transferred to the palate by way of an outline, so that a graft of the correct size and shape can be harvested. If gingival augmentation is required, the pocket is created on the labial aspect. For the correction of fistulas and defects, the pocket is prepared in such a way that the graft will block the fistula and will span beyond the margins of the fistula. In both cases, one or more sutures are used to draw the connective tissue graft into the correct position. Additional sutures are used to keep it secure.

#### Preparation of the Donor Site

A single incision made parallel to the ridge crest, or two incisions at right angles to each other creating an 'L' shape, may be used to gain access to the subepithelial connective tissue. The sequence of incisions is depicted below in Fig 17-57.

## Composite Graft

Composite grafts are essentially connective tissue grafts that have had a proportion of the keratinised epithelium harvested with the subepithelial connective tissue. Establishing the vascularity of the graft will depend on the size of the surface area of the non-epithelialised connective tissue, as it is through this area that revascularisation will be achieved.

### Applications
#### Creating Keratinised Tissue

A band of keratinised tissue can be created around the cervical margin of an implant. The graft is obtained from the palate and inserted into a pocket on the labial aspect of the implant requiring soft tissue augmentation. The graft is inserted into the pocket with the help of a suture and secured with finer sutures to precisely position the keratinised band. The graft obtains its blood supply from the interface between the connective tissue and the surrounding vascularised tissues.

## Pedicle Flap

The pedicle flap described here is a subepithelial vascularised flap, which is obtained from the palate and mobilised to the area where it is required in two different ways (lateral or inverted). The choice of technique will depend on the availability of tissue. However, the blood supply to the pedicle will play a significant part in the design.

Pedicle flaps can be used for the closure of fistulas (e.g. oro-antral fistula), for the creation of soft tissue bulk and for the creation of attached keratinised tissue.

### Applications for the Closure of Epithelial Continuity Defects
#### Oro-antral Fistulas

Pedicle flaps provide an excellent and predictable way of closing oro-antral fistulas without the loss of attached tissue, which would occur if a buccal advancement flap is used. The viability of the flap, coupled with its insertion into a subepithelial pocket surrounding the defect, offers predictable closure of the defect without anatomical compromise. Subsequent procedures to repair any bony defects can easily be carried out.

### Socket Closure after Immediate Implant Placement

Immediate placement of implants at the time of extraction may well be coupled with immediate loading or transgingival healing. However, where adequate stability of the implant has not been achieved, delayed loading becomes necessary. The pedicle flap can very effectively provide soft tissue coverage over the resultant socket without the loss of attached tissue. In addition, the bulk of the labial soft tissues can effectively be increased.

This procedure may be indicated where immediate placement of the implants is desired but the soft tissue contours need to be improved. A pedicle flap will improve the soft tissue contours and enable the loading to be commenced six weeks after implantation.

### Closure over Bone Grafts

Where there are palatal bone deficiencies and a crestal incision has been used to gain access to the bony crest, closure of the wound may be difficult to achieve. In these cases, a pedicle flap may be used.

### Closure over Implants

Closure over implants may become necessary where additional hard or soft tissue augmentation procedures need to be carried out after implant exposure. This may occur after the completion of the prosthetic phase. Closure over the implant can be predictably achieved without palatal repositioning of any labial keratinised mucosa.

### Applications for Increasing Soft Tissue Bulk
### Creating Interdental Papillae

Interdental papillae can be created with a pedicle flap provided that there is adequate bone support. The vascularity of the flap results in a sustainable increase in papillary height.

### Creating Labial Soft Tissue Bulk

Increasing the bulk of the soft tissue on the labial aspect of the implant can be achieved using this technique prior to implant exposure. However, if this procedure is carried out after exposure of the implant, the treatment will involve removal of the abutment and closure over the implant. The use of an interim provisional restoration will then be necessary while the graft heals, and the implant will be exposed at a later stage. It may be necessary to use a different abutment if the recurrence of recession is to be avoided.

### Surgical Technique

The design of the flap should comply with two basic principles:
- maintenance of an adequate blood supply
- mobilisation of sufficient tissue to successfully meet the objective.

Access to the subepithelial connective tissue is gained by elevating the palatal epithelium using a split-thickness flap. The incision design will depend on the location of the recipient site and the type of flap that is to be used. The shape of the connective tissue required for the flap is incised, often to include the periosteum. This is elevated and transferred to the recipient site, maintaining an intact blood supply. The insertion of the connective tissue flap must be subepithelial and must not overlie any region of epithelium. Attachment of the connective tissue to the recipient site can then be assured.

A suture (3-0 Vicryl) may be used to draw the edge of the flap into the subepithelial pocket that has been created. Additional fine sutures (6-0 Vicryl) may be used to approximate the margins more precisely. The split-thickness epithelial flap is then repositioned and sutured over the donor site and a proportion of the flap.

### Lateral Pedicle Flap

The lateral pedicle flap is most commonly used in the second premolar and molar regions for either of the purposes described above. This type of flap is extremely reliable as it can be designed to receive an abundant blood supply from the greater palatine vessels. There is usually sufficient tissue present in the anterior part of the maxilla to allow it to be displaced laterally over the recipient site.

The incision is made within the socket or fistula that requires coverage. The split-thickness incision is extended anteriorly along the crest of the ridge adjacent to any remaining teeth. The anterior extent of the incision will be limited by the thickness of the tissue under the rugae and by the anterior teeth.

Planning for surgery will, therefore, require the thickness of the tissues to be measured preoperatively. Local anaesthetic needles provide an atraumatic and effective way of doing this. At the anterior extent of this incision, a perpendicular split-thickness incision provides access to the subepithelial connective tissue. The incision is then extended distally as required. The split-thickness flap is elevated carefully, ensuring that no perforation of the connective tissue through to the bone takes place.

The outline of the pedicle flap is incised using two parallel incisions running mesiodistally. A perpendicular incision is then made at the anterior to limit the length of the flap. The parallel incisions may need to be extended distal to the defect to provide sufficient mobility of the flap.

The flap can be elevated as required and rotated laterally to cover the defect or bulk the labial tissue. The flap must not cross the epithelium and must be inserted into a pocket created within the subepithelial tissue on the labial aspect of the defect. The graft is drawn into the pocket and secured with 3-0 Vicryl sutures, while 6-0 Vicryl sutures can be used to fix the graft precisely and to reposition the split-thickness epithelial flap.

### Inverted Pedicle Flap

The inverted pedicle flap is most commonly used in the incisor or canine regions. This is often because there is limited tissue available for lateral transposition in these areas. Although there are occasions when tissue can be transferred across the midline, this is generally not possible because of the thin tissue in the midline and the compromised blood and sensory nerve supply.

The incision for the split-thickness epithelial flap is made within the margins of the socket or fistula that requires covering. The distal extension of the incision is made alongside the alveolar crest so that the maximum benefit is derived from the palatal blood supply. Access may be extended as far back as the distal aspect of the second molar, provided that the incision is not in close proximity to the midline. If a broader graft is required, the distal extension should not go beyond the distal aspect of the first molar to ensure that there is no interruption of the neurovascular supply from the greater palatine foramen.

The pedicle is incised using two parallel incisions running along mesiodistally. The distal incision perpendicular to the parallel incisions will interrupt the blood supply from the greater palatine vessels. The success of the pedicle graft will, therefore, depend on the collateral blood supply and will require a large area of attachment to the underlying bone on the anterior aspect of the pedicle flap. Typically, for one unit of the pedicle flap that will remain attached to the underlying bone, two units of pedicle will be required. It should be borne in mind that, of the two units of the inverted flap, one will overlay the attached portion and only one unit will be available for the required purpose.

## Corrective Soft Tissue Surgery: Clinical Cases

### Case 1: Vestibuloplasty and Free Gingival Graft

This case study demonstrates the use of vestibuloplasty and a free gingival graft to recreate a sulcus following bone graft surgery.

A 60-year-old woman presented with extensive hard and soft tissue deficiencies. These were corrected using bone grafts harvested from the iliac crest. A remote palatal incision was used. Soft tissue coverage of the grafts resulted in the loss of the vestibular sulcus (Figs 17-3–17-16).

17  Corrective Soft Tissue Surgery

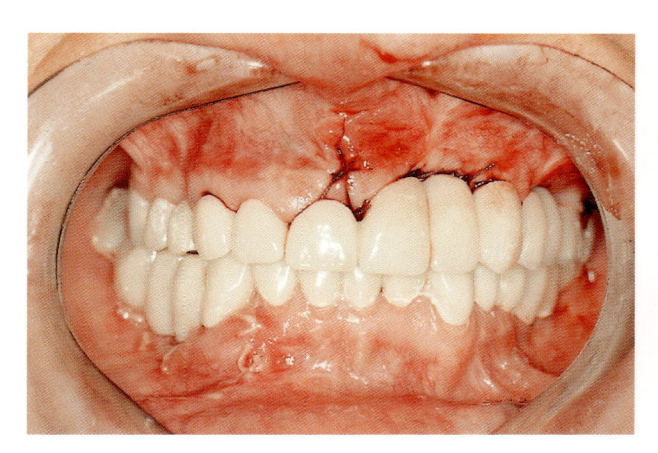

**Fig 17-3**  Labial view of the patient at the start of treatment, showing the provisional metal-acrylic bridge in situ. The extent of deficiencies on the patient's left-hand side is apparent from the increased length of the teeth.

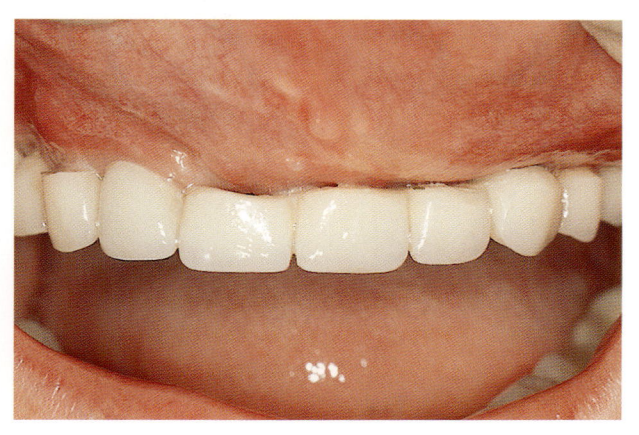

**Fig 17-4**  Labial view of the provisional maxillary restoration following bone graft surgery. The ridge has been overcontoured to compensate for the remodelling process. The reduced size of the teeth on the provisional restoration as well as the loss of sulcular height is evident. No keratinised attached tissue can be seen.

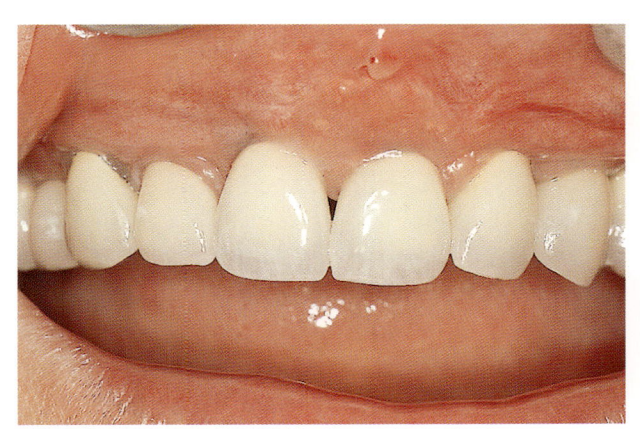

**Fig 17-5**  Labial view of the definitive maxillary metal-ceramic restoration showing good tooth form.

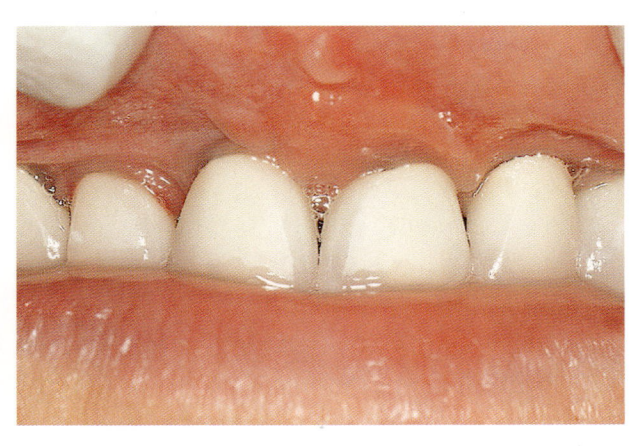

**Fig 17-6**  Close-up of the maxillary teeth emerging through non-keratinised mobile soft tissues.

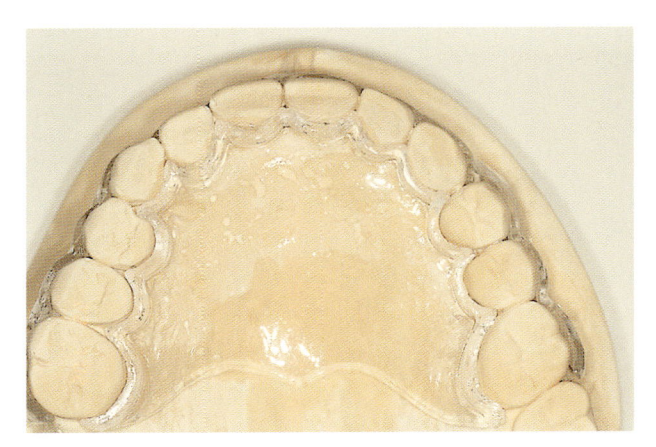

**Fig 17-7**  The laboratory cast showing a clear vacuum-formed splint for the protection of the palate following the harvesting of the keratinised soft tissue graft.

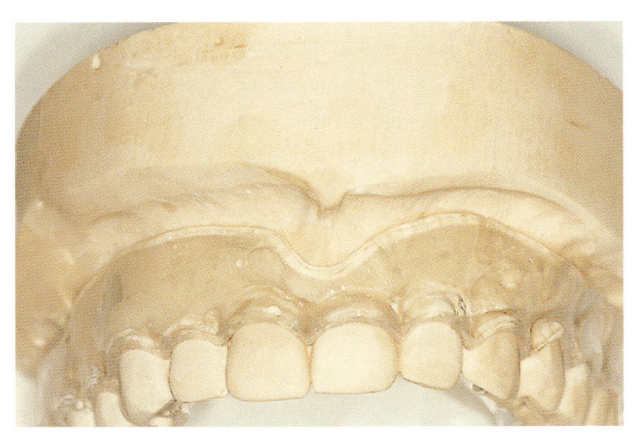

**Fig 17-8**  Laboratory cast showing a clear vacuum-formed splint designed for use on the labial aspect to provide stability for the soft tissue graft.

## III Augmentation

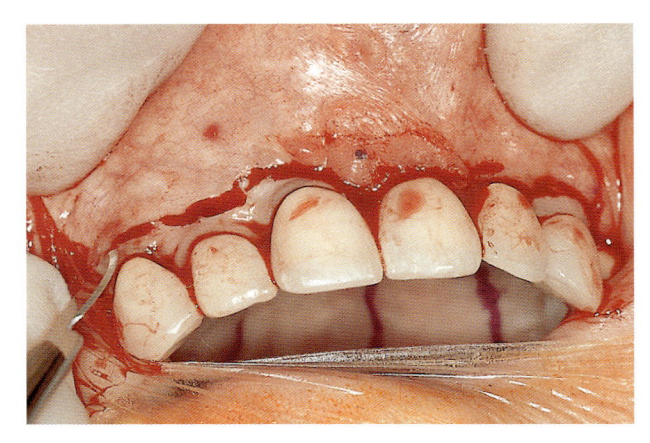

**Fig 17-9** The incision around the cervical margins of the definitive restoration can be seen being commenced. This split-thickness incision is depicted in Fig 17-1.

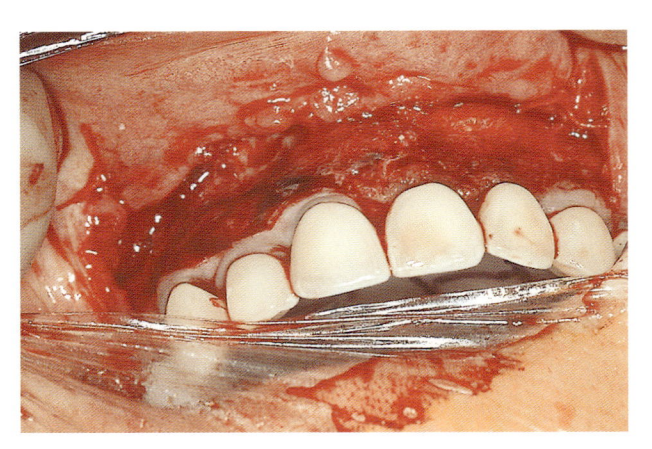

**Fig 17-10** Labial view showing the split-thickness flap reflected with the periosteum exposed. The periosteum overlying the bone graft will provide the blood supply for the proposed free gingival (epithelial) graft. The muscle attachments have been reflected for repositioning apically. The size of the graft required is measured.

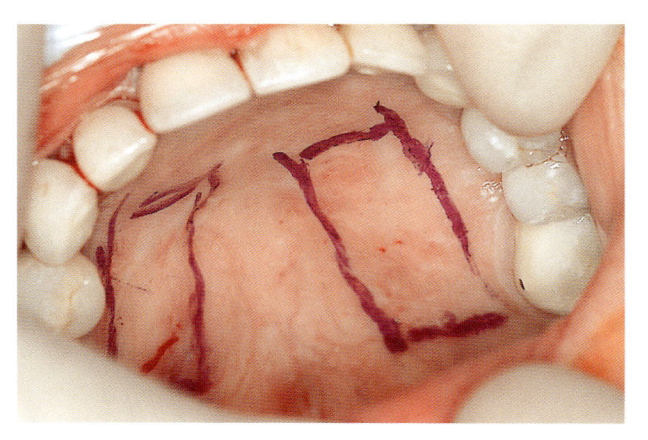

**Fig 17-11** View of the palate showing the outline of the grafts to be harvested based on the measurements made on the labial aspect.

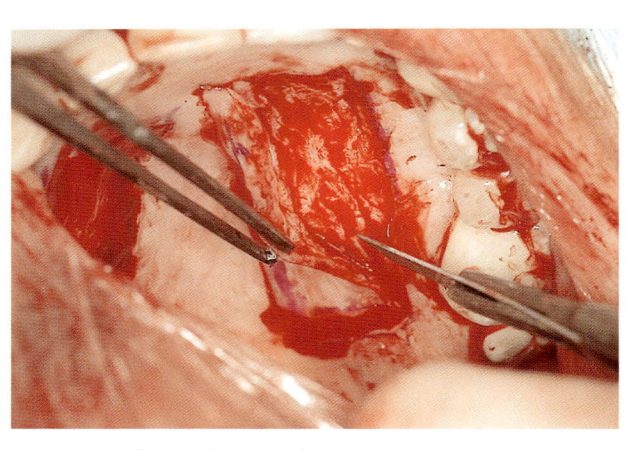

**Fig 17-12** The epithelial graft being harvested with the submucosal tissues intact, as illustrated in Fig 17-1.

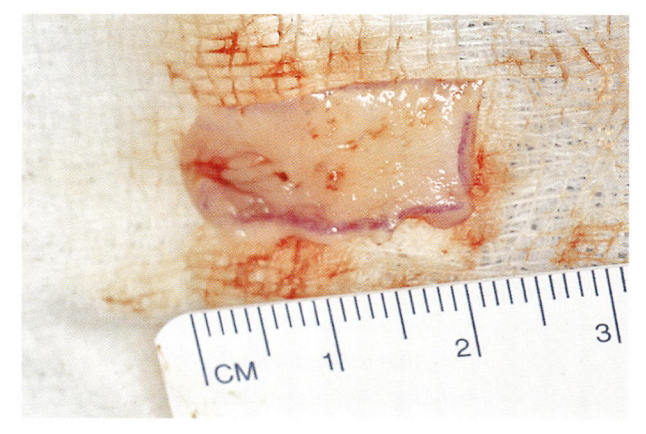

**Fig 17-13** The graft is stored on gauze soaked with sterile saline. The dimensions of the graft are confirmed.

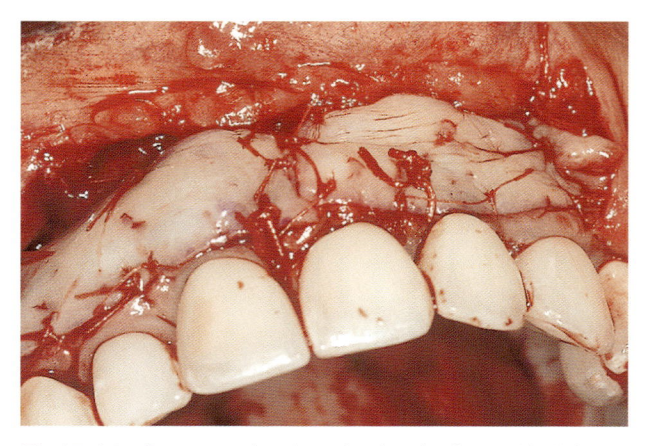

**Fig 17-14** Post-operative view showing the free epithelial grafts sutured in place.

362

## 17  Corrective Soft Tissue Surgery

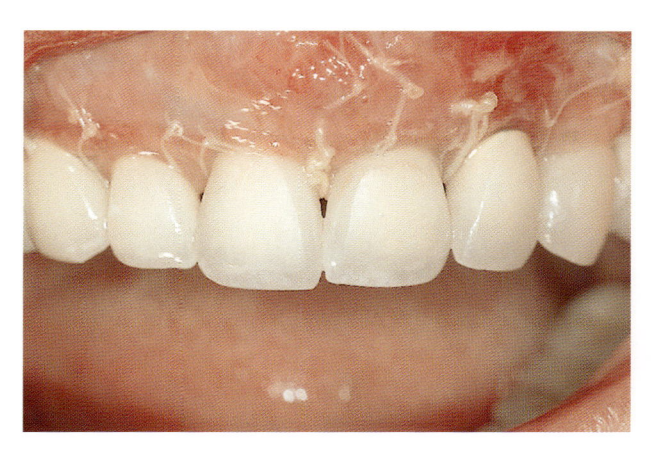

**Fig 17-15**  Labial view of the graft after the removal of the labial splint after a two-week healing period. The graft can be seen to be vascularised.

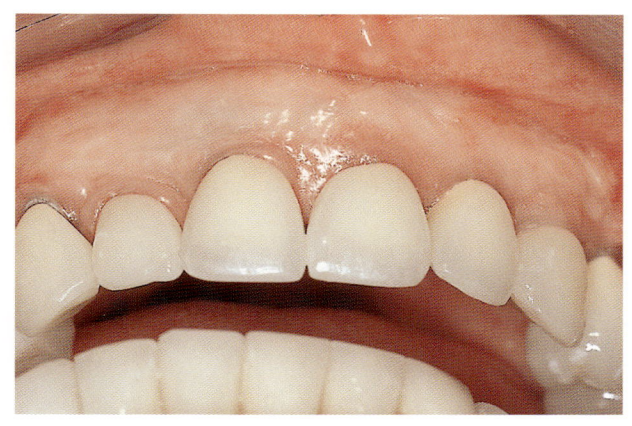

**Fig 17-16**  The post-operative view of the labial soft tissues, demonstrating the recreation of the sulcus and the presence of keratinised soft tissues.

### Case 2: Localised Vestibuloplasty and Free Gingival Graft

A young female with a high smile-line was referred following the failure of two implants and failure of the subsequent bone graft. The severe hard tissue loss and soft tissue scarring resulted in the need for careful management of the reconstruction. Reconstruction and implant placement was carried out with advancement of the scar tissue to overlie the rebuilt ridge. Advancement of the flap also resulted in muscle attachments close to the crest. Repositioning of the muscle attachments and establishment of keratinised tissue was carried out using a vestibuloplasty and a free gingival graft. The soft tissue procedure was timed to occur in the interval between implant placement and exposure as this window provided the best opportunity in terms of vascularisation of the graft and the soft tissues after graft and implant surgery. At the same time, the restorative treatment could be carried out to the stable hard and soft tissue complex (Figs 17-17–17-32).

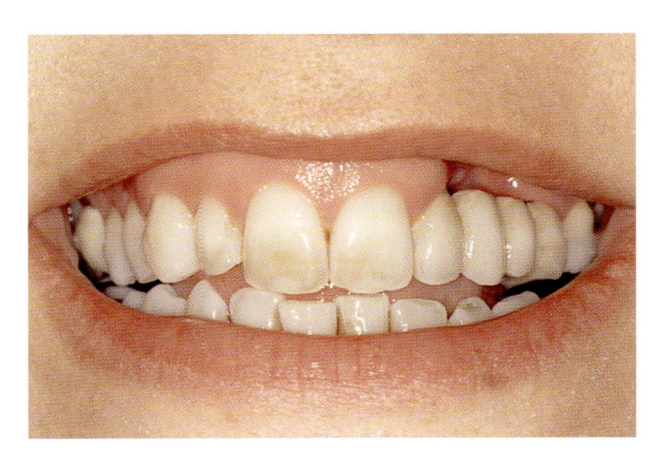

**Fig 17-17**  Anterior view of a patient smiling, showing the deficiency on the left-hand side caused by implant loss.

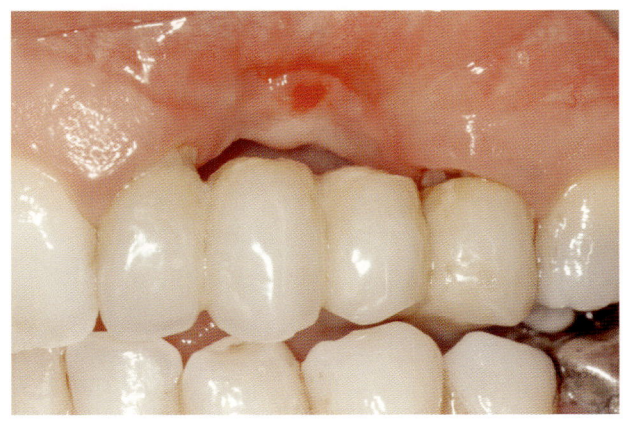

**Fig 17-18**  Intraoral view of the left side showing the deficiency in relation to the provisional prosthesis.

III  Augmentation

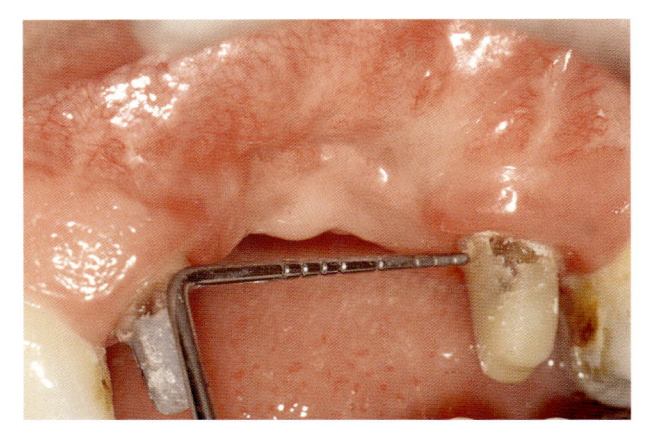

Fig 17-19  A close up of the deficiency with the periodontal probe identifying the dimensions. The deficiency in volume and nature of the soft tissue is also visible. Little or no keratinised tissue is visible.

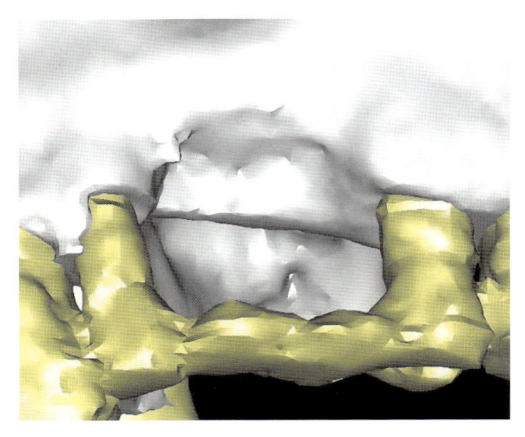

Fig 17-20  CT 3D view showing the bony deficiency.

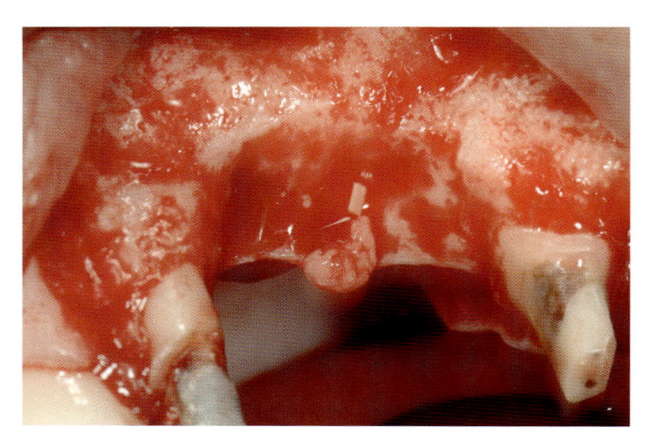

Fig 17-21  Intraoperative view of the deficiency.

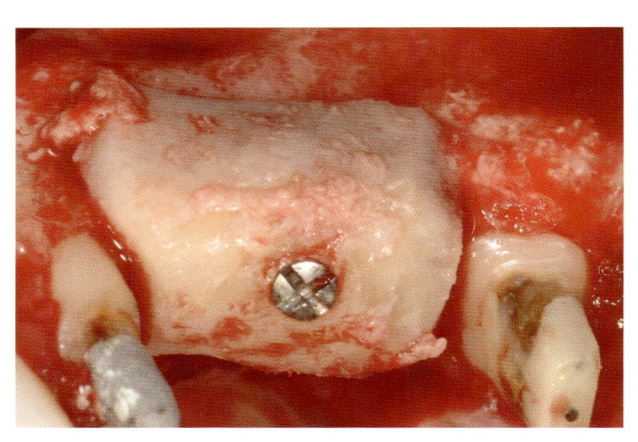

Fig 17-22  Well-adapted cortico-cancellous bone graft obtained from the iliac crest secured in place.

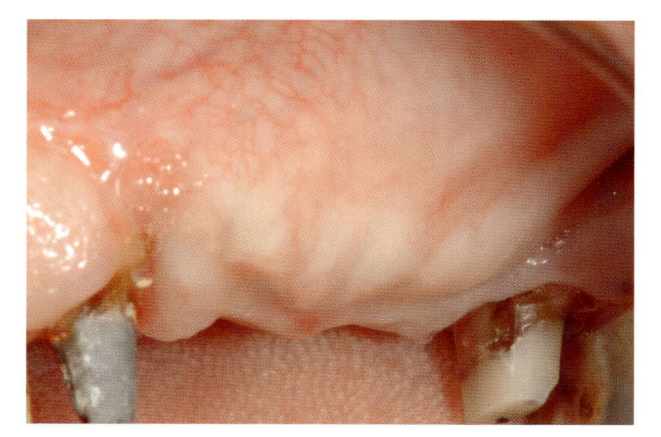

Fig 17-23  Image of the grafted site showing good coverage of the graft by the soft tissues and the bulk created. However, non-keratinised unattached tissue can be seen and, furthermore, muscle attachments are positioned close to the crest.

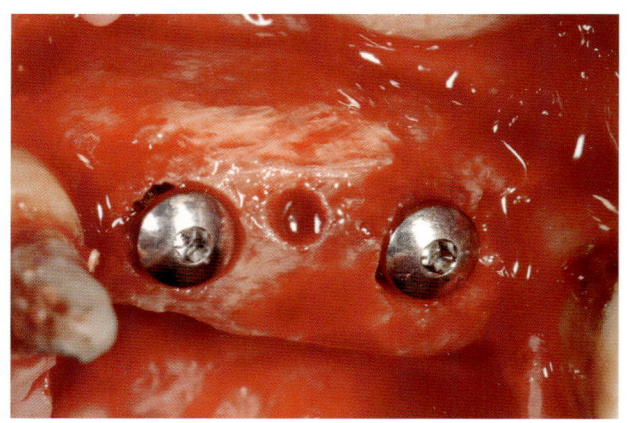

Fig 17-24  Implants (with sulcus formers) are visible, which had been inserted into mature well-vascularised healed graft.

17  Corrective Soft Tissue Surgery

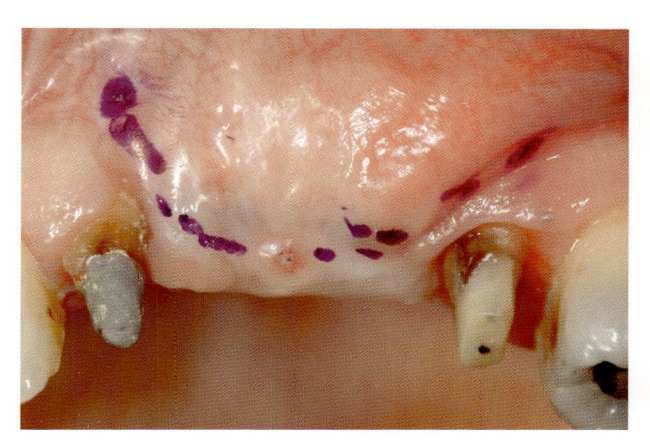

**Fig 17-25** The flap design is outlined for a vestibuloplasty and a free gingival graft.

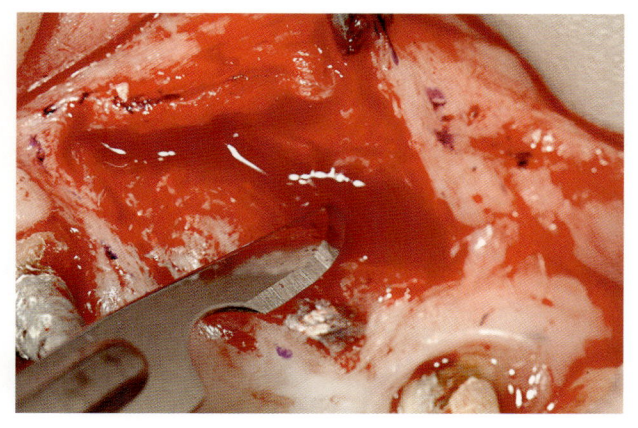

**Fig 17-26** A split-thickness flap is reflected, leaving the periosteum attached, and the muscle attachments are elevated to be re-attached apically.

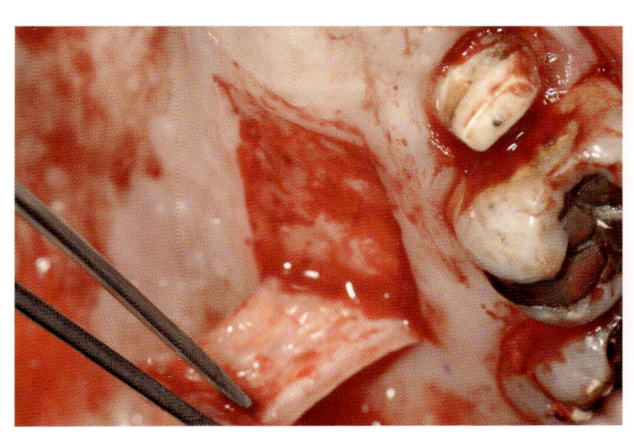

**Fig 17-27** Gingival graft being harvested from the palate.

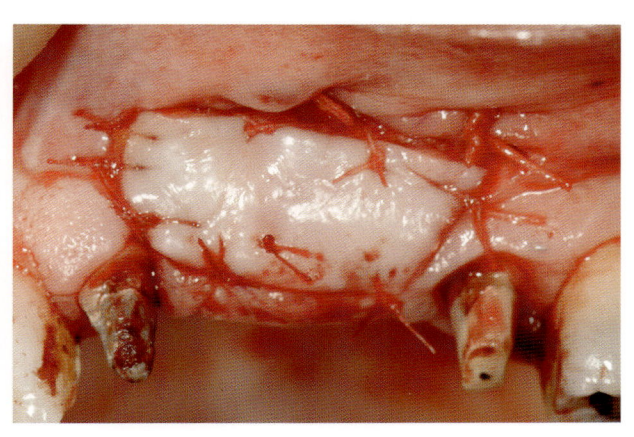

**Fig 17-28** Free gingival graft securely sutured onto the underlying periosteum. The muscles have been attached more apically.

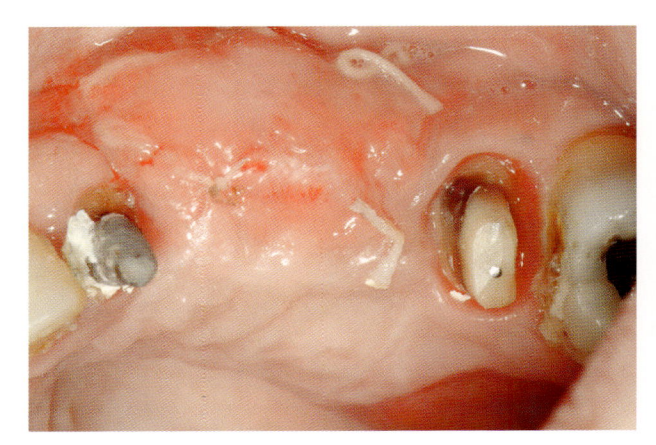

**Fig 17-29** Healing at two weeks at the suture removal appointment, showing the healed graft.

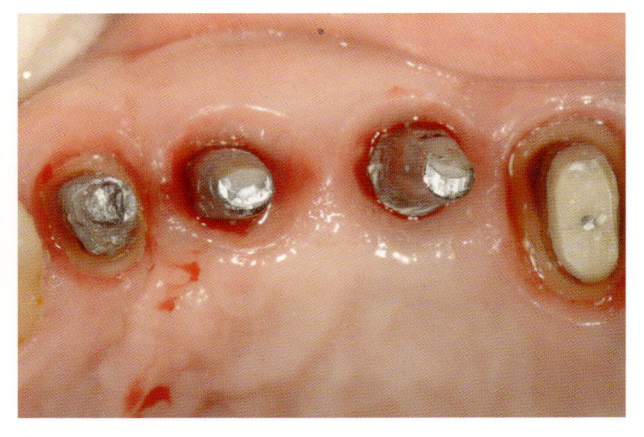

**Fig 17-30** Healing one month after surgery shows firmly attached keratinised tissue displaying a reasonably close colour match to the adjacent tissues.

III   Augmentation

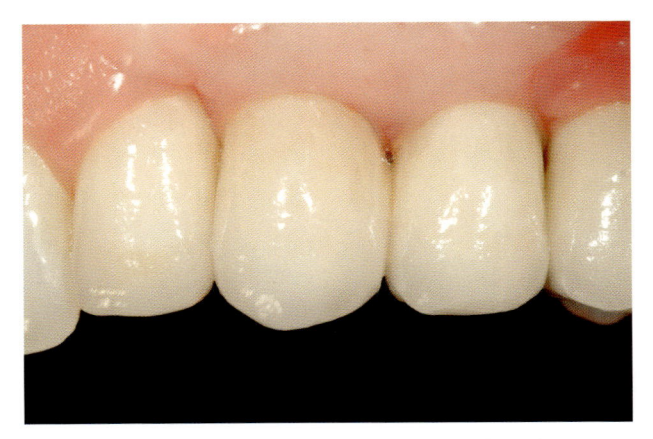

**Fig 17-31**   The definitive restoration emerging from the naturally contoured attached keratinised tissue.

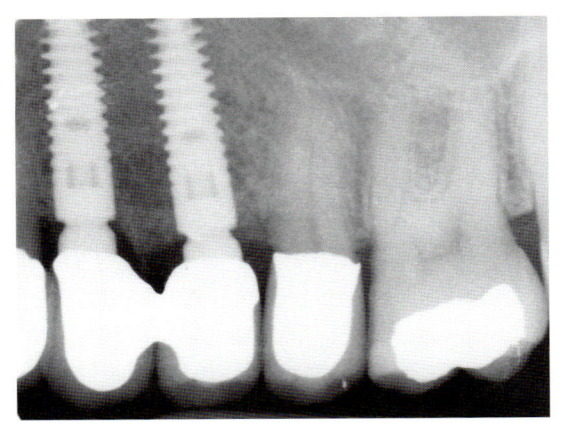

**Fig 17-32**   Post-operative radiograph of the implants, showing the stable bone levels that will be responsible for providing soft tissue support.

## Case 3: Lateral Pedicle Flap

This case study demonstrates the use of a rotational pedicle flap to close an oro-antral fistula created by the loss of a hydroxyapatite-coated implant 10 years after insertion through uncontrollable peri-implantitis (Figs 17-33–17-43).

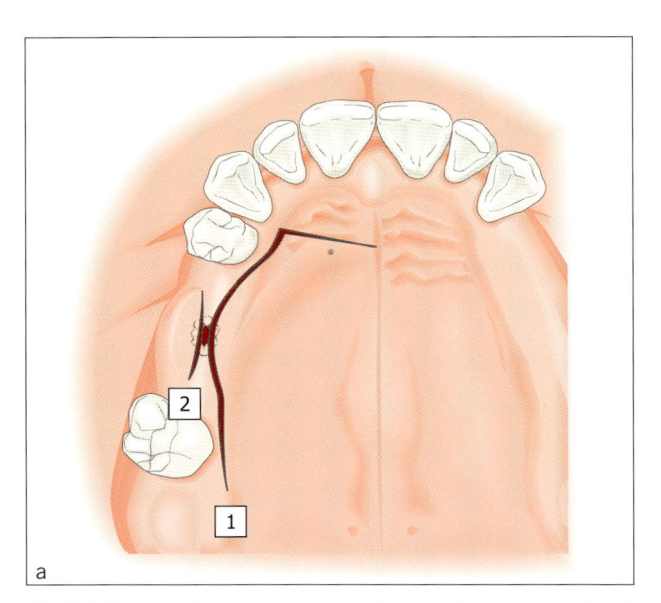

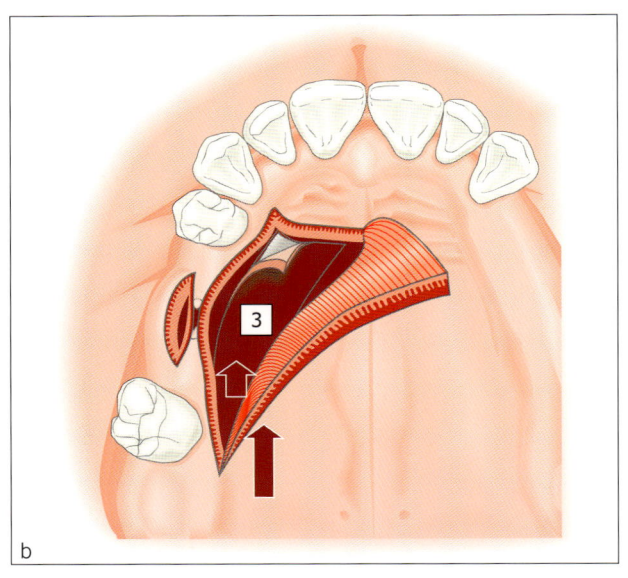

**Fig 17-33**   The four stages for creation of a lateral or rotational pedicle flap to repair a fistula in the maxillary molar region.
(a) Stage 1. A split-thickness incision is made in the palate and an epithelial flap is elevated to expose the underlying subepithelial mucosal and periosteal layer. Stage 2. A split-thickness incision is made on the labial aspect of the fistula creating a pocket into which the subepithelial flap will be secured.
(b) Stage 3. A full-thickness incision is made down to the periosteum to create a subepithelial connective tissue flap. Consideration must be given to the blood supply to the pedicle, which is indicated in this illustration by means of an arrow.

17 Corrective Soft Tissue Surgery

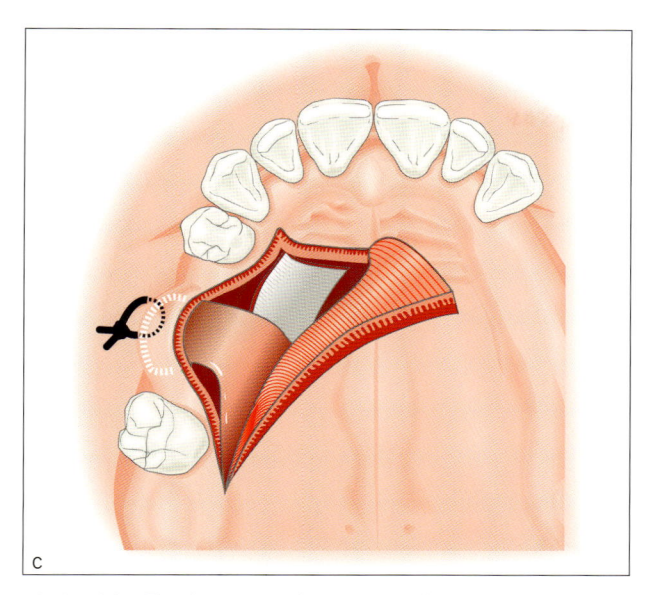

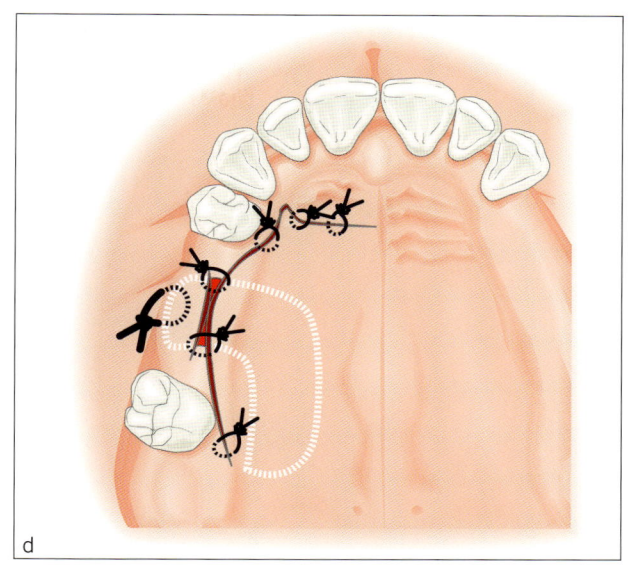

**Fig 17-33** The four stages for creation of a lateral or rotational pedicle flap to repair a fistula in the maxillary molar region.
(c) Stage 4. The pedicle flap can be seen mobilised and inserted into the pocket on the labial aspect of the fistula by means of a suture. The vascularised and viable pedicle thus closes the fistula.
(d) The epithelial flap is then sutured (using 6-0 Vicryl sutures). Closure of the epithelium over the fistula provides two-layer closure.

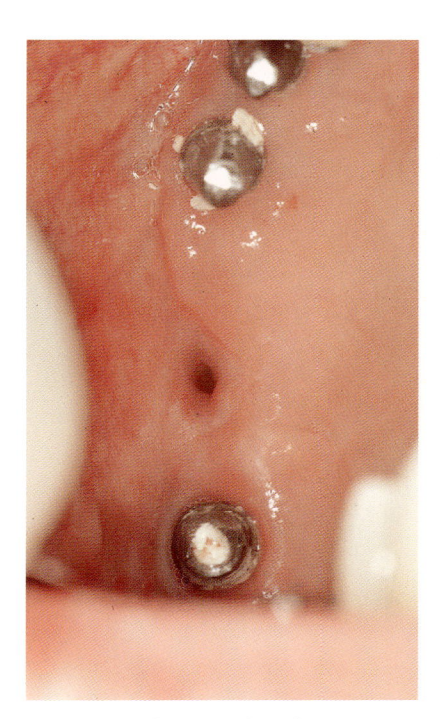

**Fig 17-34** Occlusal view of the oro-antral fistula in the first molar region.

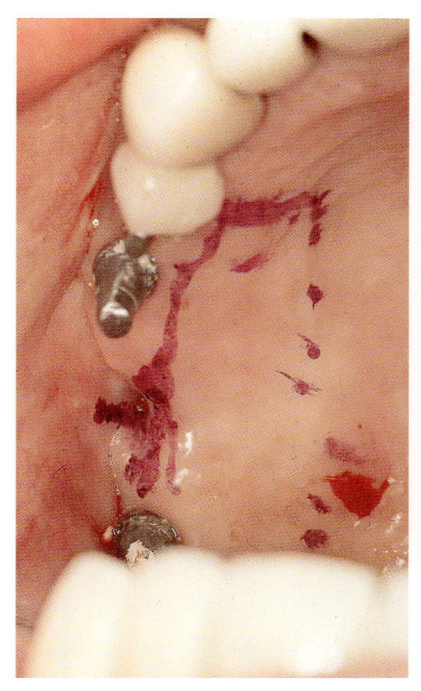

**Fig 17-35** Occlusal view of the outline of the palatal partial-thickness flap, which is designed to include the marginal tissue of the fistula. The labial subepithelial pocket is also commenced at the margin of the fistula (see Fig 17-33).

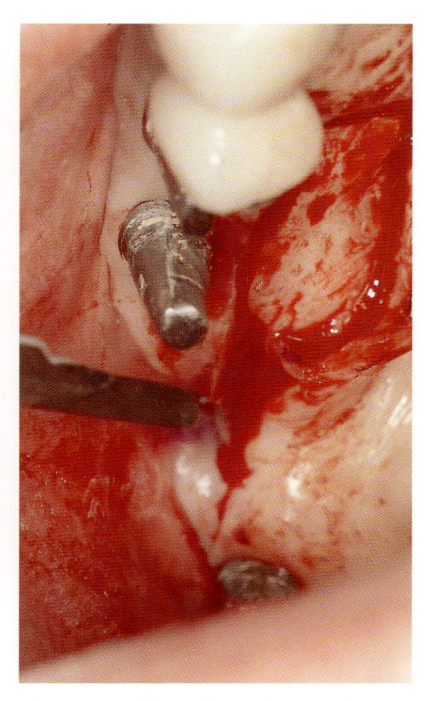

**Fig 17-36** The split-thickness epithelial flap can be seen reflected. This exposes the underlying connective tissue (see Fig 17-33).

III Augmentation

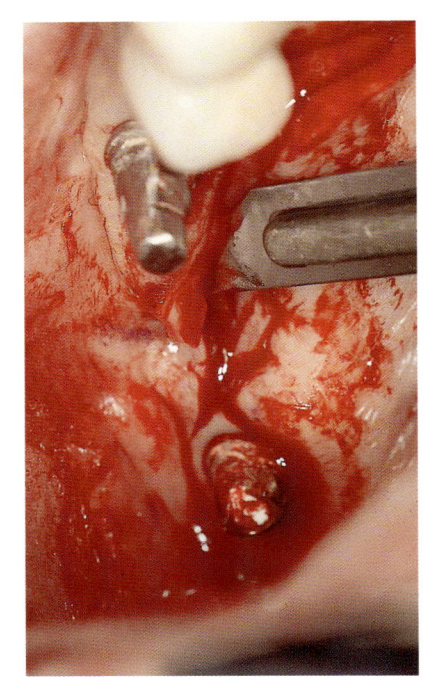

**Fig 17-37** Occlusal view of the labial subepithelial pocket being created, commencing within the marginal tissue of the fistula (see Fig 17-33).

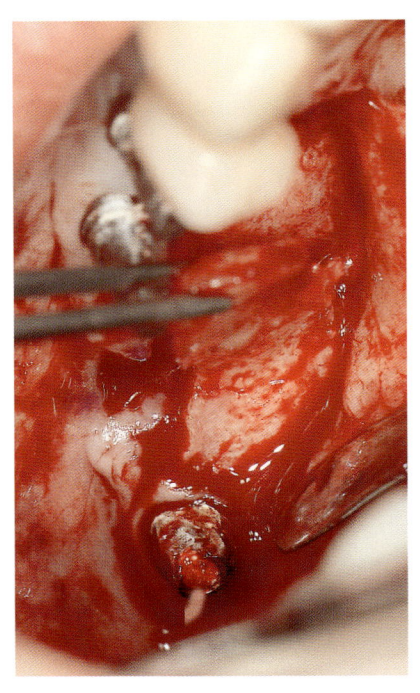

**Fig 17-38** The pedicle flap can be seen being mobilised, as demonstrated in Fig 17-33.

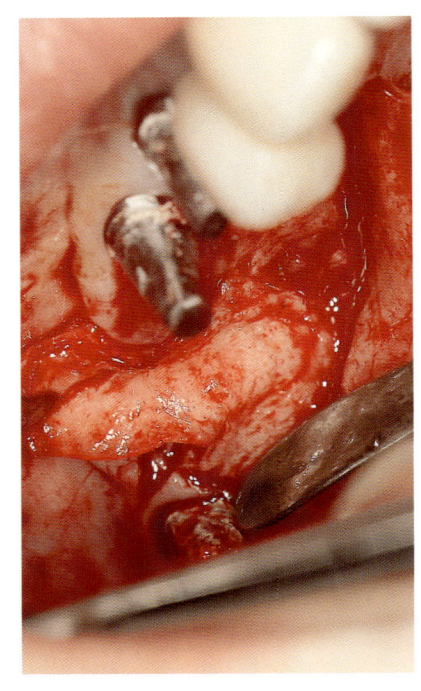

**Fig 17-39** The pedicle flap can be seen being rotated to ensure that adequate mobility has been achieved for coverage of the fistula and insertion into the labial pocket.

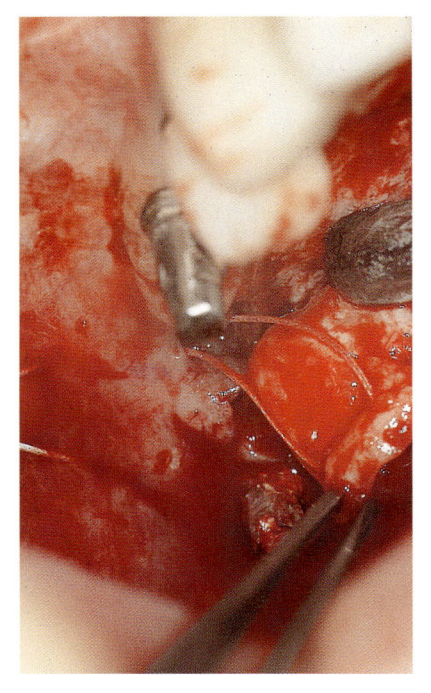

**Fig 17-40** Intraoral view showing the suture drawing the flap into the subepithelial pocket (see Fig 17-33).

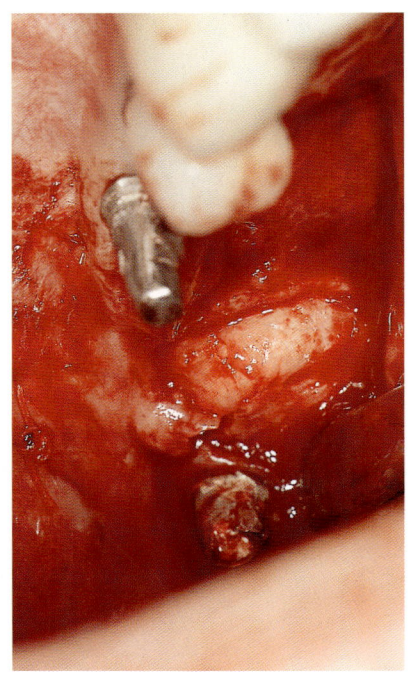

**Fig 17-41** The flap is sutured, secured by the drawing suture. A complete coverage of the fistula with a viable vascularised flap can be seen.

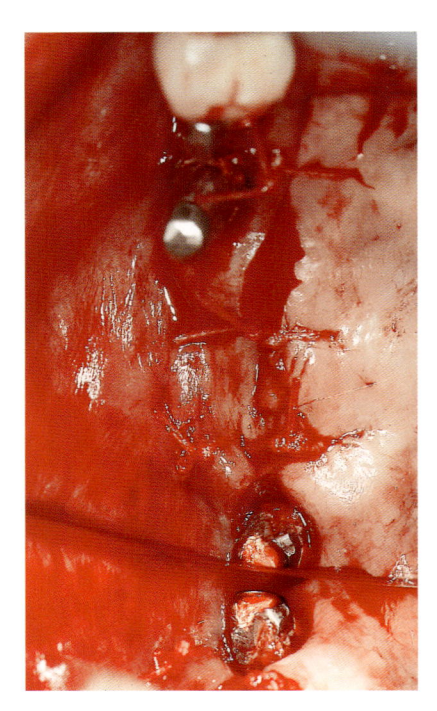

**Fig 17-42** The split-thickness epithelial flap is sutured to provide a two-layer closure.

## 17 Corrective Soft Tissue Surgery

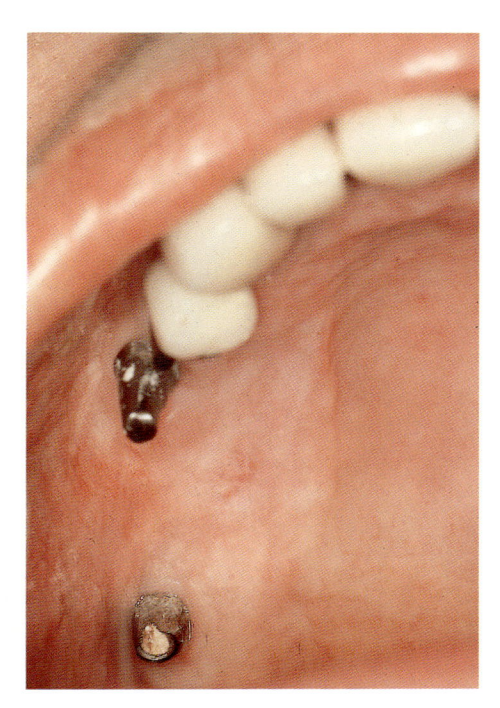

**Fig 17-43** Occlusal view showing the healed site one month after surgery.

### Case 4: Inverted Pedicle Flap

This case study illustrates the use of an inverted pedicle flap for the correction of gingival marginal discrepancy. A 35-year-old man presented with a transitional acrylic resin crown on a recently inserted implant. A discrepancy of approximately 3 mm with respect to the gingival margin of the adjacent teeth was noted. A decision was made to attempt to correct the discrepancy using soft tissue surgery. The alternatives of either a bone graft or the repositioning of the alveolar segment were also considered. The treatment proposed involved the removal of the abutment, followed by the closure of the residual fistula by means of an inverted pedicle flap. Increase in the bulk of soft tissues on the labial aspect was also planned. On completion of the soft tissue healing, exposure of the implant and the attachment of a new abutment was planned, followed by the construction of a definitive crown (Figs 17-44–17-56).

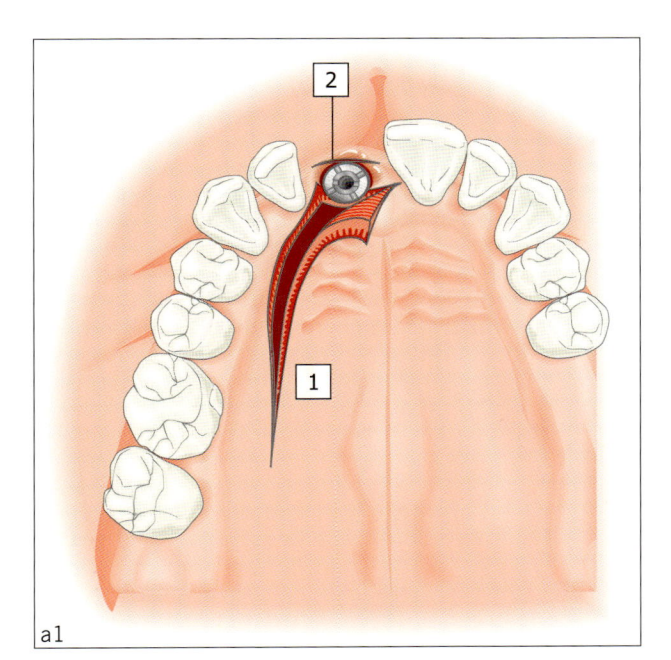

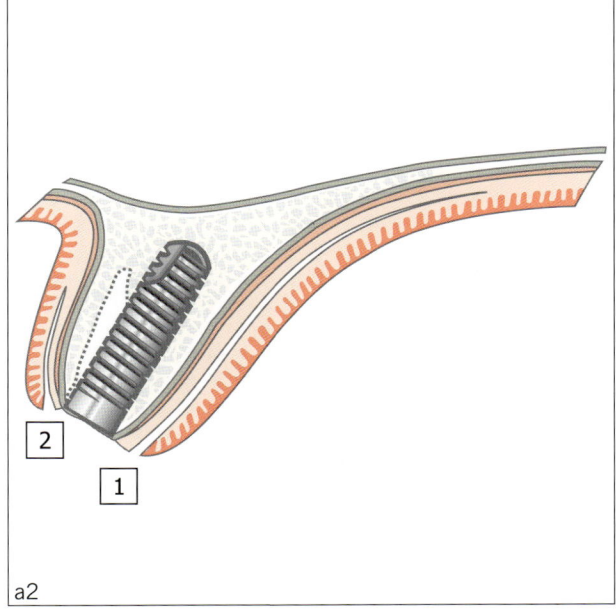

**Fig 17-44** The inverted pedicle flap technique, which may be used in the anterior region to close over an implant placed immediately into an extraction socket or for any other defects requiring closure.
(a1) Occlusal view outlining the incisions. Stage 1. Split-thickness incision in the palate to reflect a split-thickness epithelial flap, leaving attached the mucosa and periosteum. Stage 2. Split-thickness incision on the labial aspect, creating a subepithelial pocket.
(a2) Cross-sectional diagram. Stage 1: split-thickness incision. Stage 2: split-thickness incision to create subepithelial recipient site.

### III  Augmentation

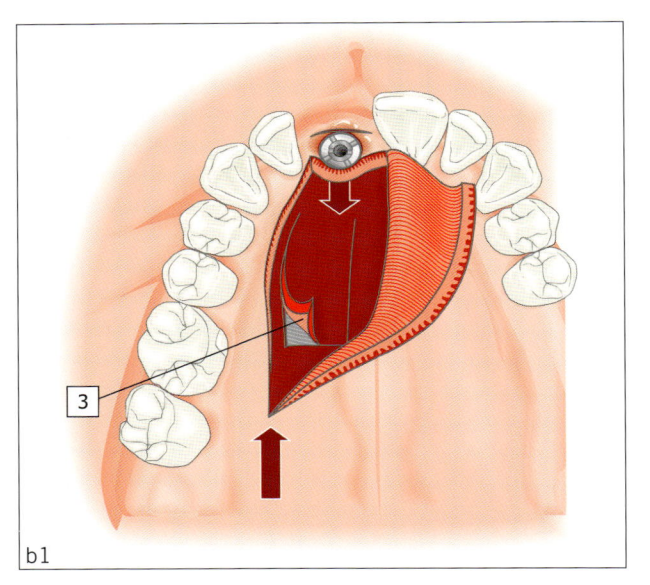

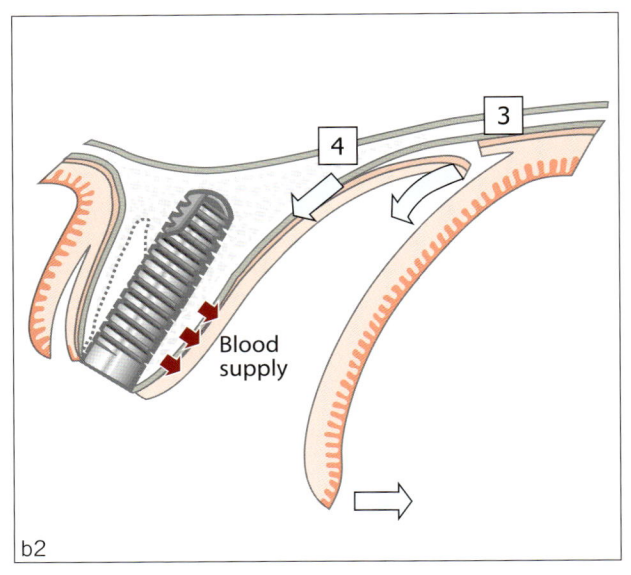

**Fig 17-44** The inverted pedicle flap technique, which may be used in the anterior region to close over an implant placed immediately into an extraction socket or for any other defects requiring closure.
(b1) Occlusal view showing the reflected split-thickness epithelial flap exposing the mucosal tissues. The full-thickness incision (3) can be seen creating an anteriorly pedicled flap. The arrow indicates the blood supply to the pedicled flap based on a collateral blood supply.
(b2) Cross-sectional diagram showing the incisions to create a pedicled flap. The blood supply (arrows), full-thickness incision (3) and reflection of the flap (4) can be seen.

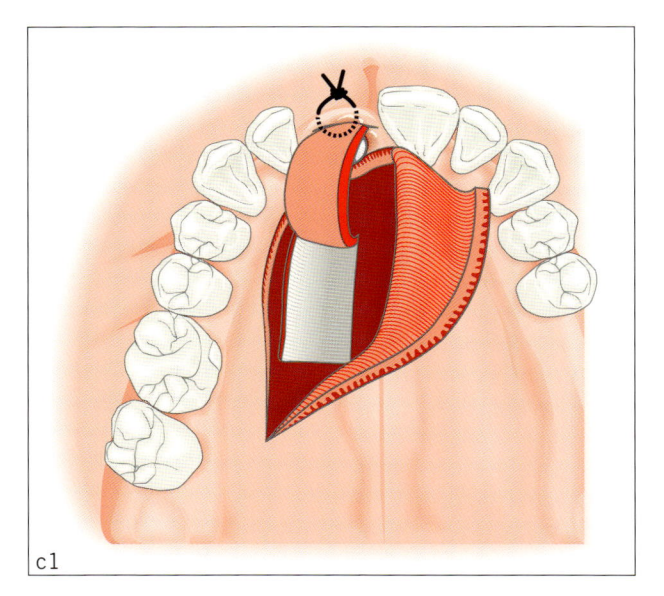

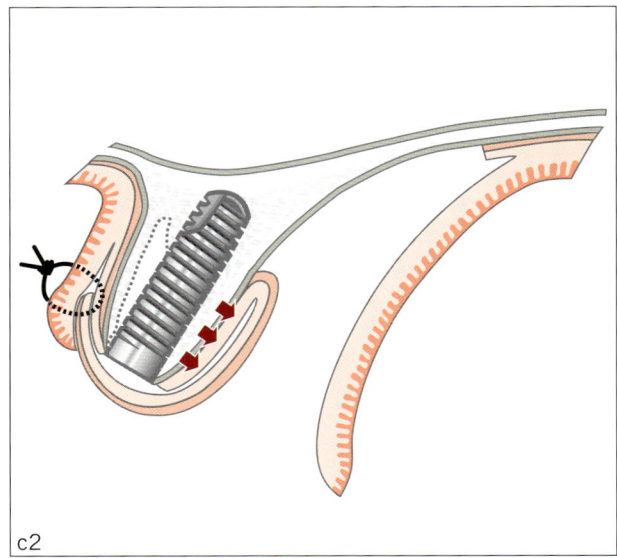

**Fig 17-44** (c1) Occlusal view showing the manner in which the flap is inverted to cover the extraction site and its insertion into the subepithelial pocket created on the labial aspect of the socket. A 3-0 Vicryl suture is used to draw the flap into the subepithelial pocket and hold it in position.
(c2) Cross-sectional diagram showing the inverted flap covering the socket and its insertion into the labial pocket. The relative proportions of the attached portion and the inverted portion are visible. Blood supply to the flap is obtained from the attached portion. This is indicated by the arrows.

17 Corrective Soft Tissue Surgery

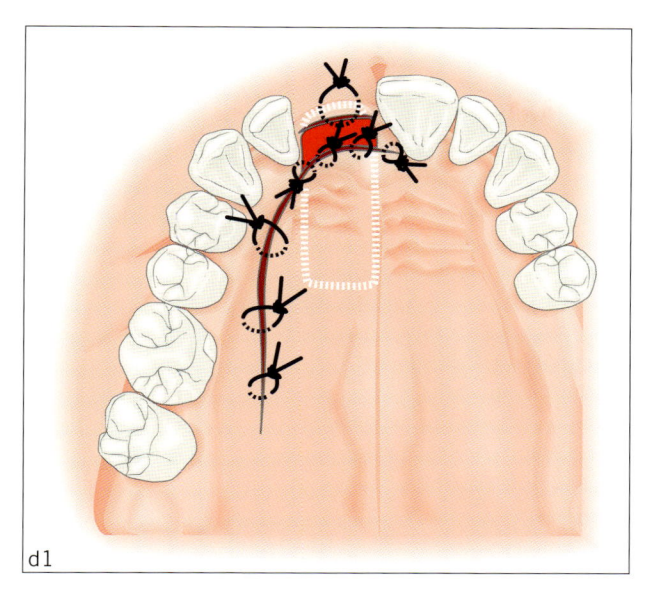

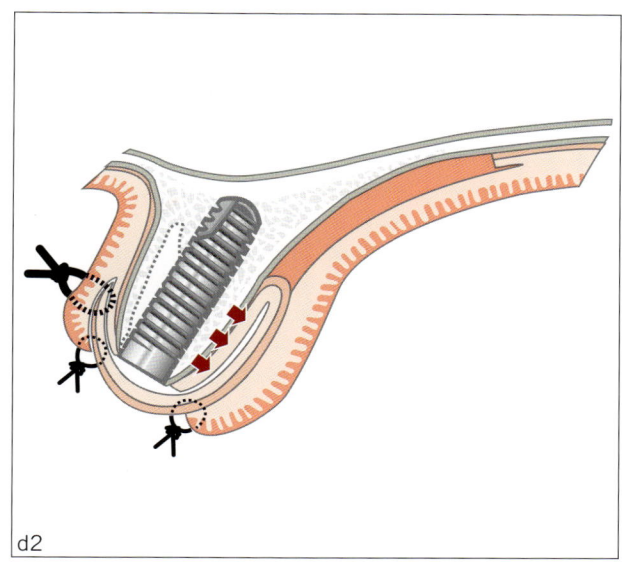

**Fig 17-44** (d1) Occlusal view of the completed inverted flap. The partial-thickness epithelial flaps are closed using 6-0 Vicryl sutures. The vascularised and viable flap can be seen covering the socket.
(d2) Cross-sectional view of sutured inverted pedicle flap.

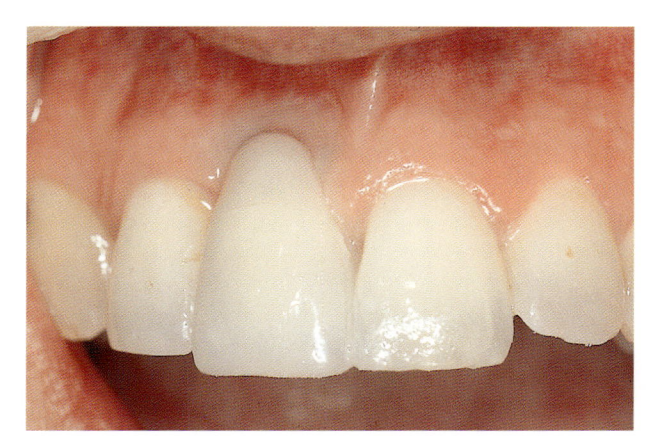

**Fig 17-45** Labial view of the transitional acrylic resin crown, showing the gingival marginal discrepancy and the thin tissue overlying the abutment.

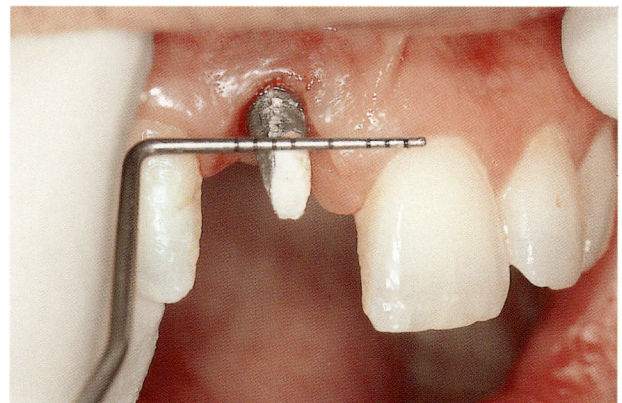

**Fig 17-46** Clinical view of the abutment of incorrect angle following the removal of the transitional crown. The abutment was also considered to be too short to provide adequate retention for a cement-retained crown.

### III  Augmentation

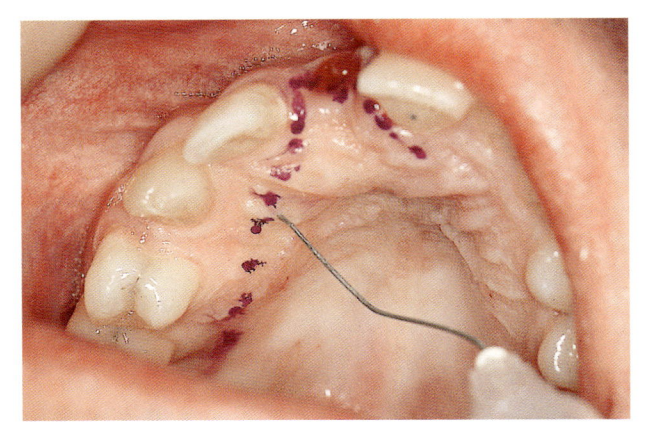

**Fig 17-47**  Occlusal view of the outline of the incision for the reflection of a partial-thickness epithelial flap to expose the subepithelial connective tissue. The use of local anaesthetic solution inflates the soft tissues and facilitates the reflection of the partial-thickness flap (see Fig 17-44).

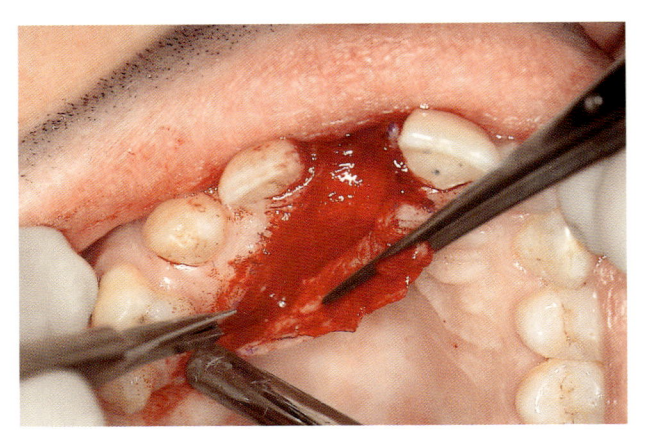

**Fig 17-48**  Reflection of the partial-thickness flap exposing the subepithelial mucosa.

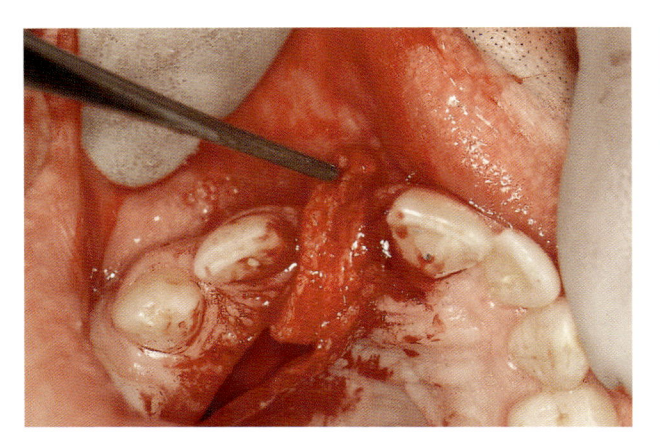

**Fig 17-49**  The mobilised inverted pedicle flap being tried in to ensure that it will cover the deficiency and fit into the labial subepithelial pocket.

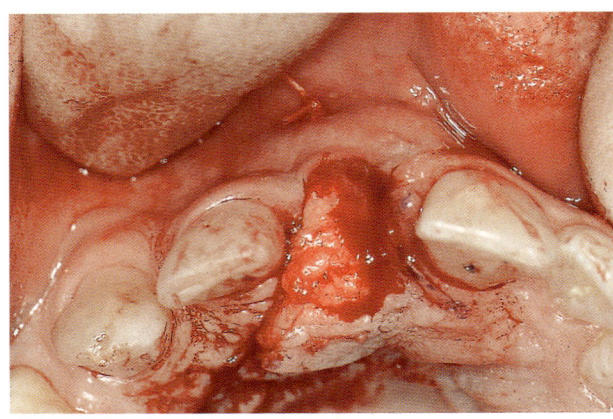

**Fig 17-50**  The pedicle flap secured by the drawing suture into the subepithelial pocket.

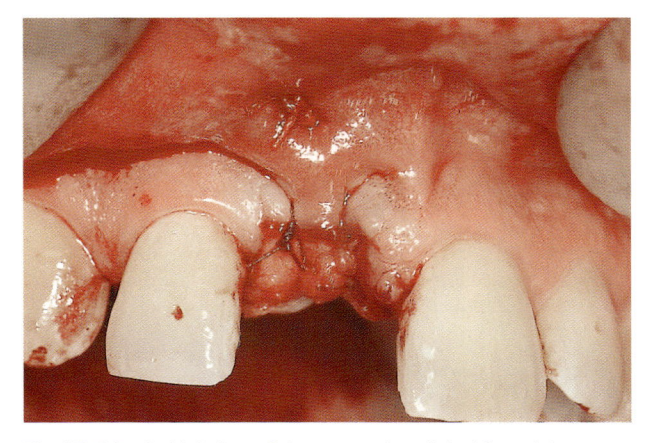

**Fig 17-51**  Labial view of the sutured pedicled flap. Adequate bulk of soft tissue on the labial aspect of the deficiency can be seen.

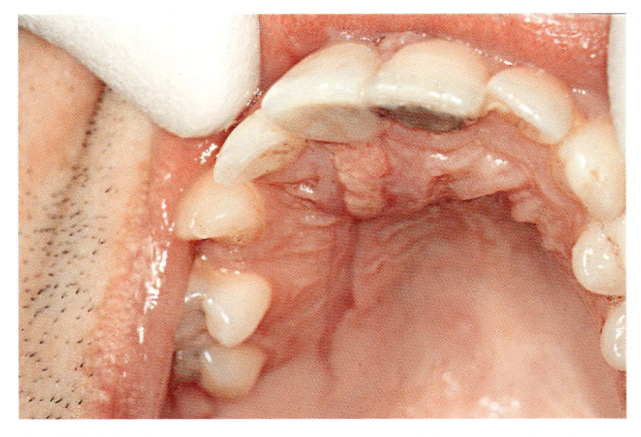

**Fig 17-52**  Post-operative view of the palate two weeks after surgery, showing good healing.

17 Corrective Soft Tissue Surgery

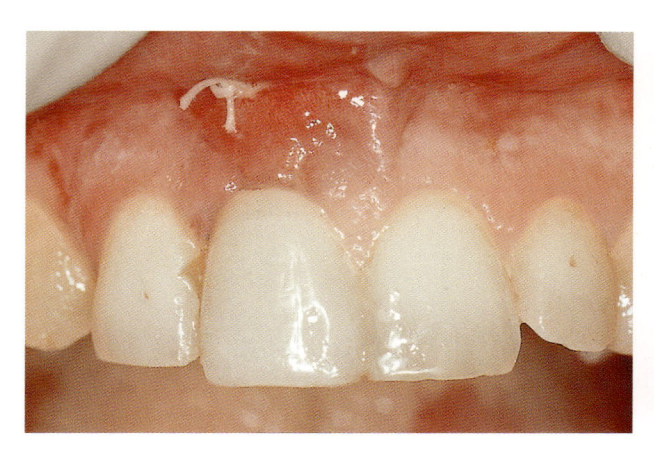

**Fig 17-53** Labial view two weeks after surgery showing adequate soft tissue height and thickness. The provisional metal-acrylic Rochette bridge provides a good indication of the eventual outcome.

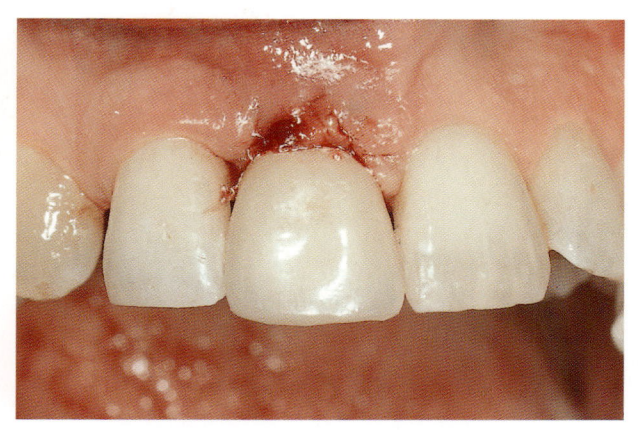

**Fig 17-54** The soft tissues are allowed to heal and mature over a period of six weeks prior to the exposure of the implant and attachment of the abutment. The figure shows the transitional restoration supported by the new abutment. Note the level of the gingival margin.

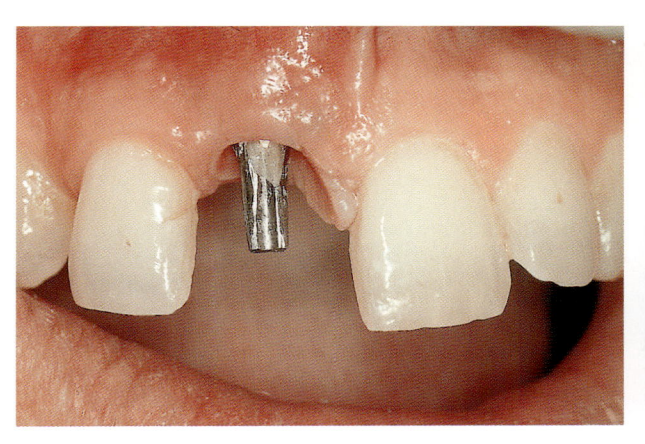

**Fig 17-55** Labial view of the new abutment emerging from the healed soft tissues.

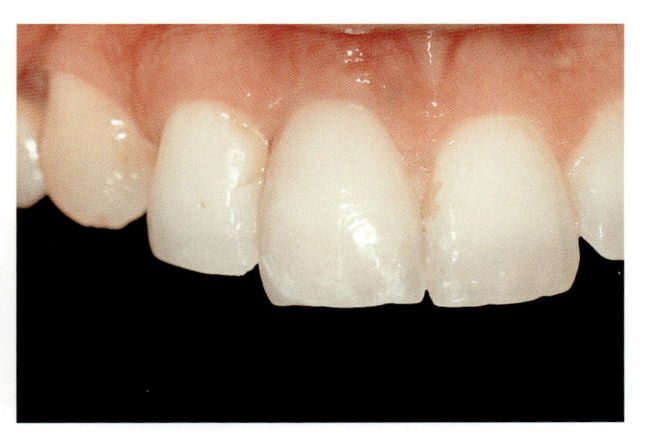

**Fig 17-56** The definitive restoration in situ with improved gingival contours, both in terms of height and thickness.

## Case 5: Subepithelial Connective Tissue Graft

A subepithelial connective tissue graft was used to increase the height and thickness of the gingival marginal tissues. A 24-year-old man had had an implant inserted using the technique of maxillary ridge expansion. Following the exposure of the implant and attachment of the abutment, the cervical margin was observed to be composed of thin keratinised tissue. The level of the gingival margin was considered to be higher than that of the adjacent teeth. A decision was made to carry out a connective tissue graft before completion of the definitive restoration to reduce the chances of further recession, which may have exposed the abutment (Figs 17-57–17-73).

III  Augmentation

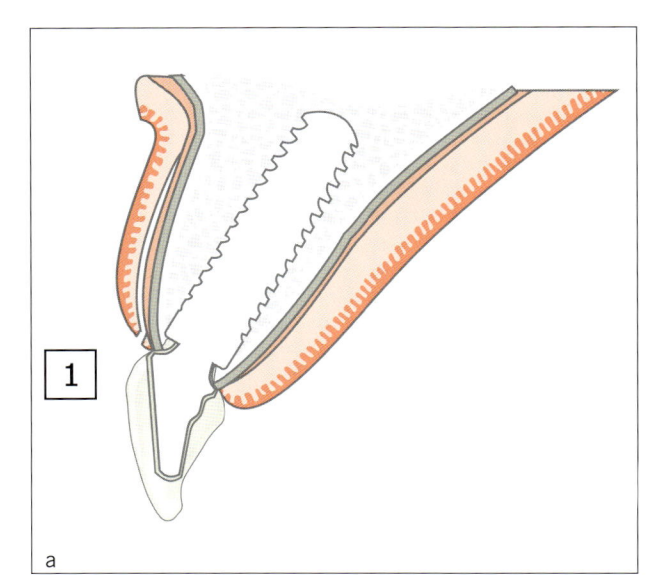

**Fig 17-57** The use of either connective tissue or composite epithelium-connected tissue grafts for the purpose of increasing the thickness of the cervical margin or altering its level to cover any exposed components. (a) Stage 1. A split-thickness incision is made to create a pocket to receive the graft. The incision is made between the epithelium and periosteum (1).

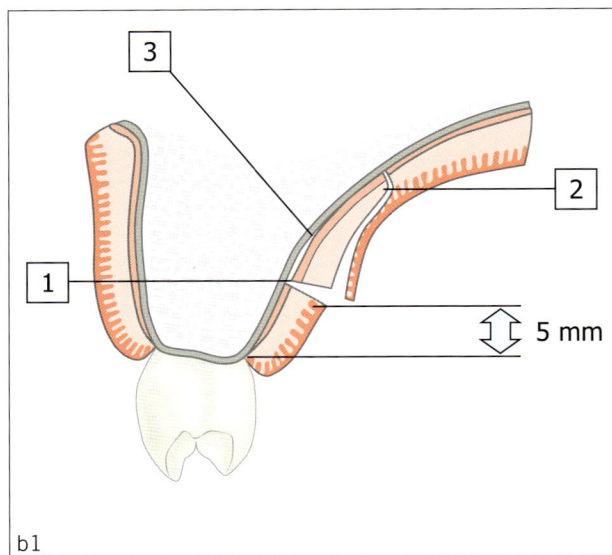

**Fig 17-57** (b1) Stage 1. An incision is made down to periosteum parallel to and approximately 5 mm from the cervical margins of the teeth in the region of the premolars and the first molar.
Stage 2. A split-thickness incision cuts through the periosteum at the selected level apical to the incision (1). Care must be taken not to sever the neurovascular vessels in this area. Two parallel incisions perpendicular to incisions 1 and 2 are made on the mesial and distal aspects to define the length of the graft (not shown). Stage 3. The graft is elevated from the bone.

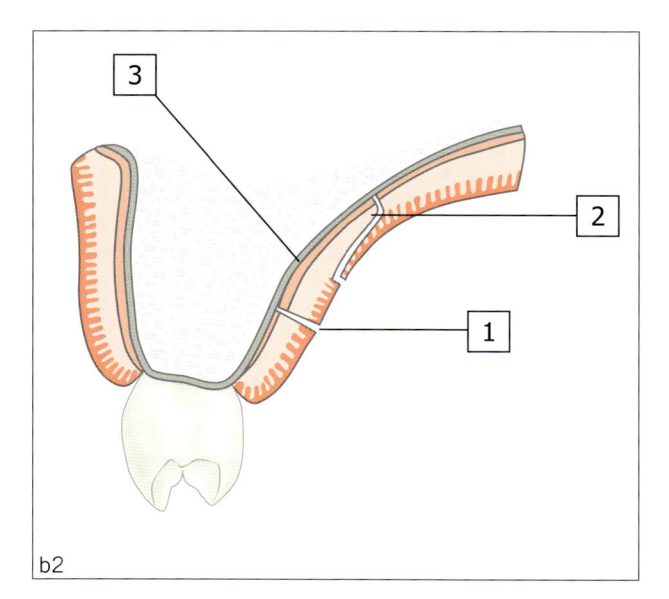

**Fig 17-57** (b2) The same sequence of incisions is used as in (b1), with the exception that an epithelial portion is included as part of the graft. Incision (2) is, therefore, made at the desired distance from incision (1).

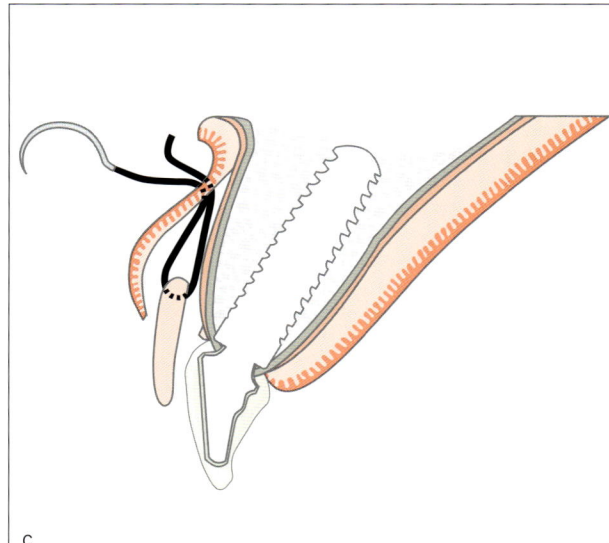

**Fig 17-57** (c) The suturing technique for both types of graft requires the graft to be drawn into the pocket created in the subepithelial tissues. This provides the primary anchorage. The same technique may be used for pedicle flaps. The sequence in which the suture is used to secure the graft is depicted. A 22-mm needle using a 3-0 Vicryl suture is suitable for this procedure.

374

17 Corrective Soft Tissue Surgery

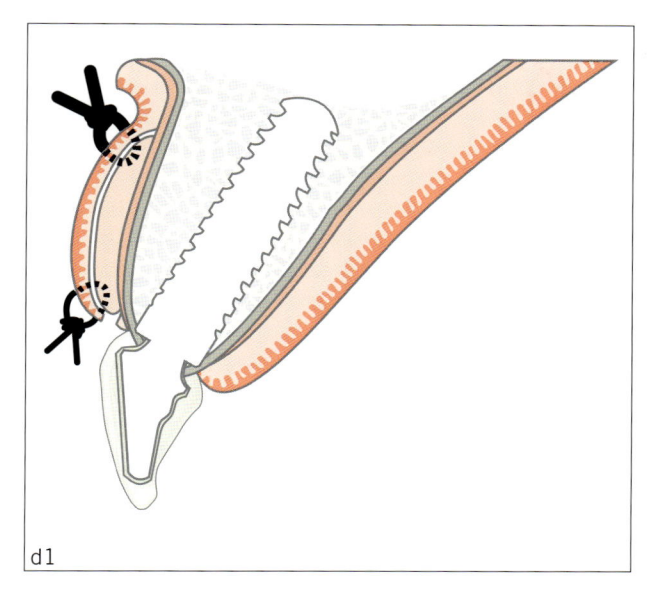

**Fig 17-57** (d1) The subepithelial connective tissue graft sutured into place. Finer sutures (6-0 Vicryl) may be used to secure the margins of the graft, positioning it to provide the required level of additional marginal height.

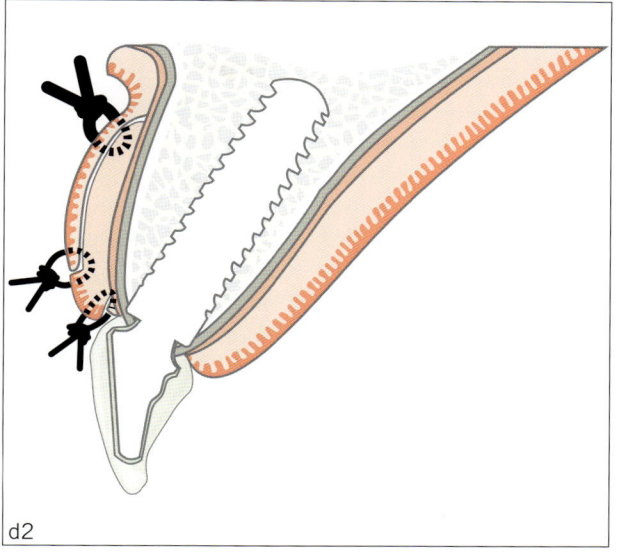

**Fig 17-57** (d2) A composite subepithelial connective tissue graft can be seen sutured into position. The epithelial portion is sutured to the margins, increasing the amount of keratinised tissue. The subepithelial connective tissue portion adds thickness as well as providing a large surface area for the establishment of a blood supply.

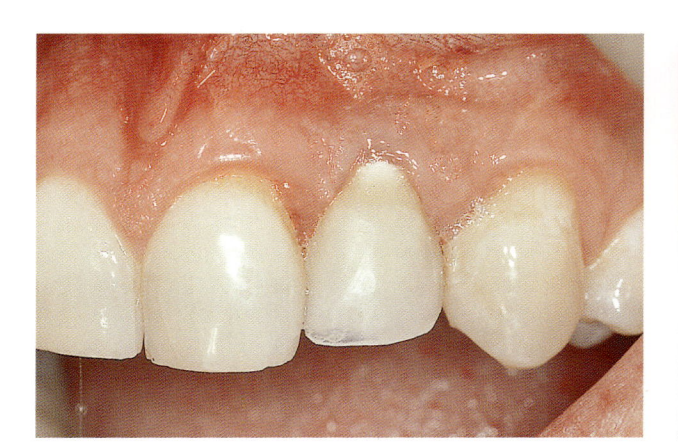

**Fig 17-58** Labial view of the lateral incisor showing the provisional restoration with its margin visible. The delicate nature of the gingival tissue is apparent (see Fig 17-57).

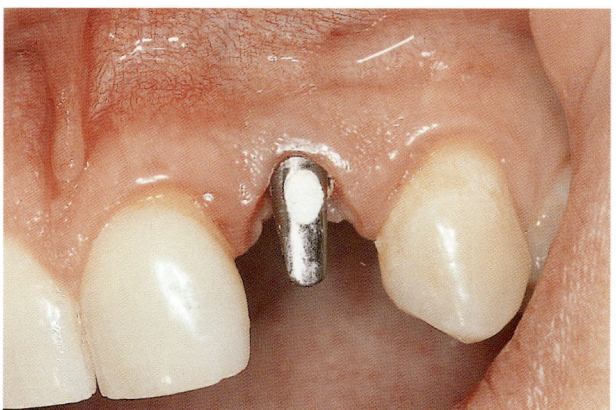

**Fig 17-59** Labial view of the abutment with the transitional crown removed, demonstrating the thin labial tissue.

375

III    Augmentation

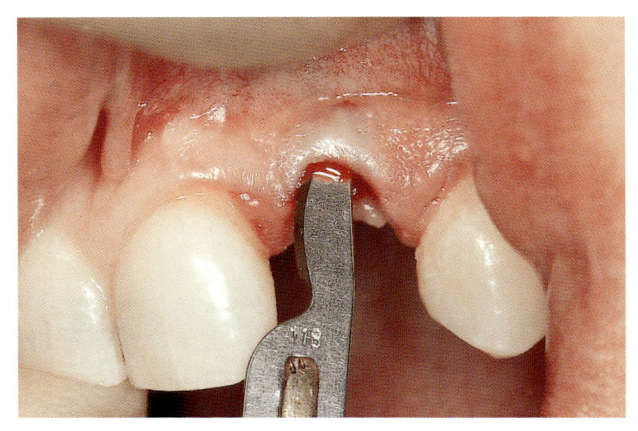

**Fig 17-60**  The split-thickness incision being carried out using a number 15C scalpel blade to create a pocket for the connective tissue graft (see Fig 17-57a).

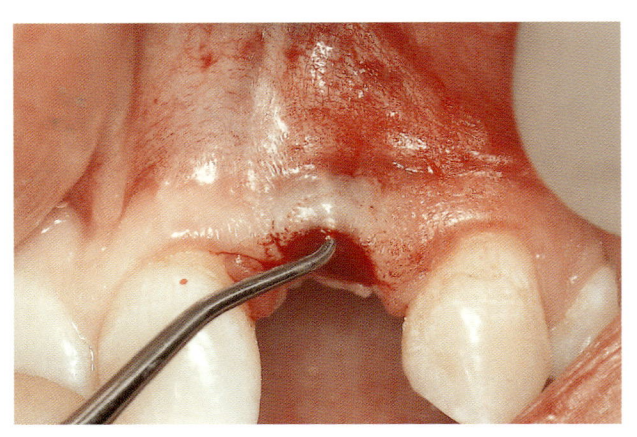

**Fig 17-61**  A small excavator being used to further separate the epithelium from the periosteum in order to create space for the connective tissue graft.

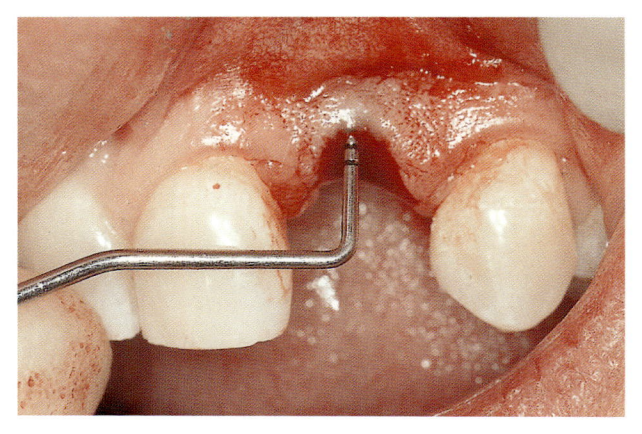

**Fig 17-62**  The dimensions of the pocket created are measured so that they can be transferred to the palate for the harvesting of the graft.

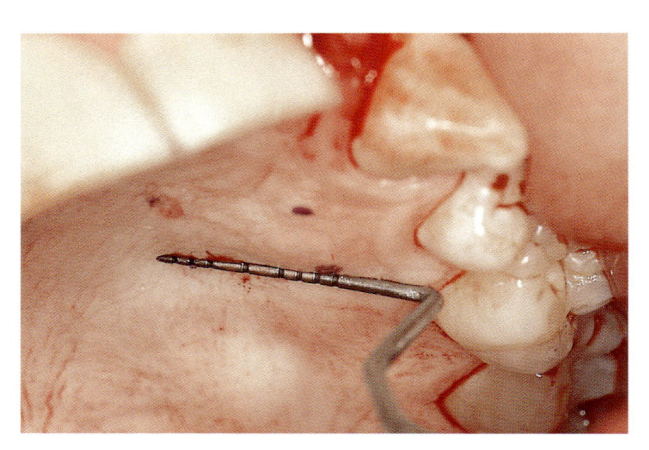

**Fig 17-63**  Clinical view of the donor site being marked in the palate adjacent to the premolar tooth.

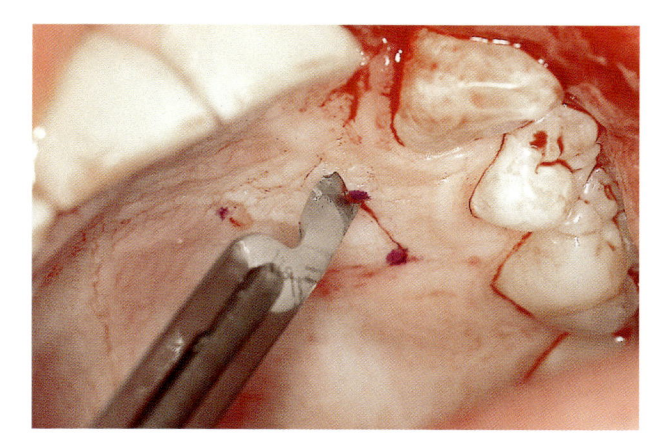

**Fig 17-64**  The first (full-thickness) incision being made to harvest the graft (see Fig 17-57b1).

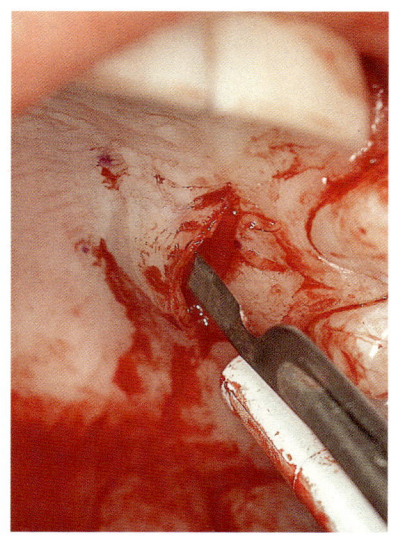

**Fig 17-65**  The remainder of the full-thickness incision (3) being carried out on completion of the bevelled split-thickness incision (2) (see Fig 17-57b1).

17   Corrective Soft Tissue Surgery

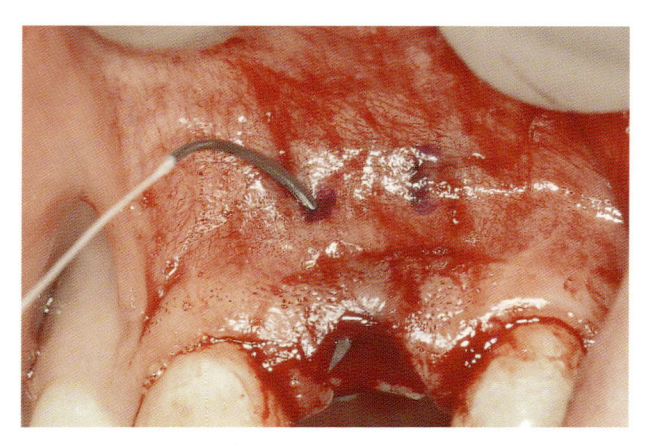

**Fig 17-66**   The needle for the drawing suture being inserted on the labial aspect of the subepithelial pocket using a 3-0 Vicryl suture.

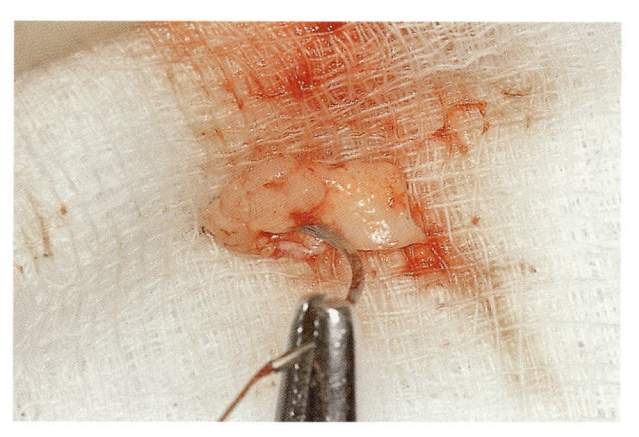

**Fig 17-67**   The harvested connective tissue graft, placed on gauze dampened with sterile saline, is picked up using the needle.

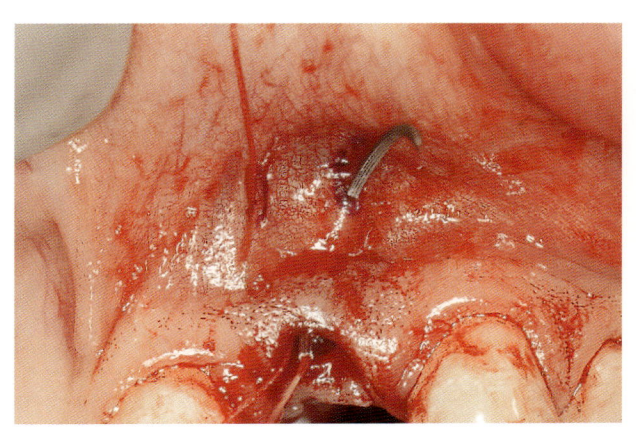

**Fig 17-68**   The needle is reinserted through the subepithelial pocket to emerge through the tissues on the labial aspect of the ridge.

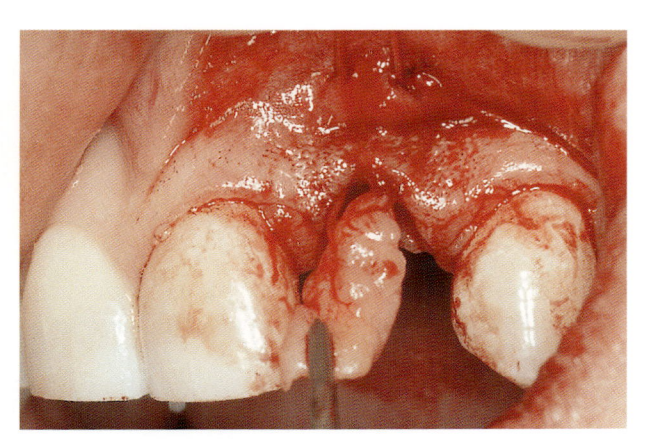

**Fig 17-69**   Both ends of the suture are pulled to draw the connective tissue graft into the pocket. The suture will secure the graft in position.

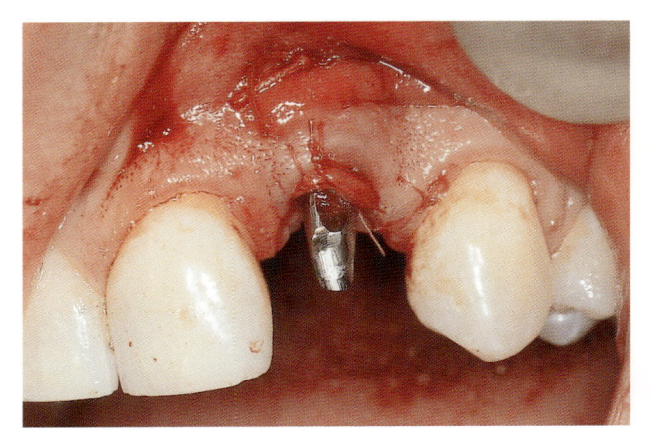

**Fig 17-70**   Labial view of the graft in situ being held in place with the drawing suture. Additional sutures using 6-0 Vicryl are placed to precisely position the graft in relation to the gingival margin.

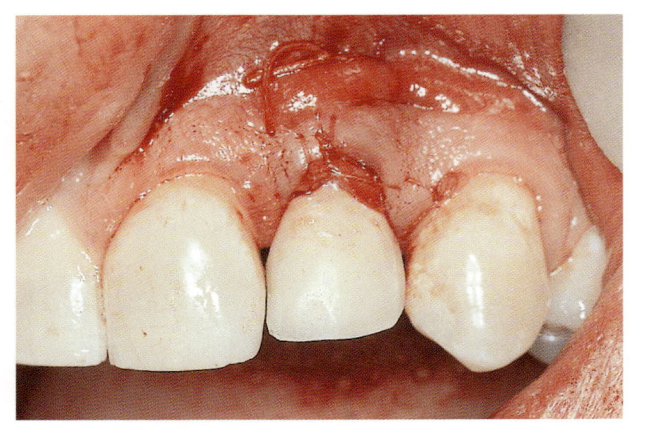

**Fig 17-71**   The transitional crown has been re-cemented. Note the increased thickness of soft tissues.

III  Augmentation

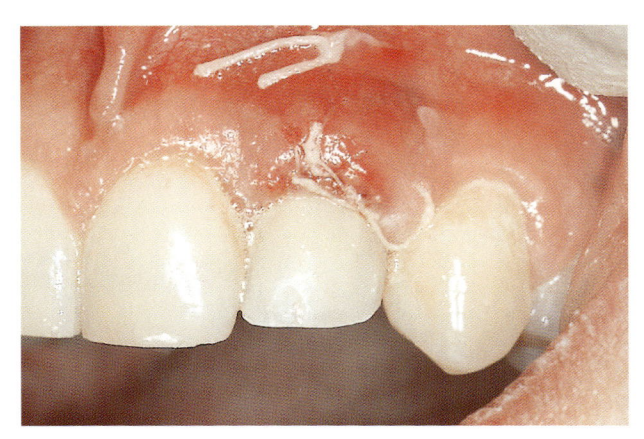

**Fig 17-72** Labial view of the site two weeks after surgery, showing some soft tissue hypertrophy.

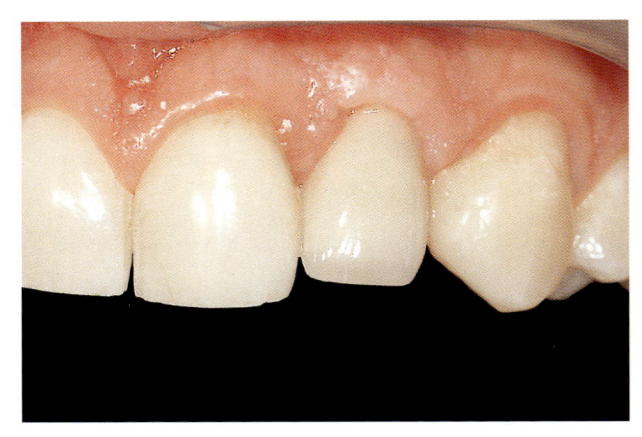

**Fig 17-73** The definitive restoration in situ six months after surgery, showing a stable, thick gingival margin at a height consistent with the adjacent teeth.

## Case 6: Connective Tissue Graft to Eliminate an Amalgam Tattoo

The advancement of a mucoperiosteal flap to cover a graft shifted the position of an amalgam tattoo from previous apicectomies from a coronal position to a more visible position. A connective tissue graft was used to avoid the contrast between the palatal and the residual buccal tissues.

The procedure required a split-thickness flap to be elevated; the removal of the amalgam resulted in the perforation of the flap and the need to repair the perforations. This was carried out by underlaying a sheet of subepithelial connective tissue. The host epithelial tissue was then able to migrate onto the connective tissue to produce a uniform colour (Figs 17-74–17-83).

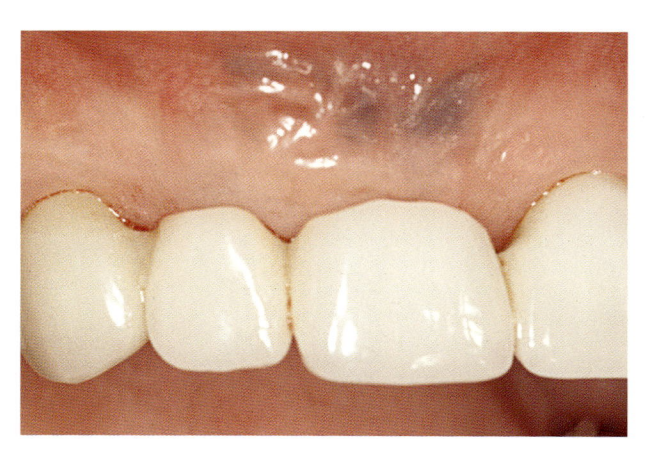

**Fig 17-74** Labial view of the central and lateral incisor region following a bone graft to reconstruct a deficient ridge. The amalgam tattoo, from previous apicectomies, is apparent.

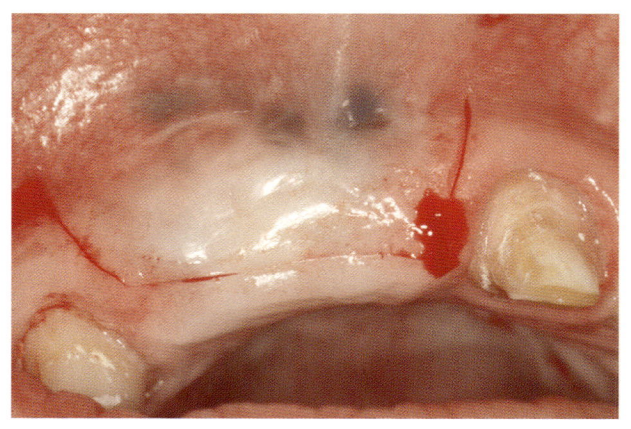

**Fig 17-75** Incision commenced for a split-thickness flap.

17 Corrective Soft Tissue Surgery

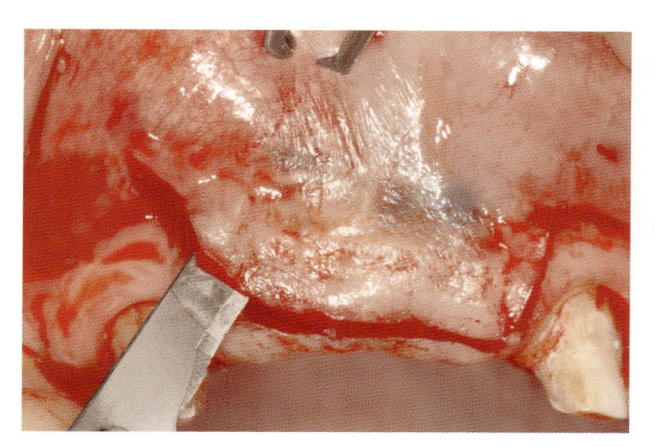

**Fig 17-76** Split-thickness flap being elevated.

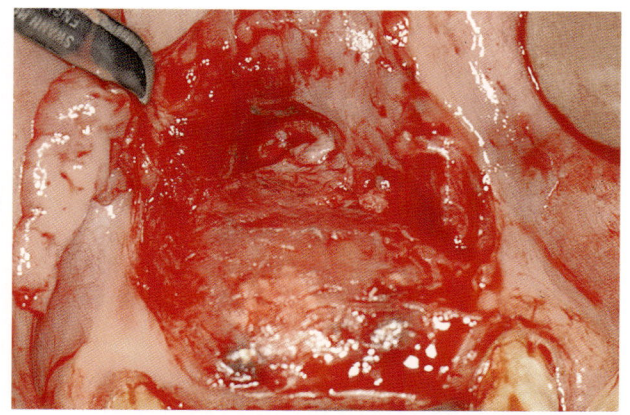

**Fig 17-77** The split-thickness epithelial soft tissue flap elevated leaving the periosteum attached to the bone. Tissue containing the amalgam is removed from the overlying flap as well as from the periosteum. Perforations in the epithelial flap and the periosteum result requiring repair.

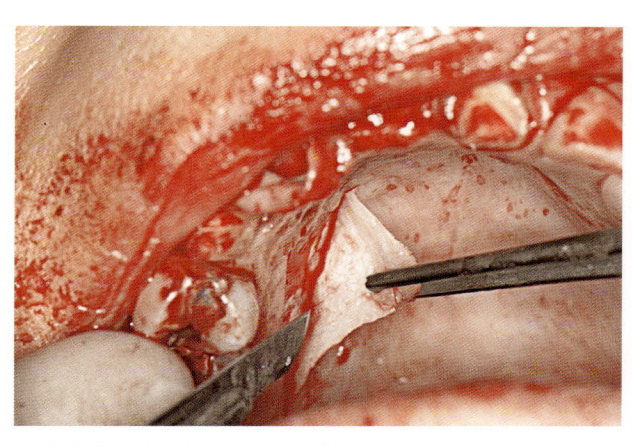

**Fig 17-78** Split-thickness flap is seen being elevated from the palatal donor site. The underlying connective tissue will be harvested for grafting on the labial aspect.

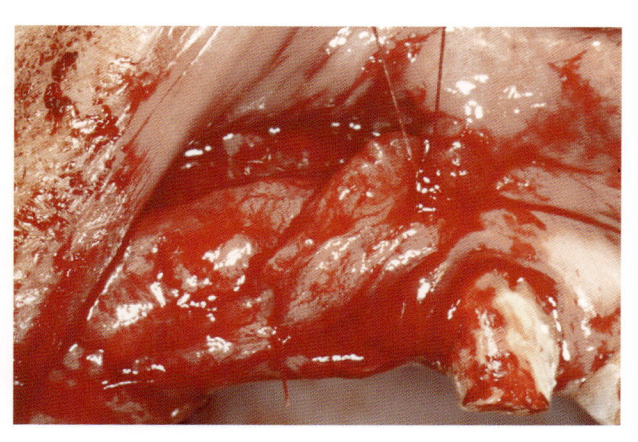

**Fig 17-79** The connective tissue graft is sutured onto the periosteum, ensuring a lack of mobility.

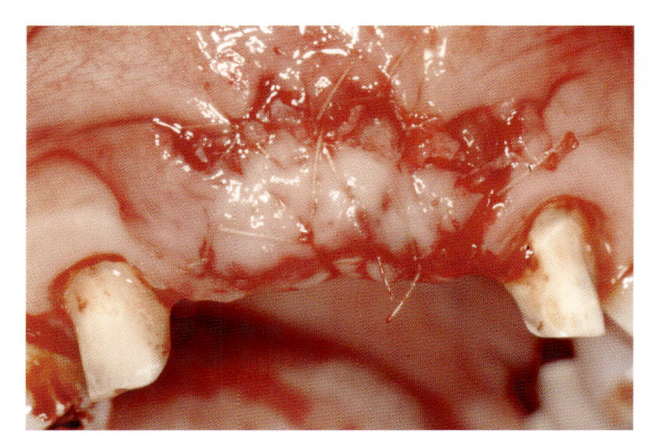

**Fig 17-80** The labial split-thickness flap is then sutured to overlie the connective tissue graft. The perforations overlie the connective tissue graft, which will be vascularised from the underlying periosteum and the overlying epithelial flap.

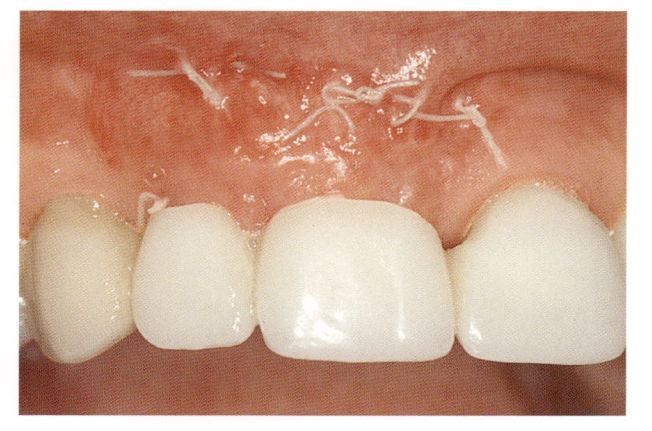

**Fig 17-81** Healing at two weeks.

379

III   Augmentation

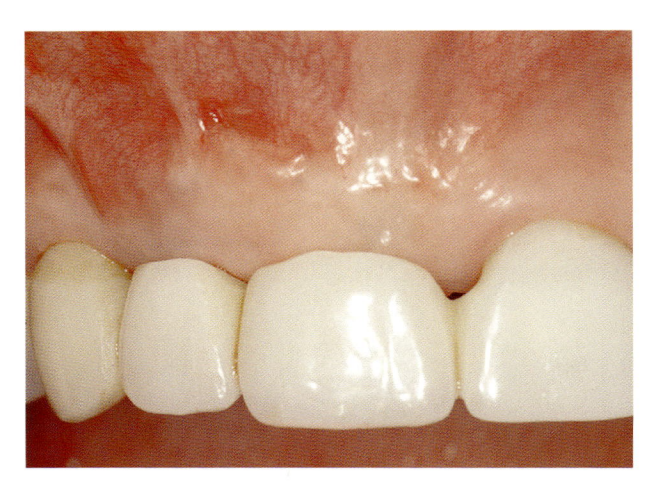

Fig 17-82   Healing at four weeks and prior to the exposure of the implants. A good colour match can be seen.

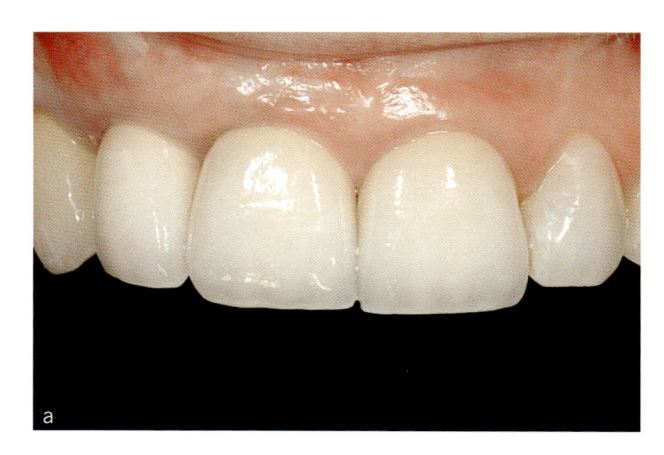

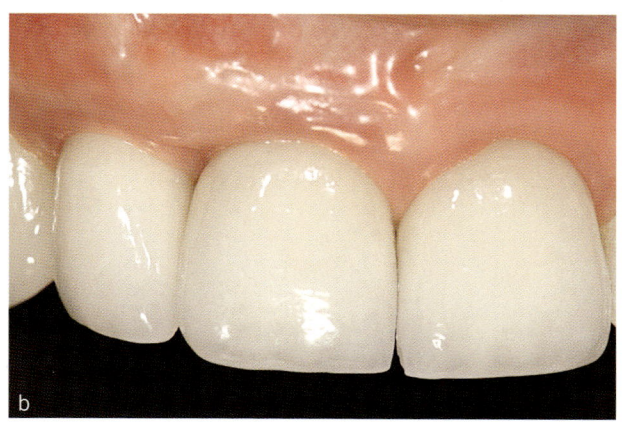

Fig 17-83   (a and b) Final views.

## Conclusions

Implant dentistry is a rapidly changing field, fraught with an abundance of information that is often not based on sound preclinical and clinical validation. There is need for academic institutions to publish new research data. The clinical relevance of experimental data needs to be validated prior to clinical application. The focus of sponsors of research is primarily to provide support for a product. This does not encourage publication of data pertaining to failures and complications, which would be of benefit to the profession. Regardless of all the difficulties that occur in sifting out relevant data, the need to define valid techniques does not diminish but becomes more urgent.

Techniques described in the literature are proliferating rapidly. It is hoped that the techniques contained in this book will remain valid as they are based on clinical observation supported by relevant literature and refined over the past 32 years.

After all, what we do as surgeons is to create an injury and depend on the body's capacity to heal. Observation of the healing process in the short and long term validates or condemns the technique.

There is no environment less forgiving for the practise of an invalid or unpredictable technique than that of private practice, where the monitoring is carried out by highly critical, well-informed assessors – namely our patients.

By the same token, there is no environment more rewarding than private practice for the execution of techniques that are predictable and can be relied on to produce an outcome planned together with our patients to meet their realistic expectations and needs.

The clinical environment in our modern society requires a high degree of documentation for the safety of our patients and to ensure that data are available for governance and peer review.

Nevertheless, the ultimate aim of our endeavours must be to conscientiously review the science-based changes and developments in our understanding of the biology of healing and maintenance of health. Armed with this we can use our judgement and intuition in the pursuit of the art that is fundamental to this field.

# References

1. Adell R, Lekholm U, Roskler BJ, Brånemark PI. A 15-year study of osseointegrated implants in the treatment of the edentulous jaw. Int J Oral Surg 1981;10:387–416.
2. Albrektsson T, Dahl E, Enbom L, Engevall S, Engquist B, Eriksson AR, et al. Osseointegrated oral implants. A Swedish multicenter study of 8139 consecutively inserted Nobelpharma implants. J Periodontol 1988;59:287–296.
3. Buser D, Mericske-Stern R, Bernard JP, Behneke A, Behneke N, Hirt HP, et al. Long-term evaluation of non-submerged ITI implants. Part 1: 8-year life table analysis of a prospective multi-center study with 2359 implants. Clin Oral Implants Res 1997;8:161–172.
4. Gomez-Roman G, Kruppenbacher M, Weber H, Schulte W. Immediate postextraction implant placement with root-analog stepped implants: surgical procedure and statistical outcome after 6 years. Int J Oral Maxillofac Implants 2001;16:503–513.
5. Gomez-Roman G, Schulte W, d'Hoedt B, Axman-Krcmar D. The Frialit-2 implant system: five-year clinical experience in single-tooth and immediately postextraction applications. Int J Oral Maxillofac Implants 1997;12:299–309.
6. Sethi A, Kaus T, Sochor P. The use of angulated abutments in implant dentistry: five-year clinical results of an ongoing prospective study. Int J Oral Maxillofac Implants 2000;15:801–810.
7. Sethi A, Kaus T, Sochor P, Axmann-Krcmar D, Chanavaz M. Evolution of the concept of angulated abutments in implant dentistry: 14-year clinical data. Implant Dent 2002;11:41–51.
8. Smith DE, Zarb GA. Criteria for success of osseointegrated endosseous implants. J Prosthet Dent 1989;62:567–572.
9. Nentwig GH. Ankylos implant system: concept and clinical application. J Oral Implantol 2004;30:171–177.
10. Morris HF, Ochi S, Crum P, Orenstein IH, Winkler S. AICRG, Part I: A 6-year multicentered, multidisciplinary clinical study of a new and innovative implant design. J Oral Implantol 2004;30:125–133.
11. Doring K, Eisenmann E, Stiller M. Functional and esthetic considerations for single-tooth Ankylos implant-crowns: 8 years of clinical performance. J Oral Implantol 2004;30:198–209.
12. Hayter JP, Cawood JI. Oral rehabilitation with endosteal implants and free flaps. Int J Oral Maxillofac Surg 1996;25:3–12.
13. Kaus T, Engel E, Cornelius CP, Ehrenfeld M. Implantatprothetische Versorgung von Patienten nach Tumoroperation. ZMK 1997;13:23–24.
14. Riediger D. Restoration of masticatory function by microsurgically revascularized iliac crest bone grafts using enosseous implants. Plast Reconstr Surg 1988;81:861–877.
15. Weber H, Schmelzle R. Prothetische Rehabilitation von osteoplastisch rekonstruierten Defektpatienten mit Hilfe von implantatgetragenem. Z Zahnarztl Implantol 1986;II:61–64.
16. Weber H, Schmelzle R, Schwenzer N. Optimierung von Rehabilitationsergebnissen bei kiefer- und gesichtschirurgisch versorgten Patienten durch implantologisch-prothetische Massnahmen. Z Zahnarztl Implantol 1988;IV:182–187.
17. Davis DM, Fiske J, Scott B, Radford DR. The emotional effects of tooth loss: a preliminary quantitative study. Br Dent J 2000;188:503–506.
18. Davis DM, Fiske J, Scott B, Radford DR. The emotional effects of tooth loss in a group of partially dentate people: a quantitative study. Eur J Prosthodont Restorative Dent 2001;9:53–57.
19. Scott BJ, Leung KC, McMillan AS, Davis DM, Fiske J. A transcultural perspective on the emotional effect of tooth loss in complete denture wearers. Int J Prosthodont 2001;14:461–465.
20. Blomberg S, Brånemark PI, Zarb GA, Albrektsson T. Psychological Response. Tissue-Integrated Prostheses: Osseointegration in Clinical Dentistry. Chicago: Quintessence, 1985:165–174.
21. Carr AB, Laney WR. Maximum occlusal force levels in patients with osseointegrated oral implant prostheses and patients with complete dentures. Int J Oral Maxillofac Implants 1987;2:101–108.
22. Engel E, Weber H. Treatment of edentulous patients with temporomandibular disorders with implant-supported overdentures. Int J Oral Maxillofac Implants 1995;10:759–764.
23. Lundqvist S, Haraldson T. Oral function in patients wearing fixed prosthesis on osseointegrated implants in the maxilla: 3-year follow-up study. Scand J Dent Res 1992;100:279–283.
24. Lundqvist S, Haraldson T, Lindblad P. Speech in connection with maxillary fixed prostheses on osseointegrated implants: a three-year follow-up study. Clin Oral Implants Res 1992;3:176–180.

## References

25. Chanavaz M. Patient screening and medical evaluation for implant and preprosthetic surgery. J Oral Implantol 1998; 24:222–229.
26. Misch CE. Medical Evaluation. Contemporary Implant Dentistry. St. Louis: Mosby, 1993:51–102.
27. Sugerman PB, Barber MT. Patient selection for endosseous dental implants: oral and systemic considerations. Int J Oral Maxillofac Implants 2002;17:191–201.
28. Cawood JI, Howell RA. Reconstructive preprosthetic surgery. I. Anatomical considerations. Int J Oral Maxillofac Surg 1991;20:75–82.
29. Gibbs CH, Mahan PE, Mauderli A, Lundeen HC, Walsh EK. Limits of human bite strength. J Prosthet Dent 1986;56:226–229.
30. Pingitore G, Chrobak V, Petrie J. The social and psychologic factors of bruxism. J Prosthet Dent 1991;65:443–446.
31. Smith BG, Knight JK. A comparison of patterns of tooth wear with aetiological factors. Br Dent J 1984;157:16–19.
32. Smith BG, Knight JK. An index for measuring the wear of teeth. Br Dent J 1984;156:435–438.
33. Smith BG, Robb ND. The prevalence of toothwear in 1007 dental patients. J Oral Rehabil 1996;23:232–239.
34. Karanicolas PJ, Smith SE, Kanbur B, Davies E, Guyatt GH. The impact of prophylactic dexamethasone on nausea and vomiting after laparoscopic cholecystectomy: a systematic review and meta-analysis. Ann Surg 2008;248:751–762.
35. Sistla S, Rajesh R, Sadasivan J, Kundra P. Does single-dose preoperative dexamethasone minimize stress response and improve recovery after laparoscopic cholecystectomy? Surg Laparosc Endosc Percutan Tech 2009;19:506–510.
36. Dula K, Mini R, van der Stelt PF, Buser D. The radiographic assessment of implant patients: decision-making criteria. Int J Oral Maxillofac Implants 2001;16:80–89.
37. Harris D, Buser D, Dula K, Grondahl K, Jacobs R, Lekholm U, et al. E.A.O. guidelines for the use of diagnostic imaging in implant dentistry. A consensus workshop organized by the European Association for Osseointegration in Trinity College Dublin. Clin Oral Implants Res 2002;13:566–570.
38. Todd AD, Gher ME, Quintero G, Richardson AC. Interpretation of linear and computed tomograms in the assessment of implant recipient sites. J Periodontol 1993;64:1243–1249.
39. Norton MR, Gamble C. Bone classification: an objective scale of bone density using the computerized tomography scan. Clin Oral Implants Res 2001;12:79–84.
40. Koong B. Cone beam imaging: is this the ultimate imaging modality. Clin Oral Impl Res 2010;21:1201–1208.
41. Swennen GR, Schutyser F. Three-dimensional cephalometry: spiral multi-slice vs cone-beam computed tomography. Am J Orthod Dentofacial Orthop 2006;130:410–416.
42. Bauer J, Schaich M, Kaus T, Grunert T, Fleiter T, Niemaier R, et al. Erzeugung anatomischer Modelle durch Verarbeitung tomographischer Bilddaten mit einem CAD-System. Min Invas Med 1995;4:171–175.
43. Kaus T, Bauer J, Schaich M, Grunert T, Claussen CD, Weber H. CT-data based construction of a surgical template for dental implant surgery. [IADR Abstracts] J Dent Res 1999;78:375–375.
44. Sethi A. Precise site location for implants using CT scans: a technical note. Int J Oral Maxillofac Implants 1993;8:433–438.
45. Gray CF, Redpath TW, Smith FW. Pre-surgical dental implant assessment by magnetic resonance imaging. J Oral Implantol 1996;22:147–153.
46. Gray CF, Redpath TW, Smith FW. Magnetic resonance imaging: a useful tool for evaluation of bone prior to implant surgery. Br Dent J 1998;184:603–607.
47. Wilson DJ. Ridge mapping for determination of alveolar ridge width. Int J Oral Maxillofac Implants 1989;4:41–43.
48. Atwood DA. Reduction of residual ridges: a major oral disease entity. J Prosthet Dent 1971;26:266–279.
49. Atwood DA. Reduction of residual ridges in the partially edentulous patient. Dent Clin North Am 1973;17:747–754.
50. Cawood JI, Howell RA. A classification of the edentulous jaws. Int J Oral Maxillofac Surg 1988;17:232–236.
51. Lekholm U, Zarb GA, Brånemark PI, Albrektsson T. Patient Selection and Preparation. Tissue-integrated Prostheses: Osseointegration in Clinical Dentistry. Chicago: Quintessence, 1985:199–209.
52. Misch CE. Divisions of available bone in implant dentistry. Int J Oral Implantol 1990;7:9–17.
53. Misch CE. Density of bone: effect on treatment plans, surgical approach, healing, and progressive bone loading. Int J Oral Implantol 1990;6:23–31.
54. Misch CE. Density of Bone: Effect on Treatment Planning, Surgical Approach, and Healing. Contemporary Implant Dentistry. St. Louis: Mosby, 1993:469–485.
55. Trisi P, Rao W. Bone classification: clinical–histomorphometric comparison. Clin Oral Implants Res 1999;10:1–7.
56. Tallgren A. The continuing reduction of the residual alveolar ridges in complete denture wearers: a mixed-longitudinal study covering 25 years. J Prosthet Dent 1972;27:120–132.
57. Enlow DH, Bianco HJ, Eklund S. The remodeling of the edentulous mandible. J Prosthet Dent 1976;36:685–693.
58. Stella JP, Tharanon W. A precise radiographic method to determine the location of the inferior alveolar canal in the posterior edentulous mandible: implications for dental implants. Part 2: clinical application. Int J Oral Maxillofac Implants 1990;5:23–29.
59. Schulte W, d'Hoedt B, Axmann D, Gomez-Roman G. 15 Jahre Tübinger Implantat und seine Weiterentwicklung zum Frialit-2 System. [15-year Tübingen implant and its development into the Frialit-2 system.] Z Zahnarztl Implantol 1992;VIII:77–96.
60. Schulte W, Heimke G. Das Tübinger Sofort-Implantat. [The Tübingen immediate implant.] Quintessenz 1976;27:17–23.
61. Schulte W, Kleineikenscheidt H, Lindner K, Schareyka R. Das Tübinger Sofortimplantat in der klinischen Prüfung. [The Tübingen immediate implant in clinical studies.] Dtsch Zahnarztl Z 1978;33:348–359.

# References

62. Crespi R, Capoare P, Gherlone E, Romanos GE. Immediate versus delayed loading of dental implants placed in fresh extraction sockets in the maxillary esthetic zone: a clinical comparative study. Int J Oral Maxillofac Implants 2008;23:753–758.

63. Ledermann PD. Stegprothetische Versorgung des zahnlosen Unterkiefers mit Hilfe plasmabeschichteter Titanschraubimplantaten. Dtsch Zahnarztl Z 1979;34:907–911.

64. Szmukler-Moncler S, Piattelli A, Favero GA, Dubruille JH. Considerations preliminary to the application of early and immediate loading protocols in dental implantology. Clin Oral Implants Res 2000;11:12–25.

65. Szmukler-Moncler S, Salama H, Reingewirtz Y, Dubruille JH. Timing of loading and effect of micromotion on bone–dental implant interface: review of experimental literature. J Biomed Mater Res 1998;43:192–203.

66. Degidi M, Scarano A, Piattelli M, Perrotti V, Piattelli A. Bone remodeling in immediately loaded and unloaded titanium dental implants: a histologic and histomorphometric study in humans. J Oral Implantol 2005;31:18–24.

67. Piattelli A, Corigliano M, Scarano A, Costigliola G, Paolantonio M. Immediate loading of titanium plasma-sprayed implants: an histologic analysis in monkeys. J Periodontol 1998;69:321–327.

68. Piattelli A, Ruggeri A, Franchi M, Romasco N, Trisi P. An histologic and histomorphometric study of bone reactions to unloaded and loaded non-submerged single implants in monkeys: a pilot study. J Oral Implantol 1993;19:314–320.

69. Barone A, Covani U, Cornelini R, Gherlone E. Radiographic bone density around immediately loaded oral implants. Clin Oral Implants Res 2003;14:610–615.

70. Romanos GE, Toh CG, Siar CH, Swaminathan D. Histologic and histomorphometric evaluation of peri-implant bone subjected to immediate loading: an experimental study with *Macaca fascicularis*. Int J Oral Maxillofac Implants 2002;17:44–51.

71. Novaes Jr AB, Novaes AB. Immediate implants placed into infected sites: a clinical report. Int J Oral Maxillofac Implants 1995;10:609–613.

72. Novaes Jr AB, Vidigal Jr GM, Novaes AB, Grisi MF, Polloni S, Rosa A. Immediate implants placed into infected sites: a histomorphometric study in dogs. Int J Oral Maxillofac Implants 1998;13:422–427.

73. Marcaccini AM, Novaes Jr AB, Souza SL, Taba Jr M, Grisi MF. Immediate placement of implants into periodontally infected sites in dogs. Part 2: A fluorescence microscopy study. Int J Oral Maxillofac Implants 2003;18:812–819.

74. Novaes Jr AB, Marcaccini AM, Souza SL, Taba Jr M, Grisi MF. Immediate placement of implants into periodontally infected sites in dogs: a histomorphometric study of bone-implant contact. Int J Oral Maxillofac Implants 2003;18:391–398.

75. Papalexiou V, Novaes Jr AB, Grisi MF, Souza SS, Taba Jr M, Kajiwara JK. Influence of implant microstructure on the dynamics of bone healing around immediate implants placed into periodontally infected sites. A confocal laser scanning microscopic study. Clin Oral Implants Res 2004;15:44–53.

76. Novaes Jr AB, Papalexiou V, Grisi MF, Souza SS, Taba Jr M, Kajiwara JK. Influence of implant microstructure on the osseointegration of immediate implants placed in periodontally infected sites. A histomorphometric study in dogs. Clin Oral Implants Res 2004;15:34–43.

77. Quayle AA. Atraumatic removal of teeth and root fragments in dental implantology. Int J Oral Maxillofac Implants 1990;5:293–296.

78. Schlegel KA, Kloss FR, Kessler P, Schultze-Mosgau S, Nkenke E, Wiltfang J. Bone conditioning to enhance implant osseointegration: an experimental study in pigs. Int J Oral Maxillofac Implants 2003;18:505–511.

79. Wiltfang J, Schultze-Mosgau S, Schlegel KA. Einfluss von Implantatbett und Implantatlager auf die Osseointegration. Zahnarztl Mitt 2001:44–49.

80. Darveau RP, Tanner A, Page RC. The microbial challenge in periodontitis. Periodontol 2000 1997;14:12–32.

81. Hart TC, Kornman KS. Genetic factors in the pathogenesis of periodontitis. Periodontol 2000 1997;14:202–215.

82. Kornman KS, Page RC, Tonetti MS. The host response to the microbial challenge in periodontitis: assembling the players. Periodontol 2000 1997;14:33–53.

83. Page RC, Offenbacher S, Schroeder HE, Seymour GJ, Kornman KS. Advances in the pathogenesis of periodontitis: summary of developments, clinical implications and future directions. Periodontol 2000 1997;14:216–248.

84. Salvi GE, Lawrence HP, Offenbacher S, Beck JD. Influence of risk factors on the pathogenesis of periodontitis. Periodontol 2000 1997;14:173–201.

85. Schwartz Z, Goultschin J, Dean DD, Boyan BD. Mechanisms of alveolar bone destruction in periodontitis. Periodontol 2000 1997;14:158–172.

86. Ericsson I, Persson LG, Berglundh T, Marinello CP, Lindhe J, Klinge B. Different types of inflammatory reactions in peri-implant soft tissues. J Clin Periodontol 1995;22:255–261.

87. Gross M, Abramovich I, Weiss EI. Microleakage at the abutment-implant interface of osseointegrated implants: a comparative study. Int J Oral Maxillofac Implants 1999;14:94–100.

88. Hermann JS, Schoolfield JD, Nummikoski PV, Buser D, Schenk RK, Cochran DL. Crestal bone changes around titanium implants: a methodologic study comparing linear radiographic with histometric measurements. Int J Oral Maxillofac Implants 2001;16:475–485.

89. Quirynen M, van der Mei HC, Bollen CM, Schotte A, Marechal M, Doornbusch GI, et al. An in vivo study of the influence of the surface roughness of implants on the microbiology of supra- and subgingival plaque. J Dent Res 1993;72:1304–1309.

90. Piattelli A, Scarano A, Paolantonio M, Assenza B, Leghissa GC, Di Bonaventura G, et al. Fluids and microbial penetration in the internal part of cement-retained versus screw-retained implant–abutment connections. J Periodontol 2001;72:1146–1150.

# References

91. Rimondini L, Marin C, Brunella F, Fini M. Internal contamination of a 2-component implant system after occlusal loading and provisionally luted reconstruction with or without a washer device. J Periodontol 2001;72:1652–1657.

92. Mairgünther R, Nentwig GH. Das Dichtigkeitsverhalten des Verbindungssystems beim zweiphasigen NM-Implantat. [The tightness behavior of the connection system of the 2-phase Ankylos implant.] Z Zahnarztl Implantol 1992;VIII:50–53.

93. Hermann JS, Schoolfield JD, Schenk RK, Buser D, Cochran DL. Influence of the size of the microgap on crestal bone changes around titanium implants. A histometric evaluation of unloaded non-submerged implants in the canine mandible. J Periodontol 2001;72:1372–1383.

94. Zipprich H, Weigl P, Lange B, Lauer HC. Erfassung, Ursachen und Folgen von Mikrobewegungen am Implantat–Abutment-Interface. Implantologie 2007;15:31–46.

95. Harder S, Dimaczek B, Acil Y, Terheyden H, Freitag-Wolf S, Kern M. Molecular leakage at implant–abutment connection: in vitro investigation of tightness of internal conical implant-abutment connections against endotoxin penetration. Clin Oral Investig 2010;14:427–432.

96. Aloise JP, Curcio R, Laporta MZ, Rossi L, da Silva AM, Rapoport A. Microbial leakage through the implant–abutment interface of Morse taper implants in vitro. Clin Oral Implants Res 2010;21:328–335.

97. Davies JE. Mechanisms of endosseous integration. Int J Prosthodont 1998;11:391–401.

98. Davies JE. Understanding peri-implant endosseous healing. J Dent Educ 2003;67:932–949.

99. Wennerberg A, Albrektsson T. Effects of titanium surface topography on bone integration: a systematic review. Clin Oral Implants Res 2009;20(Suppl 4):172–184.

100. Chen ST, Darby IB, Reynolds EC. A prospective clinical study of non-submerged immediate implants: clinical outcomes and esthetic results. Clin Oral Implants Res 2007;18:552–562.

101. Akimoto K, Becker W, Persson R, Baker DA, Rohrer MD, O'Neal RB. Evaluation of titanium implants placed into simulated extraction sockets: a study in dogs. Int J Oral Maxillofac Implants 1999;14:351–360.

102. Wilson Jr TG, Schenk R, Buser D, Cochran D. Implants placed in immediate extraction sites: a report of histologic and histometric analyses of human biopsies. Int J Oral Maxillofac Implants 1998;13:333–341.

103. Tarnow DP, Cho SC, Wallace SS. The effect of inter-implant distance on the height of inter-implant bone crest. J Periodontol 2000;71:546–549.

104. Tarnow DP, Magner AW, Fletcher P. The effect of the distance from the contact point to the crest of bone on the presence or absence of the interproximal dental papilla. J Periodontol 1992;63:995–996.

105. Subbiahdoss G, Kuijer R, Grijpma DW, van der Mei HC, Busscher HJ. Microbial biofilm growth vs. tissue integration: "the race for the surface" experimentally studied. Acta Biomater 2009;5:1399–1404.

106. Lima LA, Fuchs-Wehrle AM, Lang NP, Hammerle CH, Liberti E, Pompeu E, et al. Surface characteristics of implants influence their bone integration after simultaneous placement of implant and GBR membrane. Clin Oral Implants Res 2003;14:669–679.

107. Meredith N. Assessment of implant stability as a prognostic determinant. Int J Prosthodont 1998;11:491–501.

108. Degidi M, Piattelli A, Gehrke P, Carinci F. Clinical outcome of 802 immediately loaded 2-stage submerged implants with a new grit-blasted and acid-etched surface: 12-month follow-up. Int J Oral Maxillofac Implants 2006;21:763–768.

109. Romanos GE, Nentwig GH. Immediate loading using cross-arch fixed restorations in heavy smokers: nine consecutive case reports for edentulous arches. Int J Oral Maxillofac Implants 2008;23:513–519.

110. Ellingsen JE. Surface configurations of dental implants. Periodontol 2000 1998;17:36–46.

111. Schenk RK, Buser D. Osseointegration: a reality. Periodontol 2000 1998;17:22–35.

112. Sykaras N, Iacopino AM, Marker VA, Triplett RG, Woody RD. Implant materials, designs, and surface topographies: their effect on osseointegration. A literature review. Int J Oral Maxillofac Implants 2000;15:675–690.

113. Chaushu G, Chaushu S, Tzohar A, Dayan D. Immediate loading of single-tooth implants: immediate versus non-immediate implantation. A clinical report. Int J Oral Maxillofac Implants 2001;16:267–272.

114. Canullo L, Rasperini G. Preservation of peri-implant soft and hard tissues using platform switching of implants placed in immediate extraction sockets: a proof-of-concept study with 12- to 36-month follow-up. Int J Oral Maxillofac Implants 2007;22:995–1000.

115. Tahmaseb A, De Clerck R, Wismeijer D. Computer-guided implant placement: 3D planning software, fixed intraoral reference points, and CAD/CAM technology. A case report. Int J Oral Maxillofac Implants 2009;24:541–546.

116. Tahmaseb A, van de Weijden JJ, Mercelis P, De Clerck R, Wismeijer D. Parameters of passive fit using a new technique to mill implant-supported superstructures: an in vitro study of a novel three-dimensional force measurement-misfit method. Int J Oral Maxillofac Implants 2010;25:247–257.

117. Komiyama A, Pettersson A, Hultin M, Nasstrom K, Klinge B. Virtually planned and template-guided implant surgery: an experimental model matching approach. Clin Oral Implants Res 2011;22:308–313.

118. D'Haese J, van de Velde T, Komiyama A, Hultin M, De Bruyn H. Accuracy and complications using computer-designed stereolithographic surgical guides for oral rehabilitation by means of dental implants: a review of the literature. Clin Implant Dent Relat Res 2010.

119. Barros RR, Novaes Jr AB, Muglia VA, Iezzi G, Piattelli A. Influence of interimplant distances and placement depth on peri-implant bone remodeling of adjacent and immediately loaded Morse cone connection implants: a histomorphometric study in dogs. Clin Oral Implants Res 2010;21:371–378.

120. Sethi A, Sochor P. Predicting esthetics in implant dentistry using multiplanar angulation: a technical note. Int J Oral Maxillofac Implants 1995;10:485–490.

121. Rochette AL. Attachment of a splint to enamel of lower anterior teeth. J Prosthet Dent 1973;30:418–423.

122. Banerji S, Sethi A, Dunne SM, Millar BJ. Clinical performance of Rochette bridges used as immediate provisional restorations for single unit implants in general practice. Br Dent J 2005;199:771–775.

123. Chang JC, Koh SH, Powers JM, Duong JH. Tensile bond strengths of composites to a gold–palladium alloy after thermal cycling. J Prosthet Dent 2002;87:271–276.

124. Haselton DR, Diaz-Arnold AM, Dunne Jr JT. Shear bond strengths of 2 intraoral porcelain repair systems to porcelain or metal substrates. J Prosthet Dent 2001;86:526–531.

125. Ozcan M, Niedermeier W. Clinical study on the reasons for and location of failures of metal–ceramic restorations and survival of repairs. Int J Prosthodont 2002;15:299–302.

126. Dahl BL, Krogstad O. The effect of a partial bite raising splint on the occlusal face height. An X-ray cephalometric study in human adults. Acta Odontol Scand 1982;40:17–24.

127. Lundskog J. Heat and bone tissue. An experimental investigation of the thermal properties of bone and threshold levels for thermal injury. Scand J Plast Reconstr Surg 1972;9:1–80.

128. Kirschner H, Meyer W. Entwicklung einer Innenkühlung für chirurgische Bohrer. Dtsch Zahnarztl Z 1975;30:436–438.

129. Kirschner H, van Steenberghe D. Thermometric investigation of internally cooled burs and cutters in animal experiments and in intraoral and implantation surgery. Tissue Integration in Oral and Maxillofacial Reconstruction. Amsterdam: Excerpta Medica, 1986:101–117.

130. Lavelle C, Wedgwood D. Effect of internal irrigation on frictional heat generated from bone drilling. J Oral Surg 1980;38:499–503.

131. Balshi TJ, Ekfeldt A, Stenberg T, Vrielinck L. Three-year evaluation of Brånemark implants connected to angulated abutments. Int J Oral Maxillofac Implants 1997;12:52–58.

132. Kallus T, Henry P, Jemt T, Jorneus L. Clinical evaluation of angulated abutments for the Brånemark system: a pilot study. Int J Oral Maxillofac Implants 1990;5:39–45.

133. Krekmanov L. Placement of posterior mandibular and maxillary implants in patients with severe bone deficiency: a clinical report of procedure. Int J Oral Maxillofac Implants 2000;15:722–730.

134. Krekmanov L, Kahn M, Rangert B, Lindstrom H. Tilting of posterior mandibular and maxillary implants for improved prosthesis support. Int J Oral Maxillofac Implants 2000;15:405–414.

135. Kaus T, Sethi A. Voraussagbare Ästhetik mit dentalen Implantaten: Abformung während der Implantatinsertion. ZWR 2001;110:22–26.

136. Knode H. Rehabilitation with implant-supported suprastructures at the time of the abutment surgery: a case report. Pract Periodont Aesthet Dent 1995;7:67–73.

137. Rosenlicht JL. Advanced surgical techniques in implant dentistry: contemporary applications of early techniques. J Dent Symp 1993;1:16-9–16-19.

138. Sethi A. Refining the art: impressions at 1st stage surgery. 2nd International Symposium: Changing Faces, London UK.

139. Sethi A, Sochor P. First stage surgery impressions. Independ Dent 1998:78–85.

140. Firtell DN, Moore DJ, Pelleu GB, Jr. Sterilization of impression materials for use in the surgical operating room. J Prosthet Dent 1972;27:419–422.

141. Samaranayake LP, Hunjan M, Jennings KJ. Carriage of oral flora on irreversible hydrocolloid and elastomeric impression materials. J Prosthet Dent 1991;65:244–249.

142. Coppi C, Paolinelli Devincenzi C, Bortolini S, Consolo U, Tiozzo R. A new generation of sterile and radiopaque impression materials: an in vitro cytotoxicity study. J Biomater Appl 2007;22:83–95.

143. Roberta T, Federico M, Federica B, Antonietta CM, Sergio B, Ugo C. Study of the potential cytotoxicity of dental impression materials. Toxicol In Vitro 2003;17:657–662.

144. Abrahamsson I, Berglundh T, Lindhe J. The mucosal barrier following abutment dis/reconnection. An experimental study in dogs. J Clin Periodontol 1997;24:568–572.

145. Binon P. Evaluation of machining accuracy and consistency of selected implants, standard abutments, and laboratory analogs. Int J Prosthodont 1995;8:162–178.

146. Kaus T, Benzing U. Machining accuracy of selected implant abutments. [IADR Abstracts] J Dent Res 1996;75:184.

147. Kim S, Nicholls JI, Han CH, Lee KW. Displacement of implant components from impressions to definitive casts. Int J Oral Maxillofac Implants 2006;21:747–755.

148. Ma T, Nicholls JI, Rubenstein JE. Tolerance measurements of various implant components. Int J Oral Maxillofac Implants 1997;12:371–375.

149. Palacci P. A management des tissus peri-implantaires interet de la regeneration des papilles. Real Clin 1992;3:381–387.

150. Assif D, Fenton A, Zarb G, Schmitt A. Comparative accuracy of implant impression procedures. Int J Periodontics Restorative Dent 1992;12:112–121.

151. Carr AB. Comparison of impression techniques for a five-implant mandibular model. Int J Oral Maxillofac Implants 1991;6:448–455.

152. Carrotte PV, Johnson A, Winstanley RB. The influence of the impression tray on the accuracy of impressions for crown and bridge work: an investigation and review. Br Dent J 1998;185:580–585.

153. de la Cruz JE, Funkenbusch PD, Ercoli C, Moss ME, Graser GN, Tallents RH. Verification jig for implant-supported prostheses: a comparison of standard impressions with verification jigs made of different materials. J Prosthet Dent 2002;88:329–336.

154. Humphries RM, Yaman P, Bloem TJ. The accuracy of implant master casts constructed from transfer impressions. Int J Oral Maxillofac Implants 1990;5:331–336.

## References

155. Sorrentino R, Gherlone EF, Calesini G, Zarone F. Effect of implant angulation, connection length, and impression material on the dimensional accuracy of implant impressions: an in vitro comparative study. Clin Implant Dent Relat Res 2010;12(Suppl 1):e63–e76.

156. Spector MR, Donovan TE, Nicholls JI. An evaluation of impression techniques for osseointegrated implants. J Prosthet Dent 1990;63:444–447.

157. Thongthammachat S, Moore BK, Barco MT, Hovijitra S, Brown DT, Andres CJ. Dimensional accuracy of dental casts: influence of tray material, impression material, and time. J Prosthodont 2002;11:98–108.

158. Valderhaug J, Floystrand F. Dimensional stability of elastomeric impression materials in custom-made and stock trays. J Prosthet Dent 1984;52:514–517.

159. Kucey BK, Fraser DC. The Procera abutment: the fifth generation abutment for dental implants. J Can Dent Assoc 2000;66:445–449.

160. Lewis SG, Llamas D, Avera S. The UCLA abutment: a four-year review. J Prosthet Dent 1992;67:509–515.

161. Marchack CB. A custom titanium abutment for the anterior single-tooth implant. J Prosthet Dent 1996;76:288–291.

162. Kerstein RB, Radke J. A comparison of fabrication precision and mechanical reliability of 2 zirconia implant abutments. Int J Oral Maxillofac Implants 2008;23:1029–1036.

163. Bahat O, Fontanesi RV, Preston J. Reconstruction of the hard and soft tissues for optimal placement of osseointegrated implants. Int J Periodont Restorative Dent 1993;13:255–275.

164. Buser D, Bragger U, Lang NP, Nyman S. Regeneration and enlargement of jaw bone using guided tissue regeneration. Clin Oral Implants Res 1990;1:22–32.

165. Buser D, Dula K, Belser U, Hirt HP, Berthold H. Localized ridge augmentation using guided bone regeneration. 1. Surgical procedure in the maxilla. Int J Periodontics Restorative Dent 1993;13:29–45.

166. Buser D, Dula K, Belser UC, Hirt HP, Berthold H. Localized ridge augmentation using guided bone regeneration. II. Surgical procedure in the mandible. Int J Periodontics Restorative Dent 1995;15:10–29.

167. Fugazzotto PA. Report of 302 consecutive ridge augmentation procedures: technical considerations and clinical results. Int J Oral Maxillofac Implants 1998;13:358–368.

168. Nevins M, Mellonig JT. Enhancement of the damaged edentulous ridge to receive dental implants: a combination of allograft and the GORE-TEX membrane. Int J Periodontics Restorative Dent 1992;12:96–111.

169. Shanaman RH. The use of guided tissue regeneration to facilitate ideal prosthetic placement of implants. Int J Periodontics Restorative Dent 1992;12:256–265.

170. Shanaman RH. A retrospective study of 237 sites treated consecutively with guided tissue regeneration. Int J Periodontics Restorative Dent 1994;14:292–301.

171. Simion M, Jovanovic SA, Trisi P, Scarano A, Piattelli A. Vertical ridge augmentation around dental implants using a membrane technique and autogenous bone or allografts in humans. Int J Periodontics Restorative Dent 1998;18:8–23.

172. Simion M, Trisi P, Piattelli A. Vertical ridge augmentation using a membrane technique associated with osseointegrated implants. Int J Periodontics Restorative Dent 1994;14:496–511.

173. Mattout P, Mattout C. Conditions for success in guided bone regeneration: retrospective study on 376 implant sites. J Periodontol 2000;71:1904–1909.

174. Buser D, Dula K, Hirt HP, Schenk RK. Lateral ridge augmentation using autografts and barrier membranes: a clinical study with 40 partially edentulous patients. J Oral Maxillofac Surg 1996;54:420–432.

175. Gongloff RK, Cole M, Whitlow W, Boyne PJ. Titanium mesh and particulate cancellous bone and marrow grafts to augment the maxillary alveolar ridge. Int J Oral Maxillofac Surg 1986;15:263–268.

176. Stringer DE, Boyne PJ. Modification of the maxillary step osteotomy and stabilization with titanium mesh. J Oral Maxillofac Surg 1986;44:487–488.

177. von Arx T, Hardt N, Wallkamm B. The TIME technique: a new method for localized alveolar ridge augmentation prior to placement of dental implants. Int J Oral Maxillofac Implants 1996;11:387–394.

178. von Arx T, Kurt B. Implant placement and simultaneous peri-implant bone grafting using a micro titanium mesh for graft stabilization. Int J Periodont Restorative Dent 1998;18:117–127.

179. von Arx T, Kurt B. Implant placement and simultaneous ridge augmentation using autogenous bone and a micro titanium mesh: a prospective clinical study with 20 implants. Clin Oral Implants Res 1999;10:24–33.

180. von Arx T, Wallkamm B, Hardt N. Localized ridge augmentation using a micro titanium mesh: a report on 27 implants followed from 1 to 3 years after functional loading. Clin Oral Implants Res 1998;9:123–130.

181. Becker W, Schenk R, Higuchi K, Lekholm U, Becker BE. Variations in bone regeneration adjacent to implants augmented with barrier membranes alone or with demineralized freeze-dried bone or autologous grafts: a study in dogs. Int J Oral Maxillofac Implants 1995;10:143–154.

182. Buser D, Ruskin J, Higginbottom F, Hardwick R, Dahlin C, Schenk RK. Osseointegration of titanium implants in bone regenerated in membrane-protected defects: a histologic study in the canine mandible. Int J Oral Maxillofac Implants 1995;10:666–681.

183. Misch CM. Ridge augmentation using mandibular ramus bone grafts for the placement of dental implants: presentation of a technique. Pract Periodont Aesthet Dent 1996;8:127–135.

184. Misch CM. Comparison of intraoral donor sites for onlay grafting prior to implant placement. Int J Oral Maxillofac Implants 1997;12:767–776.

185. Misch CM, Misch CE. The repair of localized severe ridge defects for implant placement using mandibular bone grafts. Implant Dent 1995;4:261–267.
186. Sethi A, Kaus T. Ridge augmentation using mandibular block bone grafts: preliminary results of an ongoing prospective study. Int J Oral Maxillofac Implants 2001;16:378–388.
187. Lekholm U, Wannfors K, Isaksson S, Adielsson B. Oral implants in combination with bone grafts. A 3-year retrospective multicenter study using the Brånemark implant system. Int J Oral Maxillofac Surg 1999;28:181–187.
188. Lundgren S, Rasmusson L, Sjostrom M, Sennerby L. Simultaneous or delayed placement of titanium implants in free autogenous iliac bone grafts. Histological analysis of the bone graft–titanium interface in 10 consecutive patients. Int J Oral Maxillofac Surg 1999;28:31–37.
189. Aparicio C, Jensen OT. Alveolar ridge widening by distraction osteogenesis: a case report. Pract Proc Aesthet Dent 2001;13:663–668.
190. Chiapasco M, Romeo E, Casentini P, Rimondini L. Alveolar distraction osteogenesis vs. vertical guided bone regeneration for the correction of vertically deficient edentulous ridges: a 1–3-year prospective study on humans. Clin Oral Implants Res 2004;15:82–95.
191. Chiapasco M, Romeo E, Vogel G. Vertical distraction osteogenesis of edentulous ridges for improvement of oral implant positioning: a clinical report of preliminary results. Int J Oral Maxillofac Implants 2001;16:43–51.
192. Chin M, Toth BA. Distraction osteogenesis in maxillofacial surgery using internal devices: review of five cases. J Oral Maxillofac Surg 1996;54:45–53.
193. Jensen OT, Cockrell R, Kuhike L, Reed C. Anterior maxillary alveolar distraction osteogenesis: a prospective 5-year clinical study. Int J Oral Maxillofac Implants 2002;17:52–68.
194. Rachmiel A, Srouji S, Peled M. Alveolar ridge augmentation by distraction osteogenesis. Int J Oral Maxillofac Surg 2001;30:510–517.
195. Zechner W, Bernhart T, Zauza K, Celar A, Watzek G. Multidimensional osteodistraction for correction of implant malposition in edentulous segments. Clin Oral Implants Res 2001;12:531–538.
196. Holtzclaw D, Toscano N, Eisenlohr L, Callan D. The safety of bone allografts used in dentistry: a review. J Am Dent Assoc 2008;139:1192–1199.
197. McAllister DR, Joyce MJ, Mann BJ, Vangsness Jr CT. Allograft update: the current status of tissue regulation, procurement, processing, and sterilization. Am J Sports Med 2007;35:2148–2158.
198. Vangsness Jr CT. Soft-tissue allograft processing controversies. J Knee Surg 2006;19:215–219.
199. Hurzeler MB, Kirsch A, Ackermann KL, Quinones CR. Reconstruction of the severely resorbed maxilla with dental implants in the augmented maxillary sinus: a 5-year clinical investigation. Int J Oral Maxillofac Implants 1996;11:466–475.
200. Marx RE, Carlson ER, Eichstaedt RM, Schimmele SR, Strauss JE, Georgeff KR. Platelet-rich plasma: growth factor enhancement for bone grafts. Oral Surg Oral Med Oral Pathol Oral Radiol Endod 1998;85:638–646.
201. Tadjoedin ES, De Lange GL, Holzmann PJ, Kulper L, Burger EH. Histological observations on biopsies harvested following sinus floor elevation using a bioactive glass material of narrow size range. Clin Oral Implants Res 2000;11:334–344.
202. Tong DC, Rioux K, Drangsholt M, Beirne OR. A review of survival rates for implants placed in grafted maxillary sinuses using meta-analysis. Int J Oral Maxillofac Implants 1998;13:175–182.
203. de Carvalho PS, Vasconcellos LW, Pi J. Influence of bed preparation on the incorporation of autogenous bone grafts: a study in dogs. Int J Oral Maxillofac Implants 2000;15:565–570.
204. Sethi A, Kaus T. Maxillary ridge expansion with simultaneous implant placement: 5-year results of an ongoing clinical study. Int J Oral Maxillofac Implants 2000;15:491–499.
205. Sethi A, Sochor P, Hills G. Implants and maxillary ridge expansion. Independ Dent 1998:80–90.
206. Tatum H, Jr. Maxillary and sinus implant reconstructions. Dent Clin North Am 1986;30:207–229.
207. Duncan JM, Westwood RM. Ridge widening for the thin maxilla: a clinical report. Int J Oral Maxillofac Implants 1997;12:224–227.
208. Engelke WG, Diederichs CG, Jacobs HG, Deckwer I. Alveolar reconstruction with splitting osteotomy and microfixation of implants. Int J Oral Maxillofac Implants 1997;12:310–318.
209. Frisch E, Pehrsson K, Jacobs HG. Implantation mit gleichzeitigem segmentalen Bone-Splitting. Z Zahnarztl Implantol 1994;10:7–11.
210. Handtmann S, Gomez-Roman G, Axmann-Krcmar D, Schulte W, Lukas D. Vergleich von Implantationen mit und ohne simultane Kieferkammspreizung bei Frialit-2 und Tübinger Implantaten. Z Zahnarztl Implantol 1998;14:21–29.
211. Handtmann S, Gomez-Roman G, Wuest AK, Axmann-Krcmar D, Schulte W. Alveolar extension splastik bei gleichzeitiger Implantation. Z Zahnarztl Implantol 1995;11:158–164.
212. Simion M, Baldoni M, Zaffe D. Jawbone enlargement using immediate implant placement associated with a split-crest technique and guided tissue regeneration. Int J Periodont Restorative Dent 1992;12:462–473.
213. Chanavaz M. Anatomy and histophysiology of the periosteum: quantification of the periosteal blood supply to the adjacent bone with 85Sr and gamma spectrometry. J Oral Implantol 1995;21:214–219.
214. Penarrocha-Diago M, Rambla-Ferrer J, Perez V, Perez-Garrigues H. Benign paroxysmal vertigo secondary to placement of maxillary implants using the alveolar expansion technique with osteotomes: a study of 4 cases. Int J Oral Maxillofac Implants 2008;23:129–132.
215. Saker M, Ogle O. Benign paroxysmal positional vertigo subsequent to sinus lift via closed technique. J Oral Maxillofac Surg 2005;63:1385–1387.

## References

216. De Marco AC, Jardini MA, Lima LP. Revascularization of autogenous block grafts with or without an e-PTFE membrane. Int J Oral Maxillofac Implants 2005;20:867–874.

217. Bell RB, Blakey GH, White RP, Hillebrand DG, Molina A. Staged reconstruction of the severely atrophic mandible with autogenous bone graft and endosteal implants. J Oral Maxillofac Surg 2002;60:1135–1141.

218. Shin YK, Han CH, Heo SJ, Kim S, Chun HJ. Radiographic evaluation of marginal bone level around implants with different neck designs after 1 year. Int J Oral Maxillofac Implants 2006;21:789–794.

219. Chanavaz M. Maxillary sinus: anatomy, physiology, surgery, and bone grafting related to implantology: eleven years of surgical experience (1979–1990). J Oral Implantol 1990;16:199–209.

220. Chanavaz M. Sinus grafting related to implantology. Statistical analysis of 15 years of surgical experience (1979–1994). J Oral Implantol 1996;22:119–130.

221. Krennmair G, Ulm CW, Lugmayr H, Solar P. The incidence, location, and height of maxillary sinus septa in the edentulous and dentate maxilla. J Oral Maxillofac Surg 1999;57:667–671; discussion 671–662.

222. Penarrocha M, Carrillo C, Boronat A. Retrospective study of 68 implants placed in the pterygomaxillary region using drills and osteotomes. Int J Oral Maxillofac Implants 2009;24:720–726.

223. Valeron JF, Valeron PF. Long-term results in placement of screw-type implants in the pterygomaxillary-pyramidal region. Int J Oral Maxillofac Implants 2007;22:195–200.

224. Balshi SF, Wolfinger GJ, Balshi TJ. Analysis of 164 titanium oxide-surface implants in completely edentulous arches for fixed prosthesis anchorage using the pterygomaxillary region. Int J Oral Maxillofac Implants 2005;20:946–952.

225. Balshi TJ, Wolfinger GJ, Balshi SF, 2nd. Analysis of 356 pterygomaxillary implants in edentulous arches for fixed prosthesis anchorage. Int J Oral Maxillofac Implants 1999;14:398–406.

226. Bedrossian E, Stumpel LJ, III. Immediate stabilization at stage II of zygomatic implants: rationale and technique. J Prosthet Dent 2001;86:10–14.

227. Stevenson AR, Austin BW. Zygomatic fixtures: the Sydney experience. Ann Roy Aust Coll Dent Surg 2000;15:337–339.

228. Davo R. Zygomatic implants placed with a two-stage procedure: a 5-year retrospective study. Eur J Oral Implantol 2009;2:115–124.

229. Balshi SF, Wolfinger GJ, Balshi TJ. A retrospective analysis of 110 zygomatic implants in a single-stage immediate loading protocol. Int J Oral Maxillofac Implants 2009;24:335–341.

230. Parel SM, Brånemark PI, Ohrnell LO, Svensson B. Remote implant anchorage for the rehabilitation of maxillary defects. J Prosthet Dent 2001;86:377–381.

231. Sato FR, Sawazaki R, Berretta D, Moreira RW, Vargas PA, de Almeida OP. Aspergillosis of the maxillary sinus associated with a zygomatic implant. J Am Dent Assoc 2010;141:1231–1235.

232. Reychler H, Olszewski R. Intracerebral penetration of a zygomatic dental implant and consequent therapeutic dilemmas: case report. Int J Oral Maxillofac Implants 2010;25:416–418.

233. Bothur S, Garsten M. Initial speech problems in patients treated with multiple zygomatic implants. Int J Oral Maxillofac Implants 2010;25:379–384.

234. Chow J, Wat P, Hui E, Lee P, Li W. A new method to eliminate the risk of maxillary sinusitis with zygomatic implants. Int J Oral Maxillofac Implants 2010;25:1233–1240.

235. Bahat O. Osseointegrated implants in the maxillary tuberosity: report on 45 consecutive patients. Int J Oral Maxillofac Implants 1992;7:459–467.

236. Jaffin RA, Berman CL. The excessive loss of Brånemark fixtures in type IV bone: a 5-year analysis. J Periodontol 1991;62:2–4.

237. Summers RB. A new concept in maxillary implant surgery: the osteotome technique. Compendium 1994;15:152, 154–156, 158.

238. Renner PJ, Romanos GE, Nentwig GH. Die Knochenspreizung bei der Implantation im reduzierten Alveolarfortsatz des Oberkiefers. [Bone spreading during the implantation in the reduced maxillary ridge.] Dtsch Zahnnarztl Z 1996;51:118–120.

239. Summers RB. Sinus floor elevation with osteotomes. J Esthet Dent 1998;10:164–171.

240. Boyne PJ, James RA. Grafting of the maxillary sinus floor with autogenous marrow and bone. J Oral Surg 1980;38:613–616.

241. Tatum Jr OH, Lebowitz MS, Tatum CA, Borgner RA. Sinus augmentation. Rationale, development, long-term results [see comments]. N Y State Dent J 1993;59:43–48.

242. Zerbo IR, Bronckers AL, de Lange G, Burger EH. Localisation of osteogenic and osteoclastic cells in porous beta-tricalcium phosphate particles used for human maxillary sinus floor elevation. Biomaterials 2005;26:1445–1451.

243. Kieser J, Kuzmanovic D, Payne A, Dennison J, Herbison P. Patterns of emergence of the human mental nerve. Arch Oral Biol 2002;47:743–747.

244. Mardinger O, Chaushu G, Arensburg B, Taicher S, Kaffe I. Anterior loop of the mental canal: an anatomical–radiologic study. Implant Dent 2000;9:120–125.

245. Rosenquist B. Is there an anterior loop of the inferior alveolar nerve? Int J Periodont Restorative Dent 1996;16:40–45.

246. Carter RB, Keen EN. The intramandibular course of the inferior alveolar nerve. J Anat 1971;108:433–440.

247. Chuang SK, Wei LJ, Douglass CW, Dodson TB. Risk factors for dental implant failure: a strategy for the analysis of clustered failure–time observations. J Dent Res 2002;81:572–577.

248. Friberg B, Jemt T, Lekholm U. Early failures in 4641 consecutively placed Brånemark dental implants: a study from stage 1 surgery to the connection of completed prostheses. Int J Oral Maxillofac Implants 1991;6:142–146.

249. Wheeler SL. Eight-year clinical retrospective study of titanium plasma-sprayed and hydroxyapatite-coated cylinder implants. Int J Oral Maxillofac Implants 1996;11:340–350.

# References

250. Bartling R, Freeman K, Kraut RA. The incidence of altered sensation of the mental nerve after mandibular implant placement. J Oral Maxillofac Surg 1999;57:1408–1412.
251. Garg AK, Morales MJ. Lateralization of the inferior alveolar nerve with simultaneous implant placement: surgical techniques. Pract Periodont Aesthet Dent 1998;10:1197–1204.
252. Hirsch JM, Brånemark PI. Fixture stability and nerve function after transposition and lateralization of the inferior alveolar nerve and fixture installation. Br J Oral Maxillofac Surg 1995;33:276–281.
253. Rosenquist B. Fixture placement posterior to the mental foramen with transpositioning of the inferior alveolar nerve. Int J Oral Maxillofac Implants 1992;7:45–50.
254. Sethi A. Inferior alveolar nerve repositioning in implant dentistry: clinical report. Implant Dent 1993;2:195–197.
255. Sethi A. Step-by-step instructions for nerve repositioning and implant placement. Dent Implantol Update 1994;5:22–24.
256. Sethi A. Repositioning the contents of the inferior alveolar canal to accommodate the root-form implants. Dent Implantol Update 1994;5:21–22.
257. Sethi A. Inferior alveolar nerve repositioning in implant dentistry: a preliminary report. Int J Periodont Restorative Dent 1995;15:474–481.
258. Lundborg G. Nerve Injury and Repair. Edinburgh: Churchill Livingstone, 1988.
259. Mozsary PG, Syers CS. Microsurgical correction of the injured inferior alveolar nerve. J Oral Maxillofac Surg 1985;43:353–358.
260. Svane TJ, Wolford LM, Milam SB, Bass RK. Fascicular characteristics of the human inferior alveolar nerve. J Oral Maxillofac Surg 1986;44:431–434.
261. Campbell Z, Simons AM, Giordano JR. Soft tissue grafting and vestibuloplasty technique in association with endosseous implants. J Mich Dent Assoc 1993;75:26–29.
262. Simons AM, Baima RF. Free gingival grafting and vestibuloplasty with endosseous implant placement: clinical report. Implant Dent 1994;3:235–238.
263. ten Bruggenkate CM, Krekeler G, van der Kwast WA, Oosterbeek HS. Palatal mucosa grafts for oral implant devices. Oral Surg Oral Med Oral Pathol 1991;72:154–158.
264. Thies RM, Sager RD. Lipswitch vestibuloplasty in conjunction with implant placement. Compendium 1991;12:456, 458, 460.
265. Edel A. Clinical evaluation of free connective tissue grafts used to increase the width of keratinised gingiva. J Clin Periodontol 1974;1:185–196.
266. Harris RJ. The connective tissue and partial thickness double pedicle graft: a predictable method of obtaining root coverage. J Periodontol 1992;63:477–486.
267. Langer B, Calagna LJ. The subepithelial connective tissue graft. A new approach to the enhancement of anterior cosmetics. Int J Periodont Restorative Dent 1982;2:22–33.
268. Nelson SW. The subpedicle connective tissue graft. A bilaminar reconstructive procedure for the coverage of denuded root surfaces. J Periodontol 1987;58:95–102.
269. Silverstein LH, Kurtzman D, Garnick JJ, Trager PS, Waters PK. Connective tissue grafting for improved implant esthetics: clinical technique. Implant Dent 1994;3:231–234.
270. Burkhardt R, Joss A, Lang NP. Soft tissue dehiscence coverage around endosseous implants: a prospective cohort study. Clin Oral Implants Res 2008;19:451–457.
271. Wiesner G, Esposito M, Worthington H, Schlee M. Connective tissue grafts for thickening peri-implant tissues at implant placement. One-year results from an explanatory split-mouth randomised controlled clinical trial. Eur J Oral Implantol 2010;3:27–35.
272. Cornelini R, Barone A, Covani U. Connective tissue grafts in postextraction implants with immediate restoration: a prospective controlled clinical study. Pract Proc Aesthet Dent 2008;20:337–343.
273. Covani U, Marconcini S, Galassini G, Cornelini R, Santini S, Barone A. Connective tissue graft used as a biologic barrier to cover an immediate implant. J Periodontol 2007;78:1644–1649.

# Glossary of Terms

*This glossary of terms relates to the use of specific phrases within the context of this book. It is not intended as a dictionary.*

**Abutment position transfer**
Technique for transferring the abutment position to the laboratory resulting in a cast with an accurately positioned replica of the abutment. Alterations of the abutment in the mouth or its replica in the laboratory should not be carried out.

**Anti-rotation**
A feature that prevents rotation of the abutment in relation to the implant and may be provided by an irregularity (e.g. hexagon, octagon etc) or a high precision conical connection.

**Bone expansion**
Bone manipulation where a narrow bony ridge is widened by separating the two cortical plates for the insertion of an implant or biomaterial into the space created.

**Bone manipulation**
Technique for locally transpositioning bone to either alter (increase) height, width or density.

**Containment**
Method of containing particulate material in proximity to the deficient site to prevent its displacement by the use of a membrane or a mesh.

**Diagnostic preview**
Diagnostic set-up of teeth in wax, plastic or other diagnostic medium arranged in optimal aesthetic and functional position. It enables the ideal tooth position to be related to residual ridge, proposed bone graft or implant position.

**Diagnostic template**
Hollow prosthetic envelope constructed from diagnostic preview, which enables the clinician to relate the ideal tooth position to the mouth for assessing the need for augmentation, selecting implant position and the abutment.

**Direct (conventional) impressions**
Impressions of the abutment, which can be cast to reproduce a dimensionally accurate model of the mouth. Impressions of implant abutments may be cast using die stone or epoxy resins for the direct construction of the restoration.

**Free gingival graft**
Keratinised epithelial tissue that is transplanted from the donor site (often the palate) to the recipient site, which has been denuded to expose the periosteum to provide a source of revascularisation.

**Frenectomy**
Removal of a frenal attachment.

**Graft**
Transpositioning of either hard- or soft-tissues from a donor site remote from the recipient site. It has to re-establish a blood supply at the recipient site (this definition specifically differentiates it from a flap. It does not address the source of the graft e.g. autogenous, xenograft etc).

**Hybrid retention**
Retention that is achieved using two different retentive mechanisms, such as a screw and cement.

**Implant position transfer**
Technique for transferring the implant position to the laboratory, resulting in a cast with an accurately positioned replica of the implant.

**Impressions at first stage surgery**
Impressions taken at time of implant placement to transfer implant position to the laboratory for the construction of a cast containing an accurately positioned implant replica. It permits modification and/or fabrication of abutments, transitional restorations and superstructures during the healing phase.

**Indexed abutment**
An abutment that restricts the number of rotational positions in which it can be connected to the implant. The indexing (e.g. hexagon, octagon or other irregularities) is often used as anti-rotation.

# Glossary of Terms

**Lateral screw**
A small screw that is inserted through the prosthesis or superstructure into a recess in the abutment or a coping attached to the abutment. This provides resistance to displacement of the prosthesis or superstructure.

**Metal-acrylic hybrid bridge**
Provisional restoration retained by a resin bonded Rochette wing as well as a conventionally cemented abutment crown/partial crown.

**Metal-acrylic Rochette bridge**
Provisional restoration consisting of the retainer as a perforated wing constructed from metal providing mechanical retention using resin bonding for ease of attachment and reattachment. The acrylic pontic permits easy adjustment both in terms of reduction and addition.

**Metal-acrylic spring cantilever bridge**
Provisional restoration retained by an abutment tooth distant from the pontic site where teeth are present in between. The connector normally transverses over the palatal or lingual mucosa.

**Metal-acrylic spring cantilever Rochette bridge**
Provisional restoration retained by an abutment tooth distant from the pontic site where teeth are present in between. The connector normally transverses over the palatal or lingual mucosa. The retainer on the abutment is a perforated metal wing/wings on the palatal, occlusal and/or buccal aspects of the abutment tooth.

**Morphological manipulation**
Manipulation of the hard or soft tissues to alter the shape of the anatomical structure without compromising the function.

**Non-indexed abutment**
An abutment that connects to the implant in an infinite number of rotational positions. Anti-rotation can be provided by frictional fit.

**Pedicle flap**
A flap that remains connected at its base to maintain its blood supply and which may be repositioned to alter the morphology of a remote site.

**Provisional restoration**
Restoration used to replace missing tooth/teeth from the commencement of treatment until the construction of the transitional or definitive restoration. Additionally it is used to assess and confirm aesthetic and functional parameters.

**Ridge mapping**
Method of determining the width of the bony ridge underlying the soft tissues by a calibrated device that penetrates the soft tissue. Pointed calipers or calibrated probes may be used to gather the data, which is recorded appropriately.

**Sinus floor manipulation**
Bone manipulation using osteotomes (bone condensers) to deform the sinus floor through the osteotomy without creating a perforation thus increasing the height available for an implant.

**Sinus lift – subantral augmentation**
Elevation of the sinus lining from the floor and the walls of the maxillary sinus through a bony window (commonly through the lateral wall of the maxillary sinus). This permits the placement of biomaterials to increase the height of bone available for implant placement.

**Sub-epithelial connective tissue graft**
Soft tissue graft obtained from the soft-tissues underneath the epithelial layer. Most commonly this is obtained from the palate.

**Sulcus former**
A transgingival component that is attached to the implant following its exposure or at the time of implant placement to establish access to the implant for subsequent attachment of the definitive abutment.

**Transitional restoration**
Restoration used after abutment attachment until the fitting of the definitive restoration. The transitional restoration is connected to the implant and may be used to confirm the parameters for the definitive restoration.

**Vestibuloplasty**
Alteration of the morphology of the vestibule to increase the depth by repositioning the muscular attachments apically.

# Index

## A

abutment connection 85
abutments
   attachment 66–73, 162–164
   direct impressions of 173–178
   fabrication 186–187
   indexed 57
   modification 186–187
   position transfer 178–182, 196–199
   selection 66–73, 186–187
aesthetically critical zone, immediate placement 75–76
aesthetics, and augmentation 207
allogenic grafts 210, 211
alloplastic materials 211
amalgam tattoo, elimination 378–380
anaesthesia 17–18
anatomical variations 31–42
anterior mandible 37–38
anterior maxilla 32–34
   reconstruction following trauma 274–280
anti-rotation 158, 164
atrophy 31
   classification of degree of 262–264
augmentation categories 208–211
   clinical cases 280–285, 287–294, 295–300
   decision-making process 218
   indications 207–208
   *see also* bone expansion; grafting of tissues; manipulation of tissues; posterior mandible; posterior maxilla
autogenous grafts 209–210
   *see also* block bone grafts; extensive bone grafts; localised onlay bone grafts

## B

biomaterials 75–76
biomechanics, and augmentation 207
block bone grafts 210, 218
   *see also* localised onlay bone grafts
bone condensers 228, 233, 310
bone deficiencies
   assessment of localised 239–240
   causes 206–207
   measurement 246
bone expanders 225–227, 232
bone expansion 219–237
   clinical cases 230–237
      labial plate re-contouring 230–231
      multiple implants 236–237
      single implant 231–235
   healing phase 230
   implant insertion 228
   impressions at first-stage surgery 229
   restorative phase 230
   surgical protocol 223–229
bone manipulation 77, 124
bone quality 31–32
   manipulation 84–85
bone spreaders 307–308
bridgework 110

## C

'C'-shaped incision 162
CAD/CAM technology, in restoration design 196–199
Caldwell–Luc procedure 302, 306
closed tray technique 182, 186, 187
composite grafts 358
computed tomography (CT) 10, 20–22, 23, 52–53, 222, 303–304, 334–337
computer-guided surgery 85–87
   clinical cases using 87–102
      complex restorative case 95–98
      full arch immediate placement and loading 87–95
      immediate full mouth rehabilitation 98–102
      restorative phase 87
cone beam CT 22–23, 334
congenital deficiencies 206
connective tissue grafts 357–358
   clinical cases 373–380
containment 248, 250, 329
continuous full-thickness incision 159–162
conventional tomography 20
corrective soft tissue surgery 353–380
   *see also* composite grafts; frenectomy; pedicle flaps; subepithelial connective tissue grafts; vestibuloplasty
crestal ridge
   height 221–222
   morphology 222
   width 222
   *see also* ridge mapping

# Index

## D

delayed loading
  clinical cases, delayed placement with 132–141
  clinical management 64–67, 128–130
  incision for 118
  see also implant exposure
delayed placement
  advantages 103
  clinical assessment 107
  clinical cases 132–152
    with delayed loading 132–141
    with immediate loading 141–143, 144–152
    with transgingival healing 144
  implant placement 118–131
    abutment selection 127
    implant insertion 125–126
    impressions at first-stage surgery 127–128
    osteotomy preparation 122–124
  preoperative stage 108–117
  radiographic assessment 108
  restorative phase 131
  dental panoramic tomograph (DPT) 20, 52, 108, 303, 334
dentures 109
diagnostic imaging 19–20
diagnostic preview 29
diagnostic templates 109
direction indicators 228, 234
drill guides 86, 109

## E

extensive bone grafts 261–300
  assessment 262–264
  clinical cases 267–300
    anterior maxilla reconstruction following trauma 274–280
    augmentation of both jaws 295–300
    bone graft from iliac crest for class V ridge 272–274
    bone graft from iliac crest for ridge reconstruction 267–272
    management of edentulous patient with ridge augmentation 287–294
    management of periodontally compromised patient requiring augmentation 280–285
    replacement of failing teeth with implants 286–287
  donor sites 261–262
  planning of treatment 264
  posterior mandible 339
  surgery 265–267
extraoral donor sites 241

## F

financial considerations 7
fistulas, closure 357–359
flowcharts
  abutment transfer impression 179
  assessment
    for bone expansion 220
    for bone grafts 243
    for immediate or delayed loading 106
    for immediate or delayed placement 45–47, 50
    of possible augmentation 216–217
    of posterior mandible 352
    for sinus lift procedure and sinus manipulation 308–309
  bone expansion and labial recontouring 223
  clinical signs for delayed placement 120–121
  conventional impressions for restorative phase 175
  corrective soft tissue surgery 354–355
  immediate placement and loading 56–57
  implant exposure 154
  implant position transfer impression 184
  impressions at first-stage surgery 170
  ridge assessment for delayed placement 104
free gingival graft 356
  clinical cases 360–366
frenectomy 356
full mouth rehabilitation 98–102, 173–174, 176, 182, 192–195
full-thickness flaps 162

## G

GBR see guided bone regeneration
general health assessment 9–10
graft failure 207
grafting of tissues 209–211
  general principles 211–218
  see also allogenic grafts; autogenous grafts; xenogeneic grafts
  guided bone regeneration (GBR) 205, 209, 211–212
  clinical case 212–215
guided tissue regeneration (GTR) 209

## H

'H'-shaped incision 155–159
hybrid bridges 117

## I

iliac crest, as donor site 261
  clinical cases 267, 272, 274, 280, 286, 287
immediate loading
  clinical cases
    delayed placement with 141–143, 144–152
    full arch immediate placement and 87–95
  clinical management 66–75, 130

# Index

abutment selection and attachment 66–73
  restorative phase 73–75
  transitional restoration 73
considerations specific to 118
incision for 118–119
primary stability principles 84–85
immediate placement
  assessment checklist 54
  clinical assessment 50–52
  clinical variations 75–85
    aesthetically critical zone 75–76
    multiple adjacent implants 83–84
    posterior mandible 78–82
    posterior maxilla 76–77
    radiographic assessment 52–53
  treatment sequence 53–64
    extraction 54–58
    implant insertion 60–64
    implant placement 58
    impressions at first-stage surgery 64
    osteotomy preparation 58–60
    preoperative stage 54
  *see also* computer-guided surgery; delayed loading; immediate loading
implant design 85
implant exposure 153–165
  abutment attachment 162–164
  chairside fabrication 165
  continuous full-thickness incision 159–162
  localised bone grafts 252
  minimal exposure incision 154–159
  preoperative planning 154
  transitional restoration 165
implant failure 331
implant position transfer 182, 184
infection 331
  as bone loss cause 206
infectivity, of grafts 211

inferior alveolar nerve 333
  repositioning
    with onlay bone graft 348–351
    with simultaneous implant placement 342–348
informed consent 8, 306
interdental papillae, creating 359
intermaxillary relationship, recording 177
intraoral examination 10–12

## J

jaw registration bkocks 177

## L

labial soft tissue bulk, creating 359
lateral cephalography 20, 21
lateral fixation screws 168, 176, 192–195
lip line 13
load, and augmentation 207–208
localised onlay bone grafts 239–259
  bone deficiency assessment 239–240
  bone healing assessment 249–250
  clinical cases 253–259
    bone graft from ramus 254, 255–256
    bone graft from symphysis 253–254, 256–259
  corrective soft tissue surgery 252
  donor site assessment 241
  implant exposure 252
  implant insertion 250
  posterior mandible 339–342, 348–351
  restorative phase 252–253
  surgical protocol 242–249
    donor site access 246
    graft fitting 247–248
    graft harvesting 246–247
    recipient site access 242–246
    wound closure 248–249
  treatment sequence 242

## M

magnetic resonance imaging (MRI) 27
manipulation of tissues 208–209
medical evaluation 15–16
mucoceles 305
multiple units 176–177, 182, 186, 192–195

## N

neoplasm 206
non-vascularised grafts 66

## O

occlusal load 84
occlusive membranes 66, 250
onlay bone grafts *see* extensive bone grafts; localised onlay bone grafts
open tray technique 182, 185–186
oro-antral fistulas 331, 358–359
orthopantomography (OPG) *see* dental panoramic tomograph
osteotomy probe 228

## P

patient assessment 9–13
patient expectations 7–8
patient management 17–18
pedicle flaps 160–161, 358–360
  inverted 360
    clinical case 369–373
  lateral 359–360
    clinical case 366–369
periapical bone loss 206
periapical radiography 20, 52, 108, 222, 249, 334
peri-implant bone loss 207
periodontal bone loss 206–207
piezosurgery 346
pilot bone condenser 227–228
pilot osteotomy bur 228
polyps 305
position marker 58, 122, 224–225

# Index

posterior mandible 38–42, 333–352
  assessment 334–337
  clinical assessment 337
  immediate placement 78–82
  insufficient bone, treatment options 339–342
  nerve repositioning with onlay bone graft 348–351
  nerve repositioning with simultaneous implant placement 342–348
  surgical protocol, adequate bone 337–339
posterior maxilla 34–37, 301–332
  anatomy 302
  assessment of available bone and maxillary sinus 303–304
  assessment of load 306
  assessment of pathology 304–306
  bone quality 34, 301
  clinical cases 323–327
    subantral augmentation with intraoral block graft 323–324
    subantral augmentation with onlay bone graft 324–327
  clinical protocols 306–318
    increasing available bone 310–318
    manipulating bone of low density 307–310
    using available bone 306–307
  complications 327–331
  features characterising 301
  immediate placement 76–77
  planning of treatment 306
  sequence for implant insertion and sinus lift 318–323
prefabricated angled ceramic abutments 73
prefabricated angled titanium abutments 67–72
prosthetic protocols 167–199
  abutment position transfer 178–182, 196–199

abutment selection, modification or fabrication 186–187
  clinical cases 187–199
  direct impressions of abutment 173–178
  implant position transfer 182–186, 196
  impressions at first-stage surgery 64, 127–128, 169–173, 187
  restoration finishing 187

## R

ramus
  access to 246
  assessment 241
  graft harvesting 247
  wound closure 249
rapid prototyping 23–27
record keeping 8
remote palatal incision 224
restorative phase
  bone expansion 230
  computer-guided surgery 87
  delayed placement 131
  immediate loading 73–75
  localised bone grafts 252–253
  procedures and sequences 174
  prostheses *see* prosthetic protocols
rib, as donor site 262
ridge mapping 27–29, 222
risk classification 9
Rochette bridge 110–116, 274

## S

'S'-shaped incision 160–162
scalpel, scoring with 224
sedation 17–18
sensory tests 348
sinus floor manipulation 310–312
sinus lift
  lateral approach 312–318
  one-stage approach 322–323
  two-stage approach 318–322
  *see also* posterior maxilla

skull, as donor site 261
socket integrity 52
soft tissue, preserving architecture 64
soft-tissue health 52
specialist referral 16–17
spring cantilever bridges 112, 113, 115
study casts 29, 334, 337
subepithelial connective tissue grafts 357–358
  clinical cases 373–380
sulcus formers 64, 128–131, 182, 338
support, and augmentation 208
symphysis
  access to 246
  assessment 241
  graft harvesting 246–247
  wound closure 249
synthetic materials 211

## T

tele-medicine 8
three-dimensional interactive software 23–27
tibia, as donor site 261
tooth wear 12–13
transfer caps, multiple-purpose 182
transgingival healing 118–119, 130–131, 144
transmucosal approach 338
trauma 206

## V

vascularised pedicled flaps 64–66
vestibuloplasty 353–356
  clinical cases 360–363, 363–366

## W

wound closure 64–66, 128–131, 165, 229, 248–249, 252, 348

## X

xenogeneic grafts 210–211